Lecture Notes in Business Information Processing

503

Series Editors

Wil van der Aalst, *RWTH Aachen University, Aachen, Germany*

Sudha Ram, *University of Arizona, Tucson, AZ, USA*

Michael Rosemann, *Queensland University of Technology, Brisbane, QLD, Australia*

Clemens Szyperski, *Microsoft Research, Redmond, WA, USA*

Giancarlo Guizzardi, *University of Twente, Enschede, The Netherlands*

LNBIP reports state-of-the-art results in areas related to business information systems and industrial application software development – timely, at a high level, and in both printed and electronic form.

The type of material published includes

- Proceedings (published in time for the respective event)
- Postproceedings (consisting of thoroughly revised and/or extended final papers)
- Other edited monographs (such as, for example, project reports or invited volumes)
- Tutorials (coherently integrated collections of lectures given at advanced courses, seminars, schools, etc.)
- Award-winning or exceptional theses

LNBIP is abstracted/indexed in DBLP, EI and Scopus. LNBIP volumes are also submitted for the inclusion in ISI Proceedings.

Johannes De Smedt · Pnina Soffer
Editors

Process Mining Workshops

ICPM 2023 International Workshops
Rome, Italy, October 23–27, 2023
Revised Selected Papers

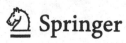

Editors
Johannes De Smedt ⓘ
KU Leuven
Leuven, Belgium

Pnina Soffer ⓘ
University of Haifa
Haifa, Israel

ISSN 1865-1348   ISSN 1865-1356 (electronic)
Lecture Notes in Business Information Processing
ISBN 978-3-031-56106-1   ISBN 978-3-031-56107-8 (eBook)
https://doi.org/10.1007/978-3-031-56107-8

This Springer imprint is published by the registered company Springer Nature Switzerland AG
The registered company address is: Gewerbestrasse 11, 6330 Cham, Switzerland

Paper in this product is recyclable.

Preface

The International Conference on Process Mining (ICPM), inaugurated four years ago, functions as a convergence point for process mining researchers, practitioners, and tool vendors representing diverse spheres, including academia and industry. This forum facilitates collaborative exploration and discussion concerning the latest advancements in process mining research and practice, encompassing theoretical frameworks, algorithmic innovations, and practical application challenges. Despite its relatively brief existence, the ICPM conference series has garnered notable research contributions of exceptional quality, evidencing the collaborative endeavors of esteemed scholars and industrial researchers.

ICPM 2023 unfolded in the city of Rome, Italy, where the conference coincided with co-located workshops on October 23, 2023. The workshops, each characterized by a distinct and focused scope, collectively presented a diverse array of outstanding research ideas still in their nascent stages, coupled with exemplary paper presentations. Moreover, these workshops were augmented with substantive contributions from keynote speakers, round-table panels, and poster sessions, creating an intellectually stimulating forum for rigorous discussions and interactions within the broader academic and industrial community.

ICPM 2023 featured six workshops, each focusing on particular aspects of process mining, either a particular technical aspect or a particular application domain:

- 4th International Workshop on Event Data and Behavioral Analytics (EDBA)
- 4th International Workshop on Leveraging Machine Learning in Process Mining (ML4PM)
- 6th International Workshop on Process-Oriented Data Science for Healthcare (PODS4H)
- 8th International Workshop on Process Querying, Manipulation, and Intelligence (PQMI)
- 2nd International Workshop on Education Meets Process Mining (EduPM)
- 2nd International Workshop on Collaboration Mining for Distributed Systems (COMINDS)

The proceedings present and summarize the work that was discussed during the workshops. In total, the ICPM 2023 workshops received 85 full-paper submissions of which 38 papers were accepted for publication after a single-blind review process in which submissions on average each received three reviews, leading to a total acceptance rate of about 45%, next to an additional 17 short-paper/abstract/poster submissions. Supported by ICPM, each workshop also granted a best workshop paper award. Finally, it is worth mentioning that selected papers will also be invited to a journal special issue.

We would like to thank all the people from the ICPM community who helped to make the ICPM 2023 workshops a success. We particularly thank the entire organization committee for delivering such an outstanding conference. We are also grateful to the workshop organizers, the numerous reviewers, and, of course, the authors for their contributions to the ICPM 2023 workshops.

October 2023

Johannes De Smedt
Pnina Soffer

Organization

IEEE Task Force Steering Committee

Boudewijn van Dongen (Chair)	Eindhoven University of Technology, The Netherlands
Wil van der Aalst (Vice-chair)	RWTH Aachen University, Germany
Moe Wynn (Vice-chair)	Queensland University of Technology, Australia
Rafael Accorsi	Accenture, Switzerland
Peter Blank	PricewaterhouseCoopers, Switzerland
Andrea Burattin	Technical University of Denmark, Denmark
Jochen De Weerdt	KU Leuven, Belgium
Claudio Di Ciccio	Sapienza University of Rome, Italy
Philipp Herrmann	Horn & Company, Germany
Micke Jans	Hasselt University, Belgium
Julian Lebherz	Standard Chartered Bank, Singapore
Marco Montali	Free University of Bozen-Bolzano, Italy
Jorge Munoz-Gama	Pontificia Unversidad Católica de Chile, Chile
Artem Polyvyanyy	University of Melbourne, Australia
Pnina Soffer	University of Haifa, Israel

Workshop Chairs

Johannes De Smedt	KU Leuven, Belgium
Pnina Soffer	University of Haifa, Israel

General Chairs

Claudio Di Ciccio	Sapienza University of Rome, Italy
Andrea Marrella	Sapienza University of Rome, Italy

Proceedings Chair

Giuseppe Perelli	Sapienza University of Rome, Italy

Publicity Chairs

Francesca Zerbato   University of St. Gallen, Switzerland
Simone Agostinelli   Sapienza University of Rome, Italy

Workshop Organizers

4th International Workshop on Event Data and Behavioral Analytics (EDBA)

Benoît Depaire   Hasselt University, Belgium
Dirk Fahland   Eindhoven University of Technology,
                              The Netherlands
Francesco Leotta   Sapienza University of Rome, Italy
Xixi Lu   Utrecht University, The Netherlands

4th International Workshop on Leveraging Machine Learning in Process Mining (ML4PM)

Annalisa Appice   Università degli studi di Bari Aldo Moro, Italy
Sylvio Barbon Junior   University of Trieste, Italy
Paolo Ceravolo   Università degli studi di Milano, Italy

6th International Workshop on Process-Oriented Data Science for Healthcare (PODS4H)

Carlos Fernandez-Llatas   Universitat Politècnica de València, Spain
Owen Johnson   University of Leeds, UK
Niels Martin   Hasselt University, Belgium
Jorge Munoz-Gama   Pontificia Universidad Católica de Chile, Chile
Marcos Sepulveda   Pontificia Universidad Católica de Chile, Chile

8th International Workshop on Process Querying, Manipulation, and Intelligence (PQMI)

Antonella Guzzo   University of Calabria, Italy
Artem Polyvyanyy   University of Melbourne, Australia
Renuka Sindhgatta   IBM Research, Australia
Arthur ter Hofstede   Queensland University of Technology, Australia

2nd International Workshop on Education Meets Process Mining (EduPM)

Gert Janssenwillen	Hasselt University, Belgium
Jorge Munoz-Gama	Pontificia Universidad Católica de Chile, Chile
Wil van der Aalst	RWTH Aachen University, Germany
Francesca Zerbato	University of St. Gallen, Switzerland

2nd International Workshop on Collaboration Mining for Distributed Systems (COMINDS)

Mahsa Pourbafrani	RWTH Aachen University, Germany
Andrea Delgado	Universidad de la República, Uruguay
Lorenzo Rossi	University of Camerino, Italy

Program Committee

Rafael Accorsi	Accenture Switzerland, Switzerland
Simone Agostinelli	Sapienza University of Rome, Italy
Davide Aloini	University of Pisa, Italy
Daniel Amyot	University of Ottawa, Canada
Burattin Andrea	Technical University of Denmark, Denmark
Robert Andrews	Queensland University of Technology, Australia
Annalisa Appice	Università degli studi di Bari Aldo Moro, Italy
Michael Arias	Universidad de Costa Rica, Costa Rica
Abel Armas Cervantes	University of Melbourne, Australia
Ahmed Awad	British University in Dubai, UAE
Mahsa Pourbafrani	RWTH Aachen University, Germany
Barbara Re	University of Camerino, Italy
Sylvio Barbon Junior	University of Trieste, Italy
Irene Bedilia Estrada Torres	University of Seville, Spain
Iris Beerepoot	Utrecht University, The Netherlands
Elisabetta Benevento	University of Pisa, Italy
Robin Bergenthum	FernUniversität in Hagen, Germany
Yannis Bertrand	KU Leuven, Belgium
Mitchel Brunings	Eindhoven University of Technology, The Netherlands
Andrea Burattin	Technical University of Denmark, Denmark
Cristina Cabanillas	University of Seville, Spain
Daniel Calegari	Universidad de la República, Uruguay
Daniel Capurro	University of Melbourne, Australia
Michelangelo Ceci	Università degli Studi di Bari Aldo Moro, Italy

Paolo Ceravolo	Università degli studi di Milano, Italy
Thomas Chatain	École Normale Supérieure Paris-Saclay, France
Ioannis Chatzigiannakis	Sapienza University of Rome, Italy
Marco Comuzzi	Ulsan National Institute of Science and Technology, South Korea
Carl Corea	University of Koblenz, Germany
Jonas Cremerius	HPI, University of Potsdam, Germany
Cristina Cabanillas	University of Seville, Spain
Benjamin Dalmas	Centre de Recherche Informatique de Montréal, Canada
René de la Fuente	Pontificia Universidad Católica de Chile, Chile
Massimiliano de Leoni	University of Padua, Italy
Johannes De Smedt	KU Leuven, Belgium
Jochen De Weerdt	KU Leuven, Belgium
Adela del Río Ortega	University of Seville, Spain
Andrea Delgado	Universidad de la República, Uruguay
Pavlos Delias	International Hellenic University, Greece
Benoît Depaire	Hasselt University, Belgium
Claudio Di Ciccio	Sapienza University of Rome, Italy
Gemma Di Federico	Technical University of Denmark, Denmark
Chiara Di Francescomarino	University of Trento, Italy
Remco Dijkman	Eindhoven University of Technology, The Netherlands
Onur Dogan	İzmir Bakırçay University, Turkey
Marlon Dumas	University of Tartu, Estonia
Gamal Elkoumy	Apromore, Estonia
Joerg Evermann	Memorial University of Newfoundland, Canada
Fabrizio Maria Maggi	Free University of Bozen-Bolzano, Italy
Dirk Fahland	Eindhoven University of Technology, The Netherlands
Stephan Fahrenkrog-Petersen	Humboldt-Universität zu Berlin, Germany
Marcelo Fantinato	University of São Paulo, Brazil
Bettina Fazzinga	University of Calabria, Italy
Carlos Fernandez-Llatas	Universitat Politècnica de València, Spain
Corradini Flavio	University of Camerino, Italy
Francesco Folino	ICAR, National Research Council of Italy (CNR), Italy
Marco Franceschetti	University of St. Gallen, Switzerland
Tiezzi Francesco	Università di Firenze, Italy
Walid Gaaloul	Télécom SudParis, France
Avigdor Gal	Technion, Israel
Luciano García-Bañuelos	Tecnológico de Monterrey, Mexico

Dragan Gasevic	Monash University, Australia
Roberto Gatta	Università Cattolica S. Cuore, Italy
Laura Genga	Eindhoven University of Technology, The Netherlands
Jerome Geyer-Klingeberg	Celonis SE, Germany
Kanika Goel	Queensland University of Technology, Australia
Oscar González-Rojas	Universidad de los Andes, Colombia
Joscha Grüger	University of Trier, Germany
Gianluigi Greco	University of Calabria, Italy
Daniela Grigori	University Paris-Dauphine, France
Antonella Guzzo	University of Calabria, Italy
Marwan Hassani	Eindhoven University of Technology, The Netherlands
Emmanuel Helm	Upper Austria University of Applied Sciences, Austria
Luciano Hidalgo	Pontificia Universidad Católica de Chile, Chile
Gema Ibañez Sanchez	UPV-ITACA, Spain
Sander J. J. Leemans	RWTH Aachen University, Germany
Mieke Jans	Hasselt University, Belgium
Gert Janssenswillen	Hasselt University, Belgium
Owen Johnson	University of Leeds, UK
Martin Kabierski	Humboldt-Universität zu Berlin, Germany
Anna Kalenkova	University of Adelaide, Australia
Agnes Koschmider	University of Bayreuth, Germany
Orlenys López Pintado	University of Tartu, Estonia
Manuel Lama Penin	University of Santiago de Compostela, Spain
Julian Lebherz	A.P. Moller-Maersk, Denmark
Henrik Leopold	Kühne Logistics University, Germany
Francesco Leotta	Sapienza University of Rome, Italy
Rong Liu	Stevens Institute of Technology, USA
Irina Lomazova	HSE University, Russia
Xixi Lu	Utrecht University, The Netherlands
Mario Luca Bernardi	University of Sannio, Italy
Rafiei Majid	RWTH Aachen University, Germany
Felix Mannhardt	Eindhoven University of Technology, The Netherlands
Ronny Mans	VitalHealth Software, The Netherlands
Sarajane Marques Peres	University of São Paulo, Brazil
Gabriel Marques Tavares	Università degli Studi di Milano, Italy
Niels Martin	Hasselt University, Belgium
Raimundas Matulevicius	University of Tartu, Estonia
Massimo Mecella	Sapienza University of Rome, Italy

Renata Medeiros de Carvalho	Eindhoven University of Technology, The Netherlands
Jan Mendling	Humboldt-Universität zu Berlin, Germany
Giovanni Meroni	Technical University of Denmark, Denmark
Alex Mircoli	Università Politecnica delle Marche, Italy
Marco Montali	Free University of Bozen-Bolzano, Italy
Jorge Munoz-Gama	Pontificia Universidad Católica de Chile, Chile
Emerson Paraiso	Pontifícia Universidade Católica do Paraná, Brazil
Poizat Pascal	Université Paris Nanterre and LIP6, France
Vincenzo Pasquadibisceglie	Università degli Studi di Bari Aldo Moro, Italy
Marco Pegoraro	RWTH Aachen University, Germany
Artem Polyvyanyy	University of Melbourne, Australia
Luigi Pontieri	ICAR, National Research Council of Italy (CNR), Italy
Simon Poon	University of Sydney, Australia
Domenico Potena	Università Politecnica delle Marche, Italy
Luise Pufahl	TU Munich, Germany
Ricardo Quintano	Philips Research, The Netherlands
Maximilian Röglinger	University of Bayreuth/Fraunhofer FIT, Germany
Majid Rafiei	RWTH Aachen University, Germany
Jana-Rebecca Rehse	University of Mannheim, Germany
Hajo Reijers	Utrecht University, The Netherlands
Peter Reimann	University of Sydney, Australia
Shangping Ren	San Diego State University, USA
Manuel Resinas	University of Seville, Spain
Stefanie Rinderle-Ma	Technical University of Munich, Germany
Eric Rojas	Universidad Católica de Chile, Chile
Lorenzo Rossi	University of Camerino, Italy
Sareh Sadeghianasl	Queensland University of Technology, Australia
Flavia Santoro	UERJ, Brazil
Rafael Seidi Oyamada	Università degli studi di Milano, Italy
Thomas Seidl	Ludwig-Maximilians-Universität München, Germany
Arik Senderovich	York University, Canada
Fernando Seoane	Karolinska Institutet, Sweden
Marcos Sepulveda	Pontificia Universidad Católica de Chile, Chile
Estefanía Serral	KU Leuven, Belgium
Natalia Sidorova	Eindhoven University of Technology, The Netherlands
Renuka Sindhgatta	IBM Research, Australia
Tijs Slaats	University of Copenhagen, Denmark
Pnina Soffer	University of Haifa, Israel

Minseok Song	Pohang University of Science and Technology, South Korea
Alessandro Stefanini	University of Pisa, Italy
Emilio Sulis	University of Turin, Italy
Ernest Teniente	UPC, Spain
Arthur ter Hofstede	Queensland University of Technology, Australia
Maria Teresa Gómez López	University of Seville, Spain
Moe Thandar Wynn	Queensland University of Technology, Australia
Pieter Toussaint	Norwegian University of Science and Technology, Norway
Vicente Traver	Universitat Politècnica de València, Spain
Florian Tschorsch	TU Berlin, Germany
Zoe Valero Ramón	Universitat Politècnica de València, Spain
Stef van den Elzen	Eindhoven University of Technology, The Netherlands
Han van der Aa	University of Mannheim, Germany
Wil van der Aalst	RWTH Aachen University, Germany
Jan Martijn van der Werf	Utrecht University, The Netherlands
Boudewijn van Dongen	Eindhoven University of Technology, The Netherlands
Greg van Houdt	Hasselt University, Belgium
William van Woensel	University of Ottawa, Canada
Sebastiaan van Zelst	Fraunhofer FIT/RWTH Aachen University, Gemany
Seppe Vanden Broucke	KU Leuven, Belgium
Eric Verbeek	Eindhoven University of Technology, The Netherlands
Pablo Villarreal	UTN Santa Fe, Argentina
Eugenio Vocaturo	University of Calabria, Italy
Hagen Voelzer	University of St. Gallen, Switzerland
Barbara Weber	University of St. Gallen, Switzerland
Matthias Weidlich	Humboldt-Universität zu Berlin, Germany
Mathias Weske	HPI, University of Potsdam, Germany
Karolin Winter	Eindhoven University of Technology, The Netherlands
Nicola Zannone	Eindhoven University of Technology, The Netherlands
Bruno Zarpelao	State University of Londrina, Brazil
Francesca Zerbato	University of St. Gallen, Switzerland

Additional Reviewers

Milda Aleknonyte-Resch
Kaan Apaydin
Andrei Buliga
Qifan Chen
Graziella De Martino
Francesco Folino
Frederik Fonger
Massimo Guarascio

Ruihua Guo
Arvid Lepsien
Yang Lu
Antonio Pellicani
Sara Pettinari
Pietro Sabatino
Yorck Zisgen

Unraveling the Fabric of Intertwined Processes: How Object-Centric Process Mining is Changing the Way We Improve Operational Processes (Invited Paper)

Wil M.P. van der Aalst[1,2] (iD)

[1] Process and Data Science (PADS), RWTH Aachen University, Germany
wvdaalst@pads.rwth-aachen.de
[2] Celonis, München, Germany

Abstract. While traditional process mining is powerful and effective, it also has its limitations. The extraction and transformation of data can be both time-consuming and repetitive, especially when changing viewpoints. Traditional event logs do not capture interactions between objects (such as sales orders, items, shipments, invoices, etc.), making it challenging to analyze these interactions using conventional methods. Yet, these interactions are often the source of problems. Additionally, fitting data into classical case-based event logs leads to the well-known convergence and divergence issues. Object-Centric Process Mining (OCPM) and the newly introduced OCEL 2.0 standard are designed to address these challenges. This extended abstract, derived from a keynote presented at the Workshop on Collaboration Mining for Distributed Systems (COMINDS 2023), offers insights into these recent advancements.

Keywords: Object-centric process mining · Concurrency · Object-centric event data · Rainbow Spaghetti · OCEL 2.0.

1 A Brief History of Process Mining

Process mining started in the late 1990-ties and initially focused on control-flow discovery, e.g., creating Directly-Follows Graphs (DFGs) or Petri nets describing the sequences of events seen in the databases of an organization [1].

In the period 2004–2011, the "golden age of process mining", many elements were added (see Fig. 1). The scope was extended to include conformance checking, decision mining, predictive analytics, process recommendations, and the automatic creation of simulation models. Also, the temporal, data, and resource perspectives were added.

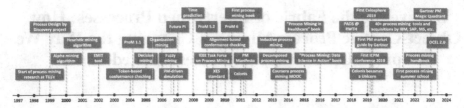

Fig. 1. A timeline of process mining showing important milestones.

In 2011, the "Process Mining Manifesto" was published [5] and the first version of the XES standard (cf. xes-standard.org) was released. Also, many process mining companies were founded (e.g., Celonis) leading to the over 40 commercial process mining products available today (see processmining.org).

In recent years, we have witnessed the uptake of process mining with thousands of organizations using it to improve their processes [3]. Although the process mining discipline has matured (see for example successful annual conferences such as ICPM and Celosphere) and there are many success stories, we can also see the limitations of the initial assumption that there is a single case notion and each event refers to precisely one case. This triggered the development of *Object-Centric Process Mining* (OCPM) [2] discussed next.

2 A New Standard for Object-Centric Event Data

Object-Centric Event Logs (OCELs) form the basis for Object-Centric Process Mining (OCPM). OCEL 1.0 was first released in 2020 and triggered the development of a range of OCPM techniques. OCEL 2.0 forms the new, more expressive standard, allowing for more extensive process analyses while remaining in an easily exchangeable format.

In contrast to the first OCEL standard, OCEL 2.0 can depict changes in objects, provide information on object relationships, and qualify these relationships to other objects or specific events (see Fig. 2). Compared to XES, it is more expressive, less complicated, and better readable. OCEL 2.0 offers three exchange formats: a relational database (SQLite), XML, and JSON format. See [4] for the specification and [6] for datasets and tool support.

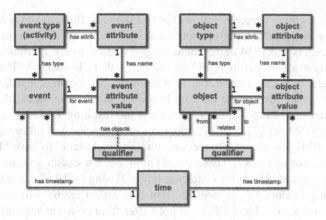

Fig. 2. The OCEL 2.0 Meta Model [2, 4, 6].

3 Advantages of Using Object-Centric Process Mining

For a basic introduction to Object-Centric Process Mining (OCPM) and an overview of literature, we refer to [2]. Here we limit ourselves to discussing the advantages of using OCEL 2.0 and related OCPM techniques.

Real-life processes can be seen as "Rainbow Spaghetti" where each strand of Spaghetti (called "Spaghetto" in Italian) corresponds to the lifecycle of an object and the color refers to the type. Often, it is not sufficient to limit the view to one object type, because the root causes of problems often involve multiple objects of different types. Therefore, classical process mining involves mapping multiple object types on a single case notion.

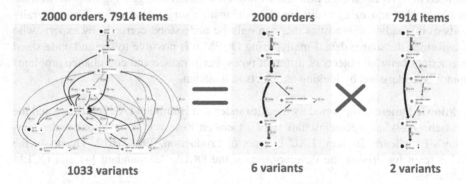

Fig. 3. Example showing the drawbacks of mapping different types of objects onto a single case notion. Although the handling of orders and items in isolation is highly structured, the combined model using a single-case notion is complex and misleading.

Figure 3 shows three Directly-Follows Graphs (DFGs). The two DFGs on the right-hand side show that the handling of orders and items in isolation is simple. In a data set with 2000 orders and 7914 items, there are just 6 respectively 2 variants. However, if both are combined, we get the DFG on the left with 1033 variants. The combined DFG uses orders as a case notion, but also includes the activities that happened for the items in the order. Orders get delayed by items being out of stock; therefore, we need to consider also these activities. However, the resulting DFG has convergence and divergence problems [2]. Statistics related to frequencies and times are distorted. Moreover, the DFG also shows connections such as "pick item" followed by "reorder item" and "item out of stock". These connections are not causal and are created by squeezing two types of objects into one case notion. Using OCEL 2.0 and OCPM, one can avoid such problems. Object-centric event data reflect reality without distortions and the discovered multi-object DFGs do not suffer from convergence and divergence problems.

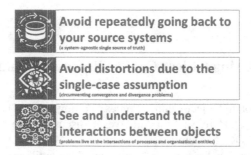

Fig. 4. Overview of the three main reasons to use OCPM.

Figure 4 summarizes the three main advantages of OCPM. Using OCEL 2.0, one can store object and event data in a system-agnostic manner. Therefore, extraction does not need to be repeated each time the view or case notion changes. Figure 3 showed the problems when squeezing reality into a model using a single-case notion. This generally leads to misleading diagnostics that can only be understood correctly by experts who transformed the source data. Finally, using OCPM it is possible to see and understand interactions between objects of different types. Performance and compliance problems cannot be understood by looking at objects in isolation.

Acknowledgments. Supported by the Alexander von Humboldt (AvH) Stiftung and the Deutsche Forschungsgemeinschaft (DFG, German Research Foundation) under Germany's Excellence Strategy, EXC Internet of Production, 390621612. Thanks to the PADS team for driving the development of the OCEL 2.0 standard [4] and OCPM techniques.

References

1. van der Aalst, W.: Process Mining: Data Science in Action. Springer, Heidelberg (2016). https://link.springer.com/book/10.1007/978-3-662-49851-4
2. van der Aalst, W.: Object-centric process mining: unraveling the fabric of real processes. Math. **11**(12), 2691 (2023)
3. van der Aalst, W., Carmona, J.: Process Mining Handbook. Lecture Notes in Business Information Processing, vol. 448. Springer, Cham (2022). https://link.springer.com/book/10.1007/978-3-031-08848-3
4. Berti, A., et al.: OCEL (Object-Centric Event Log) 2.0 Specification (2023). https://www.ocel-standard.org/2.0/ocel20_specification.pdf
5. IEEE Task Force on Process Mining: Process Mining Manifesto (2011). https://www.tf-pm.org/resources/manifesto
6. Process and Data Science Group: Object-Centric Event Log (OCEL 2.0) Website Providing Data Sets, Software, Etc. (2023) . https://www.ocel-standard.org/

Contents

**4th International Workshop on Leveraging Machine Learning for
Process Mining (ML4PM 2023)**

**6th International Workshop on Process-Oriented Data Science for
Healthcare (PODS4H 2023)**

2nd International Workshop Education Meets Process Mining (EduPM 2023)

Fourth International Workshop on Event Data and Behavioral Analytics (EdbA 2023)

Fourth International Workshop on Event Data and Behavioral Analytics (EdbA 2023)

Over the past decades, capturing, storing, and analyzing event data has gained attention in domains such as process mining, clickstream analytics, IoT analytics, online gaming analytics, website traffic analytics, and preventive maintenance. The interest in event data lies in its analytical potential as it captures the dynamic behavior of people, objects, and systems at a fine-grained level.

Behavior often involves multiple entities, objects, and actors to which events can be correlated in various ways. In these situations, a unique, straightforward process notion does not exist or is unclear, or different processes or dynamics may be recorded in the same data set.

The objective of the Event Data & Behavioral Analytics (EdbA) workshop series is to provide a forum for practitioners and researchers to study a quintessential, minimal notion of events as the common denominator for records of discrete behavior in all its forms. The workshop aims to stimulate the development of new techniques, algorithms, and data structures for recording, storing, managing, processing, analyzing, and visualizing event data in various forms. To this end, different types of submissions are welcome such as original research papers, case study reports, position papers, idea papers, challenge papers, and work-in-progress papers on event data and behavioral analytics.

The fourth edition of the EdbA workshop attracted 18 submissions of which ten were accepted for a full-paper presentation and are included in the proceedings. This year's papers cover a broad spectrum of topics, which can be organized into three main themes: event data formats and pre-processing, making sense of complex behavior, and finding patterns in processes.

Throughout the workshop, the topic of object-centricity emerged as a focal point in numerous discussions. This theme was further explored during the final plenary session, where participants engaged in a comprehensive debate. They presented various perspectives on several key issues, including: *(i)* the significance of relationships between objects compared to the sequence of steps in a process; *(ii)* the core principles of processes in the context of object-centricity and behavioral analytics; *(iii)* the contribution of object-centric data to process analysis; and *(iv)* the necessity of defining specific 'task definitions' for process mining and event data analytics.

The organizers wish to thank all the people who submitted papers to the EdbA 2023 workshop, the many participants who created fruitful discussions and shared insights, and the EdbA 2023 Program Committee members for their valuable work in reviewing the submissions. A final word of thanks goes out to the organizers of ICPM 2023 for making this workshop possible.

October, 2023

Benoît Depaire
Dirk Fahland
Francesco Leotta
Xixi Lu

Organization

Workshop Chairs

Benoît Depaire	Hasselt University, Belgium
Dirk Fahland	Eindhoven University of Technology, The Netherlands
Francesco Leotta	Sapienza University of Rome, Italy
Xixi Lu	University of Utrecht, The Netherlands

Program Committee

Yannis Bertrand	Katholieke Universiteit Leuven, Belgium
Andrea Burattin	Technical University of Denmark, Denmark
Ioannis Chatzigiannakis	Sapienza University of Rome, Italy
Massimiliano de Leoni	University of Padua, Italy
Jochen De Weerdt	Katholieke Universiteit Leuven, Belgium
Gemma Di Frederico	Technicial University of Rome, Italy
Chiara Di Francescomarino	University of Trento, Italy
Bettina Fazzinga	University of Calabria, Italy
Laura Genga	Eindhoven University of Technology, The Netherlands
Marwan Hassani	Eindhoven University of Technology, The Netherlands
Gert Janssenswillen	Hasselt University, Belgium
Agnes Koschmider	University of Bayreuth, Germany
Felix Mannhardt	Eindhoven University of Technology, The Netherlands
Niels Martin	Hasselt University, Belgium
Massimo Mecella	Sapienza University of Rome, Itally
Jan Mendling	Humboldt-Universität zu Berlin, Germany
Marco Pegoraro	RWTH Aachen University, Germany
Estefanía Serral	Katholieke Universiteit Leuven, Belgium
Stef van den Elzen	Eindhoven University of Technology, The Netherlands
Greg Van Houdt	Hasselt University, Belgium
Francesca Zerbato	University of St. Gallen, Austria

Analysing the Foraging Behaviour of Bees Using Process Mining: A Case Study

Zahra Ahmadi[1](✉) [iD], Yannis Bertrand[1] [iD], María Isabel Pozo Romero[2] [iD],
and Estefanía Serral[1] [iD]

[1] LIRIS, KU Leuven, Brussels, Belgium
{zahra.ahmadi,yannis.bertrand,estefania.serralasensio}@kuleuven.be
[2] ETSIAA, Universidad de Valladolid, Valladolid, Spain
mariaisabel.pozo@uva.es

Abstract. In this paper, we present a novel case study for the application of process mining (PM) on data captured by Internet of Things (IoT) devices. In this case study, IoT sensors in robotic flowers are employed to gather a comprehensive dataset on bee colony behaviour through a series of experiments conducted under various conditions. The primary objective of this paper is to investigate the applicability of PM to analyse the collected sensor data, map bee colony behaviour, and uncover the learning patterns exhibited by the bees during these experiments. Encouraging results have emerged from this research, demonstrating the feasibility of converting the collected sensor data into event logs that can produce insights on bees foraging behaviour using a PM tool. This case study serves as a solid foundation for future research endeavours on the application of PM to similar processes that can be monitored using IoT devices.

Keywords: Internet of Things · IoT · Process mining · Process Discovery · Bees · Foraging behaviour · Case study

1 Introduction

Bees being one of the most important insect pollinators for our ecosystem [13], numerous authors have extensively studied their behaviour. The observation of bees has traditionally relied on manual and time-intensive methods. Researchers were required to be physically present for live observations or meticulously review recorded video footage within a specific time frame to track bee behaviour. This approach yielded a restricted amount of data and was prone to errors stemming from the human element [5].

The latest innovations of the IoT have made it possible to create robotic flowers that can collect detailed information about bees' actions [14]. These flowers record very precisely and at second-level frequency the visits of the bees on such flowers. This fine-granular and rich data can be translated into a higher-level event log usable for PM [7,17].

PM has shown to be a very powerful tool to enable the automatic discovery and visualisation of actual process flows based on event data. It provides

J. De Smedt and P. Soffer (Eds.): ICPM 2023 Workshops, LNBIP 503, pp. 5–18, 2024.
https://doi.org/10.1007/978-3-031-56107-8_1

a detailed understanding of how processes are executed, revealing the actual paths and their variations. The application of PM to sensor data is challenging, although it has been increased recently, however, most of the existing literature focusing on deriving process models of human behaviour from sensor logs in smart spaces [3].

In this paper, we present a very novel case study where we apply PM to obtain new insights on the foraging behaviour of bees. We ran 4 experiments to capture data on 8 bees' colonies using 16 robotic flowers per experiment. Using these data, we use PM to compare the behaviour and the learning capabilities of healthy bees versus sick bees. Understanding this behaviour could reveal insights on the pollination process which could be used to increase bees survival chances and maximise honey production. We focused on understanding the collective behaviour (behaviour for each colony) and since the behaviour routine can be separated into multiple activities, we considered studying the behaviour changes within process notation.

The rest of the paper is structured as follows. Section 2 summarizes the related literature focusing on 1) PM with IoT data and 2) previous methods used to understand foraging behaviour. Section 3 describes the case study. In Sect. 4, we apply PM to the case study, dealing with the challenges that sensor data analysis pose for PM. The results of the analysis are discussed in Sect. 5. Finally, Sect. 6 concludes the paper and proposes directions for future work.

2   Related Work

2.1   Process Mining Using Sensor Data

Although PM has never been applied to understand the foraging behaviour of bees, it has been used to investigate sensor logs (see [4,7,9,16,19] for some representative examples). One of the most frequent domains where PM was applied to sensor data is smart spaces, namely to perform habit mining. Habit mining consists of analysing and modelling human routines and activities of daily living using IoT data collected in smart spaces [18]. Various approaches exist to create models of human behaviour based on IoT data collected smart spaces; see [2] for an overview of these approaches.

To apply PM to sensor data, different challenges need to be addressed [2], including:

1. The low-level nature of sensor data compared to process data, requiring event abstraction. A typical sensor log contains measurements of sensors that do not necessarily match with activities, e.g., a contact sensor merely indicates whether contact with the sensor is detected.
2. The definition of cases and the log segmentation following that. A sensor log contains sensor measurements that may not match with one process execution.

2.2 Analyses of Foraging Behaviour

Within the bio-engineering domain, it is frequent to use several insects as study subjects in dual-choice experiments, where two conditions are offered simultaneously in a cage or enclosure. Typical tests on such experiments collect two sets of variables: number of visits to a given group (one or more flowers), and the duration of the visit.

Number of visits is recalculated as a proportion of visits to each group. Two options are often used to compare the proportions of visits to each condition (see [14] for a representative example). On the one hand, a two-sample test for equality of proportions with a continuity correction (Pearson's chi-squared test) compares the proportion of visits to each category, already calculated by a contingency table. On the other hand, a generalised linear model can be used to determine preferences, e.g., coding one group as success and the other as failure, thus setting the response variable as binomial.

The second variable, visit duration, may indicate preference to stay or a higher intake. To investigate whether visit time differed significantly between treatments, generalised linear models are often used to compute the model-adjusted average of that time and the model-adjusted error for each experimental group. Significance arises when averages plus/minus error do not overlap. The main problem in analysing this variable is to get the right distribution of the response variable. When the number of observations is high, it is assumed the data will approach a Gaussian distribution, but data collected with IoT technologies already showed otherwise.

Note that these analyses are not focusing on foraging behaviour as a process but as individual variables: number of visits and their duration. PM can therefore bring a new perspective into play and provide an alternative or complementary way to analyse behavioural aspects.

3 Case Study Description

We focus our analysis on better understanding the foraging behaviour of bumblebees (from now on referred to as bees or foragers). Normally, bee foraging behaviour comprises flower visits of different lengths, and this length correlates with different biological activities: probing, eating (ingesting pollen/nectar provided by flowers), resting, and sleeping. Foragers are attracted to the flowers because they often provide nectar and pollen, used to fuel their flight activities and to rear their offspring. As such, foragers try to maximise their energy intake while spending the least amount of energy to forage [15]. The biggest cost to a forager is the amount of time and energy spent on landing on, entering, and probing flowers [11]. Hence, in theory, foragers will focus their efforts on nectar-rich flowers [11]. The flower colour may play a role as well in attracting a bee.

According to the optimal foraging theory, pollinators are expected to discriminate high-quality nectar resources from less valuable resources [8,10]. However, floral nectar is often rich in plant secondary compounds [1]. About 1/3 of these compounds have a medicinal influence on the colony. They have a different taste, color and odour than floral nectar, and as such they are typically avoided by most pollinators. This case study focuses on investigating if such avoidance still applies when the colony status changes, i.e. when colonies become sick. In such cases, sick bees may focus their foraging efforts on flowers that contain a medicine capable to cure them. We are interested in understanding and comparing the foraging behaviour of sick bees vs. healthy bees. We will focus on understanding the collective behaviour, i.e., behaviour for each colony, rather than the behaviour for each individual bee, as foragers mostly collect the sugar water to feed the offspring, and not to satisfy their own nutritional demands.

4   Process Mining Application: Gathering Insights on Foraging Behaviour

In order to understand bees' foraging behaviour, we follow a typical PM methodology [20] and adapt it for IoT data. First, we identify the hypotheses to be studied. Second, we collect the necessary data to test those hypotheses using IoT sensors. Third, we preprocess the collected data to deal with quality issues. Fourth, we convert the IoT data into event logs ready to be used by PM tools. Fifth, we perform an iterative analysis to confirm or reject the hypotheses by applying PM and evaluating the results.

4.1   Hypothesis Formulation

Previous research having demonstrated that bees learn and adapt their foraging behaviour, the case study focuses on investigating whether bees adapt their foraging behaviour when they are sick. It was expected that the bees would explore and thus probe from all types of flowers equally at first, and progressively learn and increase their eating activities on flowers offering a more rewarding diet: sick colonies would prefer treated sugar water containing a medicinal compound (treatment); while healthy colonies would naturally show deterrence towards the medicinal compound and prefer untreated sugar water (control). Based on this prior research and expert knowledge, the following hypotheses were formulated:

H1: Foragers will learn and adapt their foraging behaviour over time. This is further subdivided in two hypotheses:
H1a: Sick colonies will eat more and more from flowers that contain medicine.
H1b: Foragers from healthy colonies will eat more and more from flowers that do not contain medicine.
H2: Foragers visit more flowers that are closer to their nest to minimise energy expenditure (i.e., collect more nectar using less energy).

4.2   Data Collection

Four experiments were performed to collect data on the behaviour of bees. Two experiments, namely E1 and E2, were run with healthy bees, and two experiments, namely E3 and E4, were run with sick bees.

In each experiment, two identical greenhouse tents (namely left cage -L- and right cage -R-) were used. In each tent, a colony of around 30 workers and one queen was placed and 8 robotic flowers were deployed. The robotic flowers were presented in [6] with the purpose of measuring flower visit rates and duration per visit (in seconds) using a wireless transmission. The flowers are equipped with an infrared sensor located in the feeding hole that records when a bee visits it and the duration of the visit. In addition, sugar water is offered by the flowers in discrete amounts to simulate the natural availability of nectar and stimulate foraging in floral patches. Half of the flowers provided regular sugar water, while the other half contained sugar water that was treated with a plant secondary compound, being able to act as a medicine to cure the disease from which the sick bees suffered.

See Fig. 1(a) for a picture of the flowers and Fig. 1(b) for a schematic representation of the experiments' setting. As Fig. 1(b) shows, flowers were distributed in 4 groups of 2 inside the tent, with 2 groups of each colour located in diagonal to minimise influences of external variables. This setting was replicated for all four experiments. Each experiment ran for 96 h (from the noon of the first day to the noon of the fifth day), a duration that is considered by experts enough time to learn behaviour patterns.

4.3 Data Preprocessing

We assumed that only one bee can sit on each flower at a time and we focused on studying the behaviour of each colony as a single entity (not individual bees).

Given that bees usually only leave their nest during the day, visits logged after 12PM and before 6AM were considered as noise and dropped. Data quality issues due to logging, such as missing data, duplicate visits and truncated visit duration, were also solved during preprocessing.

The sensor logs are not segmented in traces of execution of the process. However, identifying a case is a prerequisite to apply PM. Since our intention

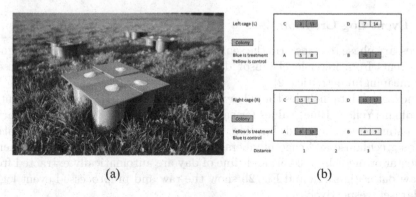

(a)   (b)

Fig. 1. (a) The robotic flowers used to collect data (picture taken outside of experiments) (b) Schema of the experimental setup to collect data on bee foraging behaviour.

is to study the collective behaviour of the bees, we considered each colony as
an individual case, i.e., experiment + left/right cage. For certain analyses, to
segment the sensor data further, we use a time window approach of 24 and 6 h.
The timestamps of each day are separated into 4 quarters, namely Quarter1
(morning), Quarter2 (afternoon), Quarter3 (evening) and Quarter4 (night) in
the intervals [6:00–12:00], [12:00–18:00], [18:00–0:00] and [0:00–6:00] respectively
(Quarter4 records are ignored). After that, data were split into 24-h time-based
windows, as follows (i represents the window number):

$$window(i) = Quarter2(i) + Quarter3(i) + Quarter1(i+1)$$

In the end, for each colony from each experiment, we have data distributed
within four 24-h windows and three-quarters per window. This step yielded a
sensor log containing 35092 events: 13062 from the first experiment (E1), 11120
from the second one (E2), 5046 from the third one (E3), and 5864 from the last
one (E4).

colony	hour	prob	Flower	date	trt	cage	color	disease
R2	13:51:58	6	flower6	20220404	D1	R	YELLOW	Healthy
R2	13:52:49	3	flower6	20220404	D1	R	YELLOW	Healthy
R2	13:53:10	4	flower6	20220404	D1	R	YELLOW	Healthy
R2	13:54:01	4	flower6	20220404	D1	R	YELLOW	Healthy
R2	13:53:29	5	flower6	20220404	D1	R	YELLOW	Healthy

(a)

Colony	Day	Window	Flower	StartTime	Activity	Prob	Cage	Color	Disease	Treatment	Group
R2	Day 1	Window 1	flower6	4/04/2022 13:51:58	eating	6	R	YELLOW	Healthy	D1	C
R2	Day 1	Window 1	flower6	4/04/2022 13:52:49	probing	3	R	YELLOW	Healthy	D1	C
R2	Day 1	Window 1	flower6	4/04/2022 13:53:10	eating	4	R	YELLOW	Healthy	D1	C
R2	Day 1	Window 1	flower6	4/04/2022 13:53:29	eating	5	R	YELLOW	Healthy	D1	C
R2	Day 1	Window 1	flower6	4/04/2022 13:54:01	eating	4	R	YELLOW	Healthy	D1	C

(b)

Fig. 2. A snapshot of the event logs (a) raw data and (b) preprocessed data

4.4   Event Log Creation

A necessary phase to transform the sensor log into an event log is to derive higher-
level events from lower-level sensor data, i.e., aggregating events to represent
more meaningful activities [2].

The logged data includes the colony, flower ID, cage (L/R), treatment/control
and colour (Yellow/Blue) values for each visit to a robotic flower, in association
with a start timestamp and duration. In the preprocessing, various information
such as greenhouse and cage numbers, flower identifier, flower type (whether it
has nectar or medicine), color, and time of day are automatically extracted from
the raw data. Figure 2a and Fig. 2b show the raw and preprocessed event log of
our dataset, respectively.

Then, for each captured sensor data, we created a record in the event log
containing the information mentioned in the sensor reading such as timestamp,

colony, cage and treatment and added some other processed information like group and distance. We determined the group (A/B/C/D) identifier and a distance attribute by grouping the flowers based on their distance from the nest in each cage. More specifically, we consider flowers located in groups A and C as distance 1 and flowers in groups B and D as distance 3 (see Fig. 1(b)).

In addition, we labelled the activities based on the duration of the visit of a bee on a flower. The used cutoffs were chosen based on previous research on bee behaviour [12] and expert knowledge. Events with a duration between 0 to 4 s are labelled as *Probing*, 4 to 30 as *Eating*, 30 to 200 as *Resting*, and 200 to 600 (maximum time in our experiment) as *Sleeping*.

4.5 Applying Process Mining

PM tools such as Celonis[1], Disco[2] and ProM[3] can help identify inefficiencies, bottlenecks, and opportunities for process optimization. Among the available commercial and research PM tools, we chose Disco as it is a powerful tool with a user-friendly interface and it provides the necessary functionalities to analyse the hypotheses. Using Disco, we have studied the events in the experiments and analysed the frequency, performance, and statistics of processes to confirm or reject the hypotheses. The results are next described in detail per hypothesis. Note that the activity and path parameters in Disco are set to 100% in all analyses, and that the conclusions of the analyses are drawn only for the experiments at hand.

H1: Foragers Will Learn and Adapt Their Foraging Behaviour over Time. We analysed the behaviour of bees for each colony focusing on the content provided by the flower, i.e. containing treated (D1) or untreated sugar water (CONTROL), over different time windows. In this way, we have considered colony as case in order to see in one single process model the behaviour evolution over the windows. In addition, the window, the bees' activity type and the flower content are considered all together as the activity feature in Disco. We then evaluated their eating activity on each flower content over time (the activity types are filtered and only data for *Eating* and *Probing* are used). In general, we observed for all colonies that the number of probing and eating activities on both flower contents increases over the time windows, decreasing a bit in the last window.

- H1a: Foragers from sick colonies will eat more and more from flowers that contain medicine (treated sugar water).
  To study this hypothesis, we created process maps for each sick colony (i.e., experiments E3 and E4, left and right cages). As a representative example, Figs. 3(a) and 3(b) illustrate the process maps for E3, Left colony (i.e., the

---

[1] https://www.celonis.com/.
[2] https://fluxicon.com/disco/.
[3] https://promtools.org/.

experiment and cage values are filtered to E3 and left respectively, and eating and probing activity). For each window except Window1, the number of eating activities on the medicine flowers (represented by nodes which have D1 in their labels) is higher than the flowers with untreated sugar water (nodes with control in the label). The same happens for E4 left. For the right cages, bees eat more from the control flowers in all windows, but there is a higher increase in eating activities in the treated flowers over time. This shows the sick bees' tendency to eat more and more treated sugar water, which follows our hypothesis.

- H1b: Foragers from healthy colonies will eat more and more from flowers that do not contain medicine (untreated sugar water).

  To study this hypothesis, we created process maps for each healthy colony (i.e., experiments E1 and E2, left and right cages). The discovered maps for the eating and probing behaviour of healthy bees for experiments E1, and E2 right cage, show that from the beginning to the end bees ate and probed more treated sugar water than not treated, however, both types of activities increased more in proportion over time for not treated sugar water than for treated sugar water. For E2, Left colony, bees started from Window 1 eating and probing more non-treated sugar water and kept that trend until the end (see Fig. 4(a) and Fig. 4(b)).

H2: Foragers Visit More the Flowers that Are Closer to Their Nest to Minimise Energy Expenditure. To explore this hypothesis, we considered the distance from the nest to the flowers as an attribute of the data in Disco. Then, we measured the percentage of all activities (eating, probing, resting and sleeping) for all experiments according to the distances that flowers were located at, Distance 1, and Distance 3, as shown in Table 1. We considered all the activities during different windows for each colony, to see if they change their selection of flowers based on their distance. Again, the colonies are considered as our cases in order to see in one single process model the behaviour evolution over the windows. The bees' activity type, window and distance are considered all together as the activity feature in Disco.

The discovered process maps indicate a similar pattern for the left colonies of sick bees: bees visit more remote flowers than close ones in all windows. Also, the sick bees in the right colonies started by visiting farther flowers in Window1 and changed their behaviour to visit the closer flowers afterwards. However, the behaviour of healthy bees do not follow any clearly identifiable pattern. Thus, the results do not show that bees prefer to visit closer flowers.

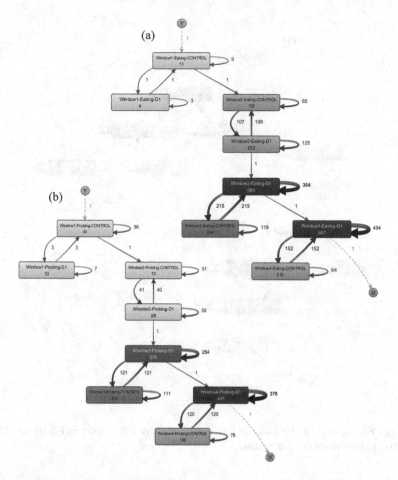

Fig. 3. (a) Eating and (b) Probing Behaviour of healthy left colony in E2 (treated (D1) and untreated (control) sugar water)

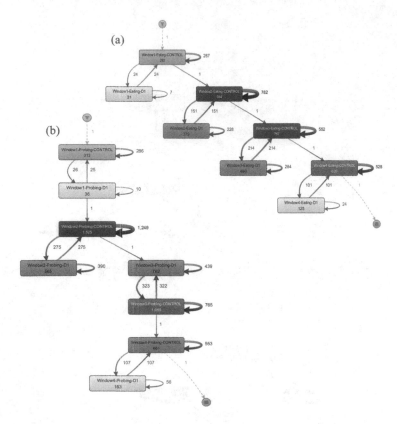

Fig. 4. (a) Eating and (b) Probing Behaviour of healthy left colony in E2 (treated (D1) and untreated (control) sugar water)

5   Discussion

Using behaviour data from 8 colonies, 4 sick and 4 healthy, we have explored the use of PM to understand the bees' behaviour and its evolution, in particular, their foraging activities and to which extent colonies learn and adapt their behaviour.

Following the successful implementations of PM in the literature mentioned in Sect. 2, we have demonstrated in our analyses that the use of a PM tool like Disco (as one of the means which can provide simplicity and understandability) is a suitable option to study the stated hypotheses and as such a valid alternative or complementary tool for the current methods used by domain experts (see Sect. 2.2). The PM techniques and tools specially can deal with the increasing amount of data that can be collected using IoT sensors and provide the domain experts with easy-to-understand interpretation in the form of DFGs with the possibility to consider all or even the most frequent activity and paths in a simpler form.

Table 1. Percentage of events based on the distance of flowers.

Distance	E1	E2	E3	E4
1	56.03	43.54	50.32	40.81
3	43.97	56.46	49.68	59.19

After preprocessing the data, their conversion into event logs by 1) abstracting the log into activities and 2) determining traces by focusing on collective behaviour (colonies), has proved capable to derive the necessary insights by applying PM. Then, the models discovered by process discovery approaches in PM techniques are used to highlight the bees' behaviour trend and their evolution over data collection period. In this way, these models are used to accept or reject the hypothesis made by domain experts. Furthermore, the models based on time windows are used to highlight the trend and evolution of bees' behaviour and activities for colonies over different days. These simple visualisations and the further interpretations made by domain experts are the results that cannot be driven with the tables and are the main point which we wanted to highlight as the application of PM.

Different process models focusing on different aspects (treatment vs control, closer or farther flowers, different activities, etc.) could easily be generated, and different analyses based on the discovered models could be performed (e.g., average or total time spent per activity). Once explained, the results are quite easily interpretable by domain experts, and the models provide helpful visuals to draw conclusions (when possible) or provide insights for further experiments. In addition, the experts in particular highlighted the benefit of visualising the transitions between the activities for each colony. The transitions between activities cannot be seen in tables, and that these transitions were given domain experts very important information on the learning process.

The visualisation of the trends over different days of an experiment or the possibility of comparing discovered models to highlight the evolution of activities for various cases in an understandable way allowed domain experts to get insights about the actual behaviours. These types of analyses are the benefits that can be enabled by PM and are the most valuable properties, which PM brings to the table and facilitates the research on natural processes.

In particular, the results allow us to draw the following insights:

- H1: while H1a is confirmed (sick bees have a tendency to eat more and more from treated sugar water), this increasing trend is not observed for healthy bees. Hence, we can state that H1b is rejected: healthy bees tend to keep their eating behaviour over time regarding the choice between treated or untreated sugar water. More experiments should therefore be carried out to reach conclusive results for confirming or rejecting H1.
- H2 can be rejected. We can conclude that the distances in our experiments did not seriously affect the preference of bees for certain flowers. However, this may be due to the relative small distances between flowers (considering

the greenhouse space limitations) compared to the areas that bees can cover for foraging in the nature.

The above insights on the behavioural differences between sick and healthy bee colonies can be used in real scenarios to test in vivo the efficacy of drugs against bee pathogens. Also, by monitoring the activity level of the bees at real-time, it may be possible to identify the discovered differences between sick and healthy colonies to determine the existence of a disease in the hive and treat the bees on time.

It is important to note that the rejection of the hypotheses in some aspects or the need to perform further experiments could be attributed to the complexity of the processes representing the behaviour of living beings, together with the involvement of multiple interacting variables that may not fully be captured by the initial setup. Next to this, we think that illumination may have caused differences in the bees' behaviour as well. The analyses enabled by PM allowed us to determine that colonies monitored in the right cages were in general less active than in the left cages. Although the experiments having mirrored cages tried to be performed under the same environmental conditions, after getting this insight from the PM analysis, the experts realised that the right cage was a bit further from the external light. The domain experts will try to minimise this difference in the next experiments. Furthermore, it is important to note that our findings only apply to the collected data. In order to obtain a more accurate understanding of bee behaviour and generalize our findings, it is necessary to perform more experiments under diverse environmental conditions.

Finally, although the chosen cut-offs to derive the high-level activities are based on previous research and expert knowledge, they should be investigated further as a difference in a few seconds could output very different process maps and as such different conclusions, specially for H1. Another approach that could be followed to be certain on the cut-offs is to install a weight scale in the flowers that monitors at real time the exact amount of sugar water that is eaten in each visit.

6   Conclusions and Future Work

In this paper, we have presented a novel case study where a PM analysis has been successfully applied to study the foraging behaviour of bees. We showed that PM, and Disco in particular, is a powerful and relatively easy-to-use tool to discover and visualise the colonies' process flows and the behaviour evolution in time, and as such it showed to be suitable to evaluate the stated hypotheses on bees' foraging behaviour. This shows the potential to use PM to study insects behaviour that can be monitored using IoT technology. It is very important however that all relevant variables are carefully determined and monitored at the right frequency in order to get insights that reflect the reality as close as possible.

As further work, we plan to use NFC or RFID tags to track the behaviour of individual bees. These data may allow us to get a better understanding on the individual behaviour and preferences of bees and their individual foraging patterns. The complexity of the bees' behaviour, together with the involvement of multiple variables, may have affected collected data and our findings. In addition, due to the limitations, the current experiments are done in the lab setting and we are going to conduct further experiments under a more realistic configuration to study the behaviour of bees under diverse environmental conditions, for longer periods of data collection and larger distances between flowers and hives, more in line with what happens in reality. Within these experiments, contextual data such as illumination will also be captured as the difference behavioural difference between the cages (left/right) may be attributed to that factor.

Acknowledgment. The work of Yannis Bertrand and Estefanía Serral was supported by the Flemish Fund for Scientific Research (FWO) with grant number G0B6922N.

References

1. Adler, L.S.: The ecological significance of toxic nectar. Oikos **91**(3), 409–420 (2000)
2. Bertrand, Y., Van den Abbeele, B., Veneruso, S., Leotta, F., Mecella, M., Serral, E.: A survey on the application of process discovery techniques to smart spaces data. Eng. Appl. Artif. Intell. **126**, 106748 (2023)
3. Bertrand, Y., De Weerdt, J., Serral, E.: Assessing the suitability of traditional event log standards for IoT-enhanced event logs. In: Cabanillas, C., Garmann-Johnsen, N.F., Koschmider, A. (eds.) BPM 2022. LNCS, vol. 460, pp. 63–75. Springer, Cham (2023). https://doi.org/10.1007/978-3-031-25383-6_6
4. Brzychczy, E., Trzcionkowska, A.: Creation of an event log from a low-level machinery monitoring system for process mining purposes. In: Yin, H., Camacho, D., Novais, P., Tallón-Ballesteros, A. (eds.) IDEAL 2018. LNCS, vol. 11315, pp. 54–63. Springer, Cham (2018). https://doi.org/10.1007/978-3-030-03496-2_7
5. Crall, J.D., Gravish, N., Mountcastle, A.M., Combes, S.A.: BEEtag: a low-cost, image-based tracking system for the study of animal behavior and locomotion. PLoS ONE **10**(9), e0136487 (2015)
6. Debeuckelaere, K., Janssens, D., Serral Asensio, E., Jacquemyn, H., Pozo, M.I.: A wireless, user-friendly, and unattended robotic flower system to assess pollinator foraging behaviour. bioRxiv (2022). https://doi.org/10.1101/2022.06.14.496104
7. Janssen, D., Mannhardt, F., Koschmider, A., van Zelst, S.J.: Process model discovery from sensor event data. In: Leemans, S., Leopold, H. (eds.) ICPM 2020. LNBIP, vol. 406, pp. 69–81. Springer, Cham (2021). https://doi.org/10.1007/978-3-030-72693-5_6
8. Knauer, A.C., Schiestl, F.P.: Bees use honest floral signals as indicators of reward when visiting flowers. Ecol. Lett. **18**(2), 135–143 (2015)
9. Koschmider, A., Janssen, D., Mannhardt, F.: Framework for process discovery from sensor data. In: EMISA, pp. 32–38 (2020)
10. MacArthur, R.H., Pianka, E.R.: On optimal use of a patchy environment. Am. Nat. **100**(916), 603–609 (1966)
11. Marden, J.H.: Remote perception of floral nectar by bumblebees. Oecologia **64**(2), 232–240 (1984)
12. Pashte, V., Shylesha, A., et al.: Pollen and nectar foraging activity of honey bees in sesamum. Indian J. Entomol. **75**(2), 124–126 (2013)

13. Patel, V., Pauli, N., Biggs, E., Barbour, L., Boruff, B.: Why bees are critical for achieving sustainable development. Ambio **50**(1), 49–59 (2021)
14. Pozo, M.I., et al.: The impact of yeast presence in nectar on bumble bee behavior and fitness. Ecol. Monogr. **90**(1), e01393 (2020)
15. Pyke, G.H.: Optimal foraging: movement patterns of bumblebees between inflorescences. Theor. Popul. Biol. **13**(1), 72–98 (1978)
16. Seiger, R., Zerbato, F., Burattin, A., Garcia-Banuelos, L., Weber, B.: Towards IoT-driven process event log generation for conformance checking in smart factories. In: EDOCW, pp. 20–26 (2020)
17. Soffer, P., et al.: From event streams to process models and back: challenges and opportunities. Inf. Syst. **81**, 181–200 (2019)
18. Sora, D., Leotta, F., Mecella, M.: An habit is a process: a BPM-based approach for smart spaces. In: Teniente, E., Weidlich, M. (eds.) BPM 2017. LNBIP, vol. 308, pp. 298–309. Springer, Cham (2018). https://doi.org/10.1007/978-3-319-74030-0_22
19. Valencia Parra, Á., Ramos Gutiérrez, B., Varela Vaca, Á.J., Gómez López, M.T., García Bernal, A.: Enabling process mining in aircraft manufactures: extracting event logs and discovering processes from complex data. In: BPM2019IF (2019)
20. van Eck, M.L., Lu, X., Leemans, S.J.J., van der Aalst, W.M.P.: PM: a process mining project methodology. In: Zdravkovic, J., Kirikova, M., Johannesson, P. (eds.) CAiSE 2015. LNCS, vol. 9097, pp. 297–313. Springer, Cham (2015). https://doi.org/10.1007/978-3-319-19069-3_19

Tiramisù: A Recipe for Visual Sensemaking of Multi-faceted Process Information

Anti Alman[1], Alessio Arleo[2], Iris Beerepoot[3][(✉)], Andrea Burattin[4],
Claudio Di Ciccio[5], and Manuel Resinas[6]

[1] University of Tartu, Tartu, Estonia
anti.alman@ut.ee
[2] TU Wien, Vienna, Austria
alessio.arleo@tuwien.ac.at
[3] Utrecht University, Utrecht, The Netherlands
i.m.beerepoot@uu.nl
[4] Technical University of Denmark, Kgs. Lyngby, Denmark
andbur@dtu.dk
[5] Sapienza University of Rome, Rome, Italy
claudio.diciccio@uniroma1.it
[6] Universidad de Sevilla, Seville, Spain
resinas@us.es

Abstract. Knowledge-intensive processes represent a particularly challenging scenario for process mining. The flexibility that such processes allow constitutes a hurdle as it is hard to capture in a single model. To tackle this problem, multiple visual representations of the same processes could be beneficial, each addressing different information dimensions according to the specific needs and background knowledge of the concrete process workers and stakeholders. In this idea paper, we propose a novel framework leveraging visual analytics for the interactive visualization of multi-faceted process information, aimed at easing the investigation tasks of users in their process analysis tasks. This is primarily achieved by an interconnection of multiple visual layers, which allow our framework to display process information under different perspectives and to project these perspectives onto a domain-friendly representation of the context in which the process unfolds. We demonstrate the feasibility of the framework through its application in two use-case scenarios in the context of healthcare and personal information management.

Keywords: Visual analytics · Process mining · Knowledge-intensive processes

1 Introduction and Background

Process mining (PM) is the discipline aimed at extracting information from events recorded by information systems executing processes [3]. The operational

J. De Smedt and P. Soffer (Eds.): ICPM 2023 Workshops, LNBIP 503, pp. 19–31, 2024.
https://doi.org/10.1007/978-3-031-56107-8_2

context of process mining is multi-variate since data potentially stems from multiple sources and pertains to diverse dimensions (control flow, time, resources, object lifecycles). As argued by the pivotal work of Beerepoot et al. [8], a critical, yet largely unaddressed, issue of process mining is the fixed-granularity level of process analysis, namely the inability to navigate through distinct, and possibly domain-specific, dimensions. This problem limits the effectiveness of process improvement investigation, as studied by Kubrak et al. [23], as it entails a partial view over an inherently complex search space, which is typical of knowledge-intensive processes [13,14]. Visual Analytics (VA) is the discipline of supporting users' analytical reasoning through the use of interactive visual interfaces [22]. VA is intended to keep the user *within* the analysis loop, so that human comprehension and perception actively contribute to generating new insights and increasing confidence with the analysis results. VA has extensively studied the problem of representing complex, multi-faceted phenomena [20,28], which is also the type of phenomena often encountered within real-life business processes.

Thus far, there has been limited cooperation between PM and VA [25] despite the remarkable achievements their interplay could bring about [19]. In this paper, we argue that VA can play a pivotal role in addressing the above limitation of fixed-granularity in process mining. And, with a cross-pollinating effect, PM can equip VA with a collection of established algorithms and techniques for the automated generation of process-oriented representations of system dynamics.

In this idea paper, we theorize a novel framework, which we call the Tiramisù approach. It relies on VA for the interactive investigation of factual evidence of process insights revolving around information mined from data sources that go under the name of *sequence event data*, to use VA's terminology, or *event logs*, as per the PM nomenclature. Our framework follows a multi-layered approach, providing end users with a context-aware visualization integrating classical PM representation elements (such as workflow nets [32], directly-follows graphs [2], or declarative process maps [4]) with additional diagrams and visual cues tailored for context-variable and metadata representations (e.g., timelines and calendars for time, geographical or building maps for space, etc.). We categorize the different data facets, discuss how and where they fit our framework, and provide representation examples, with the overarching goal of describing a design process that enables practitioners to integrate different data sources into an organic representation fitting a PM workflow. The interconnection of the different layers and their anchorage to a *backdrop* (i.e., a representation of the context, such as calendars or maps), onto which the representations are projected, provides the user with a means to foster explainability for process analysis and, eventually, enhancement. This overcomes a limitation of the few proposals that combine PM and VA [17,31], which do not consider the representation of domain-specific dimensions, thus limiting their utility for knowledge-intensive processes.

In the remainder of this paper, Sect. 2 describes our framework, incl. its key concepts and their interplay. Section 3 showcases two scenarios in the area of knowledge-intensive processes. Section 4 acknowledges some known limitations of our work, paving the way for future work discussed in the final section Sect. 5.

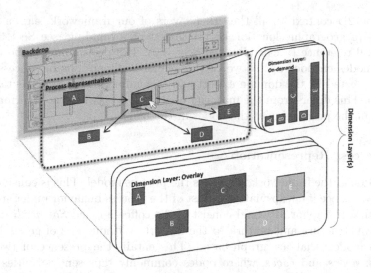

Fig. 1. An exemplification of the `Tiramisù` framework. Several dimension layers can be visualized concurrently, either overlaid on top of other layers or as an on-demand information. In this example, the backdrop resembles the one shown in Scenario 1 (see Sect. 3.1), wherein it provides the process representation within a spatial context.

2   The Tiramisù Framework

`Tiramisù` is a VA framework designed to support sensemaking when dealing with complex PM event sequences. Our goal is to augment existing process models and upgrade process maps with additional dimensions that can provide further context during the analysis, easing the generation of insights and generally providing a more comprehensive understanding of the process and phenomenon under investigation trough visualizations that better align with the mental model of the users. With this goal in mind, we design `Tiramisù` as a multi-level framework (see Fig. 1), reminiscent of the popular *tiramisù* dessert. The framework is structured with a "backdrop" providing context (see Sect. 2.1), a main layer with the process representation (Sect. 2.2), and one or more dimension layers (Sect. 2.3). We describe the individual parts of the framework in the following.

2.1   Backdrop

The backdrop (also *base*) layer acts as a common context for the process and for all the further dimensions that we include in the final interactive visualization. In the metaphor with the *tiramisù*, the backdrop would be the cream that permeates all the dessert's layers. It is designed to reflect the context of the current application, presenting the user with a familiar environment that acts as a "framing" device for the other process data and information. In PM, the idea of framing the process representation into a context that is not oriented to a specific task [12] is rather novel. From a visualization perspective, it provides a common 2D context to all the other layers of our framework, e.g., a spatial reference (a geographic location or the layout of a building, see Sect. 3.1), or a temporal reference (a calendar, see Sect. 3.2). The positioning of the process models' nodes encodes up to two of the available dimensions in process information, selected by the domain expert and depending on the analysis task (see also [31]). This differs from the majority of PM models, where no information is encoded in the positioning of the nodes in the plane.

2.2 Process Representation

This section of the framework visualizes the process model. This is considered as a core layer, since it encapsulates the gist of the process behavior under study. In the tiramisù metaphor, it would consist of the coffee-imbued *Savoiardi* biscuits, which give structure and texture to the dessert. Without loss of generality, we focus on models that are graph-based. This entails the presence of two main elements: *nodes* and *edges*, where nodes commonly represent activities of the business process and edges represent (usually temporal) relations between these activities. In our framework, nodes are anchored to the backdrop, meaning that their positioning is consistent with the context expressed in the base layer. Nodes can also encode further attributes in other visual channels, such as size, color, and transparency. Node appearance can also be encoded as glyphs, as we will see in Sect. 3.1 with Scenario 1. Similarly, visual channels related to edges can be manipulated (e.g., width, transparency, and color). Moreover, edge visualization can be explicit (i.e., visible), or implicit. In this second case, the connections between the nodes can either be extrapolated from the context without being shown, or placed in one of the dimension layers of the framework.

2.3 Dimension Layers

Our framework supports further layers to be superimposed on the first two, in a details-on-demand fashion [29]. These layers can serve different purposes, including: (i) provide contextual information on individual or arbitrarily small groups of nodes and edges in the process model (as in the scenario presented in Sect. 3); (ii) augment the backdrop visualization, such as enabling the visualization of a further dimension on the backdrop or on top of the process representation. In the tiramisù metaphor, the layers represent the different toppings, providing a distinct "character" to the dessert. In the framework, the layers are meant to expose hidden correlations between the dimensions within the auxiliary process information and the model itself. Our framework does not put any limit in the number of dimension layers. To avoid excessive visual clutter, the user can toggle the visibility of specific layers (following the details-on-demand principle). In turn, this option requires that the visualization designer knows or collaborates with a domain expert, in order to be able to rank and assign each dimension either to the backdrop or the dimension layers.

3   Use-Case Scenarios

In this section, we illustrate two scenarios that motivate our work through six user stories. We focus on two classes of knowledge-intensive processes, pertaining to healthcare [26] and personal information management [11]. Both scenarios demonstrate the capability of our solution to pinpoint deviations from the expected outcome, and investigate the cause for it in a multi-perspective fashion. The former, based on the work on [15], is described in Sect. 3.1 and illustrates the application of our solution with a particular focus on the spatial dimension. The latter, inspired by the investigation in [7], is discussed in Sect. 3.2 and involves the temporal dimension.

3.1   Behavioral Deviation Analysis in Healthcare

Healthcare is one of the most difficult, but at the same time, one of the most promising domains to tackle both in the field of PM [26] and in the field of VA [10]. Indeed, the interplay of the two research fields in this context has the potential to yield remarkable outcomes, as shown in [17]. Thus, healthcare is a natural domain for applying the Tiramisù approach. As a demonstration, we have chosen the specific task of analyzing the sleeping routine of patients suffering from dementia or other similar diseases. Naively applying the already existing process mining approaches to this task can, for example, lead to relying on simple process maps (models) where the nodes represent various activities performed by the patients, and the arcs represent dependencies or other temporal constraints among these activities [15]. While the above models may be sufficient for a process mining expert to extrapolate meaningful process insights, it can quickly become challenging for domain experts, who may lack training in interpreting these formalisms: As discussed in [15,16], the most likely users of such analysis tools would be the doctors and the nurses responsible for the care of the specific patient, and not PM experts.

When investigating this scenario in more depth, we also need to consider the types of analysis that would be relevant in this domain. To better structure our contribution, we identified the following user stories:

- **US1:** As a nurse, I want to inspect the typical sleeping routine of a patient;
- **US2:** As a nurse, I want to quickly spot the presence of deviations from the typical behavior and what these refer to;
- **US3:** As a nurse, I want to dive deeper into the context of a deviation.

As a backdrop for the above, we introduce the floor plan of the room of a specific patient, on top of which it is possible to project the activities performed by the patient in a way that more closely matches what doctors and nurses are familiar with, i.e., the environment that the patient interacts with. This backdrop can be seen on the left-hand side of Fig. 2.

As discussed in Sect. 2, the backdrop serves as a common context onto which it is possible to project process-related information. The right-hand side of Fig. 2

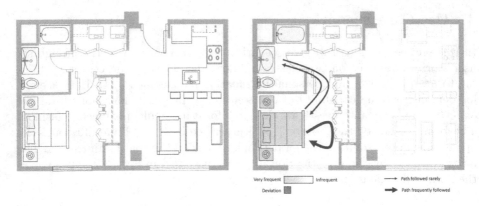

Fig. 2. The backdrop used for Scenario 1, with the floor map where patients live (left) and the backdrop overlaid with the sleeping routine of a patient (right)

depicts one such floor plan, overlaid with the sleeping routine of a patient. Instead of representing activities as "meaningless" boxes (i.e., the shape and location of the boxes does not encode any dimension), we refer directly to the parts of the room, or specific appliances/furniture, related to the corresponding activities. This approach brings visualization closer to what the analysts (i.e., nurses and doctors) are already familiar with. It also introduces an intuitive spatial dimension to representing patient behavior. This visualization, in essence, allows us to address user story **US1**. The visual encoding of nodes (i.e., the pictograms/glyphs) refers to the frequency of the activities performed by the patient (delivered via different shades of green and transparency of nodes) while the visual encoding of edges refers to the frequency of transitioning from one activity to the other (via the thickness of the nodes).

The addition of overlays will allow for the reuse of the same backdrop also for other types of analysis. For example, the overlay shown on the left-hand side of Fig. 3 would be specifically designed in a manner that allows nurses and doctors to easily spot deviations from the sleeping routine of the patient, thus answering **US2**. In this case, we use a specific color for highlighting deviations from the reference behavior of the patient. This encoding (i.e., the color) is applied to both nodes and edges.

Furthermore, as shown in Fig. 3 (right), by interacting with the visualization, doctors and nurses will have the opportunity to select specific activities in order to dive deeper into the details related to a specific deviation via a pop-up (i.e., a window that opens on top of the glyph). Following the *details on demand* principle [29], such pop-up will report details regarding the underlying process execution, such as the actual Workflow net model (possibly with colors suggesting where deviations happened) [32], a DCR model [21], and statistical aspects such as average duration, etc. This, in turn, provides a possible solution for **US3**.

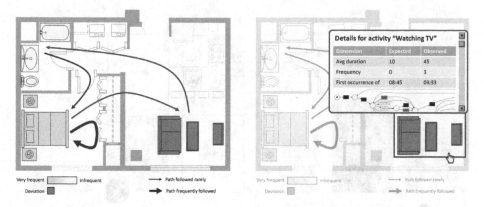

Fig. 3. The backdrop overlaid with deviations from the typical routine. The figure on the left is meant for quickly identifying the deviation, while the figure on the right represents an interaction to dive deeper into the details of a deviation.

3.2 Personal Productivity Analysis in Work Processes

Personal information management (PIM) pertains to the organization of one's own activities, contacts, etc., through the use of software on laptops and smart devices. Similarly, personal informatics systems resort to one individual's own information to pursue the objective of aiding people to collect and reflect on their personal information [24]. Several techniques can be used to collect personal information such as non-participant observations, screen recordings, and timesheet techniques, each with their own advantages and disadvantages [30]. Regardless of the technique used, collected personal information can be seen as an event log, which can be analyzed using process mining techniques to discover personal work processes [9].

Depending on the characteristics of the work, personal work processes can be knowledge-intensive and significantly unstructured, which means they present the aforementioned challenges. In this scenario, we focus on the personal work processes performed by an academic during her daily work, which involves conducting research, preparing lessons, grading students or reviewing research papers, among many other activities. Specifically, our focus is on the retrospective analysis of the influence of the personal work processes a person has followed during a certain period of time on the positive or negative outcome of some specific task (e.g., missing the deadline for submitting a review). In particular, we identify the following user stories as representative of this scenario:

- **US4:** As a researcher, I want to investigate when I was working on the reviews;
- **US5:** As a researcher, I want to shed light on the time aspects that are relevant in the context of my reviews;
- **US6:** As a researcher, I want to dive deeper into my reviewing activity on Friday afternoon to understand what caused the delay.

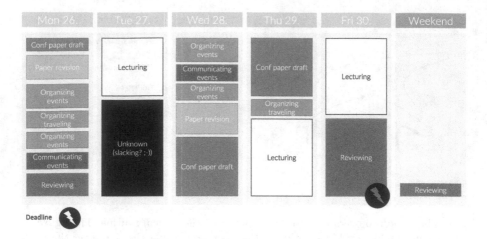

Fig. 4. The backdrop of Scenario 2 overlaid with the weekly summary of the activities and the deadlines, represented as lightning bolts

To this end, we use a calendar with a user-specified time period as the backdrop of the visual representation. This backdrop is overlaid with a summary of the activities performed during the time period, as exemplified in Fig. 4. The activities are represented as boxes with the color referring to the activity type (e.g., all lecturing activities in white, despite possibly being lectures on different topics/courses). The position and size of each box represent when the activity started and its duration, respectively. Thereby, the researcher can spot when she is reviewing the assigned papers, thus addressing **US4**. Notice the lightning bolt icon in the figure. This additional overlay signals the reviewing deadline through that glyph. The icon uses the same color code as the activities to indicate the activity the deadline refers to. Its presence helps the researcher put in a relationship the duration and allocation of work with the expected consignment time, thus catering for **US5**.

Similarly to Sect. 3.1, we use as a backdrop a representation that is intuitive to the user and specific to the scenario under analysis. However, unlike in the previous scenario, the representation refers to the time dimension (a calendar) instead of the space dimension (a floor map). This aspect illustrates that the concept of backdrop can (and must) be adapted to the dimension that best fits the scenario being addressed.

Now, as the academic wants to understand what is the cause of the delay for delivering the review (**US6**), she might want to dive deeper into the details by clicking on any of the activities of the weekly summary. For instance, let us say that the academic wants to know more details about what happened on Friday evening while performing the reviewing activity that prevented her from finishing the review on time. To this end, the academic can click on the reviewing activity of Friday evening, which will open a popup with multi-faceted details related to the activity at hand (again following the *details on demand* principle [29]),

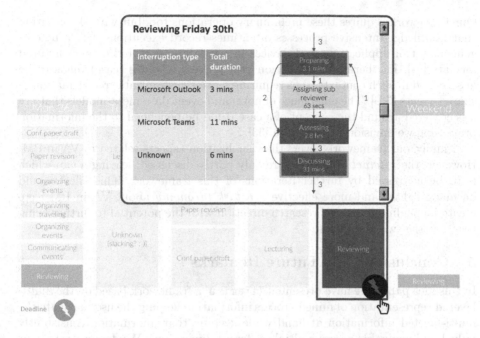

Fig. 5. The backdrop of Scenario 2 showing the details of the review activity on Friday evening.

as illustrated in Fig. 5. In this case, the details include a directly-follows graph representing the sub-activities performed as part of the reviewing activities and a summary of the interruptions that happened during that time interval.

4   Limitations

Evidence-based process discovery approaches may, in some cases, suffer from reliability issues, given that only some parts of the processes (especially in the case of knowledge-intensive processes) are recorded by computerized systems [18]. Our framework is in this sense no different. The injection of additional facts stemming from domain experts and users is complementary to this investigation and paves the path for future work.

The design of the visualizations in backdrop, and in the other layers is a challenge of its own, and should be tackled by visualization experts in close cooperation with domain experts and target users. Investigating this aspect goes beyond the scope of this paper. However, the interested reader is referred to the work of Sirgmets et al. [31], which presents a framework aimed to guide design choices for the effective visualization of analytical data, and to the paper by Munzner et al. [27], where a nested model for visualization design is presented.

Data-based process analysis tasks often involve a significant amount of time for extracting, reformatting, and filtering event logs from information systems [1].

Our framework requires these preliminary operations too, but with the addition that knowledge-intensive processes oftentimes record executions over a heterogeneous set of applications and devices in partially structured or unstructured formats [14]. Furthermore, the notion of a process instance (case) tends to be less defined in such contexts, thus requiring a prior customizable reconciliation of shared events [5,6]. The emergence of novel and event data meta-models that are less centered around the concept of a case could be beneficial to the information processing we envision in Tiramisù [33].

Finally, our framework covers the visualization aspects related to VA in PM. However, the *interaction* aspects are only partly discussed, leaving a gap which is to be addressed by further iterations of this framework. This effort would be made lighter and more effective if a *task taxonomy* about VA in PM were created, opening up a novel research direction with the potential to further bring together the two disciplines.

5   Conclusions and Future Remarks

In this idea paper, we have presented Tiramisù, a framework based on the multi-layered representation of mined process information helping the user navigate the multi-faceted information at hand while keeping that information consistently linked and navigable across multiple different dimensions. We demonstrated our solution through its application to scenarios illustrating its suitability in the context of knowledge-intensive processes.

We foresee the following research endeavors in the future originating from our current idea. An evaluation based on an empirical study involving users is in our plans to assess the efficacy and effectiveness of the Tiramisù framework. The implementation of a working prototype is crucial to this extent and is also part of our agenda. This goes in tandem with the future work of identifying the different user types and their specific visualization needs within the context of the Tiramisù framework. In connection to the previous, we envision that the customization and refactoring of layers, their aggregation rules, and backdrops will be key challenges to be addressed in the future. Finally, we observe that stepping from a multi-layered single-backdrop design to a tree-like hierarchical structure of backdrops could initiate a new path toward a significant extension of the expressive richness guaranteed by our framework.

Acknowledgments. This work was started at Schloss Dagstuhl (Leibniz-Zentrum für Informatik), seminar 23271 "Human in the (Process) Mines", and we thank the institute and the organizers for giving us the opportunity to participate. The work of A. Alman was supported by the European Social Fund via "ICT programme" measure and by the Estonian Research Council grant PRG1226. The work of C. Di Ciccio was supported by the Italian Ministry of University and Research (MUR) under PRIN grant B87G22000450001 (PINPOINT) and by project SERICS (PE00000014) under the NRRP MUR program funded by the EU-NGEU. The work of M. Resinas was partially supported by projects PID2021-126227NB-C21/ AEI/10.13039/501100011033/ FEDER, UE and TED2021-131023B-C22/ AEI/10.13039/501100011033/ Unión Europea NextGenerationEU/PRTR.

References

1. van der Aalst, W.M.P.: Process Mining - Data Science in Action, 2nd edn. Springer, Cham (2016). https://doi.org/10.1007/978-3-662-49851-4
2. van der Aalst, W.M.P.: Foundations of process discovery. In: van der Aalst and Carmona [3], pp. 37–75. https://doi.org/10.1007/978-3-031-08848-3_2
3. van der Aalst, W.M.P., Carmona, J. (eds.): Process Mining Handbook. LNBIP, vol. 448. Springer, Cham (2022)
4. Alman, A., Di Ciccio, C., Maggi, F.M., Montali, M., van der Aa, H.: RuM: declarative process mining, distilled. In: Polyvyanyy, A., Wynn, M.T., Van Looy, A., Reichert, M. (eds.) BPM 2021. LNCS, vol. 12875, pp. 23–29. Springer, Cham (2021). https://doi.org/10.1007/978-3-030-85469-0_3
5. Baier, T., Mendling, J., Weske, M.: Bridging abstraction layers in process mining. Inf. Syst. **46**, 123–139 (2014). https://doi.org/10.1016/j.is.2014.04.004
6. Bayomie, D., Di Ciccio, C., Mendling, J.: Event-case correlation for process mining using probabilistic optimization. Inf. Syst. **114**, 102167 (2023). https://doi.org/10.1016/j.is.2023.102167
7. Beerepoot, I., et al.: A window of opportunity: active window tracking for mining work practices. In: ICPM, pp. 57–64. IEEE (2023)
8. Beerepoot, I., et al.: The biggest business process management problems to solve before we die. Comput. Ind. **146**, 103837 (2023). https://doi.org/10.1016/j.compind.2022.103837
9. Bertrand, Y., Van den Abbeele, B., Veneruso, S., Leotta, F., Mecella, M., Serral, E.: A survey on the application of process mining to smart spaces data. In: Montali, M., Senderovich, A., Weidlich, M. (eds.) ICPM 2022. LNBIP, vol. 468, pp. 57–70. Springer, Cham (2023). https://doi.org/10.1007/978-3-031-27815-0_5
10. Caban, J.J., Gotz, D.: Visual analytics in healthcare - opportunities and research challenges. J. Am. Med. Inform. Assoc. **22**(2), 260–262 (2015). https://doi.org/10.1093/jamia/ocv006
11. Catarci, T., Dix, A., Katifori, A., Lepouras, G., Poggi, A.: Task-centred information management. In: Thanos, C., Borri, F., Candela, L. (eds.) DELOS 2007. LNCS, vol. 4877, pp. 197–206. Springer, Heidelberg (2007). https://doi.org/10.1007/978-3-540-77088-6_19
12. de Leoni, M., Suriadi, S., ter Hofstede, A.H.M., van der Aalst, W.M.P.: Turning event logs into process movies: animating what has really happened. Softw. Syst. Model. **15**(3), 707–732 (2016). https://doi.org/10.1007/s10270-014-0432-2
13. De Weerdt, J., Schupp, A., Vanderloock, A., Baesens, B.: Process mining for the multi-faceted analysis of business processes - a case study in a financial services organization. Comput. Ind. **64**(1), 57–67 (2013). https://doi.org/10.1016/j.compind.2012.09.010
14. Di Ciccio, C., Marrella, A., Russo, A.: Knowledge-intensive processes: characteristics, requirements and analysis of contemporary approaches. J. Data Semant. **4**(1), 29–57 (2015). https://doi.org/10.1007/s13740-014-0038-4
15. Di Federico, G., Burattin, A.: Do you behave always the same? In: Montali, M., Senderovich, A., Weidlich, M. (eds.) ICPM 2022. LNBIP, vol. 468, pp. 5–17. Springer, Cham (2023). https://doi.org/10.1007/978-3-031-27815-0_1
16. Di Federico, G., Burattin, A., Montali, M.: Human behavior as a process model: which language to use? In: ITBPM@BPM, pp. 18–25. CEUR-WS.org (2021). https://ceur-ws.org/Vol-2952/paper_293a.pdf

17. Dixit, P.M., Caballero, H.S.G., Corvò, A., Hompes, B.F.A., Buijs, J.C.A.M., van der Aalst, W.M.P.: Enabling interactive process analysis with process mining and visual analytics. In: HEALTHINF, pp. 573–584. SciTePress (2017). https://doi.org/10.5220/0006272605730584

18. Dumas, M., La Rosa, M., Mendling, J., Reijers, H.A.: Fundamentals of Business Process Management, 2nd edn. Springer, Cham (2018). https://doi.org/10.1007/978-3-662-56509-4

19. Gschwandtner, T.: Visual analytics meets process mining: challenges and opportunities. In: Ceravolo, P., Rinderle-Ma, S. (eds.) SIMPDA 2015. LNBIP, vol. 244, pp. 142–154. Springer, Cham (2017). https://doi.org/10.1007/978-3-319-53435-0_7

20. Hadlak, S., Schumann, H., Schulz, H.J.: A survey of multi-faceted graph visualization. In: EuroVis (STARs), pp. 1–20 (2015)

21. Hildebrandt, T.T., Mukkamala, R.R.: Declarative event-based workflow as distributed dynamic condition response graphs. arXiv preprint arXiv:1110.4161 (2011)

22. Keim, D., Andrienko, G., Fekete, J.D., Görg, C., Kohlhammer, J., Melancon, G.: Visual analytics: definition, process, and challenges. In: Kerren, A., Stasko, J.T., Fekete, J.D., North, C. (eds.) Information Visualization. LNCS, vol. 4950, pp. 154–175. Springer, Heidelberg (2008). https://doi.org/10.1007/978-3-540-70956-5_7

23. Kubrak, K., Milani, F., Nolte, A.: A visual approach to support process analysts in working with process improvement opportunities. Bus. Process. Manag. J. **29**(8), 101–132 (2023)

24. Li, I., Dey, A.K., Forlizzi, J.: A stage-based model of personal informatics systems. In: CHI, pp. 557–566. ACM (2010). https://doi.org/10.1145/1753326.1753409

25. Miksch, S.: Visual analytics meets process mining: challenges and opportunities. In: ICPM, pp. xiv–xiv (2021). https://doi.org/10.1109/ICPM53251.2021.9576854

26. Munoz-Gama, J., Martin, N., et al.: Process mining for healthcare: characteristics and challenges. J. Biomed. Inform. **127**, 103994 (2022). https://doi.org/10.1016/j.jbi.2022.103994

27. Munzner, T.: A nested process model for visualization design and validation. IEEE Trans. Vis. Comput. Graph. **15**(6), 921–928 (2009). https://doi.org/10.1109/TVCG.2009.111

28. Raidou, R.G.: Visual analytics for the representation, exploration, and analysis of high-dimensional, multi-faceted medical data. Biomed. Vis. **2**, 137–162 (2019)

29. Shneiderman, B.: The eyes have it: a task by data type taxonomy for information visualizations. In: VL, pp. 336–343. IEEE (1996). https://doi.org/10.1109/VL.1996.545307

30. Šinik, T., Beerepoot, I., Reijers, H.A.: A peek into the working day: comparing techniques for recording employee behaviour. In: Nurcan, S., Opdahl, A.L., Mouratidis, H., Tsohou, A. (eds.) RCIS 2023. LNBIP, vol. 476, pp. 343–359. Springer, Cham (2023). https://doi.org/10.1007/978-3-031-33080-3_21

31. Sirgmets, M., Milani, F., Nolte, A., Pungas, T.: Designing process diagrams – a framework for making design choices when visualizing process mining outputs. In: Panetto, H., Debruyne, C., Proper, H., Ardagna, C., Roman, D., Meersman, R. (eds.) OTM 2018. LNCS, vol. 11229, pp. 463–480. Springer, Cham (2018). https://doi.org/10.1007/978-3-030-02610-3_26

32. van der Aalst, W.M.P.: The application of petri nets to workflow management. J. Circuits Syst. Comput. **8**(1), 21–66 (1998). https://doi.org/10.1142/S0218126698000043

33. Wynn, M.T., et al.: Rethinking the input for process mining: insights from the XES survey and workshop. In: Munoz-Gama, J., Lu, X. (eds.) ICPM 2021. LNBIP, vol. 433, pp. 3–16. Springer, Cham (2022). https://doi.org/10.1007/978-3-030-98581-3_1

NICE: The Native IoT-Centric Event Log Model for Process Mining

Yannis Bertrand[1]([✉]) [iD], Silvestro Veneruso[2] [iD], Francesco Leotta[2] [iD], Massimo Mecella[2] [iD], and Estefanía Serral[1] [iD]

[1] Research Centre for Information Systems Engineering (LIRIS), KU Leuven, Warmoesberg 26, 1000 Brussels, Belgium
{yannis.bertrand,estefania.serral}@kuleuven.be
[2] Sapienza Universitá di Roma, Rome, Italy
{veneruso,leotta,mecella}@diag.uniroma1.it

Abstract. More and more so-called IoT-enhanced business processes (BPs) are supported by IoT devices, which collect large amounts of data about the execution of such processes. While these data have the potential to reveal crucial insights into the execution of the BPs, the absence of a suitable event log format integrating IoT data to process data greatly hampers the realisation of this potential. In this paper, we present the Native Iot-Centric Event (NICE) log, a new event log format designed to incorporate IoT data into a process event log ensuring traceability, flexibility and limiting data loss. The new format was linked to a smart spaces data simulator to generate synthetic logs. We evaluate our format against requirements previously established for an IoT-enhanced event log format, showing that it meets all requirements, contrarily to other alternative formats. We then perform an analysis of a synthetic log to show how IoT data can easily be used to explain anomalies in the process.

Keywords: Process Mining · Event Logs · IoT · Standard Format

1 Introduction

As the utilisation of Internet of Things (IoT) devices in support of business processes (BPs) becomes more frequent, there is a growing recognition of the potential to leverage the data collected by these devices for process mining (PM). Most current PM methods that can incorporate IoT data follow a similar approach: the IoT data are preprocessed with event abstraction and event-case correlation techniques to be translated into an event log in XES format (see [4,14,23,25]).

Although this is an interesting initial approach to integrate IoT data into PM and it allows for the application of existing control-flow and data-aware techniques, this method does not fully exploit the potential of IoT data. Often, the resulting high-level event log lacks contextual information (i.e., properties that can influence process execution, as explained in [4,24]) that could be derived from the IoT data, or it has limited capability to incorporate such context information. Furthermore, by separating the abstraction phase from the analysis

J. De Smedt and P. Soffer (Eds.): ICPM 2023 Workshops, LNBIP 503, pp. 32–44, 2024.
https://doi.org/10.1007/978-3-031-56107-8_3

phase, the true potential of advanced algorithms to optimise both abstraction and model discovery together cannot be harnessed. For example, the development of an IoT-enhanced decision mining algorithm requires direct access to lower-level IoT data to learn the most relevant features directly from the source data, instead of relying on an error-prone event abstraction step which might leave important information behind, at a lower granularity level [5].

This shortcoming of existing approaches is to a large extent due to limitations of the most common event log standards, i.e., the eXtensible Event Stream [10] (XES) and the Object-Centric Event Log [8] (OCEL), and has been acknowledged in the IoT PM literature [12] and beyond [2]. In a previous work [5], the authors listed ten requirements for the storage of IoT-enhanced event logs and showed that both XES and OCEL failed to meet more than half of these requirements. Building upon this paper, we present a new data format based on the conceptual model described in [4], which meets the requirements mentioned in [5]. We then describe an event log created following this format, and show that this new format greatly facilitates more in-depth analyses of IoT-enhanced BPs.

The paper is organized as follows. Section 2 introduces the previous research results that drove the development of the proposed event log format. Section 3 describes the proposed format. Section 4 validates the format by confronting it to theoretical requirements and applying it to a smart space case study. Section 5 introduces relevant related works and compare them to the proposed format. Section 6 concludes the paper and outlines future works.

2 Background

The definition of an event log suitable for IoT builds upon research and standardization efforts carried on independently in the separated fields of BPM (especially PM) and IoT. In this section we provide the background which influenced the proposed model.

2.1 Existing Standards for Event Logs

XES [10], the current standard event log model, is an XML-based model that mainly consists of the notions of event, case, and log. It proposes standard attribute types to contextualise the events, e.g. the resource executing an activity, the cost of an activity, etc. A standard activity lifecycle is defined together with XES, based on which the status of an activity can be mapped with events relating to this activity. XES also allows the definition of new data attribute types through extensions.

Recently, the gain in maturity of the PM field has increased the urge to create alternative models. Multiple propositions that relax some assumptions of XES and allow for more flexibility in event data storage have been presented, e.g., in [8,21]. Among them, the OCEL [8] was designed to be more suitable for storing event logs extracted from relational databases and is widely considered as the main challenger of XES today. It introduces the concept of object, which generalises the notion of case by allowing one event to be linked with multiple objects instead of a single case. This removes the necessity to "flatten" the event log by picking one case notion from the several potential case notions that often coexist in real-life processes.

2.2 Process Mining Using IoT Data

Challenges related to the application of PM to IoT data, and in particular to how event logs are represented are reported in [5,18]. The vast majority of the PM literature involving IoT data has focused on mining high-level events of the process from low-level IoT data to create XES event logs. Various frameworks to extract high-level logs from IoT data have been presented, e.g., [6,14–16,19, 23,26,27,29]. Traditional PM techniques can then be applied to these event logs to, e.g., discover control-flow models of the processes. A recent survey of process discovery to smart spaces, which represents a large chunk of the literature of PM applied to IoT, is provided in [3].

Although most of the existing literature is in IoT event abstraction, some other possible techniques have also been investigated. Banham et al. [1] proposes to perform data-aware process discovery with IoT-based attributes. The framework proposed requires abstracting the IoT data to integrate them in an XES event log. A second work is proposed by Rodriguez-Fernandez et al. [22], who present an approach for IoT-enhanced deviation detection in the time series data directly (in a so-called *time-series log*). Remark that all these papers bumped into the limitations of traditional event logs and had to abstract the data first or to use the raw sensor data.

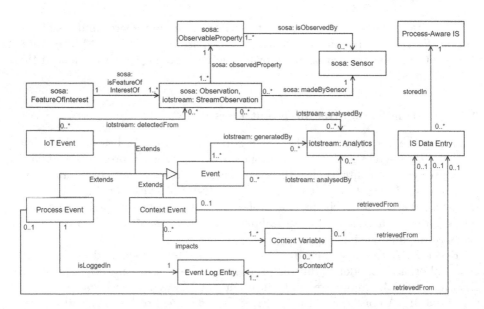

Fig. 1. Core of the bridging model for IoT and PM [4].

Another important research direction is represented by the automated segmentation of logs. Here, statistics-based techniques have been proposed [17], as well as technique based on the structure of possibly mined processes [7].

2.3 Existing Models Bridging IoT and Process Mining

A first model for bridging IoT and PM was presented in [4] (see Fig. 1). This model integrates IoT ontologies (like SOSA [13]) with typical PM concepts around the central notion of event, which is decomposed in three types of events: 1) IoT events, which correspond to events as understood in IoT systems; 2) Process events, which are events as understood in PM; 3) Context events, which correspond to changes in a parameter of the context of the process. For more information, see Sect. 3.1 or [4].

3   Format Specification

In this section, we outline the format we propose for IoT-enhanced event logs and explain how we operationalised it to generate XML-based NICE logs. It builds further upon the conceptual model presented by the authors in [4], which aimed at integrating IoT ontologies and event log models. To do so, multiple events types were defined to bridge the gap between the (physical) IoT world and the (mostly digital) PM world. In this research, in line with design science research [11], we adopted an iterative approach, moving between design and evaluation through prototyping in order to continuously improve the quality of the event log format. The evaluation step verified 1) that all constructs and relationships of the metamodel were transcribed correctly in the XML and 2) that the format was capable of representing event logs from various types of IoT-enhanced BPs.

3.1   Metamodel

At its core, our data format consists of lists of Data Sources, Objects and Events (see Fig. 2a). An Event is related to one or several Objects, which can be digital (Digital Object, e.g., an order) or physical (Feature Of Interest, e.g., a fridge), or both (e.g., a parcel). All Objects can have a collection of Properties, which can also be digital or physical (e.g., the total amount of the order, the temperature in the fridge, the weight and the value of the parcel), and represent context parameters of the process. Events are derived from one or several Data Entries or lower-level Events which are logged by a given Data Source, which can either be an information system or a Sensor. We distinguish between three types of Events, which follow the hierarchy shown in Fig. 2b:

- IoT Event: an instantaneous change in a real-world phenomenon that is monitored by a Sensor, or derived from lower-level IoT Events. E.g., the temperature in a fridge decreasing;
- Process Event: an instantaneous change of state in the transactional lifecycle of an activity (corresponding to the usual notion of event in PM). This type of event is deduced from one or more IoT Events or taken from an IS Data Entry. E.g., a product is taken from a fridge and loaded in a truck;

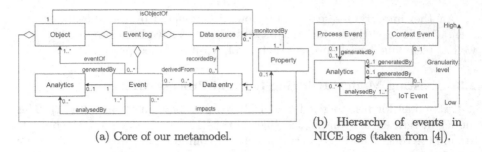

(a) Core of our metamodel.

(b) Hierarchy of events in NICE logs (taken from [4]).

Fig. 2. Metamodel for our log format.

- Context Event: an instantaneous change in a real-world phenomenon or a digital property that has an impact on the execution of a specific process instance (i.e., it impacts a Property of an Object) but does not change its control-flow state. Such an Event typically influences the path followed in a process instance, how an activity is executed, etc. This type of event is deduced from one or more IoT Events or taken from an IS Data Entry. E.g., the pressure in a tank exceeds a maximum threshold, prompting a human intervention in a chemical production process.

Higher-level Events can be derived from lower-level Events via the notion of Analytics, which represents any technique used for event abstraction (e.g., rule-based reasoning techniques like CEP, data-driven models). IoT Events can cascade until a deduced event has a direct relationship with the process, i.e., it is a Process Event or a Context Event.

3.2   Implementation

In this section, we describe how we translated the model in Fig. 2a into an XML format for NICE logs. XML was chosen for its flexibility and its popularity, though the model could also be transcribed in other languages such as JSON or YAML. The XML schema of the processed log is structured as follows: the EventLog tag is the root and contains three main elements, identified respectively by the tags:

1. ObjectList. This element contains a list of Objects. In IoT-enhanced BPs, different Objects interact and an Event can involve a combination of Objects (e.g., users, locations). The Properties of Objects are represented as attributes, which can be updated by Context Events.
2. DataSourceList. This element contains a list of Data Sources available within the observed environment. We distinguish between two types of data sources: (*i*) physical Data Sources, typically sensors, that monitor physical Properties, e.g., the opening of a door or the temperature; and (*ii*) digital Data Sources, like process-aware information systems (PAISs), recording digital Properties and Process Events.

```
 1    ...
 2    <IoTEvent id="66" timestamp="2020–01–01T00:31:58" objectID="objID_1,objID_2">
 3    <Observation id="obs_66" resultTime
           ="2020–01–01T00:31:58" value="Go_bathroom_sink" featureOfInterest="objID_24"/>
 4    <Analytics itGenerates="eventID_66" itAnalysesEvents="eventID_62,eventID_65">
 5           <Methods> <Method name="CEP"/> </Methods>
 6           </Analytics>
 7    </IoTEvent>
 8    ...
 9    <IoTEvent id="86" timestamp="2020–01–01T05:36:18" caseID="objID_1,objID_2">
10    <Observation id="obs_86"
           resultTime="2020–01–01T05:36:18" value="Go_bed" featureOfInterest="objID_26"/>
11    <Analytics itGenerates="eventID_86" itAnalysesEvents
           ="eventID_68,eventID_70,eventID_75,eventID_78,eventID_80,eventID_85">
12           <Methods> <Method name="CEP"/> </Methods>
13           </Analytics>
14    </IoTEvent>
15    ...
16    <IoTEvent id="88" timestamp="2020–01–01T05:36:22" objectID="objID_1,objID_2,objID_23">
17    <Observation id="obs_88" resultTime
           ="2020–01–01T05:36:22" value="OFF" sensor="s3" featureOfInterest="objID_23"/>
18    </IoTEvent>
19    <IoTEvent id="89" timestamp="2020–01–01T05:40:52" objectID="objID_1,objID_2,objID_23">
20    <Observation id="obs_89" resultTime
           ="2020–01–01T05:40:52" value="ON" sensor="s3" featureOfInterest="objID_23"/>
21    </IoTEvent>
22    <IoTEvent id="90" timestamp="2020–01–01T05:40:52" objectID="objID_1,objID_2">
23    <Observation id="obs_90" resultTime
           ="2020–01–01T05:40:52" value="Go_in_bed" featureOfInterest="objID_23"/>
24    <Analytics itGenerates="90" itAnalysesEvents="88,89">
25           <Methods><Method name="CEP"/></Methods>
26           </Analytics>
27    </IoTEvent>
28    <ProcessEvent id="91" timestamp="2020–01–01T05:40:52" objectID="objID_1,objID_2">
29           <Activity value="Sleeping"/>
30           <LifecyclePhase value="complete"/>
31           <Analytics itGenerates="91" itAnalysesEvents="66,86,90">
32                 <Methods><Method name="CEP"/></Methods>
33           </Analytics>
34    </ProcessEvent>
35    ...
```

Fig. 3. Example of Events connected by the `Analytics` element. In particular, in this portion of the log, there are five `IoTEvents` and one `ProcessEvent`. The mixed-level `IoTEvent` with ID 90, that represents the atomic action *Go_in_bed*, is generated by the analysis of the low-level `IoTEvents` with IDs 88 and 89, with the `Method` called CEP. The high-level `ProcessEvent` with ID 90, that completes the Event *Sleeping*, is generated by the analysis of the mixed-level `IoTEvents` with IDs 66, 86, and 90, with the `Method` called CEP. The derivation of Events with IDs 66 and 86 follows the same principle, but the lower-level `IoTEvents` from which they are derived are not shown for brevity.

3. **EventList.** This element contains a list of Events. There are three types of events: `IoTEvent`, `ContextEvent` and `ProcessEvent`. `IoTEvent` is used to represent low-level types of Events, such as raw sensor measurements, and, if relevant, mixed-level types of Events, such as the aggregation of lower-level `IoTEvents` into *actions*, i.e., atomic interactions with the environment or a part of it (e.g., sitting on a chair, opening the fridge). A `ContextEvent` represents a change in the value of a Property of an Object which impacts the execution of the process (e.g., influence a decision). It is related to an Object and the Property it updates, and contains this Property's new value. Finally,

ProcessEvent is used to represent high-level types of Events, e.g., groups of human atomic interactions with the environment that are performed with a common goal. It represents an execution of a business activity (e.g., prepare dinner, register an order).

Each Event is associated with an identifier, a timestamp, and one or more objectIDs. An IoTEvent has an additional child element called Observation that contains the raw sensor value or the action, if available. While a ProcessEvent has two child elements that refer to the name of the related Activity and its LifeCyclePhase (e.g., start, complete).

These three levels of Events are connected through the Analytics element that references the lower-level Events that generate a higher level of Event, and the Method used. For instance, the mixed-level IotEvent called "open the fridge" in its Analytics has references to the lower-level Events related to the opening of the fridge door and the triggered motion sensors near the fridge. The higher-level ProcessEvent related to the activity "cook", in its Analytics, has the references of the mixed-level Events that all together compose the activity "cook", including the mixed-level IotEvent "open the fridge". Figure 3 shows examples of Analytics elements used to derive mixed-level IoT Events and Process Events.

For our experiments, the simulator presented in [28], which was originally designed to produce logs in the XES format, has been adapted to generate NICE logs. Using a Python script, the synthetic log produced was then processed to fit the meta-model proposed in this article, following the XML structure described above. The Python script and the resulting log are available in this repository: https://github.com/silvestroveneruso/NiceParsingTool.git.

4 Format Validation

In this section, we evaluate our new format from two angles: 1) theoretically, we compare it with the requirements outlined in [5]; 2) in practice, by showing how it can be used to gain a better understanding of a process.

4.1 Theoretical Requirements Fulfilment

In this section, we confront our model with the requirements outlined in [5]. These requirements were structured along four challenges for IoT-enhanced logs: Data granularity (C1); Control-flow - context perspective convolution (C2); Scope of relevance (C3) and Data dynamicity (C4):

- R1 (Store high-level events, C1): Obtained with process and context events
- R2 (Store low-level events, C1): Obtained with IoT events
- R3 (Store intermediary events, C1): Obtained with IoT events derived from others
- R4 (Enable traceability between high-level and low-level events, C1): Achieved with the concept of Analytics, which links derived events with the events they are derived from

- R5 (Represent context at event level, C3): Done with the properties of the objects linked to an event
- R6 (Represent context at activity level, C3): Done with properties of the objects linked to the events of an activity; an additional activity object could link events together for convenience (link the events to the activity object, and the context to the activity object)
- R7 (Represent context at case/object level, C3): Context is represented at object level with the object properties, case is a special object type
- R8 (Represent context at process level, C3): This requirement can be completed with a process-wide object (e.g., the house in a smart home log)
- R9 (Update context parameters independently from process events, C2): Context parameters (Properties) are updated by context events and not by process events
- R10 (Update context parameters at a higher frequency (than process events), C4): This requirement is achieved together with R9, as context events can happen at any rate, distinguished from process events.

4.2 Log Analysis

Log Description. To showcase the usability of the data format, we generated a log simulating the behaviour of two users living in a smart home for four weeks, executing activities such as *Cook_and_eat, Do_the_dishes, Drink, Eat_cold, Eat_warm, Exercise, Go_work, Sleep, Rest, Shop, Use_Computer, Watch_tv* and *Wc*, recorded as process events, and interacting with 30 motion sensors and a temperature sensor (each change in sensor value being recorded as an IoT event). The simulator was programmed so that during one week, the users show a different behaviour, i.e., they stay at home the whole day instead of going to work in the morning and coming back home in the evening during weekdays. This change in behaviour is due to extremely high outside temperatures during that week, which are tracked by temperature sensors and logged as IoT events.

Analysis. Based on these IoT events, a context event is derived when the temperature exceeds the maximum acceptable temperature for work (set to 32.5° for office workers in Belgium) and sets a property 'Temperature suitable for work' to False. When the temperature decreases below the threshold again, another context event is generated, which sets 'Temperature suitable for work' back to True. Figure 4 contrasts directly-follows graphs (DFGs) while the 'Temperature suitable for work' property was False (Fig. 4a) and over the whole log (Fig. 4b). From the figure we can see that the behaviour of the users differs in both circumstances, as the activity Go_work is not performed during the heatwave period and more activities are recorded at home.

These context events make the change in the behaviour of the users easy to explain, as the days of anomalous behaviour are flagged with context events and characterised by a value of 'Temperature suitable for work' equal to True. This way, all relevant information is stored in the log and is easily traceable, as lower-level IoT events are still present. Moreover, this approach makes it possible to set

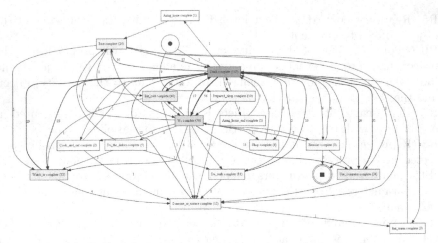

(a) DFG of the behaviour of the users during the heatwave.

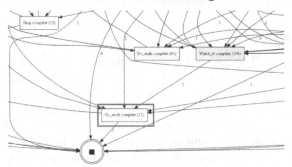

(b) Zoom in on the 'Go_work' activity in the DFG of
the behaviour of the users over the whole log.

Fig. 4. DFGs of the behaviour of the users in the simulated log.

or mine different thresholds for 'Temperature suitable for work', e.g., for users
working in different sectors, and to create one context parameter for each user,
with different rules, which would be much more difficult in traditional event log
formats. Once clearly identified with the context events, deviating behaviour can
be removed from the log or treated separately simply by removing the events
recorded between the two context events. Finally, storing the low-level data in
the log enables the use of, e.g., decision mining or trace clustering techniques to
mine the finer-grained rules behind the break from work from the low-level data
directly, which is not possible in a XES or OCEL log.

5   Related Works

In the last years, several data formats have been adapted to IoT-enhanced event logs [10,20,22,28]. In this section, we present these new alternatives and compare them to our data format with respect to the requirements identified in [5].

Of these models, the least tailored one to IoT-enhanced logs is D-OCEL [10]. It is an extension of the OCEL [8] which introduces dynamic attributes, thereby solving one of the main issues faced by OCEL for IoT-enhanced event logs.

In [20], authors present the XES DataStream extension, which aims at facilitating the storage of IoT data in XES logs. DataStream introduces, among others, the notions of *point* and *datastream*, which respectively represent individual sensor observations and group together points that belong to a same event or trace. This enables the storage of all IoT data in the log, together with the impacted events or traces.

Another format based on XES is described in [28] and represents IoT-enhanced logs generated by the smart home simulator used in this paper. It generates multiple files: a segmented high-level event log, an unsegmented high-level event log and a sensor log.

Finally, the TS-log, a model which is completely independent from existing standards like XES and OCEL, was presented in [22]. This model is designed exclusively for TS data which are collected around a process and can be used to derived the execution of activities (i.e., process events). A TS-log therefore contains a set of variable names, a domain function for each variable, an index and a function recording the value of each variable at each timestamp.

Comparing our model to related works, the NICE log format is the most flexible and balanced and the only one fulfilling all requirements expressed in [5] (see Table 1). OCEL does neither allow data attribute updates nor traceability and only has one event type. XES and D-OCEL have the same limitations, except that they allow for data attribute updates, but only with (process) events. XES with DataStream does much better, but still requires all sensor data points to be linked with one process event, and the support for mixed-level events is uncertain. The simulation tool does not support all context representation and enables only limited traceability (and information is scattered in multiple files). Finally, TS logs focus fully on low-level data, and cannot store traditional process data.

Compared to the conceptual model presented by the authors in [4], the format of the NICE logs differs in several aspects. Primarily, NICE logs rely on the concept of object instead of the concept of case. This is because objects offer more flexibility and can be used to precisely define the scope of context parameters as object properties. Then, while the original conceptual model gave a more detailed description of IoT concepts than of process concepts, NICE logs harmonise both perspectives with overarching concepts. Finally, attention has been given to reducing the redundancy between some concepts and attributes.

Table 1. Comparison of different solutions with respect to the Requirements.

		XES [10]	OCEL [8]	D - OCEL [9]	DS [20]	Simu- lator [28]	TS log [22]	NICE log
Requirements	R1: Store high-level events	✓	✓	✓	✓	✓		✓
	R2: Store low-level events				✓	✓	✓	✓
	R3: Store intermediary/mixed-level events					✓		✓
	R4: Enable traceability between high-level and low-level events				✓			✓
	R5: Represent context at event level	✓	✓	✓	✓	✓		✓
	R6: Represent context at activity level			✓	✓			✓
	R7: Represent context at case/object level	✓	✓	✓	✓			
	R8: Represent context at process level	✓		✓		✓		✓
	R9: Update context parameters independently from process events					✓	✓	✓
	R10: Update context parameters at a higher frequency				✓	✓	✓	✓

6   Conclusion

In this paper, we presented a new format for IoT-enhanced event logs. This format combines the different event types presented in [4] with the notion of object from OCEL to form a very flexible format, capable of integrating IoT data with process data with a minimal information loss. The format was evaluated in Sect. 4, where we gave evidence of its theoretical robustness and its practical usefulness. In Sect. 5, we also compared our new format with existing alternatives and showed that it is the only one fulfilling the requirements in [5]. Moreover, a first practical application demonstrated how generating a log following our format enables process analyses integrating IoT data.

Some limitations of our work include the still experimental implementation so far and the potential amplifying effect of multiple event abstraction steps on sensor data quality issues. To cope for these limitations, in future works, we first plan to further develop the format by creating more tool support to generate and manipulate logs. Next to this, we would like to design new analysis techniques taking advantage of the capabilities of the new format, e.g., for IoT-enhanced trace clustering, IoT-enhanced predictive process monitoring. As such, looking into the compatibility of NICE logs with the OCEL 2.0 format could help leveraging existing techniques and tools.

Acknowledgments. The work of Yannis Bertrand and Estefanía Serral was supported by the Flemish Fund for Scientific Research (FWO) with grant number

G0B6922N. The work of Francesco Leotta and Silvestro Veneruso was supported by the Sapienza University of Rome with grant number RM120172B3B5EC34.

References

1. Banham, A., Leemans, S.J., Wynn, M.T., Andrews, R., Laupland, K.B., Shinners, L.: xPM: enhancing exogenous data visibility. AI Med. **133**, 102409 (2022)
2. Beerepoot, I., et al.: The biggest business process management problems to solve before we die. Comput. Ind. **146**, 103837 (2023)
3. Bertrand, Y., Van den Abbeele, B., Veneruso, S., Leotta, F., Mecella, M., Serral, E.: A survey on the application of process discovery techniques to smart spaces data. EAAI **126**, 106748 (2023)
4. Bertrand, Y., De Weerdt, J., Serral, E.: A bridging model for process mining and IoT. In: Munoz-Gama, J., Lu, X. (eds.) ICPM 2021. LNBIP, vol. 433, pp. 98–110. Springer, Cham (2022). https://doi.org/10.1007/978-3-030-98581-3_8
5. Bertrand, Y., De Weerdt, J., Serral, E.: Assessing the suitability of traditional event log standards for IoT-enhanced event logs. In: Cabanillas, C., Garmann-Johnsen, N.F., Koschmider, A. (eds.) BPM 2022. LNBIP, vol. 460, pp. 63–75. Springer, Cham (2022). https://doi.org/10.1007/978-3-031-25383-6_6
6. Dimaggio, M., Leotta, F., Mecella, M., Sora, D.: Process-based habit mining: experiments and techniques. In: UIC 2016, pp. 145–152. IEEE (2016)
7. Esposito, L., Leotta, F., Mecella, M., Veneruso, S.: Unsupervised segmentation of smart home logs for human habit discovery. In: IE 2022, pp. 1–8. IEEE (2022)
8. Ghahfarokhi, A.F., Park, G., Berti, A., van der Aalst, W.M.P.: OCEL: a standard for object-centric event logs. In: Bellatreche, L., et al. (eds.) ADBIS 2021. CCIS, vol. 1450, pp. 169–175. Springer, Cham (2021). https://doi.org/10.1007/978-3-030-85082-1_16
9. Günther, C.W., Verbeek, E.: XES standard definition (2014)
10. Goossens, A., De Smedt, J., Vanthienen, J., van der Aalst, W.M.: Enhancing data-awareness of object-centric event logs. In: Montali, M., Senderovich, A., Weidlich, M. (eds.) ICPM 2022. LNBIP, vol. 468, pp. 18–30. Springer, Cham (2022). https://doi.org/10.1007/978-3-031-27815-0_2
11. Hevner, A.R., March, S.T., Park, J., Ram, S.: Design science in information systems research. MIS Q. 75–105 (2004)
12. Janiesch, C., et al.: The internet of things meets business process management: a manifesto. IEEE Syst. Man Cybern. Mag. **6**(4), 34–44 (2020)
13. Janowicz, K., Haller, A., Cox, S.J.D., Le Phuoc, D., Lefrançois, M.: SOSA: a lightweight ontology for sensors, observations, samples, and actuators. Jo. Web Semant. **56**, 1–10 (2019)
14. Janssen, D., Mannhardt, F., Koschmider, A., van Zelst, S.J.: Process model discovery from sensor event data. In: Leemans, S., Leopold, H. (eds.) ICPM 2020. LNBIP, vol. 406, pp. 69–81. Springer, Cham (2021). https://doi.org/10.1007/978-3-030-72693-5_6
15. Koschmider, A., Janssen, D., Mannhardt, F.: Framework for process discovery from sensor data. In: EMISA, p. 8 (2020)
16. Koschmider, A., Mannhardt, F., Heuser, T.: On the contextualization of event-activity mappings. In: Daniel, F., Sheng, Q.Z., Motahari, H. (eds.) BPM 2018. LNBIP, vol. 342, pp. 445–457. Springer, Cham (2019). https://doi.org/10.1007/978-3-030-11641-5_35

17. de Leoni, M., Pellattiero, L.: The benefits of sensor-measurement aggregation in discovering IoT process models: a smart-house case study. In: Marrella, A., Weber, B. (eds.) BPM 2021. LNBIP, vol. 436, pp. 403–415. Springer, Cham (2022). https://doi.org/10.1007/978-3-030-94343-1_31
18. Leotta, F., Mecella, M., Mendling, J.: Applying process mining to smart spaces: perspectives and research challenges. In: Persson, A., Stirna, J. (eds.) CAiSE 2015. LNBIP, vol. 215, pp. 298–304. Springer, Cham (2015). https://doi.org/10.1007/978-3-319-19243-7_28
19. Leotta, F., Mecella, M., Sora, D.: Visual process maps: a visualization tool for discovering habits in smart homes. JAIHC **11**(5), 1997–2025 (2020)
20. Mangler, J., et al.: DataStream XES extension: embedding IoT sensor data into extensible event stream logs. Future Internet **15**(3), 109 (2023)
21. Popova, V., Fahland, D., Dumas, M.: Artifact lifecycle discovery. arXiv:1303.2554 [cs] (2013)
22. Rodriguez-Fernandez, V., Trzcionkowska, A., Gonzalez-Pardo, A., Brzychczy, E., Nalepa, G.J., Camacho, D.: Conformance checking for time-series-aware processes. IEEE TII **17**(2), 871–881 (2021)
23. Seiger, R., Zerbato, F., Burattin, A., Garcia-Banuelos, L., Weber, B.: Towards IoT-driven process event log generation for conformance checking in smart factories. In: EDOCW, pp. 20–26 (2020)
24. Serral, E., De Smedt, J., Vanthienen, J.: Making business environments smarter: a context-adaptive petri net approach. In: UIC 2014, pp. 343–348 (2014)
25. Soffer, P., et al.: From event streams to process models and back: challenges and opportunities. Inf. Syst. **81**, 181–200 (2019)
26. Trzcionkowska, A., Brzychczy, E.: Practical aspects of event logs creation for industrial process modelling. MAPE **1**(1), 77–83 (2018)
27. Valencia-Parra, A., Ramos-Gutierrez, B., Varela-Vaca, A.J., Gomez-Lopez, M.T., Bernal, A.G.: Enabling process mining in aircraft manufactures: extracting event logs and discovering processes from complex data, pp. 166–177 (2019)
28. Veneruso, S., Bertrand, Y., Leotta, F., Serral, E., Mecella, M.: A model-based simulator for smart homes: enabling reproducibility and standardization. JAISE **15**(2), 143–166 (2023)
29. van Zelst, S.J., Mannhardt, F., de Leoni, M., Koschmider, A.: Event abstraction in process mining: literature review and taxonomy. Granular Comput. **6**, 719–736 (2021)

CaseID Detection for Process Mining:
A Heuristic-Based Methodology

Roberta De Fazio[1]([⊠]) [iD], Antonio Balzanella[1] [iD], Stefano Marrone[1] [iD],
Fiammetta Marulli[1] [iD], Laura Verde[1]([⊠]) [iD], Vincenzo Reccia[2],
and Paolo Valletta[2]

[1] Dipartimento di Matematica e Fisica, Università della Campania "Luigi Vanvitelli",
viale Lincoln, 7, Caserta, Italy
{roberta.defazio,antonio.balzanella,stefano.marrone,
fiammetta.marulli,laura.verde}@unicampania.it
[2] Gematica srl, via Diocleziano 107, Naples, Italy
{v.reccia,p.valletta}@gematica.com

Abstract. Process Mining is getting a growing interest in many contexts where performance bottlenecks are critical for the business. Unfortunately, real cyber-physical systems are usually not implemented to easily address these techniques. One of the most frequent problems to face is transforming acquired data, often heterogeneous and unlabeled to allow the application of Process Mining technique. In this study, we propose an automatised and unsupervised methodology for extracting *CaseIDs* from an unlabeled event log. The proposed detection of *CaseIDs* is based on the definition of appropriate heuristic metrics, able to highlight the correlation between events that are part of the same process instance, according to temporal and topological features (e.g., kinds of functionally-related devices, topological distance, etc.). These features constitute the inputs for a clustering technique, which has been used to extract different cases. The performance of the proposed methodology was evaluated on a real diagnostic management system to support the decisions in maintenance operations in railway infrastructures. The system has been reproduced and tested in Gematica's laboratory for simulating the data used in this work.

Keywords: Unlabeled Event Log · CaseID detection · Event Data ·
K-Means Clustering · Predictive Maintenance · Railway Infrastructure

1 Introduction

The massive use of information technologies and the development of the Internet of Things (IoT) have produced a huge amount of data in different contexts: from smart cities to Industrial Internet of Things (IIoT) and Supervisory Control And Data Acquisition (SCADA) systems. This change is driving the need to extract valuable insights from this data. Nowadays, Data Mining is a mature

© The Author(s), under exclusive license to Springer Nature Switzerland AG 2024
J. De Smedt and P. Soffer (Eds.): ICPM 2023 Workshops, LNBIP 503, pp. 45–57, 2024.
https://doi.org/10.1007/978-3-031-56107-8_4

body of knowledge and methods, proposing new techniques applicable to real-life problems. Process Mining is affirming as one of the most valuable set of techniques able to extract explicit, useful knowledge from real data, bridging computational intelligence and process modelling [20].

Process Mining (PM) has found multiple applications throughout the years [9]. Critical infrastructures like transportation, public health, and telecommunication networks can enhance their reliability and security with the support of Process Mining. The extracted models offer monitoring capabilities, detecting anomalies and cyber-attacks. They also enhance understanding of system criticality, boosting resilience, and reducing vulnerabilities [14].

The event logs constitute the starting point for PM: an event log involves a set of cases, stored in a multiple-record table. Each case is a sequence of events executed in a single process instance. Each record has a precise structure in which the key attribute groups are clearly prescribed. First, all the events belonging to the same case are marked by a *CaseID*, which constitutes one of the discriminant features of an event log. Moreover, an event is, usually, characterized by other attributes such as a *timestamp*, a corresponding *activity*, and some *resources* involved in the logged event [17]. However, this well-defined data structure is difficult to meet in real-world applications [5,15]. In this context, several works in literature, face the issue of *CaseID* detection [2–4], i.e., the identification of events belonging to the same process instance: the event logs in which the values of this attribute are not a-priori determined are named *unlabelled event logs* [2]. Erroneous or invalid values of *CaseID* can damage the accuracy and reliability of the model [8].

This work is framed in the general context of the PM application for Predictive Maintenance (PdM) of Cyber-Physical System (CPS). Such systems are often characterized by a high level of heterogeneity and coexistence of people, legacy hardware and software, and natural and external events that affect the performance and availability of the systems themselves. As an example, if we consider a smart building, many of the different interactions between the users and the building itself cannot be accurately tracked.

To this aim, having a post-processing tool able to understand which events are related to the same case, is of paramount importance to effectively run PM algorithms. The specific topic here argued is related to the pre-processing issues, due to the lack of real system preparedness in hosting these techniques.

Several approaches can be adopted to detect appropriate CaseIDs in an unlabeled event log [4,11,15]. In this paper, we introduce a heuristic-based methodology for the determination of *CaseIDs* in unlabeled datasets, necessary to define a PM model. In particular, we propose the application of a specifically addressed clustering technique in an unsupervised approach. The core of this methodology is the definition of metrics, based on heuristics that model guidelines and insights provided by domain experts. In this context, the *CaseID* represents a system failure - i.e. a sequence of faults that are correlated and lead to the delivery of an incorrect service. The metrics, that quantify the distance between couples of events, are designed in order to catch the characteristics of a process instance (for example the time frame, the location of the faults' chain in the infrastructure or the functional dependencies among the components involved) hidden among the events' attributes. A case study considering a monitoring system for transportation and distribution infrastructures is used to demonstrate the potentiality of the proposed methodology. In detail, railway infrastructure monitoring is used as a test bench for the approach.

The rest of the paper is organized as follows. Sections 2 and 3 describe, respectively, the main existing approaches of *CaseID* detection for PM processes and background. Section 4 describes the proposed methodology to determine these cases automatically, while Sect. 5 describes its application to a concrete monitoring system. Conclusions are drawn in Sect. 6.

2   Related Work

Recently, PM has found several applications in different fields involving real-life contexts from business informatics to critical infrastructures, moving from academia towards the industry. Many scientific papers consider the event logs already structured and labelled. However, in real-life problems, it may be difficult to have event logs properly defined with all the key attributes [17]. Hence, the pre-processing constitutes a fundamental phase to achieve an accurate and reliable analysis [13]. The quality of the input, in fact, affects the performances of the algorithms, the readability of the process model and the interpretation of the results [7,13]. In [2], an approach called Deduce Case IDs (DCI) has been introduced, which oversees generating labelled events from cyclic processing defined by a relation matrix derived from the process model. In [8], the authors propose an approach for identifying a *CaseID*, knowing only the sequence of the activities. Bayomie et al., propose an approach that infers the *CaseID* by solving a multi-level optimization problem, using the fitness metrics calculated from the unlabeled logs and the process model, and looking for the nearest optimal correlated log [3]. Other authors extract this knowledge using association rules and defining cost functions on the base of these rules [4]. However, all these approaches require information about the performed activities and how they are related in the model to build. All the required inputs could be unavailable in real case studies, especially if considering a complex CPS. In fact, in this class of systems, people and things interact together, letting complex behaviours emerge. In these situations, the mechanism of labelling each action with a specific *CaseID* is often unfeasible.

Some works provide methodologies that do not require a process model as input: in [5], the authors define a methodology for *CaseID* detection, based on the correlation between different activities that show the same values for that so-called decorative attributes—i.e. that are not strictly required for applying PM technique—of the event logs. Although they start from the assumption that the *CaseID* is a combination of these attributes and their values depend on the type of activity in the respective log entry. Lichtenstein et al., instead, propose an approach where the *CaseID* is identified in an unlabeled event log without any information about the process model. They introduce a strategy based on the division of the event log into several classes of data models defined by an activity-attribute relationship diagram [11].

Most of the studies existing in the literature propose methodologies relying on supervised approaches; the present work assumes that in a real context, this hypothesis we should not be done, due to some issues related to CPS context. In this study, we propose a bottom-up strategy: starting from every single event, a set of events is clustered in different cases using some metrics defined considering guidelines that enhance the meaning of the domain attributes. In other words, the strategy proposed is formulated without using any supervision by a process model or any kind of control flow, although guided by some knowledge of the domain experts able to catch the peculiarities of the considered domain.

3   Background

The proposed methodology aims at identifying an automatised and unsupervised way, based on domain-oriented heuristics, to extract *CaseIDs* from an event log in which they are not provided. The heuristics should be defined with the support of domain experts. Before describing such an approach, a general introduction of the application domain is due. Figure 1 puts at the centre of the study a communication network, composed of Network Agents that are the elements (e.g., a router, a switch, a Base Transceiver Station (BTS) in case of wireless communication) of the network enabling the communication of domain-specific ends. Examples of these ends are trains, trackside controllers, rail switches (railway); smart Heating, Ventilation and Air Conditioning (HVAC), lighting systems, connected healthcare equipment (smart hospitals); infotainment car systems, roadside equipment, Smart Road Centres (smart vehicles).

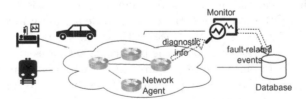

Fig. 1. Monitored system structure.

As these systems are in operation, the interaction between such elements solicits the Network Agents that exchange messages according to the adopted communication protocol. To monitor the correct functioning of the network, a Monitor is responsible for periodically polling Network Agents and for auditing for specific diagnostic messages detecting failures or performance degradations. The Monitor is responsible for populating an On-line Transaction Processing (OLTP)-level Database (DB) (i.e., the *Database*) with these fault-related events.

Among these events, there are faults, system failures, performance degradation, repair actions, and returning to full operation. The structure of the dataset is assumed to be shaped by a traditional event-log structure, with the presence of the elements proper of the PM methods (e.g., *CaseID*, activity name, timestamp, involved resources and other valuable data). Since we are interested in the problem of case identification in this work, we assume that all fields are present in the dataset except the *CaseID*.

4   Methodology

The workflow of the proposed methodology, depicted in Fig. 2, is divided into four phases.

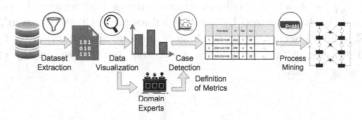

Fig. 2. The proposed workflow.

Starting from the *Database*, two preparatory phases are related to the extraction of valuable features from the Database itself into a dataset on which proper visualisation actions are performed. These phases are respectively *Dataset Extraction* and *Data Visualization*, they are performed to capture evident relationships between the considered features, allowing the Domain Experts to design a concrete playground for the definition of heuristics. It should be taken into account that these phases are very dependent on the system analyzed. The most challenging part, which constitutes the core of the formalized methodology, refers to the third phase: the *Case Detection* phase. It aims at inferring the cases from both the considered dataset and the metrics determined by the Domain Experts. The last phase, the *Process Mining*, applies common PM algorithms and toolchains to extract readable and explicit models of the PdM models.

4.1   The Case Detection Phase

The basic steps constituting the *CaseID Detection* are depicted in Fig. 3. In particular, the first step is devoted to the definition of the entities: a process instance is meant as a system failure and the metrics are defined to measure similarity between events in terms of process features. In this scenario, the event is meant as a fault of a system component characterized by fixed features such as a timestamp, the device involved with its attributes and the description of the fault. After that, it has been defined a mathematical model to formalize all the concepts.

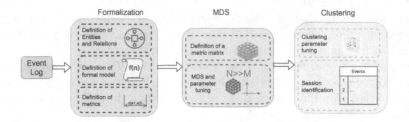

Fig. 3. The Case Detection phase workflow.

In detail, let $\mathcal{D} = \{d_1, d_2, \ldots, d_m\}$ be the set of the monitored devices, and let $E = \{e_1, e_2, \ldots, e_n\}$ be the set of the events of interest. Moreover, let $\mathcal{A} = \{a_1, a_2, \ldots, a_k\}$ be a set of attributes characterizing the devices. In this way, each device d_i is characterized by a set of values for each attribute in $\mathcal{A}$. The function $\mathcal{R}$, defined according to Eq. 1, is a non-bijective function that relates events and devices; in fact, some devices may not be involved in any event as well as in many events.

$$\mathcal{R} : E \to \mathcal{D} \tag{1}$$

Equation 2 defines another function, which assigns a timestamp to every event; this function is not bijective, since more than one event could occur at the same time. The range of this function is the set of real numbers because the timestamp is meant as its conversion to a float number.

$$\mathcal{T} : E \to \mathbb{R} \tag{2}$$

For each $a_s \in \mathcal{A}$, a function φ_{a_s} is defined as in Eq. 3.

$$\varphi_{a_s} : \mathcal{D} \to \vartheta(a_s) \subseteq \mathbb{R} \tag{3}$$

$\vartheta(a_s)$ is the set of all the possible values for the attribute a_s. $\varphi_{a_s}(d_i)$ is then used to assign actual values to the device d_i for the attribute a_s.

Indeed, the core of the entire approach is based on the definition of a domain-aware metric, quantifying the distance between two events in terms of process instance's attributes, such as time frame or location of the failure in the infrastructure.

It is possible to define:

$$\mathbf{m} : E \times E \to \mathbb{R} \mid (e_i, e_j) \to m_{i,j} \tag{4}$$

where the $\mathbf{m}$ function is used to build the distance matrix M, and $m_{i,j} = \mathbf{m}(e_i, e_j)$ for all $i, j \in \{0, \ldots, n\}$. It is important to underline that despite being very general, this formalization allows the definition of metrics that should quantify the crucial aspect of the specific application domain and more in particular the case study. Indeed, it is possible to model some aspects strictly dependent on domain knowledge, providing more consciousness of the context. One of the metrics that can be generally adopted in all the applications is the *time metric*: given two events e_i and e_j where their timestamps are, respectively, $\mathcal{T}(e_i) = t_i, \mathcal{T}(e_i) = t_j \in \mathbb{R}$ then it is defined as:

$$m_{i,j} = |t_i - t_j| \qquad (5)$$

and it is easy to derive the properties of symmetry and the zero diagonal of M. It should be generically adopted starting from the assumption that the events that belong to the same time frame should be part of the same process instance.

However, this only assumption could not satisfy all the requirements of the problem; for example, two separated components of a CPS could fail at the same time for completely different reasons, generating events belonging to two different process instances, but this metric is not able to detect this distinction by itself. A possible solution could be to adopt more than one metric to evaluate different aspects of the cases and quantify their distances under different points of view (i.e. lexical, topological.). The second step of the proposed methodology involves the implementation of one or more matrices in which every event is described in terms of distances by the others events and identified by a row in every matrix. These will be the input for the following operations. For the sake of simplicity, here we consider only one matrix M, but in the following section, we will present the implementation taking into account two different matrices obtained from two metrics.

The first operation we propose consists of using the proximity relations in M to represent the events as points on q-dimensional Cartesian axis. We utilize the Multidimensional Scaling (MDS) algorithm [6], which takes as input a number of components q, and the matrix of distances M whose dimensions are $n \times n$, with $q \ll n$. The MDS algorithm calculates the coordinates of the points in an $\mathbb{R}^q$ space by minimizing a loss function that ensures the preservation of distances between objects as much as possible. The aim of this operation is twofold: it supports visualization of the events where the distances between points in the scatter plot correspond to the dissimilarities between the original objects, allowing the domain expert to understand the proximity relation among events; it supports the use of centroid-based clustering methods for the partitioning of events into homogeneous groups. It is important to underline that in case of using more than one metric, the MDS will be performed on each resulting matrix separately, obtaining q coordinates for every transformed matrix and finally using all these features as input for the following steps, as reported in the following section. Every event is then identified by q coordinates in a $\mathbb{R}^q$ space:

$$\mathbf{MDS} : \mathbb{R}^{n \times n} \to \mathbb{R}^{n \times q} \mid M \to \mathbf{MDS}(M) \qquad (6)$$

Let $\mathcal{B} = \mathbf{MDS}(M)$ where $b_{i,j} \in \mathcal{B}$. We can then assign a tuple of q values to each event, as in Eq. 7.

$$\psi : E \to \mathbb{R}^q , \; e_i \to \psi(e_i) = (b_{i,1}, b_{i,2}, \ldots, b_{i,q}) \qquad (7)$$

The dataset is now composed of a set of n tuples $S = \{\psi(e_1), \ldots, \psi(e_n)\}$ where $\psi(e_i) \in \mathbb{R}^q$. This dataset serves as input for the last step of the methodology: the application of a clustering algorithm that partitions the events into homogeneous groups, evaluating the distances between events described by the q attributes provided by the previous MDS step. K-means is chosen as the method for this clustering phase [12] because it provides, as output, the partition of events and a set of centroids. The latter is a useful synthesis of the data as they describe the average behaviour of events in each cluster. K-means requires as input the dataset and the number of clusters k we want to obtain, the output is a n dimensional vector of the label, one for each row of the input data set, and the set of cluster centroids. Since K-means optimizes a within-cluster heterogeneity criterion, the value of k is typically determined using rules that evaluate within-cluster and/or between-cluster variability for various values of k. Among these rules, the most common include the Elbow method [18], the Average Silhouette method [16], and the Gap Statistic method [19]. Equation 8 defines the function:

$$\mathbf{KM} : \mathbb{R}^{n \times q} \times \mathbb{N} \to \mathbb{R}^n \ , \ (S, k) \to \mathbf{KM}(S, k) = (l_1, l_2, \ldots, l_n) \tag{8}$$

The labels l_i represent for each event the values of the *CaseID*: the dataset can now be processed by PM techniques.

$$\mathcal{C} : E \to \mathbb{R}^2 \times \mathcal{D} \ , \ e_i \to \mathcal{C}(e_i) = (l_i, \mathcal{T}(e_i), \mathcal{R}(e_i)) \tag{9}$$

5   Case Study

The reliability of the proposed methodology for detecting correctly *CaseID* from an unlabeled dataset was evaluated in a case study involving cyber-physical infrastructure activities. In detail, a monitoring infrastructure is analysed with the support of Gematica[1] company, which has developed solid expertise in complex communication systems and Information Technology (IT) infrastructure management solutions in heterogeneous domains—e.g., railway, automotive, building management. Gematica has realized a test bed in their laboratories where the data used in this paper has been collected. In particular, by modelling a railway infrastructure for a simple plant, data coming from trains, stations, waysides, and a control centre were collected into a monitoring centre. In this scenario, the events are messages characterized by different features, arising from the devices which compose the railway infrastructure. They are mapped on three kinds of triggering events: (1) *fault events*, which are associated with a severity code from 1 to 3; (2) *resolving events*, whose severity code is equal to 4, which logs the clearing of an error situation by the end of a maintenance action; and *information events*, associated to severity code 5, which is limited to reporting non-fault-related events worth to be logged. In our preliminary tests, 56 fault events with high-level severity and 106 fault events with medium-level severity were considered. The dataset extracted comprises several rows, every of which represents an event with its details: event ID, timestamp, event description, severity, IP of the device involved, and three attributes that topologically locate the device involved within the infrastructure, as shown in Table 1.

---

[1] https://gematica.com/.

Table 1. An excerpt of the dataset.

id	timestamp_event	description_event	severity_event	Level1	Level2	Level3	device_id	device_ip_address
320897	2023-05-09 11:47:59+02:00	Link Down FastEthernet0/5	2	1	342	538	3844	192.168.231.253
320898	2023-05-09 11:48:08+02:00	Device Down	2	1	342	538	3846	192.168.231.120
320903	2023-05-09 12:10:13+02:00	Link Down	2	2	345	542	3862	192.168.220.253

The *CaseID* to infer represents the identifier for all the fault events correlated and generated from the same cause in a way that they could be assigned to the same failure process. Therefore, we have: $n = 162$ events (E); $m = 19$ devices $(\mathcal{D})$; and $k = 21$ attributes $(\mathcal{A})$. After this *Data Extraction* phase, the *Data Visualization* phase has led to the possible choice of the features for the metrics definition, using MDS algorithm as a visualization technique. Its application allowed us to plot the temporal distribution among the events and their topological distribution within the infrastructure. The visualization of the events' distribution under those features, helps the domain experts to consider the usage of these attributes for defining the metrics. In detail, from the set of attributes, we selected those useful in our methodology and PM application, as indicated in Table 1: the topological features *Level1*, *Level2*, *Level3*, *IP* and *time*, i.e. timestamp converted in second. During the *CaseID Detection* phase, we could assign a device and a timestamp to each event, as stated respectively in Eq. 1 and Eq. 2. Moreover, we could define the function in Eq. 3 for each device's attribute that specifies where it is located in the overall infrastructure- i.e. the topological attributes.

Successively, the metrics, necessary to quantify the distance between two events, were calculated. The proposed methodology is a very general approach that allows applying this formalism to different case studies in multiple domains, giving high flexibility to the technique. The definition and calculation of these metrics were suggested by the guidelines of domain experts. Experts can contribute insights and knowledge that may not automatically emerge from the analysis of data, improving the reliability of the proposed approach. In our context, we defined the metric following the approach proposed in [10]: we started from the assumption that faults caused by the same root event should be "near" in terms of time and topology. The temporal distance was calculated as stated in Eq. 5, as it is reasonable to assume that two temporally "close" events are related, but this assumption is not sufficient as stated in the previous Sect. 4. Therefore, another metric was added: topological distance. This metric is strictly dependent on the context information because is defined by the functional and topological dependencies among events related to the same system failure, suggested by the knowledge of domain experts. The topological distance was defined as follows: let be subset $\mathcal{A}' = \{Level1,\ Level2,\ Level3,\ IP\text{-}Group\} \subseteq \mathcal{A}$, it is possible to use the function in Eq. 3 in the one in Eq. 10, for assigning to each device the values of the attributes selected for the metric, such as:

$$\mathcal{L} : \mathcal{D} \to \mathbb{R}^4$$
$$d_j \to \mathcal{L}(d_j) = (\varphi_{Level1}(d_j), \varphi_{Level2}(d_j), \varphi_{Level3}(d_j), \varphi_{IP-Group}(d_j)) \tag{10}$$

According to the Eq. 4 for all $i, j \in \{1, \ldots, n\}$, we define

$$m_{i,j} = d(\mathcal{L}(\mathcal{R}(e_i)), \mathcal{L}(\mathcal{R}(e_j))) \tag{11}$$

where the function is computed as in Fig. 4. The topological distance can vary from 0 (i.e., two events involving devices in the same IP-Group) to 4 (two events occurred in different settings of the infrastructure). After the metrics definition, it is possible to calculate the two distance matrices M_t and M_l, in which every event is described by a row, in terms of distances—respectively temporal and topological—from the others. Starting from these non-euclidean distances, it is possible to assign to the events, coordinates in a $\mathbb{R}^q$ space with $q \ll n$ whose Cartesian distances match that stored in the matrix, as stated in the Eq. 7. To obtain this, the Eq. 6 is applied to the matrix M_t by choosing $q_t = 5$ and to the matrix M_l with $q_l = 2$, obtaining acceptable results, in terms of stress. Now, it is possible to identify every event with $q_t = 5$ coordinates that locate itself in time and $q_l = 2$ in space. After that, K-Means is performed on these $q = q_t + q_l$ features obtained for each event. The choice of the number of clusters has been performed according to the Elbow rule applied to the Within-Cluster Sum of Squares for $\mathbf{k} = 2, \ldots, 40$. Consistently with this criterion, we set $\mathbf{k} = 27$.

Scikit-learn 1.2.2[2] is used for the K-Means algorithm.

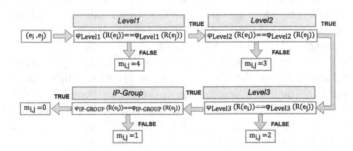

Fig. 4. Definition of the topological distance between two events.

In order to assess the effectiveness of the proposed methodology and its ability to accurately detect *CaseIDs*, an evaluation of its reliability was conducted. Since the faults were simulated we were aware, supported by domain experts, of the interconnection among the components so we can exactly reconstruct the sequence of events in each process instance, labelling and comparing the cases with that inferred by the methodology.

---

[2] https://scikit-learn.org/stable/modules/generated/sklearn.cluster.KMeans.html.

The performance of clustering was evaluated in terms Silhouette (S) coefficient [1] which is an internal clustering validity index that evaluates cluster compactness and separability, and Rand Index (RI), Adjusted Rand Index (ARI), Precision and Recall, which are external clustering validity indexes based on comparing the obtained partition with the a-priori one. RI and ARI were introduced to determine whether the cluster results are similar to each other. While precision evaluates the percentage of correctly labelled events according the true label indicated by the experts. Recall, instead, measures the percentage of all correctly labelled events. Precision and recall were calculated by defining True Positive (TP) (i.e., the number of events in which the *CaseID* predicted matches with the true label indicated by the experts), False Positive (FP) (i.e., number of events in which the *CaseID* predicted does not match with the true label indicated by the experts), and False Negative (FN) (i.e., number of events in which the *CaseID* does not exist in the labelled log obtained applying the proposed approach) [2].

The results are reported in the Table 2, showing the proposed approach achieves a precision of about 81%.

Table 2. Evaluation metrics obtained with the proposed methodology.

Rand Index	Adjusted Rand Index	Silhouette	Precision	Recall
0.973	0.649	0.738	81.0%	88.1%

6   Conclusions

In recent years, the use of PM in day-to-day business process management has increased significantly. The present paper moves from the necessity to improve the case detection in the unlabeled event log, which is a precondition to the application of PM algorithms.

This work proposes an approach based on the analysis of temporal and topological features, which are considered to aggregate faulty events. The K-Means clustering technique is used to group together similar event log entries. The approach has been tested on a railway infrastructure monitoring system, equipped in the laboratories of Gematica company.

The proposed methodology was tested by evaluating unlabeled event logs of the infrastructure monitoring system, achieving the expected results. It is important to underline, that in this preliminary phase, simulated data were adopted in experiments. In prospect, we will explore the performance of the proposed methodology by using real data with a more homogeneous distribution in time and in the types of faults involved. Moreover, in a real context, the metrics calculated could be improved by considering other context information, such as, for example, functional and non-functional dependence between devices, improving the expressive power of such methodology. Another future perspective could be that of comparing the results obtained by using the proposed methodology for applying traditional PM techniques with those obtained using Object-centric Process Mining metamodels, aiming to gain more insights for PdM tasks.

Acknowledgements. The research has been supported by the DARWINIST project, funded by Universitá della Campania "L. Vanvitelli", D.R. 834 30-09-2022. The work of Roberta De Fazio is granted by PON Ricerca e Innovazione 2014/2020 MUR—Ministero dell'Università e della Ricerca (Italy)—with the PhD program XXXVII cycle D.M. N.1061 "Dottorati e contratti di ricerca su tematiche dell'Innovazione". The work of Laura Verde is granted by the "Predictive Maintenance Multidominio (Multidomain predictive maintenance)" project, PON "Ricerca e Innovazione" 2014–2020, Asse IV-Azione IV.4 #B61B21005470007.

References

1. Al-Mhairat, A.M., Alabbadi, R., Shaban, R., AlQudah, A.: Performance evaluation of clustering algorithms (2019)
2. Bayomie, D., Awad, A., Ezat, E.: Correlating unlabeled events from cyclic business processes execution. In: Nurcan, S., Soffer, P., Bajec, M., Eder, J. (eds.) CAiSE 2016. LNCS, vol. 9694, pp. 274–289. Springer, Cham (2016). https://doi.org/10.1007/978-3-319-39696-5_17
3. Bayomie, D., Di Ciccio, C., La Rosa, M., Mendling, J.: A probabilistic approach to event-case correlation for process mining. In: Laender, A.H.F., Pernici, B., Lim, E.-P., de Oliveira, J.P.M. (eds.) ER 2019. LNCS, vol. 11788, pp. 136–152. Springer, Cham (2019). https://doi.org/10.1007/978-3-030-33223-5_12
4. Bayomie, D., Revoredo, K., Di Ciccio, C., Mendling, J.: Improving accuracy and explainability in event-case correlation via rule mining. In: 2022 4th International Conference on Process Mining (ICPM), pp. 24–31 (2022)
5. Burattin, A., Vigo, R.: A framework for semi-automated process instance discovery from decorative attributes. In: 2011 IEEE Symposium on Computational Intelligence and Data Mining (CIDM), pp. 176–183 (2011)
6. Carroll, J.D., Arabie, P.: Multidimensional scaling. Measur. Judgment Decis. Mak. 179–250 (1998)
7. Emamjome, F.F., Andrews, R., ter Hofstede, A.H., Reijers, H.A.: Alohomora: unlocking data quality causes through event log context. In: European Conference on Information Systems (2020)
8. Ferreira, D.R., Gillblad, D.: Discovering process models from unlabelled event logs. In: Dayal, U., Eder, J., Koehler, J., Reijers, H.A. (eds.) BPM 2009. LNCS, vol. 5701, pp. 143–158. Springer, Heidelberg (2009). https://doi.org/10.1007/978-3-642-03848-8_11
9. dos Santos Garcia, C., et al.: Process mining techniques and applications - a systematic mapping study. Expert Syst. Appl. **133**, 260–295 (2019)
10. Gayo-Avello, D.: A survey on session detection methods in query logs and a proposal for future evaluation. Inf. Sci. **179**(12), 1822–1843 (2009)
11. Lichtenstein, T., Bano, D., Weske, M.: Attribute-driven case notion discovery for unlabeled event logs. In: Marrella, A., Weber, B. (eds.) BPM 2021. LNBIP, vol. 436, pp. 111–122. Springer, Cham (2022). https://doi.org/10.1007/978-3-030-94343-1_9
12. Likas, A., Vlassis, N., Verbeek, J.J.: The global k-means clustering algorithm. Pattern Recogn. **36**(2), 451–461 (2003)

13. Marin-Castro, H.M., Tello-Leal, E.: Event log preprocessing for process mining: a review. Appl. Sci. **11**(22) (2021)
14. Myers, D., Suriadi, S., Radke, K., Foo, E.: Anomaly detection for industrial control systems using process mining. Comput. Secur. **78**, 103–125 (2018)
15. Pourmirza, S., Dijkman, R., Grefen, P.: Correlation mining: mining process orchestrations without case identifiers. In: Barros, A., Grigori, D., Narendra, N.C., Dam, H.K. (eds.) ICSOC 2015. LNCS, vol. 9435, pp. 237–252. Springer, Heidelberg (2015). https://doi.org/10.1007/978-3-662-48616-0_15
16. Rousseeuw, P.J.: Silhouettes: a graphical aid to the interpretation and validation of cluster analysis. J. Comput. Appl. Math. **20**, 53–65 (1987)
17. Suriadi, S., Andrews, R., ter Hofstede, A., Wynn, M.: Event log imperfection patterns for process mining: towards a systematic approach to cleaning event logs. Inf. Syst. **64**, 132–150 (2017)
18. Thorndike, R.L.: Who belongs in the family? Psychometrika **18**(4), 267–276 (1953)
19. Tibshirani, R., Walther, G., Hastie, T.: Estimating the number of clusters in a data set via the gap statistic. J. R. Stat. Soc.: Ser. B **63** (2001)
20. van der Aalst, W., et al.: Process mining manifesto. In: Daniel, F., Barkaoui, K., Dustdar, S. (eds.) BPM 2011. LNBIP, vol. 99, pp. 169–194. Springer, Heidelberg (2012). https://doi.org/10.1007/978-3-642-28108-2_19

Parallelism-Based Session Creation to Identify High-Level Activities in Event Log Abstraction

Onur Dogan[1,2] and Massimiliano de Leoni[1(✉)]

[1] Department of Mathematics, University of Padua, 35121 Padua, Italy
`onur.dogan@unipd.it, deleoni@math.unipd.it`
[2] Department of Management Information Systems, Izmir Bakircay University,
35665 Izmir, Turkey
`onur.dogan@bakircay.edu.tr`

Abstract. Process mining utilizes event data to gain insights into the execution of processes. While techniques are valuable, their effectiveness may be hindered when dealing with highly complex processes that have a vast number of variants. Additionally, because the recorded events in information systems are at a low-level, process mining techniques may not align with the higher-level concepts understood at the business level. Without abstracting event sequences to higher-level concepts, the outcomes of process mining, such as discovering a model, can become overly complex and challenging to interpret, rendering them less useful. Some research has been conducted on event abstraction, often requiring significant domain knowledge that may not be readily accessible. Alternatively, unsupervised abstraction techniques may yield less accurate results and rely on stronger assumptions. This paper introduces a technique that addresses the challenge of limited domain knowledge by utilizing a straightforward approach. The technique involves dividing traces into batch sessions, taking into account relationships between subsequent events. Each session is then abstracted as a single high-level activity execution. This abstraction process utilizes a combination of automatic clustering and visualization methods. The proposed technique was evaluated using a randomly generated process model with high variability. The results demonstrate the significant advantages of the proposed abstraction in effectively communicating accurate knowledge to stakeholders.

Keywords: Event log abstraction · Parallel relationships · Clustering · Visual analytics · Process discovery

1 Introduction

In today's data-driven business landscape, organizations have access to vast amounts of event data generated by their information systems. This event data captures valuable insights into how processes are executed in the organization. Process mining techniques have emerged as powerful tools to analyze and leverage this event data to gain valuable insights into process execution. However, as processes become more complex and exhibit a large number of variants, the effectiveness of traditional process mining techniques is diminished [14]. Moreover, the low-level nature of the recorded events in information systems often fails to capture the higher-level concepts known at the

J. De Smedt and P. Soffer (Eds.): ICPM 2023 Workshops, LNBIP 503, pp. 58–69, 2024.
https://doi.org/10.1007/978-3-031-56107-8_5

business level, further complicating the analysis and interpretation of process mining results.

The need to abstract low-level event sequences into higher-level activities has been recognized as a crucial step in enhancing the usability and interpretability of process mining outcomes [11]. Traditional approaches to event abstraction often rely on significant domain knowledge, which may not be readily available or feasible to obtain. Thus, there is a pressing need to develop a technique that enables effective event abstraction without relying on extensive domain knowledge and with improved accuracy.

Existing approaches assume that each low-level sequence that is abstracted to one high-level activity does not interleave with other low-level sequences. In other words, there are no parallel high-level activities. This is a strong assumption because parallel activities are performed simultaneously, and the execution order changes in different traces.

This paper puts forward a technique that detects parallel low-level sequences by leveraging a combination of clustering and visualization methods. The proposed technique first identifies session creation rules by evaluating the time threshold and the parallel relationship between subsequent low-level events. Events having parallel relationships are assigned into different sessions to catch the parallelism. Then, it encodes the sessions as vectors, with each dimension representing an activity associated with a low-level event. A clustering algorithm groups the vectors of similar low-level sequences into clusters, where each cluster includes a set of parallel events. An abstracted model is generated using high-level event sequences. Then, each cluster, including sub-logs, is discovered for sub-models, and sub-models are replaced with the corresponding high-level activity on the abstracted model. After this replacement, the model's quality is measured with different parameter values. The parameter values giving the best quality are chosen to use for the evaluation of the abstraction technique.

The effectiveness of the proposed technique was evaluated through different synthetic processes and event logs. The results showed that the abstraction technique enables to mining process models with a better balance of fitness and precision.

2   Motivation

This section motivates the importance to consider the interleaving of low-level sequences. The discussion is based on the work by de Leoni et al. [8], but a similar reasoning applies when employing other techniques that overlook the parallelism of high-level activities [14]. The event-log abstraction technique in [8] divides traces into sessions, where each session represents the smallest subsequences within a trace. A session is determined based on a user-defined threshold, which is the time difference between the last event in a session and the first event in the subsequent session.

Let us consider the model in Fig. 1 to motivate the importance of consider parallelism of high-level activities. The model consists of three parallel branches, each of which corresponds to one high-level activities. High-level activities A and B consists of the sequence of three low-level ones, in the model represented by the sequences $\langle A1, A2, A3 \rangle$, $\langle B1, B2, B3 \rangle$. Similarly, high-level activities C consists of the sequence of two low-level activities. The corresponding event log records the execution of these

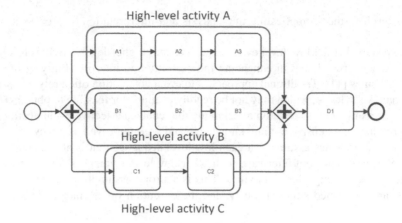

High-level activity C

Fig. 1. An illustrative model including three parallel low-level sequences corresponding three different high-level activities

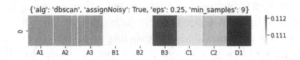

Fig. 2. Heatmap of clustering results for the technique in [8]. It highlights how each cluster has one or two evident dominant low-level activities (the cells of the darkest colors) according to the cluster centroids. There is only one cluster and the dominant low-level activities $D1, B3$, etc. (Color figure online)

the low-level activities, and no information is stored about the high-level counterparts. The timestamps of the low-level events are temporarily space out with a distance of one second from each other.

After applying the technique by de Leoni et al. [8] using a threshold of nine seconds, the outcome is one single cluster in which every low-level activity is added. This can be visualized through the heatmap in Fig. 2, which illustrates the centroid of the created cluster. The most frequent low-level activities are given darker colours.

The expectation is to obtain four clusters, namely for the low-level activities related to the high-level A, B, C and D. However, since the low-level activities are given timestamps with distance of one second against a threshold session of nine seconds, the technique assigns every low-level activities into the same session, making it impossible to create the expected clusters. This can be solved by observing that low-level activities must not be in the same cluster if they can occur in any order, namely they are parallel. This idea motivates the research work reported in this paper. The remainder will detail the techniques. When parallelism is considered, we obtain the clusters depicted in Fig. 3. The high-level activity A is covered via Cluster 0 where the most frequent low-level activities are indeed $A1$, $A2$ and $A3$. Clusters 1 and 3 incorporate the low-level activities related to the high-level activities C and B, respectively. Note the presence of clusters 2, 4 and 5, which are respectively related to high-level activities B, A and C: in these clusters, a predominant low-level activity is also $D1$, which indeed may follow

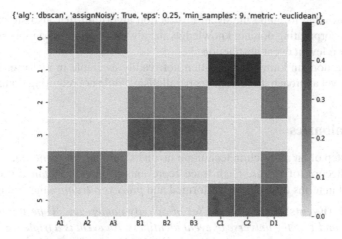

Fig. 3. Heatmap of clustering results for the proposed technique. Six clusters have different dominant low-level activities, and none of the clusters has low-level activities having a parallel relationship.

$A3$, $B3$ or $C2$. In fact, the expected cluster for high-level activity D has been merged with those for A, B and C. The approach is thus not exactly achieving the four clusters, as expected, but yet is able to approximate the expected results.

3 Related Work

The problem of event-log abstract is currently gaining momentum, but most of the techniques do not consider the parallelism among high-level activities. Bakullari and van der Aalst [3] developed a framework for generating high-level events by dividing events into time windows. Van Eck et al. [12] presented an approach for creating high-level event logs from sensor data of smart products using segmentation and clustering techniques. Similarly, Brzychczy et al. [4] employed a combination of hierarchical clustering and domain knowledge to identify process stages. Michael Mayr et al. [10] extended the approach proposed by van Eck et al. [12] by incorporating time-series-based process-state and product-state data as additional attributes in the event log. Augusto et al. [1] applied the k-th order Markovian abstraction technique to create high-level activities and then discovered process models to compare the quality of the models based on a family of fitness and precision measures.

Some techniques support high-level activities parallelism, but they rely on manual effort and domain expertise. Mannhardt and Tax [9] suggested first discovering local process models from the event log to capture the behavior of specific subsets of events. The local process models were then used to lift the event log to a higher level of abstraction. Van Houdt et al. [13] employed a method that combines local process models with behavioral pattern mining to identify event abstraction patterns, leveraging on the event-log transformation by Mannhardt and Tax [9]. Baier et al. [2] leverage on domain knowledge to guide the event abstraction algorithm that also supports parallelism. By incorporating domain knowledge, the algorithm achieves a more precise and contextually relevant event abstraction.

However, domain knowledge is often not readily available in real life. This paper presents a novel approach that considers parallelism, while not requiring domain knowledge.

4 Preliminaries

The initial step of an abstraction technique involves utilizing an *event log*, which comprises a collection of *traces*. Each trace represents a *process instance* (i.e., a *case*) manipulated in terms of *activities* performed and *process attributes* that are influenced.

Definition 1 (Events). *Let A be the set of activity names, and T be the universe of timestamps, and I be the universe of event identifiers. An event is a triple $e = (a, t, i) \in A \times T \times I$ and represents that the event with identifier i refers to the execution of an instance of activity a for at timestamp t.*

We use shortcuts $\lambda_A(e) = a, \lambda_T(e) = t, \lambda_I(e) = i$ to extract the activity name a, the timestamp t, and identifier i of any event e. Events may define several additional attributes, but they are not formalized here, to keep the notation simple. A trace refers to a sequence of events:

Definition 2 (Traces and Event Logs). *A trace σ is a sequence of events, i.e., $\sigma \in \mathcal{E}^*$. An event log L is a set of traces, i.e., $\mathcal{L} \subset \mathcal{E}^*$.*

In the remainder, for each pair (a, b) of activities and each event log $\mathcal{L}$, $|a >_{\mathcal{L}} b|$ is used to denote the number of occurrences of events for activity a followed by events for b in $\mathcal{L}$. The concept of parallelism used here is based on the dependency measured introduced within the Heuristic Miner [11]:

Definition 3 (Dependency Measure). *Let A be the set of activity names, and T be the universe of timestamps, and I be the universe of event identifiers. Let $\mathcal{E} = A \times T \times I$ be the university of events. Let $\mathcal{L} \subset \mathcal{E}^*$ be an event log. The dependency measure for each pair $(a, b) \in A \times A$ is defined as follows:*

$$a \Rightarrow_{\mathcal{L}} b = \begin{cases} \frac{|a >_{\mathcal{L}} b| - |b >_{\mathcal{L}} a|}{|a >_{\mathcal{L}} b| + |b >_{\mathcal{L}} a| + 1} & \text{if } a \neq b \\ \frac{|a >_{\mathcal{L}} a|}{|a >_{\mathcal{L}} a| + 1} & \text{if } a = b \end{cases}$$

The value of $a \Rightarrow_{\mathcal{L}} b$ is always between -1 and 1. If the absolute value of $a \Rightarrow_{\mathcal{L}} b$ is lower than a user-defined threshold, and at least once a is followed by b in $\mathcal{L}$ or the other way around, activities a and b are considered in parallel:

Definition 4 (Parallelism). *Let A be the set of activity names, and T be the universe of timestamps, and I be the universe of event identifiers. Let $\mathcal{E} = A \times T \times I$ be the university of events. Let $\mathcal{L} \subset \mathcal{E}^*$ be an event log. Given two activities $a, b \in A$ and a dependency threshold Θ, activities a and b are consider parallel:*

$$a \parallel_{\mathcal{L}, \Theta} b \Leftrightarrow |a >_{\mathcal{L}} b| + |b >_{\mathcal{L}} a| > 0 \wedge |a \Rightarrow_{\mathcal{L}} b| < \Theta$$

The use of a threshold is to be tolerant to noise. In an ideal world, activities are parallel if we see once a followed by b, and also b followed by a.

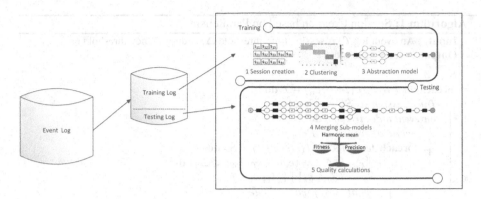

Fig. 4. Abstraction technique framework

5 Abstraction Technique

Figure 4 depicts the steps of the proposed abstraction technique. The input consists of an event log, which is split into training and testing. The training event log is used to create sessions at step 1: the events of each trace of the event log are divided into sessions. A session is a sequence of events. At step 2, sessions are clustered, where each cluster represents a high-level activities. The sessions of each cluster are the sequence of low-level activities that are mapped to the high-level activity corresponding to that cluster. At step 3, the low-level event sequences are replaced by high-level events to obtain an abstracted event log: this abstracted event log can then be used, e.g., to mine a high-level model. The sessions of each cluster can be seen as a sublog that can be used as input for process discovery: this would discover a low-level process model of how each high-level activity is mapped to the executions of low-level activities. The low-level process models can then be merged with the abstract process model to in fact obtain a hierarchical model: this is step 4. At step 5, a testing event log is used to compute the harmonic mean of fitness and precision, and thus to assess the quality of the hierarchical model.

This procedure relies on the DBSCAN clustering algorithm: the above procedure is repeated for different values of the algorithm's parameters ϵ and $min\_samples$, aiming to find those that allow mining a hierarchical model that maximizes the harmonic mean of fitness and precision.

The remainder of this section provides further details of the different steps of the proposed techniques.

5.1 Parallelism-Based Session Creation

Algorithm 1 illustrates how sessions are created. The input is the event log $\mathcal{L}$, a time threshold Δ and the dependency threshold Θ (cf. Eq. 4). Values observed for Θ in [11] are usually between 0.7 and 0.9.

As illustrated in Algorithm 1, the creation is done by trace (see line 2). For each trace $\sigma \in \mathcal{L}$, a set S_σ of the sessions of σ is created to include a session that consists

---

Algorithm 1: Session Creation based on Parallelism

Input : An event log $\mathcal{L}$, A session time-threshold Δ, A dependency threshold Θ

Output: A set S of sessions

1 $S \leftarrow \emptyset$

2 **foreach** *trace* $\sigma = \langle e_1, \cdots, e_n \rangle \in \mathcal{L}$ **do**

3 $\quad$ *Trace-session set* $S_\sigma \leftarrow \{\langle e_1 \rangle\}$

4 $\quad$ **for** *event index i=2 to n* **do**

5 $\quad\quad$ *event_assigned* $\leftarrow$ *False*

6 $\quad\quad$ **foreach** *session* $s = \langle f_1, \cdots, f_m \rangle \in S_\sigma$ **do**

7 $\quad\quad\quad$ **if** $(a \parallel_{\mathcal{L},\Theta} b \wedge (\lambda_T(e_i) - \lambda_T(f_m) < \Delta))$ **then**

8 $\quad\quad\quad\quad$ $S_\sigma \leftarrow (S_\sigma \setminus s) \bigcup \{\langle f_1, \cdots, f_m, e_i \rangle\}$

9 $\quad\quad\quad\quad$ *event_assigned* $\leftarrow$ *True*

10 $\quad\quad\quad\quad$ break

11 $\quad\quad\quad$ **end**

12 $\quad\quad$ **end**

13 $\quad\quad$ **if** *event_assigned* = *False* **then**

14 $\quad\quad\quad$ $S_\sigma \leftarrow S_\sigma \bigcup \{\langle e_i \rangle\}$

15 $\quad\quad$ **end**

16 $\quad$ **end**

17 $\quad$ $S \leftarrow S \bigcup S_\sigma$

18 **end**

19 **return** S

---

of the sequence with only the first event (see line 3). In fact, a session for a trace σ is a sequence of events of σ. The loop from line 4 to 16 iterates over all events of the trace of length n, and adds each event e_i either to an existing session or to a new session. The inner loop from line 6 to 12 iterates over the existing sessions: if any session s concludes with an event f_m that is not parallel with e_i and also the time difference between the two events is lower than the time threshold Δ (conditions at line 7), e_i is added to f_m (see line 8) and no more sessions are considered (see break of the inner loop at line 10). A special case is when the event is not added to any of the existing session because the conditions at line 7 are never both satisfied. In this case, the inner loop between 6 and 12 concludes. The boolean variable *event_assigned* stays set to false: it would become true if and only if it is added to some session (cf. line 9 where the variable is set to true). The condition at line 13 refers to this case: if the event is assigned to no session, a new session is created and added to the existing set S_δ At the end of this step, every trace is broken down into the constituent sessions, then clustered as discussed in the next step.

5.2 Clustering

Each session s is converted into a vector via an encoding function $\mathrm{ENCODE}(s)$ that abstract the behavior observed in the session. All these vectors (e.g. the sessions) are clustered. The encoding can be obtained in many ways. Here we consider $\mathrm{ENCODE}(s) = (v_{x_1}, \ldots, v_{x_n})$, where $x_1, \ldots, x_n$ are the activities observed in the log and any v_{x_i} is obtained in one of the two following alternatives:

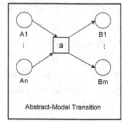
Abstract-Model Transition

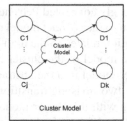
Cluster Model

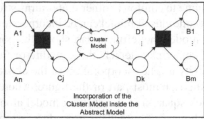
Incorporation of the
Cluster Model inside the
Abstract Model

Fig. 5. Merging one Cluster model into the Abstract Model (source [8]).

Frequency-based encoding. The value of dimension v_{x_k} is the number of events for activity x_k in s. If both starting and completion events are observed for an activity x_k, the number of events is ultimately divided by two, to prevent double counting.

Duration-based encoding. The value of dimension v_{x_k} is the average duration of instances of activity x_k in the session s (a zero value is given if x_k does not occur in s).

Once sessions are converted into vectors, they are clustered. Here, we opt for the clustering algorithm DBSCAN, which are shown to lead to better results [7,8] Clusters are visualized on the heatmap for insights into how sessions were clustered. The x-axis refers to low-level activities, whereas the y-axis indicates clusters. The intersection of the axes is colored according to the value of the dimension a in cluster c. A value of 0 is represented as white, while 1 is given as the most intense red. The cluster centroids $(c_1, \cdots, c_k)$ are normalized by dividing the sum of the centroid values $\left(\frac{c_1}{\sum_{j=1}^{k} c_j}, \cdots, \frac{c_1}{\sum_{j=1}^{k} c_k} \right)$. Varying intensities of the color red represent the centroids on the heat maps.

5.3   Creation of Abstracted Model

The third step focuses on the mining of an abstract model, namely the model consisting of the high-level activities. The input of this step is the set C of clusters of sessions. Each cluster $c \in C$ is associated with a high-level activity NAME(c). Since high-level activity names are not resulting from the clusters, we visualize the centroids of the clusters on a heatmap, which provides insights to process analysts into the names to assign to clusters, and consequently to high-level activities, in line with what discussed in [7,8]. This enables the creation of the abstract event log. For each log trace σ, we compute the sessions' sequence $\circledS_\Delta(\sigma) = \langle s_{\sigma_1}, \ldots, s_{\sigma_m} \rangle$ and then the abstract trace $\sigma_{\text{ABST}} = \langle f_{\sigma_1}^{st}, f_{\sigma_1}^{co} \cdots, f_{\sigma_n}^{st}, f_{\sigma_n}^{co} \rangle$ where, for every $1 \le i \le m$, $f_{\sigma_i}^{st}$ and $f_{\sigma_i}^{co}$ are the abstract events for session s_{σ_i}: the activity names of $\lambda_A(f_{\sigma_i}^{st})$ and $\lambda_A(f_{\sigma_i}^{co})$ are equal to the name NAME(c_i) of the cluster c_i to which s_{σ_i}. The so-constructed abstract event log can then be used to discover an abstract model.

5.4   Merging Sub-cluster Models

Each cluster $c \in C$ consists of a set of sessions, which is in fact an event log to be used as input to mine a model of the behaviour of the sessions within the cluster. Here we also assume to employ a miner that returns strongly connected Petri nets. Figure 5 illustrates how one cluster model can be incorporate into the abstract model to create the hierarchical model: the leftmost part shows the portion related to the high-level activity a where the center part depicts the structure of the model of the cluster referring to high-level activity a. The incorporation of the cluster model into the abstract model is illustrated in the rightmost part of the figure, where two invisible transitions are introduced (the black squares) in the abstract model along with the cluster model, which is connected as shown in figure. This procedure is repeated for each cluster, thus finally producing the hierarchical model. Note that often those invisible transitions are not necessary (see, e.g., the case study): in that case, the invisible transitions can finally be removed.

5.5 Computing Model Quality

Quality computing for a process model involves evaluating the discovered process model's accuracy, reliability, and usefulness. Fitness reflects how well the model aligns with the actual execution of the process, with higher fitness values indicating a closer match between the observed and modeled behavior [11]. Precision evaluates how effectively the model represents the actual process without oversimplifying or omitting essential details [11]. In particular, fitness is computed on the test event log, whereas precision considers train and test event log together for more reliability. This computation of the model quality is then returned as the harmonic means of fitness and precision, which heavily penalizes configurations where the fitness and precision values are not well balanced.

6   Evaluation

To evaluate the effectiveness of the proposed technique, we employed two artificial processes with synthetic event logs. In particular, we confronted the quality of the hierarchical model obtained using the abstraction technique introduced in this paper with the models obtained using no event-log abstractions and the technique by de Leoni et al. [8], which overlooks parallelism.

Processes and Logs Generator 2 (PLG2) was used to create the artificial models and accordant event logs [5]. PLG2 allows to generate random process models and to create accordant event logs. PLG2 also allows noise to be added, in terms of percentage of events that are randomly inserted, deleted or swapped.

Two processes were randomly generated, containing 109 and 119 activities for model 1 and 2, respectively. Initially, we generated logs with no noise: The average number of events per trace is respectively 107.41 and 105.01. Then, we also generated new event logs with 5%, 10%, 15%, 20% of noise, which were used to define the noise's probabilities of three types: trace missing head probability, trace missing tail probability, and trace missing episode probability. Because PLG2 generates a log with fixed 1-hour timestamps for each consecutive activity, we changed the timestamps randomly, considering relationships among activities.

Our technique has been implemented in in Python, whose source code is available at https://github.com/onurdogannet/ParallelismbasedEventLogAbstraction, where we also uploaded the generated models and logs.

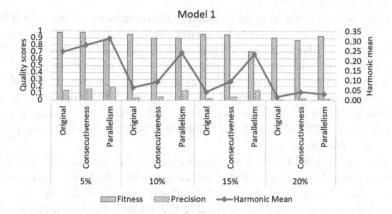

Fig. 6. Quality of Model 1 in terms of the harmonic mean of fitness and precision

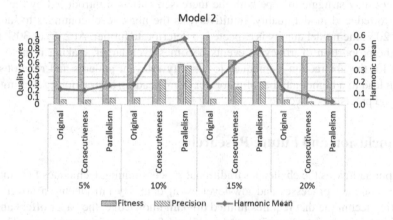

Fig. 7. Quality of Model 2 in terms of the harmonic mean of fitness and precision

Our technique leverages on a process discovery: we used Inductive Miner with a noise threshold of 0.2 [6]. The session threshold has been set to be the average time between consecutive events: this is used both for the technique proposed in this paper and for the technique reported in [7, 8]. Figures 6 and 7 provide an evaluation of process models based on their fitness, precision, and harmonic mean scores for the increasing level of noise in the event log. The models include three technique: *Original*, namely without using event-log abstraction, *Consecutiveness*, which is the technique reported in [7, 8], and *Parallelism*, which is what proposed in this paper.

The original models show high fitness scores but low precision. On the other hand, abstraction techniques based on consecutiveness and parallelism result in lower fitness scores but improved precision, in general.

Across different session creation methods (Original, Consecutiveness, Parallelism), there are variations in fitness. For example, in Model 1, the Parallelism variation tends to have lower fitness compared to the Original or Consecutiveness, especially at higher noise levels. In Model 2, the fitness of the Consecutiveness variation varies significantly with noise levels. It's important to note that Model 1 generally exhibits higher fitness scores compared to Model 2 under the same conditions and noise levels.

Precision varies across different noise levels and model names. In Model 1, the Parallelism variation tends to have higher precision compared to the other two variations across noise levels. In Model 2, the precision of the Parallelism variation is notably high, especially at 10% noise level, suggesting it is better at avoiding false positives under certain conditions.

The parallelism-based abstraction achieves a better balance between fitness and precision compared to the consecutiveness-based abstraction for both event logs, except the event logs with 20% noise. Because both abstraction methods consider noises by assigning them to the nearest cluster before creating the abstracted model, they gave better results until a certain noise level. However, after a certain level of noise, abstraction techniques may struggle to cope with the increased variation introduced by the noise, leading to reduced model quality. Intuitively, as the noise level continues to increase beyond 20%, the model quality is expected to deteriorate further. At 25% or 30% noise levels, the proportion of irrelevant events becomes even larger, making it more challenging for the abstraction techniques to identify relevant patterns and relationships. This can lead to a higher number of incorrect or misleading abstractions, resulting both fitness and precision to decline.

7   Conclusion and Future Research

This paper addresses the challenges traditional process mining techniques face in dealing with complex processes and low-level event data. By introducing a novel event abstraction technique that requires limited domain knowledge, the paper offers an approach to enhance the interpretability and usability of process mining outcomes. The proposed technique's effectiveness is validated through different noise levels, emphasizing its ability to provide accurate knowledge to stakeholders. The improved interpretability and usability of the abstracted process model enable users to gain valuable insights and make informed decisions regarding process analysis, optimization, and improvement.

For noise levels up to 20%, the abstraction techniques perform better than the not abstracted model because they can effectively filter out some noise and separate the essential patterns. The fact that parallelism is the best abstraction technique at noise levels less than 20% can be attributed to its ability to handle more diverse and complex event patterns. Parallelism captures relationships among high-level activities that can occur simultaneously. The choice of the best abstraction technique depends on the specific characteristics and noise level of the event log being analyzed.

As future work, we aim to experience alternative clustering algorithms, such as hierarchical clustering, which may lead to better clustering results, and ultimately to hierarchical models of higher quality. So do we plan to work on automatically finding a suitable time threshold for session creation.

Acknowledgements. This research is financially supported by the Department of Mathematics of the University of Padua, through the BIRD project "Web-site Interaction Discovery" (code BIRD219730/21).

References

1. Augusto, A., Armas-Cervantes, A., Conforti, R., Dumas, M., La Rosa, M.: Measuring fitness and precision of automatically discovered process models: a principled and scalable approach. IEEE Trans. Knowl. Data Eng. **34**(4), 1870–1888 (2020)
2. Baier, T., Mendling, J., Weske, M.: Bridging abstraction layers in process mining. Inf. Syst. **46**, 123–139 (2014)
3. Bakullari, B., van der Aalst, W.M.: High-level event mining: a framework. In: 2022 4th International Conference on Process Mining (ICPM), pp. 136–143. IEEE (2022)
4. Brzychczy, E., Trzcionkowska, A.: Process-oriented approach for analysis of sensor data from longwall monitoring system. In: Burduk, A., Chlebus, E., Nowakowski, T., Tubis, A. (eds.) ISPEM 2018. AISC, vol. 835, pp. 611–621. Springer, Cham (2019). https://doi.org/10.1007/978-3-319-97490-3_58
5. Burattin, A.: PLG2: multiperspective process randomization with online and offline simulations. In: Proceedings of the BPM Demo Track 2016. CEUR Workshop Proceedings, vol. 1789, pp. 1–6. CEUR-WS.org (2016)
6. Leemans, S.J.J., Fahland, D., van der Aalst, W.M.P.: Discovering block-structured process models from event logs - a constructive approach. In: Colom, J.-M., Desel, J. (eds.) PETRI NETS 2013. LNCS, vol. 7927, pp. 311–329. Springer, Heidelberg (2013). https://doi.org/10.1007/978-3-642-38697-8_17
7. de Leoni, M., Dündar, S.: Event-log abstraction using batch session identification and clustering. In: Proceedings of the 35th Annual ACM Symposium on Applied Computing, pp. 36–44 (2020)
8. de Leoni, M., Pellattiero, L.: The benefits of sensor-measurement aggregation in discovering IoT process models: a smart-house case study. In: Marrella, A., Weber, B. (eds.) BPM 2021. LNBIP, vol. 436, pp. 403–415. Springer, Cham (2022). https://doi.org/10.1007/978-3-030-94343-1_31
9. Mannhardt, F., Tax, N.: Unsupervised event abstraction using pattern abstraction and local process models. arXiv preprint arXiv:1704.03520 (2017)
10. Mayr, M., Luftensteiner, S., Chasparis, G.C.: Abstracting process mining event logs from process-state data to monitor control-flow of industrial manufacturing processes. Procedia Comput. Sci. **200**, 1442–1450 (2022)
11. Van Der Aalst, W.M.P.: Data science in action. In: Van Der Aalst, W.M.P. (ed.) Process Mining, pp. 3–23. Springer, Heidelberg (2016). https://doi.org/10.1007/978-3-662-49851-4_1
12. Van Eck, M.L., Sidorova, N., Van der Aalst, W.M.: Enabling process mining on sensor data from smart products. In: 2016 IEEE Tenth International Conference on Research Challenges in Information Science (RCIS), pp. 1–12. IEEE (2016)
13. Van Houdt, G., Depaire, B., Martin, N.: Unsupervised event abstraction in a process mining context: a benchmark study. In: Leemans, S., Leopold, H. (eds.) ICPM 2020. LNBIP, vol. 406, pp. 82–93. Springer, Cham (2021). https://doi.org/10.1007/978-3-030-72693-5_7
14. van Zelst, S.J., Mannhardt, F., de Leoni, M., Koschmider, A.: Event abstraction in process mining: literature review and taxonomy. Granular Comput. **6**, 719–736 (2021)

From OCEL to DOCEL – Datasets and Automated Transformation

Alexandre Goossens[1](✉) [iD], Adrian Rebmann[2](✉) [iD], Johannes De Smedt[1] [iD], Jan Vanthienen[1] [iD], and Han van der Aa[2] [iD]

[1] Leuven Institute for Research on Information Systems (LIRIS), KU Leuven, Leuven, Belgium
{Alexandre.Goossens,Johannes.Smedt,Jan.Vanthienen}@kuleuven.be
[2] Data and Web Science Group, University of Mannheim, Mannheim, Germany
{rebmann,han.van.der.aa}@uni-mannheim.de

Abstract. Object-centric event data represent processes from the point of view of all the involved object types. This perspective has gained interest in recent years as it supports the analysis of processes that previously could not be adequately captured, due to the lack of a clear case notion as well as an increasing amount of output data that needs to be stored. Although publicly available event logs are crucial artifacts for researchers to develop and evaluate novel process mining techniques, the currently available object-centric event logs have limitations in this regard. Specifically, they mainly focus on control-flow and rarely contain objects with attributes that change over time, even though this is not realistic, as the attribute values of objects can be altered during their lifecycle. This paper addresses this gap by providing two means of establishing object-centric datasets with dynamically evolving attributes. First, we provide event log generators, which allow researchers to generate customized, artificial logs with dynamic attributes in the recently proposed DOCEL format. Second, we propose and evaluate an algorithm to convert OCEL logs into DOCEL logs, which involves the detection of event attributes that capture evolving object information and the creation of dynamic attributes from these. Through these contributions, this paper supports the advancement of object-centric process analysis by providing researchers with new means to obtain relevant data to use during the development of new techniques.

Keywords: Object-centric processes · OCEL · DOCEL · Log Generator

1 Introduction

Organizations often operate in complex environments with multiple objects interacting and participating in the same business process. To capture these different perspectives, the concept of object-centric processes has been proposed, in which multiple object types participate over the course of a business process [1]. In recent years, object-centric process mining has gained increasing interest in the research community with the introduction of novel event log formats such as eXtensible Object-Centric (XOC) logs [16],

---

A. Goossens and A. Rebmann—Joint first authors.

J. De Smedt and P. Soffer (Eds.): ICPM 2023 Workshops, LNBIP 503, pp. 70–83, 2024.
https://doi.org/10.1007/978-3-031-56107-8_6

Object-Centric Behavioral Constraint (OCBC) models [2], and Object-Centric Event Logs (OCEL) [13]. Especially, OCEL is currently the most used object-centric event log format with its own evaluation metrics [3], visualization tool [11] and various analysis techniques [4,5].

However, OCEL has some limitations by design. Particularly, the relationships between objects and attributes are not strictly defined and attributes that can change in value over time are challenging to deal with in OCEL [14]. This makes the analysis of attribute change difficult, because it is not always clear which event or object manipulated the attribute value, e.g. whether an update event changed the quantity of an order or the price of a product. To overcome this, there have been efforts to establish a new format for object-centric event data such as Data-aware Object-Centric Event Logs (DOCEL) [14]. The main aspect DOCEL introduced is the notion of static and dynamic attributes [14]. Static attributes are attributes that do not change over the course of a business process and can either be linked to an event or to an object. Conversely, dynamic attributes are attributes that can change over the course of a business process and are linked to both an object and to an event with the use of foreign keys. As of now, no general consensus has been reached, however, regarding the exact set of entities and relationships a meta model of such a data format shall have. Currently, the Object-Centric Event Data (OCED) is under development and will surely take into account the explicit representation of object evolution and their attributes.[1]

However, despite the benefits of moving to object-centric data with dynamic attributes, no datasets are available that can actually be leveraged by researchers for the development of process mining techniques that account for such attributes. This paper addresses this issue in two ways:

1. We propose two process-specific log generators to create customized object-centric event logs in the DOCEL format [14], which also generate dynamic object attributes, i.e., they create objects with attributes that change over time.
2. We propose an algorithm that takes an existing OCEL event log and automatically transforms it into an event log in the DOCEL format. Combined with earlier work, this algorithm can also be used to transform flat XES [15] logs into DOCEL logs.

The remainder of this paper is structured as follows: Sect. 2 motivates the need for data sets with dynamic object attributes. Section 3 presents our log generators to create DOCEL logs. Section 4 then describes our algorithm to transform OCEL into DOCEL logs. Section 5 uses data sets created using our log generators to evaluate the algorithm and shows how even real-life event data captured in XES format can be transformed into DOCEL and thus be used for research on object-centric process mining. Finally, Sect. 6 reflects on related work and Sect. 7 concludes the paper.

2 Motivation

Over the course of the execution of a business process, the objects involved in its execution may undergo changes, such as creating, updating or deleting, which results in attribute values changes throughout an object's lifecycle. The eXtensible Event Stream

---

[1] https://www.tf-pm.org/resources/oced-standard.

(XES) event log format, with its traditional case-based view of processes, addresses this issue by directly linking attributes to the events that manipulate them [15]. Because each event belongs to exactly one case, it is unambiguously clear which attribute was manipulated by a specific event as well as to which trace it belongs.

However, in object-centric processes, events may refer to any number of objects [4]. In OCEL, this is implemented using an event table storing all attributes that are manipulated by events and an objects table storing all objects and their (static) attributes. Unfortunately, with OCEL it is not possible to uniquely identify to which object a dynamic attribute belongs, neither through its events table nor its objects table [14]. To illustrate this, consider the event table of an OCEL log shown in Table 1 and its objects table in Table 2, which cover the (simplified) handling of two orders. First, an order is created, then the ordered items are picked, before they are sent. Between creating an order and sending items, orders can be updated, i.e., items may be added or removed. Besides the common `EventID`, `Activity`, and `Timestamp` attributes and the references to the instances of different object types associated with each event, the log contains an additional event attribute, `Value`. While this attribute is associated with events, it is clear that it actually refers to objects. Specifically, it refers to the current value of the order the event is associated with. This is left implicit by the OCEL format making it impossible for automated process analysis techniques to properly leverage this information. For instance, by looking at event e_6, it is unclear whether the *Value* refers to the current value of the order or the value of the item that is removed. This makes analyzing attribute changes in object-centric business processes difficult using OCEL.

<table>
<tr><td colspan="6">Table 1. Events of an OCEL log.</td></tr>
<tr><td>ID</td><td>Activity</td><td>Timestamp</td><td>Orders</td><td>Items</td><td>Value</td></tr>
<tr><td>e_1</td><td>Create order</td><td>05-20 09:07</td><td>$\{o_1\}$</td><td>$\{i_1, i_2\}$</td><td>100</td></tr>
<tr><td>e_2</td><td>Pick items</td><td>05-23 14:20</td><td>$\{o_1\}$</td><td>$\{i_1, i_2\}$</td><td>100</td></tr>
<tr><td>e_3</td><td>Create order</td><td>06-03 19:17</td><td>$\{o_2\}$</td><td>$\{i_3\}$</td><td>60</td></tr>
<tr><td>e_4</td><td>Pick items</td><td>06-04 15:20</td><td>$\{o_2\}$</td><td>$\{i_3\}$</td><td>60</td></tr>
<tr><td>e_5</td><td>Update order</td><td>06-04 18:11</td><td>$\{o_1\}$</td><td>$\{i_1\}$</td><td>70</td></tr>
<tr><td>e_6</td><td>Remove item</td><td>06-05 11:48</td><td>$\{o_1\}$</td><td>$\{i_2\}$</td><td>70</td></tr>
</table>

Table 2. Objects of the log

Type	Instances
Orders	$\{o_1,$
	$o_2\}$
Items	$\{i_1(\text{Weight: } 24),$
	$i_2(\text{Weight: } 99),$
	$i_3(\text{Weight: } 10)\}$

The DOCEL format addresses this issue with the notion of static and dynamic attributes. Static attributes do not change over the course of a business process, whereas dynamic object attributes can change value over the course of a process and are linked to both an event and an object. For instance, consider the running example, where orders have a `Value` attribute. If an order changes during its lifecycle, i.e., between its first and last occurrence in the execution of a business process, e.g., because items are added later on, the value attribute changes. DOCEL explicitly links this change to the order itself and the event that caused it. Unfortunately, despite the increased interest in object-centric processes, there are currently no event logs available describing processes with dynamic attributes nor are there tools available to generate such object-centric logs.

Table 3. Object types order-to-delivery process

Object Type	Static Attributes	Dynamic Attributes
Customer	Name, Bank Account	Customer Address
Order	/	Weight, Order Price
Product Type	Product Name, Price, Weight	/
Item	Price, Weight	/
Packages	Price, Weight	/

Table 4. Object types shipping-method process

Object Type	Static Attributes	Dynamic Attributes
Customers	Name, Bank Account	/
Product Type	Value, Fragile	/
Orders	Quantity	Value, Refund, Shipping Method

3   DOCEL Dataset Generators

This section introduces the DOCEL log generators for two artificial, yet realistic processes. First, we introduce the two processes that are simulated by the log generators. These processes contain dynamic attributes as well as various AND and OR-gateways, and loops, which are also found in real-life processes. Second, we explain the log generators and their tunable parameters.

3.1   Process Descriptions

In this section, we describe the processes that serve as a basis for our log generators. The process models can be found alongside the Python notebooks that implement the generators[2]. In this paper, we limit ourselves to a textual description for space reasons.

Order-to-Delivery Process. The order-to-delivery process[3] contains 5 object types and various attributes that we summarize in Table 3.

The process starts with the customer adding items to an order which increases the value and the weight of an order. Each item is of a certain product type and inherits its weight and price. Once the order is placed, the items are picked. Before paying the order, the customer is still allowed to remove items from an order. If that is the case, the items are removed and the value and weight of an order are updated. Once the order is paid, the package is created with a weight and price and sent out. However, a customer might change their delivery address in which case the delivery fails and has to be re-executed. Moreover, every delivery has a very small chance of failing due to unforeseen circumstances. Once the package is successfully delivered, the process ends.

---

[2] Available at https://github.com/a-rebmann/ocel_to_docel/tree/main/notebooks.

[3] This process is based on the running example OCEL log available on ocel-standard.org.

Shipping-Method Process. The shipping-method process covers orders that have different shipping modes depending on various factors. It is based on the process described in [8] and contains three object types whose attributes are summarized in Table 4.

A customer places an order with a quantity for each product type. This is then received by the company which has to manually confirm the purchase at which point the value of the order is also determined. Once the purchase is confirmed, the products are retrieved from the warehouse and added to the package. In case, the product type is fragile (indicated with a binary value), the product is first wrapped with some protection. Next, the customer has to confirm the shipping information, after which the shipping method is determined. If the package contains a fragile product or its value exceeds a certain amount, the package is shipped with a courier. Otherwise the package is shipped by mail. Simultaneously, an invoice is sent to the customer. Once the package has arrived, the customer determines their satisfaction. If the customer is satisfied the process is ended after the order has been filed. In case, the customer is dissatisfied, the customer requests a refund, setting the binary refund value to 1. Next, the customer confirms the shipping information, which will be handled using an express courier. The company sends a recollect letter after which the customer returns the package. Once the package is returned, the company refunds the customer. Once the package has arrived, the customer determines their satisfaction (assumed to be positive here) after which the order is filed and the process ends.

3.2 Log Generators

To allow the research community to generate as many different logs as desired for different research needs, we propose log generators that allow users to change various parameters that influence the generated logs, as summarized in Tables 5 and 6. In both log generators, it is possible to change the amount of object instances of all the object types involved in the process as well as changing the time between events and initial time frame of a process. Beyond that, it is possible to change various probabilities of events happening in the process such as removing an item or asking for a refund. Both log generators can generate DOCEL logs in a spreadsheet format, which is intuitive to understand because every table (events, objects and dynamic attribute tables) can be stored in a separate sheet. Note that, because we provide the generators as Python notebooks, it is possible to change the logs beyond the options described in the tables with some minimal Python coding.

Finally, to be able to evaluate our automated OCEL-to-DOCEL transformation algorithm (cf. Sect. 4), we also included the option to create an OCEL log for a generated DOCEL log. If OCEL logs are created, the dynamic attributes are directly linked to the events, therefore, losing the clear information on object-attribute allocations.

Table 5. Summary of functionality in the order-to-delivery Log Generator

Tunable parameter	Description of Functionality
Customer Addresses and Names	Randomly generated for each log entry along with randomly generated bank account details.
Products	Taken from a fixed list directly obtained from the OCEL log of X.
Start Timeframe	Allows defining the start time for the process.
Time Between Events	Allows adjusting the time interval between consecutive events.
Number of Orders	Can be changed to generate logs with varying numbers of orders.
Max Number of Products	Can be adjusted to set a maximum limit for the number of products in an order.
Max Number of Items	Can be modified to set a maximum limit for the total number of items in an order.
Probability of Removing an Item	Can be adjusted to control the likelihood of an item being removed from an order. The higher the value, the more likely an item is removed.
Probability of Changing an Address	Allows changing the probability of an address being modified in the log entries. The higher the probability, the more likely the address will be changed.
Probability of Failing a Delivery	Can be altered to control the likelihood of a delivery failure occurrence. The higher the probability, the more likely the probability will be changed

Table 6. Summary of functionality in the shipping method log generator

Tunable parameters	Description of Functionality
Number of Products	Allows adding new products with custom values for the price and the possibility of fragility.
Number of Customers	Enables creating new customers with randomly generated names and bank accounts.
Lists of People Executing Activities	Allows adapting the lists of people who execute the company's activities.
Start Timeframe	Allows defining the start time for the process.
Time interval Between Events	Allows adjusting the time interval between consecutive events.
Order Value Threshold	Can be changed to determine the shipping method based on the order's value.
Number of Orders	Can be changed to generate logs with varying numbers of orders.
Probability of Refund	Can be adapted to determine the likelihood of a refund, indicating customer satisfaction with the purchase. The higher the value the more satisfied the customer is

4 Transforming OCEL to DOCEL

This section presents our proposed algorithm to transform an OCEL event log into a DOCEL formatted one, achieved by detecting dynamic object attributes and assigning them to the appropriate object instances. Our algorithm takes as input an OCEL format-ted event log L, which comprises a set of events recorded by an information system. Each event $e \in L$ is a tuple $e = (eid, act, ts, OI, AV)$, with eid the event's id, act its activity, ts its timestamp, OI a set of object instances, and AI a set of attribute-value pairs. Each object instance $oi \in OI$ is a tuple $(oid, type)$, where oid is the instance's identifier and $type$ its type, whereas each attribute-value pair $(a, v) \in AI$ relates an attribute value v to an attribute name a. We denote the set of object types that occur in L as $\mathcal{O}_T^L$ and the set of event attribute names as $\mathcal{A}_T^L$.

As visualized in Fig. 1, our algorithm applies two steps to transform an OCEL log L into a DOCEL formatted log L'. Step 1, *Dynamic object attribute detection*, aims to detect dynamic object attributes in the event attributes of the input log and match them with the object type they refer to. Based on that matching, Step 2, *Dynamic-object-attribute-to-object assignment*, creates object attributes and associates these with the individual object instances they relate to, establishing a DOCEL log that makes these relationships explicit. In the remainder of this section, we describe these steps in detail.

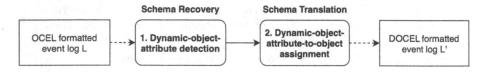

Fig. 1. Algorithm overview.

4.1 Dynamic Object Attribute Detection

This step aims to determine whether an attribute $a \in \mathcal{A}_T^L$ is a dynamic object attribute of an object type $t \in \mathcal{O}_T^L$, resulting in a set of attribute-object-type matches M.

For this step, recall that dynamic object attributes are attached to events in the OCEL format, even though they capture information about an object associated with an event rather than relate to the event itself. For instance, although an *Update order* event has a `Value` attribute in Table 1, this attribute actually captures the (new) value of the order, not of the event.

Identifying Candidate Object Types. For each attribute $a \in \mathcal{A}_T^L$, our algorithm first identifies a set of candidate object types $O_a \subseteq \mathcal{O}_T^L$. To determine if an object type $t \in \mathcal{O}_T^L$ is a candidate type for attribute a, our algorithm checks if it meets two requirements:

- *Object-attribute co-occurrence:* First, our algorithm checks if every occurrence of attribute a can be related to exactly one instance of object type t. This means that L cannot contain an event e for which $(a, v) \in e.AV$ and for which $e.OI$ either does not contain any object instance of type t or contains multiple of them. For instance, for the running example type *item* is not a candidate for attribute `Value`, since events e_1 and e_2 each refer to two items, but only contain a single `Value`.

– *Observed attribute changes:* Second, our algorithm checks if attribute a is actually dynamic (with respect to type t), i.e., if its value is observed to change during an object's lifecycle. For this, our algorithm checks if L contains (at least) two events, e and e', which both contain the same object instance of type t, but are associated with different values for attribute a.

Any object type t that passes both checks is added to the set of candidate object types O_a. If, after checking all object types in $\mathcal{O}_T^L$, O_a contains exactly one candidate type t, the match (a, t) is added to M. Instead, if O_a does not contain any candidates, then a is not a dynamic attribute, whereas, if O_a contains more than one candidate, our algorithm turns to the disambiguation procedure described next.

Disambiguating Candidate Types. An attribute a can have multiple candidate object types in O_a if certain object types always occur together for events. For example, if every event in a log L is associated with both a *customer* and an *order*, an attribute such as Value would have both of these types as a candidate, since each occurrence of Value can be associated with exactly one *customer* and one *order*.

To be able to match a to a single object type $t \in O_A$ in such cases, our algorithm employs two disambiguation strategies:

– *Relation-based selection:* Our algorithm first checks for 1:N relationships between object types in O_a, aiming to assign a to a more fine-granular candidate object type. For illustration, consider a Refund attribute and two object types, *customer* and *order* in O_{Refund}. All events with a value for Refund refer to one customer and one order. Matching Refund to *customer* would obfuscate the relation between single orders and their Refund if a customer places multiple orders. Therefore, the algorithm tries to identify cases for each $t \in O_a$, where for two events $e_1, e_2 \in L$ an instance oi_t of t occurs together with two different instances $oi_{t'_1}$ and $oi_{t'_2}$ of another type $t' \in O_a$ and, if so, removes t from the candidates. If a single candidate t remains, the match (a, t) is added to M.
– *Name-based selection:* If, after the relation-based selection, O_a still contains more than one candidate, our algorithm finds the most similar object type among the candidates based on a's name. For this, our algorithm quantifies the semantic similarity $\text{sim}(a, t) \in [0, 1]$ between a and each type $t \in O_a$ by computing the cosine similarity between sentence embeddings, obtained from a pretrained *Sentence Transformer* [18]. These embeddings are specifically designed to capture semantically meaningful representations on the level of (short) sentences rather than individual words, making them highly suitable for our purpose.
  Given these similarity scores, our algorithm determines if there is a type $t \in O_a$ for which the similarity score is distinctly higher (according to a threshold τ, set to 0.1 by default) than the scores of the other types, i.e., if $\text{sim}(a, t) > \text{sim}(a, t') + \tau$ for each $t' \in O_a \setminus \{t\}$. If such a distinctively similar type t is found, the match (a, t) is added to M, otherwise a is not matched to any object type.

The set of attribute-object-type matches M then serves as input to the next step.

4.2 Dynamic-Object-Attribute-to-Object Assignment

Based on each match $(a, t) \in M$, Step 2 creates an object attribute $a_{(e,oi)} = (vid, eid, oid, a)$ for each event e that changes oi's value for a. The algorithm first assign $a_{(e,oi)}$ a unique identifier $a_{(e,oi)}.vid$. Then it sets its attribute-value pair, $a_{(e,oi)}.a = (a, v)$ with $(a, v) \in e.AI$, its event identifier, $a_{(e,oi)}.eid = e.eid$, and its object instance identifier, $a_{(e,oi)}.oid = oi.id$ with $oi \in e.OI \wedge oi.type = t$. For the attribute Value of our running example, this creates the object attribute table visualized in Table 7.

Finally, the algorithm removes the attributes for which a match was found from the events' set of attribute-value pairs and returns the established DOCEL log. For the example, it would, therefore, remove the Value attribute from the events in Table 1 and return the resulting event table, the unchanged objects table, and the newly created object attribute table (Table 7).

Table 7. Value attribute table.

ValueID	OrderID	EventID	Value
v1	o1	e1	100
v2	o2	e3	60
v3	o1	e5	70

5   Evaluation

We implemented our algorithm in Python and performed evaluation experiments to assess our algorithm's capability to accurately transform OCEL logs into DOCEL logs (Sect. 5.1). Afterwards, we show how it can be used in combination with an existing approach to also transform XES event logs into DOCEL logs (Sect. 5.2). The implementation, evaluation data, and generated DOCEL logs are available in our repository[4].

5.1   Experiments

We assess whether our algorithm is able to correctly detect the dynamic attributes in an OCEL log and transform it into a DOCEL log.

Datasets. We use OCEL and DOCEL event logs generated using our log generators (cf. Sect. 3) by simulating the process execution for 100 orders per scenario. The OCEL logs serve as input to our algorithm, whereas the DOCEL logs serve as a gold standard, i.e., the correct transformation result. The OCEL logs obtained in this manner differ in their number of events, objects, object types, and attributes as shown in Table 8.

Setup. To assess the ability of our algorithm to correctly detect dynamic object attributes in the OCEL event logs, we conduct experiments using two settings:

(1) Original attribute names. In this setting, we use all information from the event log as input to our approach.
(2) Hidden attribute names. To assess the robustness of our algorithm, we reduce the available information by hiding event attribute names in the OCEL logs. This allows us to assess the dependency of our algorithm on its name-based check (Sect. 4.1).

---

[4] https://github.com/a-rebmann/ocel_to_docel.

Table 8. Characteristics of the OCEL logs used for the evaluation

ID	# Events	Objects	# Event att.	# Dyn. att.
Order to Delivery	6,014	Customer (44), Order (100), Item (3,559), Packages (100), Product Type (20)	7	3
Shipping Method	2,036	Customer (50), Product Type (3), Order (100)	5	3

We measure the performance in terms of precision, recall, and F_1-score with respect to the dynamic object attributes in the original DOCEL logs. Using tp to denote the dynamic attributes correctly matched to an object type fp for the dynamic attributes incorrectly matched to an object type, and fn for the dynamic attributes that were wrongly not matched to an object type, we then quantify the precision as $tp/(tp + fp)$, the recall as $tp/(tp + fn)$, and F_1-score as the harmonic mean of precision and recall.

Results. We first report on the results of attribute-to-object-type matching, which is the most challenging part, before we report on the attribute value to object assignment.

Attribute-to-Object-Type Matching. Table 9 reports on the results of the attribute-to-object-type matching per event log.

Table 9. Results of the attribute-to-object-type matching per OCEL log.

Log	Original Attribute Names				Hidden Attribute Names			
	Count	Precision	Recall	F_1	Count	Precision	Recall	F_1
Order to delivery	3	1.00	1.00	1.00	3	1.00	0.75	0.86
Shipping method	4	0.80	1.00	0.89	4	0.80	1.00	0.89
Average	3.5	0.90	1.00	0.95	3.5	0.90	0.88	0.88

We find that our approach achieves a perfect recall and good precision (0.9) in detecting dynamic object attributes and associating these with the correct object type, when all original information from the input log is available. An in-depth look shows that the only error made is the assignment of the *Resource* attribute of shipping-method process to the *order* type. While unconventional, this assignment is not necessarily problematic, since indeed each time a resource executes a process step, that step relates to a specific order. Such incorrect assignments could be easily avoided by specifying a set of names reserved for event attributes, e.g., *org:resource* or *org:role* as done in XES logs [15]. The importance of the duplicate-resolution strategy based on object lifecycles becomes clear for the shipping-method process, where *customer* and *order* are in 1:N relation. Without it, e.g., the Refund attribute would be matched to both *customer* and *order*. This strategy resolves this, correctly matching Refund only to the *order*. Note that the name-based matching strategy could not resolve this, because *refund* is semantically similar to both *customer* and *order*.

When hiding the original attribute names, we find that for shipping-method process the performance remains the same, whereas for order to delivery it drops achieving an F_1-score of 0.86 compared to 1.00 with original attribute names. The reason for this is the missing match of the Customer Address attribute to the *customer* object type, because the candidates *order* and *customer* could not be resolved solely using the relation-based disambiguation in this case.

Object-Attribute-to-Object Assignment. We also report on the results of Step 2, i.e., the assignment of object-attributes to objects, for the setting with original attribute names. We provide results for (1) when propagating false positives from Step 1 and (2) when only including object attributes that were correctly matched to object types in Table 10.

Table 10. Results of the dynamic-object-attribute-to-object assignment per OCEL log for the setting with original attribute names, with and without propagation of false positives (*fps*) from Step 1.

Log	When propagating *fps*				Without propagating *fps*			
	Count	Precision	Recall	F_1	Count	Precision	Recall	F_1
Order to delivery	3,710	1.00	1.00	1.00	3,710	1.00	1.00	1.00
Shipping method	1,886	0.23	1.00	0.37	442	1.00	1.00	1.00
Average	2,798	0.62	1.00	0.69	1,875	1.00	1.00	1.00

We find that when propagating false positives (*fps*) from Step 1, we achieve an average F_1-score of 0.69, a precision of 0.37, and a perfect recall (1.00). The lower precision is caused only by the assignment of the Resource attribute to the *order* object type for the shipping-method event log. Given that there are many more resource handovers involved than value changes to the actual object attributes this has a considerable impact on the overall performance scores. Apart from this, we achieve perfect scores, though. This can also be seen when disregarding false positives from Step 1. In this case, we achieve perfect scores for the assignment of object attributes to objects.

5.2 Application: From XES to DOCEL

Recently an approach was proposed to uncover object-centric data in a flat event log, e.g., in XES format, to automatically transform it into a log OCEL format [17]. Given the limitations of OCEL, we aim to combine our algorithm with this approach to investigate whether XES logs can be transformed into DOCEL.

To this end, we use the BPI Challenge 2017 log [9], which captures the loan application process at a financial institute and involves two main types of objects: applications and offers. For a single application, multiple offers can be made, where at some point an offer may be accepted. To make sure we have a dynamic object attribute in this log, we add an OfferAccepted attribute to each event, which is set to false when a new application is created and changes to true, when an offer associated with the application is accepted. The goal is to check if our algorithm can identify this attribute correctly as a dynamic object attribute associated with the *application* object type creating a DOCEL log from the output of the XES-to-OCEL approach.

When applying our algorithm to the transformed XES log, we find that it indeed correctly matched the `OfferAccepted` attribute to the application. Based on that it removed the corresponding event attributes and created correct object attributes linked to both the correct application and the event that writes the value. Beyond detecting the derived attribute correctly, the algorithm also detected the `EventOrigin` and the `Action` attributes as dynamic object attributes of the *application* object type. After inspecting the attribute values, the latter of these matches makes sense, because `Action` captures the status of the application, which changes throughout its lifecycle. `EventOrigin`, as its name indicates, captures the origin of the event and was, therefore, falsely associated with *application*. Nevertheless, this outcome shows the potential of our algorithm to help generate a broader variety of object-centric event logs that consider evolving objects based on available event data. The DOCEL log our algorithm created can be found in our repository linked on Page 71.

6 Related Work

The first proposed object-centric event log formats are XOC logs [16] together with OCBC models [2]. These proposals have scalability issues because of the duplication of attributes and object relations with each executed event. Next, OCEL logs were introduced which do not have such scalability issues and are currently the most used object-centric event log format [13] with a lot of dedicated research and tools such as a visualization tool [11], fitness and precision metrics [3], clustering analysis [12], or predictive object-centric process analysis [10].

The conversion of XES logs to OCEL logs has been investigated in [17]. Next to that a generic approach to extract OCEL logs from SAP systems and relational databases has also been researched in respectively [7] and [6]. Finally, the extraction of OCEL logs from virtual knowledge graphs was researched in [19].

7 Conclusion

This paper offers two problem-specific log generators and a transformation algorithm to the research community. The two paramaterizable log generators support both the widely used OCEL format and the more recent DOCEL format, which allows for dynamic attributes and consistent object-attribute allocation. To further support the creation of DOCEL logs, we also proposed an algorithm to convert OCEL logs to DOCEL logs. This algorithm not only identifies the presence of dynamic attributes, which are better represented in the DOCEL format, but also links the attributes to the correct object types. Our evaluation shows that the algorithm can accurately transform OCEL into DOCEL logs and that, in combination with previous work, it can even be used to convert XES logs to DOCEL logs. However, it cannot deal with all situations. For instance, if multiple instances of the same object type are changed by one event (batching), this cannot be handled if these instance have not previously been changed individually.

In the future, we aim to address this limitation. We also plan to develop a comprehensive user interface tool to enhance the user experience. Furthermore, we aim to transform additional XES logs that would benefit from a conversion to DOCEL logs.

References

1. van der Aalst, W.M., Barthelmess, P., Ellis, C.A., Wainer, J.: Proclets: a framework for lightweight interacting workflow processes. Int. J. Coop. Inf. Syst. **10**(04), 443–481 (2001)
2. van der Aalst, W.M., Li, G., Montali, M.: Object-centric behavioral constraints. arXiv preprint arXiv:1703.05740 (2017)
3. Adams, J.N., van der Aalst, W.: Precision and fitness in object-centric process mining. In: 2021 3rd International Conference on Process Mining (ICPM), pp. 128–135. IEEE (2021)
4. Adams, J.N., Schuster, D., Schmitz, S., Schuh, G., van der Aalst, W.M.: Defining cases and variants for object-centric event data. arXiv preprint arXiv:2208.03235 (2022)
5. Berti, A.: Filtering and sampling object-centric event logs. arXiv preprint arXiv:2205.01428 (2022)
6. Berti, A., Park, G., Rafiei, M., van der Aalst, W.: A generic approach to extract object-centric event data from relational databases (2023)
7. Berti, A., Park, G., Rafiei, M., van der Aalst, W.M.: A generic approach to extract object-centric event data from databases supporting SAP ERP. J. Intell. Inf. Syst. 1–23 (2023)
8. De Smedt, J., Hasić, F., vanden Broucke, S.K.L.M., Vanthienen, J.: Towards a holistic discovery of decisions in process-aware information systems. In: Carmona, J., Engels, G., Kumar, A. (eds.) BPM 2017. LNCS, vol. 10445, pp. 183–199. Springer, Cham (2017). https://doi.org/10.1007/978-3-319-65000-5_11
9. van Dongen, B.: BPI Challenge (2017). https://doi.org/10.4121/uuid:5f3067df-f10b-45da-b98b-86ae4c7a310b
10. Galanti, R., de Leoni, M., Navarin, N., Marazzi, A.: Object-centric process predictive analytics. arXiv preprint arXiv:2203.02801 (2022)
11. Ghahfarokhi, A.F., van der Aalst, W.: A python tool for object-centric process mining comparison. arXiv preprint arXiv:2202.05709 (2022)
12. Ghahfarokhi, A.F., Akoochekian, F., Zandkarimi, F., van der Aalst, W.M.: Clustering object-centric event logs. arXiv preprint arXiv:2207.12764 (2022)
13. Ghahfarokhi, A.F., Park, G., Berti, A., van der Aalst, W.M.P.: OCEL: a standard for object-centric event logs. In: Bellatreche, L., et al. (eds.) ADBIS 2021. CCIS, vol. 1450, pp. 169–175. Springer, Cham (2021). https://doi.org/10.1007/978-3-030-85082-1_16
14. Goossens, A., De Smedt, J., Vanthienen, J., van der Aalst, W.M.P.: Enhancing data-awareness of object-centric event logs. In: Montali, M., Senderovich, A., Weidlich, M. (eds.) ICPM 2022. LNBIP, vol. 468, pp. 18–30. Springer, Cham (2023). https://doi.org/10.1007/978-3-031-27815-0_2
15. Günther, C.W., Verbeek, H.M.W.: XES standard definition. IEEE Std (2014)
16. Li, G., de Murillas, E.G.L., de Carvalho, R.M., van der Aalst, W.M.P.: Extracting object-centric event logs to support process mining on databases. In: Mendling, J., Mouratidis, H. (eds.) CAiSE 2018. LNBIP, vol. 317, pp. 182–199. Springer, Cham (2018). https://doi.org/10.1007/978-3-319-92901-9_16
17. Rebmann, A., Rehse, J.R., van der Aa, H.: Uncovering object-centric data in classical event logs for the automated transformation from XES to OCEL. In: Di Ciccio, C., Dijkman, R., del Río Ortega, A., Rinderle-Ma, S. (eds.) BPM 2022. LNCS, vol. 13420, pp. 379–396. Springer, Cham (2022). https://doi.org/10.1007/978-3-031-16103-2_25

18. Reimers, N., Gurevych, I.: Sentence-BERT: sentence embeddings using Siamese BERT-networks. In: EMNLP. ACL (2019)
19. Xiong, J., Xiao, G., Kalayci, T.E., Montali, M., Gu, Z., Calvanese, D.: Extraction of object-centric event logs through virtual knowledge graphs. In: 35th International Workshop on Description Logics, DL 2022, Haifa, Israel, 7–10 August 2022 (2022)

Event Knowledge Graphs for Auditing: A Case Study

Eva L. Klijn[1], Dennis Preuss[2], Lulzim Imeri[2], Florin Baumann[2], Felix Mannhardt[1], and Dirk Fahland[1](✉)

[1] Eindhoven University of Technology, Eindhoven, The Netherlands
{e.l.klijn,f.mannhardt,d.fahland}@tue.nl
[2] Ernst & Young AG, Lancy, Switzerland
{dennis.preuss,lulzim.imeri,florin.baumann}@ch.ey.com

Abstract. Due to its potential benefits, process mining has become more and more embedded in financial auditing as an analysis technique to support the auditor in their assessment of internal controls executed in financially relevant processes. However, standard process mining solutions for audit are developed under the pretense of a single case notion. As a result, an auditor is presented with models and data visualizations of the process that do not accurately reflect the underlying relationship between accounting and other relevant objects in the process, posing challenges for the auditor in obtaining a precise understanding of the process and related controls. In this case study together with EY, we aim to understand requirements for improving the application of process mining in audit. After first inventorizing the current limitations, we explore on a real-life audit use case provided by EY the benefits of graph-based event data representation using an event knowledge graph, especially considering accounting related objects and events. Discussing these results with auditing experts at EY revealed insights and requirements for a process mining analysis in the context of auditing not documented in the literature before.

Keywords: financial auditing · multiple objects · knowledge graph · querying

1 Introduction

An organization's published financial statements are main trusted sources for economies and capital markets. Many stakeholder rely in their decision making upon the information published [14]. To provide assurance that the financial statements of an organization represent a true and fair view, a *financial audit* is performed. Using process mining (PM) on recorded event data in such audit has been shown to be useful in supporting an auditor in assessing the design and operating effectiveness of companies internal controls, as it provides a comprehensive and faithful view of processes [9].

© The Author(s), under exclusive license to Springer Nature Switzerland AG 2024
J. De Smedt and P. Soffer (Eds.): ICPM 2023 Workshops, LNBIP 503, pp. 84–97, 2024.
https://doi.org/10.1007/978-3-031-56107-8_7

The application of process mining for auditing and specifically financial auditing has been researched [7–9, 12–14]. Using existing process mining tools forces the auditor into an undesired trade-off decision early in the analysis when picking a case identifier to build the event log [7], e.g., in a purchasing process, the case could be chosen at the higher level of purchase order headers or each individual line item of the purchase order. Either choice has drawbacks [7] as flattening the relational source data into a sequential event log causes *convergence* (event duplication) and *divergence* (false behavioral dependencies) [1] that complicate the audit. Werner et al. [12] avoid the trade-offs and drawbacks by not flattening the data under a particular case, but directly constructing from data attributes a *graph of related events* for financial auditing. However, their resulting graph structure cannot be directly used by process mining solutions. Alternative, graph- and object-centric event data representations have been proposed [1, 4] but their application to auditing in practice has not yet been researched.

This paper reports on a case study conducted together with Ernst & Young (EY) with the objective of exploring the challenges of transitioning from a classical process mining analysis to a graph-based process mining analysis for financial auditing. We selected purchase-to-pay (P2P) as standard process and were provided with an anonymized, non-client attributed data set and process description from a real-life case (Sect. 2). Reflecting on the current use of sequential event logs, auditing experts from EY confirmed the known trade-offs and drawbacks [7] but also raised analytical challenges that future process mining solutions in audit have to overcome, specifically the need for flexible multi-perspective views on events and objects at different granularity levels is not fulfilled (Sect. 3). To explore whether graph-based event data models and visualizations meet these challenges, we transformed the ERP data of the P2P process into an Event Knowledge Graph (EKG) [4, 5] and designed a prototype visualization for auditing in an open-source graph database and visualization software (Sect. 4). We confronted the EY auditing experts with this visualization to obtain feedback whether this representation avoided the trade-offs and addressed the challenges through a more realistic and accurate view of the process from an auditing perspective (Sect. 5). We found that the graph, indeed, makes it easier for auditors to understand how business and accounting objects are interrelated and whether controls are violated. It provides the required flexibility to subset the event data for different objects and, therefore, switch between different perspectives. We reflect on the implications in Sect. 6.

2   Context and Use Case

We first recall financial auditing and its use case in process mining (Sect. 2.1) after which we introduce our use case and the ERP source data (Sect. 2.2).

2.1   Process Mining for Financial Auditing

Financial auditing is the process of examining financial statements of an organization with the purpose of providing reasonable assurance that the statements represent a true and fair view [9]. Financial audits are conducted by external auditors; larger organizations also have an internal audit department that assesses the broad scope of functioning of the organization, e.g., its operations or corporate governance.

Due to its potential benefits, *Process Mining* (PM) has become more and more embedded in financial auditing as an analysis technique to support the external auditor in their assessment of internal controls [14]. This procedure, shaped by the "International Standards on Auditing" (ISA), consists of four main phases: (1) understanding the entity, e.g., the organization, and its environment, including its internal control (ISA 315), (2) identifying and assessing the risk of material misstatement (ISA 315), (3) auditor's responses to assessed risks (ISA 330), and (4) forming an opinion and reporting on financial statements (ISA 700) [14].

In this study, we aim to understand requirements for improving the application of PM in the *first phase* of an *external* audit. Here, an auditor has to understand the entity and its environment, including the entity's internal control with the aim to asses the *design* and *operating* effectiveness of a control. The control is *effective* if it prevents the risk that a certain type of behavior or transaction results in material financial misstatement.

2.2   Use Case: Process, Data, and Controls

To understand the nature of the data and the behavior that an auditor has to understand when assessing a control, EY provided us with a use case of an anonymized, non-client attributed data set representing a real-life purchase-to-pay process (P2P) and corresponding auditing controls.

Process. A purchase-to-pay (P2P) process is a standard operational process aimed at procuring goods or services for an organization. The specific process handles *documents* of five different types that are created and updated throughout its execution.

The process starts with the creation of a purchase order (PO), a document containing one or multiple purchase order line items (POLs) detailing the goods or services being procured. From an ERP design and data perspective, a PO and a POL are considered two distinct types of entities; the PO stores information about, e.g., the vendor, purchasing organization or the total PO value and the POL stores item specific information, e.g., its quantity and price. Once created, the PO is sent to the supplier. When (part of) the goods and/or services, i.e., a number of POLs requested in the PO, are delivered, a goods receipt (GR) is created: a document stating that the goods entered the company's warehouse. Receiving and recording a supplier invoice continues the process which generates an invoice document (INV): a document detailing the goods or services rendered that need to be paid by the company. Receipt of goods and invoicing both lead to an increase in the company's inventory and liabilities it has towards its suppliers and, as such, both a goods receipt and invoice relate to an accounting document (AD). In the end, the AD related to the INV is settled through *another* AD, which is typically the payment to the supplier.

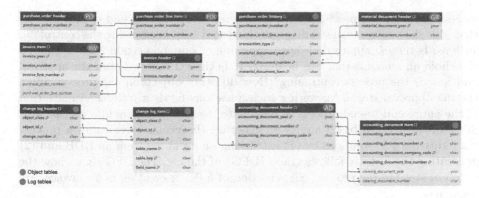

Fig. 1. Simplified database schema from source system provided by EY. Note: the change log item table has an n:1 relationship to each object table (omitted for simplicity).

Risks, Controls, and Auditing. In the example of P2P there is a risk that unauthorized procurements are charged on a company, leading to paying unjustified expenditures. To prevent that risk, companies typically define a "Purchase Order (PO) approval" control within their internal control framework that purchase orders have to be approved by authorized personnel. During the audit, auditors assess whether the control is designed in a way which addresses the above mentioned business risk. For example, if the POL quantity or price is changed then effective control design would trigger re-approval of the entire PO, as the total value of the PO changed. Similar behavior is expected if new procurements, i.e., new POLs, are added to an existing PO. Looking into the process' data records helps in assessing the control.

Data. Operational processes under audit, like the P2P process of our use case, track executions through records in a relational database (RDB). Its documents and items, jointly called *(data) objects*, are stored in uniquely identifiable information records, that are interrelated via 1:1, 1:n or n:m relations [11]. Figure 1 shows the (simplified) data schema of the P2P process in our case study, e.g., defining header and item-level objects for PO and POL (1:n relation), INV and INV item (1:n), AD and AD item (1:n). While POL refers to INV on the line item-level (1:n), INV refers to AD on the header level (1:n). If configured in the ERP system, the creation or update of an object is recorded as a timestamped *event* in a respective *change log* table (header and item-level). Each change log item table holds the object type as well as the object key that refers to the object that was updated (n:1, not shown in Fig. 1). The change log header table holds various information like the timestamp and user who performed the change.

3   Challenges of Event Data Representation in Auditing

To be able to assess a control, an auditor in phase 1 (cf. Sect. 2.1) first needs to get an overall view of the process to identify behavior that is relevant for this assessment. PM can provide a *visual overview* of the actual end-to-end process that aids the auditor in answering questions that help in assessing the control [9], such as: Is the PO approval always happening or only on certain POs? Is there a threshold on amounts that can be derived? Is the PO changed after the approval and how is the process continuing? How do other objects in the process affect the PO approval state? Answering such questions needs a *faithful* visualization of the entire end-to-end process to be able to assess the control in a precise way. State-of-the-art PM-based audits [9] generate the visual overview of a process via industrial PM solutions by (1) extracting an event log from an RDB and (2) generating the directly-follows graph (DFG) of the log. The DFG shows how the different steps in the process, e.g., creation of a PO or creation of an invoice, are sequenced.

We reviewed the current PM-based auditing practice together with experts from EY. We report our findings, which (1) confirm trade-offs in log extraction reported previously [7], and (2) detail how models derived from logs lack faithfulness to the underlying data and process – forcing auditors to compensate through additional analyses. (3) The review results in requirements for faithful event data representation and visualizations for auditing. (4) Auditing experts reviewed the state-of-the-art [9] and alternative [12,13] audit approaches and data models [3,5] against these requirements.

Event Log Extraction for PM-Based Audit: Choices and Implications.
In current PM-based audit practice, data from an RDB, e.g., of a P2P process, is first extracted into a *sequential event log* based on a specific object chosen as *case identifier*. Technically, all events (indirectly) related to the case identifier are grouped into a *trace* [2,5]. The choice of case identifier depends on the analysis goal and the cardinality of the relations between object in the process [10]. However, each of the choices has known drawbacks for auditing practice [7] that were confirmed by EY's experts.

In the use case of the P2P process (cf. Sect. 2.2), current audit practice prefers the *item-level POL object* as case identifier. The trace of one POL p contains all event records referring to p, and all event records referring to any (relevant) object o related (via other objects) to p [6]. However, as typically one AD header a is related to multiple POLs $p_1, \ldots, p_k$ via two 1:n relationships (cf. Fig. 1), a single Settle AD event e referring to a is extracted k times into the trace for each related POL $p_1, \ldots, p_k$, suggesting that k AD objects were settled (i.e., paid) instead of just 1, known as *convergence* [1].

Choosing the *header-level AD object as case identifier* avoids event duplication and would in principle allow to analyze the entire behavior leading to a payment. However, the resulting trace for a orders events of $p_1, \ldots, p_k$ (which are mutually unrelated, see Fig. 1) into a sequence, known as *divergence* [1]: it would become impossible to derive from the DFG which AD-related events relate to which POL.

Finally, the large amount of data kept within a single RDB of a large enterprise requires pre-filtering during extraction, e.g., extract only data of the company within the audit scope. The challenge for an auditor lies in the organization of change logs by object type rather than by company. To ease this, the change log is pre-filtered to changes of relevant objects within a set time frame while object-related tables are filtered based on organizational attributes.

Analytical Challenges on the DFG. The auditing experts emphasized the following limitations of standard DFG-based audits and the resulting challenges (C1-C3) for answering questions in the first phase of an audit.

Auditors in practice are not involved in the choices and transformations during event log extraction. They perceive the DFG computed from the log as the truth and are not aware of implications of convergence and divergence. This leads to challenge (C1): this requires extensive expertise to overcome leading to longer onboarding times for using PM in audit. Also, the more decisions are made in the data transformation, the more has to be explained about the audit result to the client.

The main challenges of using a single-case DFG in audit are related to the performing of the audit itself. First, an auditor needs to validate the DFG, which, in practice, is often done by reconciling the figures from the accounting related events back to the balance sheet and income statement movements. Often a single payment (i.e., the accounting relevant event) settles multiple invoices, each related to mutiple POLs. However, the preferred POL-perspective DFG duplicates the accounting relevant events, along with the payments values, for each of the POLs. (C2): As a result, it is more difficult for the auditor to reconcile, as there are now multiple events with the same payment value, but only a single entry in the accounting ledger.

Second, to assess controls, the auditor needs to understand how the process perspective is related to the accounting perspective, in particular, how a process activity can impact objects and the effect this has on the control. This involves inferring from the activities how the process flows between the different business objects (PO, POL, INV, GR) and accounting objects (AD). These accounting objects are the financial transactions leading to the financial statements. The auditor has to understand at which level of granularity (line-item level or header level), a particular attribute is located and how to relate different attributes correctly, e.g., relating amounts in a POL (line-item) to amount in PO (header). (C3): However, the DFG only shows the flows between the different activities related to the objects but not the objects themselves, nor how these are structurally related. Moreover, different controls concern different levels of granularity, while the DFG is fixed to the granularity of the chosen case identifier. Both limitations increase auditor effort. Overall, the inherent limitations of flattening event data under a single case identifier forces auditors into undesirable trade-offs and complex decisions.

Requirements. The review above resulted in the following requirements for faithful event data representation and visualizations for auditing. **(R1)** The preference of auditing experts is to avoid these trade-offs altogether and to work with the data "as-is" (no duplication, no false behavioral dependencies, i.e., address C2) which also reduces the decisions made in transforming the source system data into event data for audits (C1). **(R2)** Auditing experts prefer to explicitly visualize (and access) the objects (of different levels) related to events and require flexibility from which angle to analyze the data (any document, header or item level, i.e., C3).

Alternative Event Data Models. Reviewing the literature, the auditing experts confirmed that event-log based auditing approaches, e.g., [7,8,14], see [9] for an overview, violate R1 (due to the event log) and R2 (due to lack of visualizing related objects). Very few alternative event data models exist. Werner et al.'s [12,13] graph-based data model is based on accounting structures and patterns (instead of process events ordered by time) where characteristics and relationships of objects (accounting entries) are more important than their temporal order. According to experts, this aligns with an auditor's task, whose first focus point in an audit is to understand accounting entries and how they relate to other accounting entries which the model describes "as-is". By focusing on the accounting perspective, the model omits the process steps and their temporal order which are relevant for the auditor to understand the entity's control environment, as the control typically governs the process steps the precede the accounting entries.

Generic *graph-based* event data models were proposed in [3,4] and consolidated as *event knowledge graphs* (EKGs) in [5]. An EKG models events and objects in a process as nodes and the relationships between them as edges; a node or relationship *label* distinguishes different types; *properties* (attribute-value pairs) describe a node or edge further. An EKG specifically models which events are related to which objects, which objects (of any level) are related to each other, and which events temporally follow each other from the perspective of a specific object; see Fig. 5 for an example. By design, EKGs satisfy R1 and R2 [5]. Auditing experts perceive EKGs to provide the necessary flexibility to explore the base questions in audit (see above) and define a corresponding faithful visualization of the process that suits audit phase 1.

4   Prototyping a Graph-Based Visualization for Audit

As the potential benefits and challenges of using EKGs in first phase of an external audit have not been analyzed yet, we developed a prototype visualization based on an EKG. Instead of extracting an event log, we constructed an EKG from the ERP SAP data of the P2P process of Sect. 2 in two steps (see Fig. 2): (1) we extracted the data from the RDB into a tabular format anonymizing the data in the process (Sect. 4.1) and then (2) constructed the EKG in an open-source graph DB; we used existing tools to create a prototype visualization (Sect. 4.2).

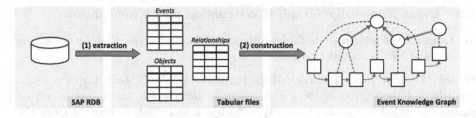

Fig. 2. Data transformation procedure.

4.1 Event Data Extraction

Our input data is stored in an ERP SAP relational database as described in
Sect. 2.2. EY's auditing experts first filtered the data to a relevant subset required
for an analysis use case as in any standard audit (as explained in Sect. 3).

To enable EKG
construction, the ERP
data (Fig. 1) is extracted
into events, objects
and relationships accord-
ing to the schema
in Fig. 3, using 5
steps. (1) We chose
the following objects

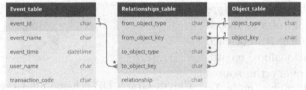

Fig. 3. Tabular data schema after DB extraction (Fig. 2 middle).

(explained in Sect. 2.2) for the use case: PO header, POL item, GR header, AD
header (invoice), AD line item. (2) We extract event records for the selected
objects by joining the object's table of the ERP data with its respective change
log table [6]. Each event record includes the foreign key to the object record
to which it was joined. All events are inserted into event table of Fig. 3. Each
activity requires its own SQL query. (3) For each extracted event, we extract
the related ERP system's object as object record (with the object type) into the
object table of Fig. 3. (4) Then we build the relationship table by joining tables
according to the ERP data model (Fig. 1). For example, the POL item is *a child
of* a PO header, or the AD header *posts* an AD line item. We add each such joins
as a record in the relationship table of Fig. 3. (5) Finally, the foreign keys in
the event records are translated into event-object relation records added to the
relationship table.

Generally, the scope of the extracted data has to be determined per project
and use case. For this study, we filtered events by timestamp to limit the data
to a three-month period that was considered sufficient for the exploration of
the concepts. For some activities additional object tables are joined to limit
extraction, e.g., we limited posting of AD line item events to those ADs related
to an INV with a related POL and PO. We obtained an *object table* with 304'777
objects of 5 different types, an *event table* with 333'358 events of 10 activities,
and a *relationship table* with 560'975 relationships.

4.2   Event Knowledge Graph Construction and Visualization

We translate the intermediate tables into an EKG in two steps, thereby extending the original EKG construction procedure of [4]:

Event, Object, and Relationship Import. While [4] only imports event records and then infers objects and relations from event attributes based on domain knowledge, we also have explicit object and relation records from the ERP export of Sect. 4.1.

Adapting the import queries of [4] we import each event record as a node with label *event*, and each object record as a node labeled with the *object_type* in the object record (see Fig. 3). For each relationship record, we query the source and target node by their type and identifier and create a corresponding edge in

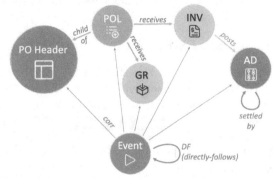

Fig. 4. Graph DB schema after event knowledge graph construction (Fig. 2 right).

the EKG. Indices on the event and object identifiers increase performance. Import of the entire dataset required 2.8 min on an Intel i5 CPU@1.6 GHz machine with 24 GB RAM. The resulting EKG models the source data "as-is" with 304'777 entity nodes, 333'358 event nodes, and 560'975 relationships. After import, we addressed data quality issues: PO and POL create events are recorded at different levels of granularity, which falsely suggested that the first POL item of PO object was created before the PO object itself. To improve data quality, we queried the EKG for the first POL node related to a PO node, matched the POL node's timestamp to the PO node's timestamp. Figure 4 shows the schema of the resulting EKG and Fig. 5 shows a sample of the EKG.

Deriving Behavioral Relationships. To model the behavior of an object, i.e., the "trace of an object", we derive the df-edges using the query from [4] that (1) retrieves all events $e_1, ..., e_k$ related to an object o (*corr* edges in Fig. 4), (2) orders them by timestamp $e_i.time$ and (3) creates a *df*-edge between each subsequent pair of event nodes e_j, e_{j+1}. In Fig. 5, this results in the df-edge from the Create POL to the Change POL event related to the top-most POL object.

To model the interactions *between* related objects, we derive df-edges from the perspective of the relation itself them using queries from [4]: (1) for each relation (of interest) between two objects o_i and o_j we create a new "derived" object $o_{i \times j}$ and relate it to o_i and o_j via relationships with label *derived*. (2) For each event e related to o_i or to o_j, we also relate e to $o_{i \times j}$ (adding *corr* edges). (3) We then order all events of $o_{i\times j}$ by time and add df-relationships as explained above. For events of different objects with the same timestamp, we sort events of header objects before item objects, e.g., to correctly sort Create PO and Create POL events. For instance, the df-edge from the Create PO to the Create POL event related to the top-most POL object in Fig. 5 is a behavioral relationship between two objects.

Prototype Visualization. In order to get feedback on the suitability of an EKG-based representation for auditing, we prototyped a visualization of the EKG using Neo4j Bloom on a subset of the data selected by EY. We queried the EKG for all documents and events related to a specific AD that was known to EY to involve the auditing challenges of Sect. 3. We visualized the 5 object types, events, and relations of the schema (Fig. 4, omitting "derived" objects) using distinct colors, icons, and node sizes, and line width to distinguish types. We laid out the graph manually (events placed beneath their related objects, events ordered horizontally according to df-relations).

Figure 5 shows the chosen subset: it contains two POs (dark blue nodes) related to three POLs (light blue nodes). Each POL receives one INV document (yellow node) that posts to one respective AD (green node); all ADs are settled by a single final AD. There are two additional sets of POLs, INVs, ADs (bottom four rows of nodes in Fig. 5) whose preceding POs are outside the extracted 3-month window. Each document has related event nodes (orange); the df-edges flow "in parallel" with the document relations and the derived df-edges (marked (2a–2b) in Fig. 5) show flow between line-item documents related to the same header. Importantly, the graph explicitly shows *each* financial transaction (ADs) of this execution as individual (green) nodes.

5   Results

Feedback. We confronted the auditing experts at EY with the prototype visualization to receive feedback on how well EKGs provide the desired visual overview of the process in the first phase of an audit (R1, R2 in Sect. 3); their feedback is summarized below.

Showing data "as-is". The experts immediately recognized that the graph matches the process description (Sect. 2.2) "as-is": Each source event record is shown as exactly one event node (orange in Fig. 5), i.e., no duplication (satisfying R1). Its right-most Settle AD event e is related to a single AD object (green node in Fig. 5); e follows (via multiple blue df-edges) 5 Enter INV events that are related to 5 INV objects, which are related to 5 AD objects that are settled by the same (final) AD object.

Multiple levels of granularity. As each event is clearly associated to a particular object on a particular level (item or header), experts find it easier to understand that approvals to POL changes happen at the header level, while a POL change happens at the item level. The df-relations between objects of different levels (via "derived objects"), reveal which PO approval relates to (i.e.,

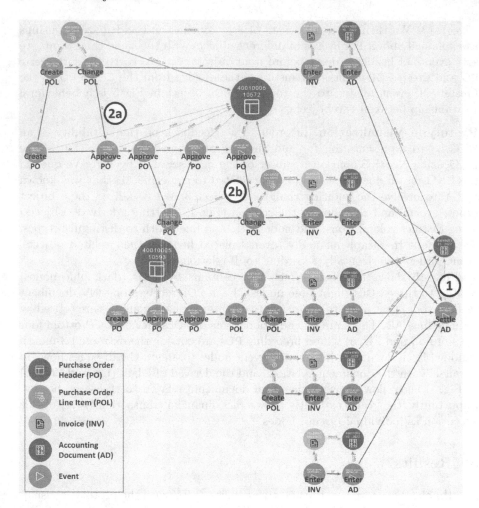

Fig. 5. Prototypical example of two PO objects and related objects.

follows) which POL changes giving a larger-scale understanding missing in a POL-oriented event log (see Sect. 3). As a result it is easier to assess whether there is a violation of this particular control. For example in Fig. 5 (2a) we see an instance where this control is working, i.e., a POL change is later approved on the PO level, whereas Fig. 5 (2b) shows a violation of this control, i.e., a POL is changed and, without further approval, an INV is entered and eventually settled.

Layout shows the process along business and accounting objects. The blue df-edges form *df-paths* from the events of the initial POL items to the event of the final AD object. As these paths run "in parallel" to objects and object-object relations, the EKG visualizes how process steps precede accounting objects, i.e., AD objects, in relation to business objects (satisfying R2). This allows an auditor to understand how the process leads to accounting entries. While in classical event logs, the auditor has the burden to mentally reconstruct these relations from the source data, the EKG visualizes the relations directly, enabling a different view and understanding of the process.

Brainstorming. Reflecting on the properties of the prototype led the auditing experts to generate further potential benefits and requirements for graph-based models in auditing which we summarize next.

Overall, the ability to read the graph from different perspectives (objects at header and item-level granularity) *opens up the possibility for header-level oriented auditing analysis* that considers larger-scale patterns without suffering from convergence/divergence errors.

Subsetting in a graph allows an auditor to quickly get to the level of detail that is tied to certain objects relevant for a control, e.g., POL amounts, vendor, company codes; in logs the relation between objects and attributes for subsetting is more implicit. But the graph potentially enables further use cases: Subsetting based on an object would allow an auditor to assess controls specific to that object, e.g., invoice approval. Subsetting based on interactions between different objects would allow an auditor to assess controls across those objects, e.g. the control of the PO approval which involves both the PO and POL object.

Aggregation wrt. particular objects, relations, or patterns would enable auditors to understand controls on a higher-level of granularity, e.g., by summarizing item-level events to the related header level.

Recognize impact on controls. If an auditor understands which object and event nodes in the graph relate to a specific control, then the graph enables an auditor to understand which objects and events impact which controls (and whether one object or event impacts multiple controls). For example, adding the user as an "object" allows to observe batch work [5] in turn enabling the auditor to assess whether controls are implemented correctly in all circumstances, e.g., also in case of batch processing 10 subsequent invoice approvals in a short timeframe. This is not possible in a DFG based on a sequential event log.

The approach enables to *inter-link multiple processes* in a single graph, enabling, for instance, to assess whether changes to master data involved in an object impacted a particular control, which is laborious in a classical setting.

6   Conclusion

This paper presents the results of a case study conducted together with EY on the application of graph-based process mining for the *first phase* of an external financial audit of a real-world P2P process: providing the auditor with a visual overview to understand the process. Reviewing the difficulties encountered when analyzing ERP system data that was transformed into single case event logs brought to the forefront a set of analytical challenges and requirements for process mining when used in financial auditing. We built a graph-based event representation using an EKG directly from the ERP system data and evaluated this representation for its suitability to meet the identified requirements.

We found that the graph-based representation shows potential in overcoming the technical and analytical challenges that arise in PM-based audits on case-based event logs. This strongly suggests that future research on PM-based auditing solutions should systematically address these challenges. Another advantage is the flexibility of using open source software like the one used in our case study. This enables companies to focus much more on the use cases and its benefits before investing in a broad process mining software implementation. Analysis and queries can be executed in an open source implementation. This helps to sharpen the audit use cases without the need for a full fledged process mining solution implementation/roll-out. Addressing the remaining audit phases requires further research, e.g., automatically checking controls on the EKG structure.

Our findings are limited by the exploration of a single process and data set, suggesting further studies for robustness. Our approach for limiting just the event extraction by a strict time frame led to objects missing events and events missing related objects which occurred outside the time frame; this can be addressed either during extraction from the source system or by extracting a larger time frame and filtering in the EKG. Moreover, the prototype visualization was based on a manually created layout that significantly helped conveying the structure of the event data. Substantial research in better visualizations in process mining is required for automation.

References

1. van der Aalst, W.M.P.: Object-centric process mining: dealing with divergence and convergence in event data. In: Ölveczky, P., Salaün, G. (eds.) SEFM 2019. LNCS, vol. 11724, pp. 3–25. Springer, Cham (2019). https://doi.org/10.1007/978-3-030-30446-1_1
2. Accorsi, R., Lebherz, J.: A practitioner's view on process mining adoption, event log engineering and data challenges. In: van der Aalst, W.M.P., Carmona, J. (eds.) Process Mining Handbook. LNBIP, vol. 448, pp. 212–240. Springer, Cham (2022). https://doi.org/10.1007/978-3-031-08848-3_7
3. Berti, A., van der Aalst, W.: Extracting multiple viewpoint models from relational databases. In: Ceravolo, P., van Keulen, M., Gómez-López, M. (eds.) SIMPDA 2018 & 2019. LNBIP, vol. 379, pp. 24–51. Springer, Cham (2020). https://doi.org/10.1007/978-3-030-46633-6_2
4. Esser, S., Fahland, D.: Multi-dimensional event data in graph databases. J. Data Semant. **10**, 109–141 (2021)
5. Fahland, D.: Process mining over multiple behavioral dimensions with event knowledge graphs. In: van der Aalst, W.M.P., Carmona, J. (eds.) Process Mining Handbook. LNBIP, vol. 448, pp. 274–319. Springer, Cham (2022). https://doi.org/10.1007/978-3-031-08848-3_9
6. Fahland, D., de Leoni, M., van Dongen, B.F., van der Aalst, W.M.P.: Behavioral conformance of artifact-centric process models. In: Abramowicz, W. (ed.) BIS 2011. LNBIP, vol. 87, pp. 37–49. Springer, Heidelberg (2011). https://doi.org/10.1007/978-3-642-21863-7_4
7. Jans, M.: Auditor choices during event log building for process mining. J. Emerg. Technol. Account. **16**(2), 59–67 (2019)

8. Jans, M., Alles, M.G., Vasarhelyi, M.A.: A field study on the use of process mining of event logs as an analytical procedure in auditing. Account. Rev. **89**(5), 1751–1773 (2014)
9. Jans, M., Eulerich, M.: Process mining for financial auditing. In: van der Aalst, W.M.P., Carmona, J. (eds.) Process Mining Handbook. LNBIP, vol. 448, pp. 445–467. Springer, Cham (2022). https://doi.org/10.1007/978-3-031-08848-3_15
10. Jans, M., Soffer, P.: From relational database to event log: decisions with quality impact. In: Teniente, E., Weidlich, M. (eds.) BPM 2017. LNBIP, vol. 308, pp. 588–599. Springer, Cham (2018). https://doi.org/10.1007/978-3-319-74030-0_46
11. Lu, X., Nagelkerke, M., van de Wiel, D., Fahland, D.: Discovering interacting artifacts from ERP systems. IEEE Trans. Serv. Comput. **8**(6), 861–873 (2015)
12. Werner, M.: Financial process mining - accounting data structure dependent control flow inference. Int. J. Account. Inf. Syst. **25**, 57–80 (2017)
13. Werner, M., Gehrke, N.: Multilevel process mining for financial audits. IEEE Trans. Serv. Comput. **8**(6), 820–832 (2015)
14. Werner, M., Wiese, M., Maas, A.: Embedding process mining into financial statement audits. Int. J. Account. Inf. Syst. **41**, 100514 (2021)

Turning Logs into Lumber: Preprocessing Tasks in Process Mining

Ying Liu, Vinicius Stein Dani⬤, Iris Beerepoot⬤, and Xixi Lu$^{(\boxtimes)}$⬤

Utrecht University, Utrecht, The Netherlands
{v.steindani,i.m.beerepoot,x.lu}@uu.nl

Abstract. Event logs are invaluable for conducting process mining projects, offering insights into process improvement and data-driven decision-making. However, data quality issues affect the correctness and trustworthiness of these insights, making preprocessing tasks a necessity. Despite the recognized importance, the execution of preprocessing tasks remains ad-hoc, lacking support. This paper presents a systematic literature review that establishes a comprehensive repository of preprocessing tasks and their usage in case studies. We identify six high-level and 20 low-level preprocessing tasks in case studies. Log filtering, transformation, and abstraction are commonly used, while log enriching, integration, and reduction are less frequent. These results can be considered a first step in contributing to more structured, transparent event log preprocessing, enhancing process mining reliability.

Keywords: Log preprocessing · Process mining · Event log

1 Introduction

In the landscape of data-driven decision-making, event logs stand as invaluable assets, capturing the execution of activities of processes and their interactions within diverse operational systems. The potential insights that can be obtained from these logs are immense, spanning process improvement, anomaly detection, performance evaluation, and strategic planning [1]. However, the axiom "garbage in, garbage out" holds particularly true in this context [36]. The presence of data quality issues underscores the vital importance of preprocessing techniques. Without proper preprocessing, the very foundation of analysis is compromised.

The importance of data quality and preprocessing in the field of process mining has been acknowledged, as evidenced by the growing attention dedicated to these subjects [36,40]. Despite the acknowledgment, the execution of log preprocessing seems to remain ad-hoc. Moreover, little support has been provided on which preprocessing tasks are possible and how to select them. Although a few process mining methodologies sketched potential preprocessing tasks, a comprehensive overview of these tasks has been notably absent. Furthermore, the way these preprocessing tasks are used in real-life has remained unclear.

Existing systematic literature reviews (SLRs) have attempted to tackle specific tasks of log preprocessing, such as event abstraction techniques [40] and data extraction [34].

© The Author(s), under exclusive license to Springer Nature Switzerland AG 2024
J. De Smedt and P. Soffer (Eds.): ICPM 2023 Workshops, LNBIP 503, pp. 98–109, 2024.
https://doi.org/10.1007/978-3-031-56107-8_8

However, a comprehensive review that covers diverse preprocessing tasks and their practical applications in real-world scenarios is lacking.

In this paper, we perform a systematic literature review to establish an initial, comprehensive overview of the preprocessing tasks and their utilization in process mining case studies. By undertaking this endeavor, we aim to create a repository of log preprocessing tasks that may provide guidance and support for researchers and practitioners.

We identified six high-level preprocessing tasks, and for four of these tasks, we observed 20 low-level preprocessing tasks described in the case studies. The results show that log filtering, transformation, and abstraction have been more frequently used in case studies, while log enriching, integration, and reduction (e.g., sampling) are much less frequently performed.

The remainder of this paper is organized as follows. In Sect. 2, we discuss related work. Next, we explain the methodology followed in Sect. 3 and present the results in Sect. 4. Finally, we conclude the paper in Sect. 5.

2 Related Work

In this section, we discuss the related work, based on which we synthesized an initial set of six high-level preprocessing tasks: (a) *log integration*, (b) *log transformation*, (c) *log reduction*, (d) *log abstraction*, (e) *log filtering*, and (f) *log enriching*, see Fig. 1.

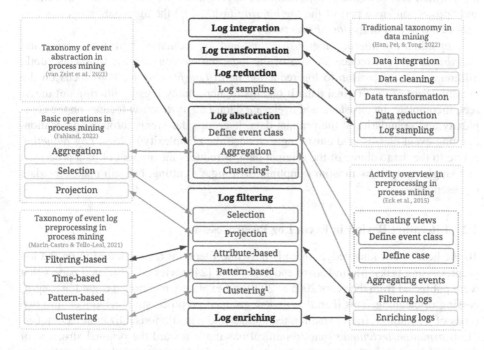

Fig. 1. Initial result of high-level log preprocessing tasks and techniques in the related work.

2.1 Taxonomy of Log Preprocessing Tasks

Han et al. [16] propose four categories of data preprocessing techniques: data cleaning, data integration, data transformation, and data reduction. Data cleaning focuses on handling missing values, identifying noise or outliers, and repairing errors. Since these subtasks are not interesting (e.g., identifying missing variable values) or not directly applicable to process mining (e.g., identifying noise/outliers in a distribution), we omit this task and decide to focus on the latter three tasks. For each, we create a corresponding log preprocessing task: *log integration*, *log transformation*, and *log reduction*.

Van Eck et al. [10] listed four tasks in the preprocessing stage, which are specifically tailored towards event logs: creating views, aggregating events, filtering logs, and enriching logs. We exclude the task "creating views" because this task assumes that there is no event log yet, while we assume we have a raw event log as input. We match the task "aggregating events" to *log abstraction*, also known as *event abstraction* that has been already surveyed [40]. The filtering of event logs ("filtering logs") is also considered a log preprocessing task within our scope, which we refer to as *log filtering*. Finally, the preprocessing task "enriching logs" is mapped to *log enriching*. As for *log enriching* and *log integration*, we consider *log integration* as creating a new event log by integrating one or more external data sources, while *log enriching* focuses on using the information within the event log to derive additional attributes.

Fahland [12] indicated that there are three basic preprocessing operations on event logs, which are: selection, projection, and aggregation. We consider the "selection" and "projection" as a part of the *log filtering* task, while the aggregation operation is considered as part of the *log abstraction*.

Regarding *log filtering*, *log abstraction*, and *log reduction*, both *log filtering* and *log abstraction* can reduce the size of the logs, but we consider the following subtle differences in comparison to log reduction here. *Log filtering* tends to focus on the quality issues of the original data. It obtains higher-quality logs by filtering out incorrect, incomplete, inconsistent, and irrelevant data. *Log abstraction* focuses on the complexity and granularity of the original data. It groups the events through aggregation, defining event classes, and clustering to reduce the complexity of logs. *Log reduction* is due to the data volume of the original data. It reduces the amount of data processed in a single analysis by random sampling, dividing, or cutting, but still makes the data representative.

2.2 Literature Review in Event Log Preprocessing

To the best of our knowledge, there is only one literature review focusing on the log preprocessing tasks: Marin-Castro and Tello-Leal [24] reviewed 70 related papers that were published from the years 2005 to 2020 and explicitly mentioned event log preprocessing or cleaning. This literature review grouped preprocessing techniques into two types of *techniques*: transformation techniques and detection-visualization techniques. *Transformation techniques* mark modifications made toward the original structure of the event log, while the events or traces that can lead to issues with data quality are identified, grouped, and isolated using *detection-visualization techniques*. In this paper, we cover six high-level *preprocessing tasks*, instead of the techniques. We include log enriching, log integration, and log reduction, which have not been discussed.

Van Zelst et al. [40] conducted a review and presented a taxonomy of event abstraction techniques. While valuable and detailed insights are provided into the event abstraction techniques, no insights are provided into their usage in practice, and no overview is provided for other preprocessing tasks. Similarly, Stein Dani et al. [34] report that preprocessing, on a high level represented by filtering-related tasks, is still a manual effort in the event log preparation phase of a process mining project. However, they mainly focus on data extraction tasks and do not provide an overview of the preprocessing tasks, including automated ones, and their usage in real-life case studies.

Currently, there is no clear overview of log preprocessing tasks and how frequently are these preprocessing tasks being used in process mining projects. Using the six high-level tasks as our scope, we conduct an SLR in order to provide insights into the usage of log preprocessing techniques in process mining case studies.

3   Systematic Literature Review

To arrive at an initial selection of relevant papers, and inspired by Kitchenham and Petersen [19,28], we applied the following search string on Scopus: ("process mining") AND ("case study" OR "case studies") within the article title, abstract, and keywords. As of December 20, 2022, we initially found 4565 papers. Figure 2 shows an overview of the paper screening process we followed. Next, we applied the exclusion and inclusion criteria in order to narrow down the scope of the review. The following exclusion criteria were defined and applied directly via the search engine: (1) the paper is published in 2021 and 2022; (2) the paper is published in conferences or journals under peer-review; (3) the paper explicitly mentions "process mining" in the keywords; and, (4) the paper is written in English. As we are particularly interested in the current trend in case studies that use process mining as the core technique, this is our inclusion criteria. Therefore, only papers meeting these criteria were selected to be further analyzed.

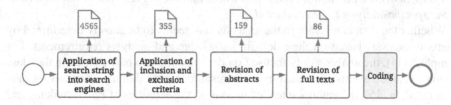

Fig. 2. Paper screening procedure.

After applying our exclusion and inclusion criteria, we obtained 355 papers. Because our focus is on log preprocessing tasks applied in real-world settings, we then read the abstracts of all these papers and filtered out the ones that did not mention collecting data from a real-world scenario. Thereafter, we obtained 159 papers to go through the full paper screening. These papers were downloaded and imported into the software Nvivo[1] for further analysis. During the full paper analysis stage, the papers that did not mention any data preprocessing steps were discarded and, finally, 86 papers were obtained as relevant papers to go through the coding stage of our work.

The following codes were defined for the analysis: high-level category, low-level category, and data domain. Next, we discuss what each one of them entails. *High-level categories* were defined based on related work and used to deductively categorize the papers. The six high-level categories are (1) log integration, (2) log reduction, (3) log abstraction, (4) log filtering, (5) log enriching, and (6) log transformation. Several *Low-level categories* within the high-level categories were inductively defined from the studied papers. Finally, in addition, we also coded the *data domain* (e.g., healthcare, education, manufacture, etc.), the analysis purpose, the PM task, and the year. Due to space limits, we do not discuss these results in this paper. The initial result of the categorization process is presented in Fig. 1.

4   Results

In this section, we present the results of coding 86 papers. The results are discussed for each high-level category. For a complete overview of the results and the detailed coding, we refer to [23].

4.1   Log Filtering

Log filtering is the most commonly performed preprocessing task, with 55 out of 86 papers performing this preprocessing task. These 55 papers mentioned filtering different objects, such as noise, outliers, redundant, duplicated cases and events, missing values, useless values, blank values, irrelevant values, and so on. Using the objects mentioned in these papers, the category log filtering is subdivided into 9 detailed low-level categories.

Filtering Irrelevant Data. We observed that 29 out of 55 papers mentioned filtering "irrelevant" data. After analyzing these papers, we define *irrelevant data* as *those resources, activities, attributes, events, and traces that are not relevant or not important for the specific analysis to be conducted.*

Whether the data is relevant to the analysis task seems to be mostly determined by experts or analysts based on their domain knowledge and analysis requirements. For example, in [4], the analysis only focused on the students who participated in the class (resource), so the events generated by other resources were defined as irrelevant data and filtered. In [15], the authors intended to analyze the activities of Ph.D. students and improve their journeys. So after a discussion by analysts and stakeholders, a filter is applied to retain the traces of full-time students who completed their Ph.D. and who withdrew (case status). The term *useless data* is also used in some of the papers to describe irrelevant data. For example, in [37], the authors mentioned "*filtering useless information such as links and marker symbols*", since the links and marker symbols (attributes) cannot make any contribution to the intended analysis and are regarded as useless data.

---

[1] https://lumivero.com/products/nvivo/.

Filtering Incomplete Data. In 16 out of 55 papers, the authors mentioned filtering incomplete data. Incomplete data can be divided into *incomplete events* and *incomplete cases*. *Incomplete events* usually refer to events having missing values or missing attributes. Incomplete events include missing case id [20], missing timestamps [9,15,27], and missing activities [7,9], missing other attribute values that are relevant to this analysis [14].

The incompleteness of a case is usually described as cases that are not completed or do not represent the end-to-end process. It means that the cases lack some events, for example, *"remove any record that may create only one event per case as it will not depict the sequence of activities and hinder the performance analysis of the model"* [29] and *"removing cases that did not cover the whole steps"* [7].

Filtering Infrequent Data. We use *infrequent data* to refer to the infrequent case variant. In 13 papers, the authors mentioned that they performed the infrequent case variants filtering as a preprocessing task. Filtering infrequent data is done to *"prevent the PM tool from returning incomprehensible or inaccurate results"* [32], and *"to improve the quality of results, and to avoid low precision and highly complex results"* [39].

Filtering Inconsistent Data. A simple example of inconsistent data is that the values are recorded in different formats, e.g., "2023-01-01" and "2023/01/01" as the attribute timestamps. This inconsistency in data format may be due to recording errors or caused by manual input. It may also be that different data sources have used different data formats. Inconsistent event labels make it difficult to assign clear semantics to the activities of a discovered process model [1], and may also bring about a dimensional explosion of the process model.

Filtering Incorrect Data. Incorrect data is erroneous or unreliable data that violates the logic of reality. For example, in the real process, activity A should be executed earlier than activity B, but in the log, the timestamp of A in a specific case is later than activity B [27].

Filtering Duplicates. Duplicates refer to repeated data. In process mining, the case ID needs to be a unique identifier, and the traces represented by different case IDs must be different, so as to ensure the accuracy of the data. However, in real life, duplicate data is usually generated due to system bugs or other reasons. For example, in [8], repeated events with the same Call-ID were excluded.

Filtering Redundant Data. Only two papers mentioned redundant data [6,7]. In [7], redundant events were included in data error: *"we conducted some data preprocessing, including handling data error (e.g., removing redundant events and eliminating multiple yield values)"*, while there was no further definition and explanation in [6]. We consider redundant events to be events that semantically are the same but not necessarily identical, while duplicates are identical events.

Filtering Outliers. In [2,3,22], the authors only mentioned *"removing outliers"* without any further explanation or definition. In [5], the authors mention *"we noticed the existence of outliers, i.e., cases that take too long, or incomplete"*; so, too long trace and incomplete data are considered outliers. In [31], *"if lecture activities in the short semester are included, it will be an outlier because it has activities that are far more than short than activities in the semester in general"*; thus, traces that are too short are also considered outliers. It seems that process analysts use the distributions of a case or event-attribute to define outliers, e.g., the number of events per case, the case duration per case, etc.

Filtering Noise. Noise is an overused word. Data that is not conducive to the analysis task is often defined as noise. An interesting point is that among the 86 papers, more than one paper mentioned noise, but only one paper described what noise is and how to filter it, *"In the original log the noisy activities were conveniently named 'Noise', so they were removed using a filter on the activity name"* [21].

4.2   Log Transformation

In 38 of the 86 papers, the authors described that they performed a *log transformation* task. The coding resulted in four data objects that are being transformed, which we use to further divide the high-level category.

Transforming Format. Among the format transformations, the transformation of the log format from CSV to XES was mentioned the most (14 out of 25 papers), such that the event logs can be used in the PM tool. This is because the log format after extraction is usually CSV, and PM tools require the log format to be imported as XES. The remaining format transformation is related to determining which columns are the key columns (such as case ID, activity name, and timestamps) after importing the log into PM tools.

Transforming Values. The difference between transforming values and transforming format is that transforming values means the change of one or more specific values in an event. For example, replacing infrequent values with the value 'other' to avoid dimension explosion, replacing missing values, replacing NaN values with 'zero', capturing data, and encrypting data.

Reordering. Reordering is the process of sorting the log by a particular timestamp. When the original log is out of order, it is essential to reorder it so that the process model displays the activities' proper execution sequence.

Transition Matrices and Encoding. In particular, transition matrices and trace encoding are used as a preprocessing for predictive process monitoring. Given that the trace encoding is a subfield itself and was not included in the search, we consider this category outside of our scope. We found two case studies mentioning this preprocessing task and coded them without further analysis.

4.3   Log Enriching

In 16 out of 86 papers, the log-enriching techniques were applied. Log enriching is split into four categories. Three of them are shown using an example in Fig. 3.

Adding Calculation Metrics. In this low-level category, the calculation metrics are computed from existing attributes in the log. For example, in [8], call center processes of a company were examined. In the original event log, each call only had attributes Start and Call Duration, but process analysis required the end time of the call. Therefore, the attribute End was obtained by adding Call Duration to Start.

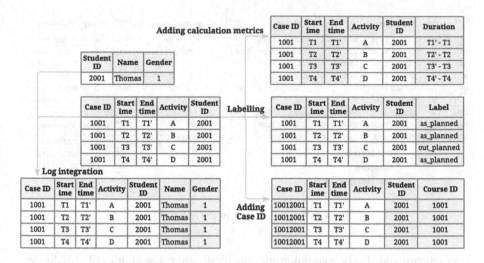

Fig. 3. Examples of three log integration tasks versus log enriching.

Labelling. Labeling is the task of assigning a tag or a class to an event or a trace. In [38], *"the cases are labeled as either successful or failed, depending on how they have been executed and their outcome"*, to further divide the log into two logs. In [26], for recording differences over time between the intended operation and the actual execution, a label was assigned to each event to indicate if the event was carried out on time or not.

Adding Case Id. Case id is a unique attribute in event logs. The data collected in some case studies did not have the attribute of case id, then the case id was created artificially in the data preprocessing stage. For example, in [35], *"the caseid is created by combining the three-digit client number (MANDT) with a ten-digit document number and a five-digit item number"*.

Adding Noise. Adding noise is not a typical preprocessing task, as just one publication described it. [33] evaluated privacy assurance of healthcare metadata. Noise-adding plugins in the tool ProM were used to make the original event logs more privacy-preserving [25].

4.4 Log Reduction

In 11 out of 86 papers, the authors used log reduction to do log preprocessing. Examples of the three log reduction tasks are shown in Fig. 4.

Dividing into Sub-logs In the example presented in Fig. 4, the original log is divided into two logs by the date in timestamp. In [11,21], IoT logs were collected in a smart house and the aim was to explore human habits. They firstly divided logs into smaller pieces by timestamps to analyse the time distribution of the activities (user habits) within a day [21].

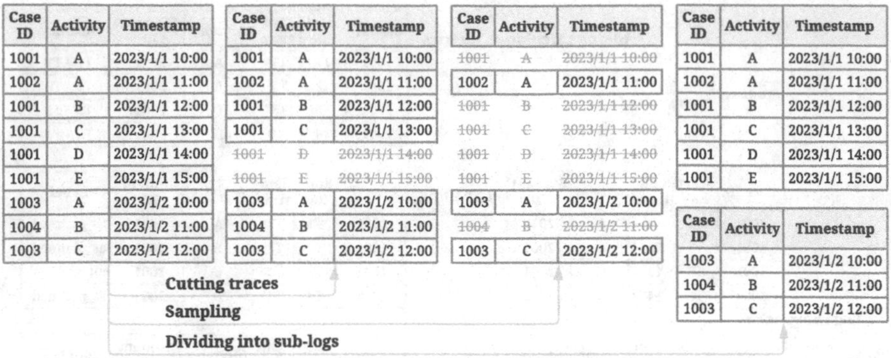

Case ID	Activity	Timestamp
1001	A	2023/1/1 10:00
1002	A	2023/1/1 11:00
1001	B	2023/1/1 12:00
1001	C	2023/1/1 13:00
1001	D	2023/1/1 14:00
1001	E	2023/1/1 15:00
1003	A	2023/1/2 10:00
1004	B	2023/1/2 11:00
1003	C	2023/1/2 12:00

Case ID	Activity	Timestamp
1001	A	2023/1/1 10:00
1002	A	2023/1/1 11:00
1001	B	2023/1/1 12:00
1001	C	2023/1/1 13:00
~~1001~~	~~D~~	~~2023/1/1 14:00~~
~~1001~~	~~E~~	~~2023/1/1 15:00~~
1003	A	2023/1/2 10:00
1004	B	2023/1/2 11:00
1003	C	2023/1/2 12:00

Case ID	Activity	Timestamp
~~1001~~	~~A~~	~~2023/1/1 10:00~~
1002	A	2023/1/1 11:00
~~1001~~	~~B~~	~~2023/1/1 12:00~~
~~1001~~	~~C~~	~~2023/1/1 13:00~~
~~1001~~	~~D~~	~~2023/1/1 14:00~~
~~1001~~	~~E~~	~~2023/1/1 15:00~~
1003	A	2023/1/2 10:00
~~1004~~	~~B~~	~~2023/1/2 11:00~~
1003	C	2023/1/2 12:00

Case ID	Activity	Timestamp
1001	A	2023/1/1 10:00
1002	A	2023/1/1 11:00
1001	B	2023/1/1 12:00
1001	C	2023/1/1 13:00
1001	D	2023/1/1 14:00
1001	E	2023/1/1 15:00

Case ID	Activity	Timestamp
1003	A	2023/1/2 10:00
1004	B	2023/1/2 11:00
1003	C	2023/1/2 12:00

Cutting traces

Sampling

Dividing into sub-logs

Fig. 4. A simple example of log reduction.

Resource could also be a common attribute for division. The authors of [30] divided the traces into subsets to model different profiles of users. Dividing original logs according to specific attributes is usually for more in-depth analysis [15].

In addition, in order to test the proposed algorithm or approach, the log was divided into training data and test data according to a certain proportion [7,17].

Sampling. The most notable characteristic of sampling is randomness. The reduction here is to reduce the trace; that is to say, the data processing needs to be in the unit of a trace. In the example shown in Fig. 4, there are four traces $[\langle A, B, C, D, E \rangle, \langle A \rangle, \langle A, C \rangle, \langle B \rangle]$. After randomly sampling 50% of the traces, the log $[\langle A \rangle, \langle A, C \rangle]$ in the lower right corner is obtained.

Cutting Traces. In the example in Fig. 4, compared to other traces, the trace $\langle A, B, C, D, E \rangle$ is obviously longer and contains more events. Cutting off the event at the end of the trace will get the processed log in the lower left corner. The purpose of this technique is to avoid bias from very long traces [13].

4.5 Log Integration

Among the 86 papers, 14 papers used log integration to combine multiple data tables. No objects of interest are repetitively mentioned, nor have we observed obvious low-level tasks. Therefore, the log integration task has not been further divided.

Figure 3 shows an example where a new event log is created by matching two data tables using the shared attribute "*student_id*". It is worth mentioning that some papers mention that additional data was added to the original event data without indicating the source, but we believe that the combination of these data is realized by log integration. According to [18], "*Besides the attributes shown in Table 4, we included the educational level of the nurses executing the activity, as well as their nursing experience/organisational role, the hospital shift and weekday on which the activities were performed, and the ward in which the shift took place*". It is reasonable to speculate that this additional information actually comes from a separate data table that stores information about all nurses.

4.6   Log Abstraction

In 37 out of the 86 papers, the authors used preprocessing techniques in log abstraction, which is the most widely performed task after log filtering and log transformation among the six preprocessing tasks. In [40], a review and taxonomy of event abstraction were presented. Therefore, we will not focus on this category here.

4.7   Discussion

The *log filtering* task emerges as the most commonly performed preprocessing task, with over 63% of the case studies mentioning that some filtering is performed. However, it's worth noting that the specifics of the log filtering tasks appear to heavily rely on domain knowledge. Moreover, more than 30 papers use somewhat ambiguous terminologies such as 'irrelevant' or 'noise'. The *log transformation* task ranks as the second most frequently employed, accounting for 44%. Currently, the majority of subtasks in the log transformation focus on fixing format-related and data-quality issues. This highlights the importance of data quality in process mining and suggests that efforts to enhance data quality should continue to be a focal point in log preprocessing.

In contrast, log enriching (18%), log integration (16%), and log reduction (12%) tasks are notably less commonly performed. One plausible explanation is the limited support for these tasks in both academic and commercial tools. Furthermore, the relatively uncommon use of log reduction can be attributed to the fact that many filtering techniques inherently reduce the log size.

5   Conclusion

In this paper, we conducted a systematic literature review, examining the use of log preprocessing tasks in process mining case studies and presented the results. We identified six high-level tasks that were synthesized from the related work discussion and 20 low-level tasks inducted from the reported case studies. The log filtering task emerges as the most frequently used preprocessing task, featured in over 63% of the case studies reviewed. The log transformation task follows closely behind, accounting for 44% of the cases. Conversely, log enriching, integration, and reduction tasks are less commonly performed, possibly due to limited tool support. Future research can delve into these preprocessing tasks, providing operational guidance. Standardization in reporting practices and greater support for less common preprocessing tasks are valuable for improving traceability and advancing the reliability of process mining results.

References

1. van der Aalst, W.M.P.: Process Mining. Springer, Heidelberg (2011)
2. Benevento, E., Aloini, D., van der Aalst, W.M.: How can interactive process discovery address data quality issues in real business settings? Evidence from a case study in healthcare. J. Biomed. Inform. **130**, 104083 (2022)

3. Birk, A., Wilhelm, Y., Dreher, S., Flack, C., Reimann, P., Gröger, C.: A real-world application of process mining for data-driven analysis of multi-level interlinked manufacturing
   processes. Procedia CIRP **104**, 417–422 (2021)
4. Cenka, B.A.N., Santoso, H.B., Junus, K.: Analysing student behaviour in a learning management system using a process mining approach. Knowl. Manage. E-Learn.: Int. J. **14**, 62–80
   (2022)
5. Chen, L., Klasky, H.B.: Six machine-learning methods for predicting hospital-stay duration
   for patients with sepsis: a comparative study. In: SoutheastCon 2022. IEEE (2022)
6. Chen, Q., Lu, Y., Tam, C.S., Poon, S.K.: A multi-view framework to detect redundant activity
   labels for more representative event logs in process mining. Future Internet **14**(6), 181 (2022)
7. Cho, M., Park, G., Song, M., Lee, J., Lee, B., Kum, E.: Discovery of resource-oriented transition systems for yield enhancement in semiconductor manufacturing. IEEE Trans. Semicond.
   Manuf. **34**(1), 17–24 (2020)
8. Dogan, O.: A process-centric performance management in a call center. Appl. Intell. **53**(3),
   3304–3317 (2022)
9. Du, L., Cheng, L., Liu, C.: Process mining for wind turbine maintenance process analysis: a
   case study. In: 2021 IEEE 5th Conference on Energy Internet and Energy System Integration
   (EI2). IEEE (2021)
10. van Eck, M.L., Lu, X., Leemans, S.J.J., van der Aalst, W.M.P.: PM^2: a process mining project
    methodology. In: Zdravkovic, J., Kirikova, M., Johannesson, P. (eds.) CAiSE 2015. LNCS,
    vol. 9097, pp. 297–313. Springer, Cham (2015). https://doi.org/10.1007/978-3-319-19069-
    3_19
11. Esposito, L., Leotta, F., Mecella, M., Veneruso, S.: Unsupervised segmentation of smart
    home logs for human habit discovery. In: 2022 18th International Conference on Intelligent
    Environments (IE). IEEE (2022)
12. Fahland, D.: Extracting and pre-processing event logs (2022)
13. Fahrenkrog-Petersen, S.A., et al.: Fire now, fire later: alarm-based systems for prescriptive
    process monitoring. Knowl. Inf. Syst. **64**(2), 559–587 (2021)
14. Gao, W., Wu, C., Huang, W., Lin, B., Su, X.: A data structure for studying 3D modeling
    design behavior based on event logs. Autom. Constr. **132**, 103967 (2021)
15. Goel, K., Leemans, S., Wynn, M.T., ter Hofstede, A., Barnes, J.: Improving PhD student
    journeys with process mining: insights from a higher education institution. In: Proceedings
    of the Industry Forum (BPM IF 2021) Co-located with 19th International Conference on
    Business Process Management (BPM 2021), pp. 39–49 (2021)
16. Han, J., Pei, J., Tong, H.: Data Mining: Concepts and Techniques. Morgan Kaufmann (2022)
17. Huda, S., Aripin, Naufal, M.F., Yudianingtias, V.M.: Identification of fraud attributes for
    detecting fraud based online sales transaction. Indian J. Comput. Sci. Eng. **12**(5), 1409–1424
    (2021)
18. van Hulzen, G.A., Li, C.Y., Martin, N., van Zelst, S.J., Depaire, B.: Mining context-aware
    resource profiles in the presence of multitasking. Artif. Intell. Med. **134**, 102434 (2022)
19. Kitchenham, B., Brereton, O.P., Budgen, D., Turner, M., Bailey, J., Linkman, S.: System-
    atic literature reviews in software engineering - a systematic literature review. Inf. Softw.
    Technol. **51**(1), 7–15 (2009)
20. Lamghari, Z.: Process mining: a new approach for simplifying the process model control
    flow visualization. Transdisc. J. Eng. Sci. **13** (2022)
21. de Leoni, M., Pellattiero, L.: The benefits of sensor-measurement aggregation in discovering
    IoT process models: a smart-house case study. In: Marrella, A., Weber, B. (eds.) BPM 2021.
    LNBIP, vol. 436, pp. 403–415. Springer, Cham (2022). https://doi.org/10.1007/978-3-030-
    94343-1_31
22. Lim, J., et al.: Assessment of the feasibility of developing a clinical pathway using a clinical
    order log. J. Biomed. Inform. **128**, 104038 (2022)

23. Liu, Y., Dani, V.S., Beerepoot, I., Lu, X.: Turning logs into lumber: preprocessing tasks in process mining. CoRR abs/2309.17100 (2023). https://doi.org/10.48550/ARXIV.2309.17100
24. Marin-Castro, H.M., Tello-Leal, E.: Event log preprocessing for process mining: a review. Appl. Sci. **11**(22), 10556 (2021)
25. Mivule, K.: Utilizing noise addition for data privacy, an overview (2013)
26. Pan, Y., Zhang, L.: Automated process discovery from event logs in BIM construction projects. Autom. Constr. **127**, 103713 (2021)
27. Pang, J., et al.: Process mining framework with time perspective for understanding acute care: a case study of AIS in hospitals. BMC Med. Inform. Decis. Making **21**(1), 1–10 (2021)
28. Petersen, K., Feldt, R., Mujtaba, S., Mattsson, M.: Systematic mapping studies in software engineering. In: EASE (2008)
29. Pradana, M.I.A., Kurniati, A.P., Wisudiawan, G.A.A.: Inductive miner implementation to improve healthcare efficiency on Indonesia national health insurance data. In: 2022 International Conference on Data Science and Its Applications (ICoDSA). IEEE (2022)
30. Ramos-Gutiérrez, B., Varela-Vaca, Á.J., Galindo, J.A., Gómez-López, M.T., Benavides, D.: Discovering configuration workflows from existing logs using process mining. Empir. Softw. Eng. **26**(1), 1–41 (2021)
31. Ridwanah, R.D., Andreswari, R., Fauzi, R.: Analysis and implementation of TELKOM university lecture business processes evaluation on heuristic miner algorithm: a process mining approach. In: ISMODE. IEEE (2022)
32. Rismanchian, F., Kassani, S.H., Shavarani, S.M., Lee, Y.H.: A data-driven approach to support the understanding and improvement of patients' journeys: a case study using electronic health records of an emergency department. Value Health **26**(1), 18–27 (2023)
33. Sohail, S.A., Bukhsh, F.A., van Keulen, M.: Multilevel privacy assurance evaluation of healthcare metadata. Appl. Sci. **11**(22), 10686 (2021)
34. Stein Dani, V., et al.: Towards understanding the role of the human in event log extraction. In: Marrella, A., Weber, B. (eds.) BPM 2021. LNBIP, vol. 436, pp. 86–98. Springer, Cham (2022). https://doi.org/10.1007/978-3-030-94343-1_7
35. Stephan, S., Lahann, J., Fettke, P.: A case study on the application of process mining in combination with journal entry tests for financial auditing (2021)
36. Suriadi, S., Andrews, R., ter Hofstede, A.H.M., Wynn, M.T.: Event log imperfection patterns for process mining: towards a systematic approach to cleaning event logs. Inf. Syst. **64**, 132–150 (2017)
37. Tang, J., Liu, Y., Lin, K., Li, L.: Process bottlenecks identification and its root cause analysis using fusion-based clustering and knowledge graph. Adv. Eng. Inform. **55**, 101862 (2023)
38. Tariq, Z., Charles, D., McClean, S., McChesney, I., Taylor, P.: Anomaly detection for service-oriented business processes using conformance analysis. Algorithms **15**(8), 257 (2022)
39. Tavakoli-Zaniani, M., Gholamian, M.R., Hashemi-Golpayegani, S.A.: Improving heuristics miners for healthcare applications by discovering optimal dependency graphs. J. Supercomput. **78**(18), 19628–19661 (2022)
40. van Zelst, S.J., Mannhardt, F., de Leoni, M., Koschmider, A.: Event abstraction in process mining: literature review and taxonomy. Granular Comput. **6**(3), 719–736 (2021)

Improving Precision in Process Trees Using Subprocess Tree Logs

Christian Rennert[✉][iD] and Wil M. P. van der Aalst[iD]

Chair of Process and Data Science (PADS), RWTH Aachen University,
Aachen, Germany
{rennert,wvdaalst}@pads.rwth-aachen.de

Abstract. Process mining is a family of techniques that provide tools
for gaining insights from processes in, for example, business, industrial,
healthcare and administrative settings. Process discovery, as a field of
process mining, aims to give a process model that describes a process
given by an event log. A process model describes an underlying process
well if it contains all behavior relevant (fitness) and if it does not model
behavior that is not contained in the event log (precision). The Inductive
Miner (IM) family provides algorithms to find process models on complex
event logs efficiently and in an easy-to-understand process model representation using process trees. Due to its characteristics, the IM family
is one of the state-of-the-art discovery algorithms and is implemented in
software of market-leading process mining vendors. Nevertheless, process
trees and in particular those discovered by the IM can have imprecise
parts. In this work, we combine existing work and present an approach
that replaces such parts with more precise parts while preserving fitness.
In addition, we demonstrate the frameworks applicability and utilization
by improving process trees discovered by the IM, using the IM itself. Further, guarantees on the preservation of fitness and precision are given.
Our experiments clearly show that our techniques can be applied to real-
life event logs and that they lead to an improvement in precision.

Keywords: Process Tree · Event Data · Process Discovery · Process
Enhancement

1 Introduction and Related Work

Information systems are widely used to collect organizational data related to processes performed. This data are so-called *event data*, where an event corresponds
to an activity that is executed for a running instance of a process. By considering
a temporal relation between events, the events of each running instance can be
translated to a case and multiple cases can be combined into an *event log*. In
general, event data may contain further attributes that are not considered in this
work. Using event logs, one can use *process mining* to derive insights, value, and
actions. Process mining can be used, to evaluate and improve processes, e.g., in
terms of sustainability, fairness, productivity or resource consumption

We thank the Alexander von Humboldt (AvH) Stiftung for supporting our research.

J. De Smedt and P. Soffer (Eds.): ICPM 2023 Workshops, LNBIP 503, pp. 110–122, 2024.
https://doi.org/10.1007/978-3-031-56107-8_9

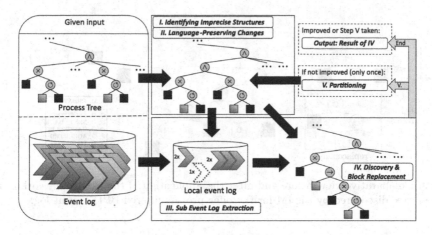

Fig. 1. Overview of process tree projection & replacement (PtR) framework.

Process discovery is a subfield of process mining that aims to discover a *process model* given an event log that can be taken as a starting point for further analysis. In general, a process model describes the possible, not necessarily sequential, flow of activities in a process. Process models are evaluated against four driving quality criteria. A process model is considered a good representation if it represents all running instances of the process seen in the event log (*fitness*), if it does not allow for running sequences unrelated to what is present in the event log (*precision*), if it is easy to understand for a reader (*simplicity*), and if it allows for running sequences not supported to what is seen in the event log but what is likely to happen as well, i.e., if it is not overfitting (*generalization*). For real-life event logs, in most cases it is not possible to satisfy all four quality criteria with one model.

In this work, we focus on *process trees* as a class of process models. Due to their block-structure, process trees are easy to understand. The Inductive Miner (IM) [5], as the state-of-the-art algorithm for discovering process trees, does not guarantee to return the most precise process tree given an event log. A process tree that is not the most precise can be improved using the property that blocks can be replaced with more precise blocks without having to consider the entire tree, improving overall precision while maintaining fitness. Existing theory is taken as a starting point for the approach presented and evaluated in this work. The introduced process tree projection & replacement (PtR) framework follows the procedure shown in Fig. 1: Given as input an (intermediate) process tree and an event log, first, imprecise structures are identified; second, if necessary, language-preserving changes are made to separate the imprecise structure from other structures; third, the sub event log for the separated imprecise structure is extracted; and fourth, it is used as input to discover a process tree that replaces the previous imprecise structure. As an additional fifth step, a partitioning based on the activities contained in the separated process tree can be

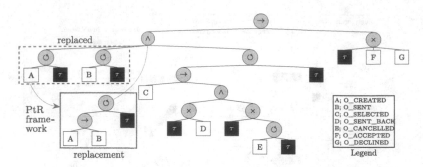

Fig. 2. Comparative view before and after the application of the PtR framework to a process tree discovered by the IM for the offer process filtered ฿PI12 event log.

applied at most once, if no improvement has occurred after the fourth step. This would result in the second through fourth steps having to be performed again.

An example for the application of the PtR framework is given in Fig. 2 visualizing a process tree discovered by the IM on the BPI12 challenge log[1] that is filtered for the events related to the offer process. Here, the replaced part of the process tree and the replacement are indicated. The application of our framework improves the precision as it restricts the process tree such that each creation of an offer is eventually followed by the offer being sent. Further, fitness is preserved by the framework.

There are different process discovery algorithms existent. Region-based discovery algorithms such as the ILP-Miner [10] or the Prime Miner [3] guarantee a strong relation between the input event log and the returned process model and therefore return process models with high precision in their class of process models but are limited by their representational bias (e.g. no use of silent transitions). Furthermore, region-based approaches tend to not handle noise and tend to have a high runtime. Here, the Inductive Miner (IM) can be put into relation as it achieves a good generalization and is computationally fast. Similar to the Split Miner [2], the IM discovers process models solely using the directly-follows relation between events in the event log and therefore reducing its complexity, which may result in less precise models than models returned by region-based techniques. Additionally, the Inductive Miner does not guarantee to discover the most precise process tree for a given event log due to its greedy approach.

The algorithms and approaches proposed in this work are related to the field of incremental process discovery [4] and to repair techniques in the field of process enhancement [6]. In particular, the work by Schuster et al. [9] is the most related to the ideas presented in this work. In their work, the authors aim to incrementally discover and adapt process trees by including traces successively into the behavior modeled. In this work, we use their proposed techniques for tree modification and sublog identification. However, we extend their work by giving a framework that tackles precision improvement in general and as we

---

[1] All event logs used in this work are taken from https://data.4tu.nl/.

give a formal reasoning on the guarantees of the techniques. Conceptually, the framework presented is related to a similar work on imprecise structure replacement in Petri nets [8]. As process trees can be translated into block-structured Petri nets, the results of this work can be taken as starting point for refining the imprecise structure replacement on Petri nets to also consider block structures.

The remainder of this work is structured as follows. Section 2 presents mathematical notations and concepts related to process mining used in this work. Section 3 introduces the framework presented in this work in detail. Section 4 describes and proves the guarantees of the steps taken in our framework. In Sect. 5, the framework is evaluated using process trees discovered on real-life events logs with the Inductive Miner without noise filtering. Lastly, in Sect. 6, this paper is concluded and outlook for future work is given.

2 Preliminaries

Basic Notations. A multiset, e.g., $[a, b, b, a, b, c] = [a^2, b^3, c]$ can contain an element multiple times. We refer to the set of multisets over a set X as $\mathbb{M}(X)$. While sets and multisets are unordered, sequences are ordered and can contain an element multiple times, e.g., $\langle a, b, a, a, c \rangle \in \{a, b, c\}^*$. We denote the projection of a sequence $\sigma \in X^*$ on a subset of activities $Y \subseteq X$ by $\sigma\restriction_Y$. For example, $\langle a, b, c, b, a \rangle\restriction_{\{a,c\}} = \langle a, c, a \rangle$. For a tuple $t = (x_1, x_2, \ldots, x_n)$ with $n \in \mathbb{N}$ and $i \in [1, n]$ we denote by π_i the selector function selecting the i-th element in a tuple, i.e., $\pi_i(t) = x_i$. For example, $\pi_3((a, b, c, d)) = c$. We uplift all functions applicable for single elements of a sequence to be applicable to the full sequence, i.e., for a function $f \colon X \to Y$ and a sequence $\sigma = \langle x_1, x_2, \ldots, x_n \rangle$ we write $f(\sigma) = \langle f(x_1), f(x_2), \ldots, f(x_n) \rangle$. Similarly, given a function applicable to two elements of two sets $X \subseteq \mathcal{X}, Y \subseteq \mathcal{Y}$, we uplift the function to all combinations of elements, i.e., for a function $\circ \colon \mathcal{X} \to \mathcal{Y}$ we write $X \circ Y = \bigcup_{x \in X, y \in Y} \{x \circ y\}$. For any two traces $\sigma \in X^*, \sigma' \in Y^*$ and for any two elements $x \in X, y \in Y$, we denote the shuffle operation $\diamond \colon (X^*, Y^*) \to (X \cup Y)^*$ recursively with: $\sigma \diamond \langle \rangle = \sigma$, $\langle \rangle \diamond \sigma' = \sigma'$ and $(\sigma \cdot x) \diamond (\sigma' \cdot y) = (((\sigma \cdot x) \diamond \sigma') \cdot \langle y \rangle) \cup ((\sigma \diamond (\sigma' \cdot y)) \cdot \langle x \rangle)$, i.e., $\langle a, b \rangle \diamond \langle c, d \rangle = \{\langle a, b, c, d \rangle, \langle a, c, b, d \rangle, \langle a, c, d, b \rangle, \langle c, a, b, d \rangle, \langle c, a, d, b \rangle, \langle c, d, a, b \rangle\}$.

Event Logs and Process Trees. The universe of activities (e.g. actions or operations) is denoted by $\mathcal{A}$. A trace $\sigma \in \mathcal{A}^*$ is a finite sequence of activities. The universe of traces is denoted by $\mathcal{T}$. A log $\log \in \mathbb{M}(\mathcal{A}^*)$ is a multiset of traces. We represent the behavior described by an event log using process trees. A process tree is an hierarchical process model. Every leaf of a process tree is labeled with an activity, while every other node is labeled with an operator $\oplus = \{\to, \wedge, \times, \circlearrowright\}$ such as the sequential operator $\to$, the parallel operator $\wedge$, the exclusive choice operator $\times$ and the loop operator $\circlearrowright$. Every operator node can have an arbitrary, non-empty set of children except for the loop operator $\circlearrowright$ that has two children exactly. For the $\to$ and $\circlearrowright$ operator, the order of children is relevant and taken into account by totally ordering the edges in the process tree. A so-called silent activity is labeled with the designated silent activity label $\tau \notin \mathcal{A}$. Further we describe process trees as follows.

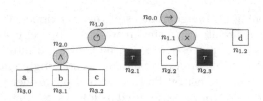

Fig. 3. Process Tree $T_p = (V_p, E_p, A_p, l_p, r_p) = (\{n_{0.0}, n_{1.0}, \ldots, n_{3.2}\}, \{(n_{0.0}, n_{1.0}),$ $(n_{0.0}, n_{1.1}), \ldots, (n_{2.0}, n_{3.2})\}, \{a, b, c, d\}, \{(n_{0.0}, \rightarrow), (n_{1.0}, \times), \ldots, (n_{3.2}, c)\}, n_{0.0}).$

Definition 1 (Process Tree). *A process tree is a directed acyclic graph defined as a quintuplet $T = (V, E, A, l, r)$, where V is a finite set of nodes, $E \subseteq V \times V$ is a totally ordered set of edges between nodes, $A \subseteq \mathscr{A}$ with $\tau \notin A$ is a set of non-silent activity labels, $l : V \rightarrow A \cup \{\tau\} \cup \oplus$ for $\oplus = \{\rightarrow, \wedge, \times, \circlearrowleft\}$, and r is the root node of the process tree. Further, the following holds:*

- *$T = (\{n\}, \emptyset, \{a\}, \{(n, a)\}, n)$ with $a \in \mathscr{A} \cup \{\tau\}$ is a process tree*
- *given $k \geq 1$ distinct process trees $T_1, T_2, \ldots, T_k$ with $T_l = (V_l, E_l, A_l, l_l, r_l)$ for $l \in [1, k]$, i.e., $\forall_{i,j \in [1,k]} : V_i \cup V_j \neq \emptyset \Rightarrow i = j$ then $T = (V, E, A, l, r)$ is a process tree for which:*
  - $V = \bigcup_{i \in [1,k]} V_i \cup \{r\}$
  - $E = \bigcup_{i \in [1,k]} (E_i \cup \{(r, r_i)\})$
  - $A = \bigcup_{i \in [1,k]} A_i$
  - $l = \bigcup_{i \in [1,k]} l_i \cup \{(r, op) \mid op \in \oplus\}$
  where $(op = \circlearrowleft \Rightarrow k = 2)$ and $\forall_{i \in [1,k]} : r \notin V_i$ holds.

A process tree given can be represented using a graphical notation, as shown in Fig. 3. Further, a process tree can also be represented textually, e.g., $T_p \hat{=} \rightarrow(\circlearrowleft(\wedge(a, b, c), \tau), \times(c, \tau), d)$ for the process tree in Fig. 3. For a process tree $T = (V, E, A, l, r)$ and a node $n \in V$ given, we denote the subtree rooted in n as $T_n = (V_n, E_n, A_n, l_n, r_n)$, i.e., $r_n = n$ holds. Further, we define a child function $ch^T(n)$ returning the children of n as a sequence according to the order of edges E by $ch^T(n) = \langle n_1, n_2, \ldots, n_k \rangle$, s.t., $\forall_{(n,n_o) \in E} : n_o \in \{n_1, n_2, \ldots, n_k\}$. For example, given the node $n_{2.0} \in V_p$ of the process tree T_p shown in Fig. 3, we conclude the subtree $T_{n_{2.0}}$ rooted in $n_{2.0}$ to be $T_{n_{2.0}} \hat{=} \wedge(a, b, c)$ and its children $ch^{T_p}(n_{2.0})$ to be $ch^{T_p}(n_{2.0}) = \{n_{3.0}, n_{3.1}, n_{3.2}\}$.

Each process tree has a non-empty set of valid sequences of node visits, so-called running sequences. A running sequence is defined recursively as follows.

Definition 2 (Process Tree Running Sequences). *Let $T = (V, E, A, l, r)$ be a process tree. We define its running sequences $\Omega_T \subseteq V \times (A \cup \{\tau, op, cl\})^*$ with $op(en), cl(ose) \notin A$ recursively as:*

- *$\Omega_T = \{\langle (r, l(r)) \rangle\}$ iff r is a leaf node, i.e., $E = \emptyset$ holds,*
- *$\Omega_T = \{\langle (r, op) \cdot \Omega_{T_{n_1}} \cdot \Omega_{T_{n_2}} \cdot \ldots \cdot \Omega_{T_{n_k}} \cdot (r, cl) \rangle\}$ for $k \geq 1$, $ch^T(r) = \langle n_1, n_2, \ldots, n_k \rangle$ iff r is labeled as sequential node, i.e., $l(r) = \rightarrow$ holds,*

- $\Omega_T = \{\langle (r, op) \cdot \bigcup_{i \in [1,k]} \Omega_{T_{n_i}} \cdot (r, cl) \rangle\}$ *for* $k \geq 1$, $ch^T(r) = \langle n_1, n_2, \ldots, n_k \rangle$
  iff r *is labeled as exclusive choice node, i.e.,* $l(r) = \times$ *holds,*
- $\Omega_T = \{\langle (r, op) \cdot (\Omega_{T_{n_1}} \diamond \Omega_{T_{n_2}} \diamond \ldots \diamond \Omega_{T_{n_k}}) \cdot (r, cl) \rangle\}$ *for* $k \geq 1$, $ch^T(r) =$
  $\langle n_1, n_2, \ldots, n_k \rangle$ *iff* r *is labeled as parallel node, i.e.,* $l(r) = \wedge$ *holds,*
- $\Omega_T = \{\langle (r, op) \cdot \sigma_1 \cdot \sigma'_1 \cdot \sigma_2 \cdot \sigma'_2 \cdot \ldots \cdot \sigma'_{m-1} \cdot \sigma_m \cdot (r, cl) \rangle \mid m \in \mathbb{N} \wedge \sigma_m \in \Omega_{T_{n_1}} \wedge$
  $\forall_{i \in [1,m-1]} \colon \sigma_i \in \Omega_{T_{n_1}} \wedge \sigma'_i \in \Omega_{T_{n_2}}\}$ *for* $ch^T(r) = \langle n_1, n_2 \rangle$ *iff* r *is labeled as*
  loop node, i.e., $l(r) = \circlearrowright$ *holds,*

Given all possible running sequences existing in a tree, we can conclude the language of the process tree $\mathcal{L}(T)$ by considering the occurrences of the leaves with non-silent activities in the running sequence.

Definition 3 (Process Tree Language). *Let* $T = (V, E, A, l, r)$ *be a process tree. We define the corresponding language by* $\mathcal{L}(T) = \{(\pi_2(\omega))\restriction_A \mid \omega \in \Omega_T\}$.

For example, the running sequences of the subprocess tree $T_{n_{1.1}} \hat{=} \times(c, \tau)$ of T_p shown in Fig. 3 are $\Omega_{T_{n_{1.1}}} = \{\langle (n_{1.1}, op), (n_{2.2}, c), (n_{1.1}, cl) \rangle, \langle (n_{1.1}, op),$ $(n_{2.2}, \tau), (n_{1.1}, cl) \rangle\}$ and the process tree language is $\mathcal{L}(T_{n_{1.1}}) = \{\langle c \rangle, \langle \rangle\}$. We say that a running sequence ω is corresponding to a trace σ if the occurrences of the leaves labeled with an activity from set of non-silent activities A_v match with the trace σ, i.e., if $(\pi_2(\omega))\restriction_{A_v} = \sigma$ holds. For a running sequence given, we can identify all subtraces modeled by a subprocess tree. The union of all such subtraces corresponds to a sub event log of the subprocess tree.

Definition 4 (Sub Event Log of a Subprocess Tree (cf. [9])). *Let* $T = (V, E, A, l, r)$ *be a process tree and* $T_s = (V_s, E_s, A_s, l_s, r_s)$ *be a subtree of* T, *i.e.,* $r_s \in V$ *holds. Further, let* ω *be a running sequence on* T. *Then we define the sub event log* $\omega\restriction_{T_s} \in \mathbb{M}(\mathcal{L}(T_s))$ *of the subprocess tree* T_s *considering the running sequence* $\omega = \langle a_1, a_2, \ldots, a_n \rangle$ *with* $n \in \mathbb{N}$ *as:*

$$\omega\restriction_{T_s} = [\pi_2(\langle a_i, a_{i+1}, \ldots, a_j \rangle \restriction_{(V_s \times A_s)}) \mid i \in [1, n-1] \wedge j \in [i+1, n] \wedge \&$$
$$\forall_{k \in [i,j]} \colon (a_k = (T_s, op) \Leftrightarrow k = i \wedge a_k = (T_s, cl) \Leftrightarrow k = j)].$$

In this work, we only consider nodes for replacement that have a common father node that is labeled with the parallel operator, i.e., we only consider concurrent (sub-)process trees to be replaced. Further, as we want to keep precise (sub-)process trees which are concurrent as well, we may not always want to find the sub event log of all concurrent (sub-)process trees, but rather the sub event log of a partition of them. Therefore, we present a technique to separate a partition of (sub-)process trees from their siblings. This is achieved using expansion rules that lower the partition while leaving their siblings unchanged.

This preserves the language of the process tree, as we show in Sect. 4.

Definition 5 (Lowering a Set of Children of a $\wedge$-Rooted Tree (cf. [9])). *Given* $T = (V, E, A, l, r)$ *a process tree and* T_n *a subprocess tree with root* $n \in V$, $ch^T(n) = \langle cn_1, cn_2, \ldots, cn_j \rangle$ *for* $j \in \mathbb{N}$ *and* $l(n) = \wedge$. *Then we can add a* node n_{low}, where $V_c = ch^{T'}(n_{low}) \subseteq ch^T(n)$ holds, while preserving the language of the tree T resulting in a process tree $T' = (V', E', A, l', r)$ where:

$$V' = V \cup \{n_{low}\}$$
$$E' = (E \setminus \{(n, cn) \mid cn \in V_c\}) \cup \{(n, n_{low})\} \cup \{(n_{low}, cn) \mid cn \in V_c\}$$
$$l' = l \cup \{(n_{low}, \wedge)\}.$$

Given the process tree $T_p \cong \rightarrow(\circlearrowleft(\wedge(a, b, c), \tau), \times(c, \tau), d)$ shown in Fig. 3, we obtain $T_p \cong \rightarrow(\circlearrowleft(\wedge(b, \wedge(a, c)), \tau), \times(c, \tau), d)$ by lowering the set $\{n_{3.0}, n_{3.2}\}$. Last, we give a comparative view on fitness and precision between process trees.

Definition 6 (Fitness and Precision Comparison). *Let* log *be an event log and* T, T' *be two process trees.* T' *is at least as fitting as* T *considering the event log* log, *if every trace* $\sigma \in$ log *that is in the language of* T *is also in the language of* T', *i.e.,* $\sigma \in \mathcal{L}(T) \Rightarrow \sigma \in \mathcal{L}(T')$. T' *is at least as precise as* T, *if every trace* $\sigma \in \mathcal{T}$ *that is in the language of* T' *is also in the language of* T, *i.e.,* $\sigma \in \mathcal{L}(T') \Rightarrow \sigma \in \mathcal{L}(T)$. T' *is more precise than* T, *if there is an additional trace* $\sigma' \in \mathcal{T} \setminus$ log *that is in the language of* T *but not of* T', *i.e.,* $\sigma' \in \mathcal{L}(T) \wedge \sigma' \notin \mathcal{L}(T')$.

3   Process Tree Projection and Replacement Framework

The Inductive Miner analyzes a log and splits the log greedily into two sublogs by projecting the current log onto two distinct sets of activities following defined rules and fall-throughs. For each log analysis, a new node is inserted into the result process tree. Here, the algorithm can be prone to find imprecise subtrees as it does not use look-ahead. An example of such an imprecise subtree is a tree in which at least two activities can be replayed in parallel and arbitrarily often, i.e., in the process tree $\wedge(\times(\tau, \circlearrowleft(a, \tau)), b, \times(\circlearrowleft(c, \tau)))$ this is the case for the subprocess trees containing activities a and c. As this kind of subprocess trees restricts the behavior only marginally, we consider such structures as most promising candidates for replacement and precision improvement.

Our presented approach is not limited to process trees discovered by the Inductive Miner as other discovery algorithms may also discover process trees with imprecise structures. However, given that there are no other known discovery algorithm for process trees, and for reasons of comprehensibility, we restrict ourselves to the Inductive Miner without noise filtering. In the following, we give a short overview of the *Process Tree Projection & Replacement Framework (PtR framework)* presented and used in this work.

PtR Framework. We follow the structure shown in Fig. 1 consisting of the following steps recursively applied to an event log log and a process tree T:
Step I - Identification: Identifying imprecise structures as candidates, e.g., multiple flower structures, choice constructs modeling optionality or loop constructs which occur in parallel can be considered.

Step II - Modification: Applying expansion rules to separate the imprecise structures as subprocess trees according to Definition 5, e.g., we lower a set of parallel nodes that are considered as imprecise candidates by adding another parallel node that is a parent of the candidate nodes, while their former parent is the parent of the new node.

Step III - Sub Event Log Extraction: Extracting and uniting all sub event log of the separated subprocess tree, which are obtained according to Definition 4. In case that a running sequence, relevant for the sub event log extraction, does not exist, we obtain a running sequence by using alignments [1].

Step IV - Discovery and Block Replacement: Discovering a replacing process tree where each trace in the sub event log is in its language and potentially replacing the separated structure if the replacement is more precise.

Step V - Partitioning (Fall-Through): If precision is not improved, a fall-through is applied that bi-partitions the children of the separated structure and considers the partitions as new candidates for improval. For each such candidate, the Steps II–IV of the framework are applied.

As an example, we consider T_1 shown in Fig. 4 which is discovered by the Inductive Miner on the log $\log[1] = [\langle a, d, a, d\rangle, \langle b\rangle, \langle b, c, c, b, c, c\rangle,$

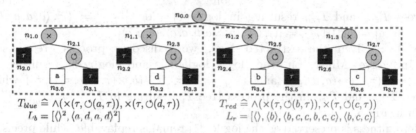

Fig. 4. Process tree T_1 discovered by the IM on the event log $\log[1]$. T_{blue} and T_{red} show two partitions and their corresponding lowered subtrees resulting from Step I and II.

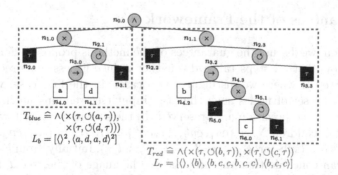

Fig. 5. Process tree T_1' resulting from applying the PtR framework to event log $\log[1]$ and the process tree T_1. The logs $\log[b]$ and $\log[r]$ correspond to the logs identified by Step III.

$\langle b, a, d, c, a, c, d \rangle]$. Here, the potential discovery of imprecise structures becomes more apparent as the language $\mathcal{L}(T_1) = \{a, b, c, d\}^*$ of the example process tree T_1 is imprecise considering the input event log log[1]. Here, the PtR framework is applicable to the process tree T_1 and the log log[1]. This results in the process tree T_1' shown in Fig. 5. In detail, the following (intermediate) results are produced:

Step I: The nodes $n_{1.0}, n_{1.1}, n_{1.2}$ and $n_{1.3}$ are in parallel and flower structures and are therefore identified as a candidate for replacement together.

Step II–V: Applying Steps II–III results in the input event log log[1] for which we rediscover the identical process tree in Step IV. Conclusively, we are in Step V as fall-through and thus bi-partition the set of nodes. For the sake of comprehensibility, we follow the optimal partitioning to be applied directly in this example. Thus, the partitioning results in a blue set of nodes $n_b = \{n_{1.0}, n_{1.1}\}$ and a red set of nodes $n_r = \{n_{1.2}, n_{1.3}\}$, both being highlighted in Fig. 4 and considered as new candidates for replacement.

Step II: We modify T_1 by applying the expansion rules to partition n_b and partition n_r, resulting in a modified process tree $T_i \hateq \wedge (T_{blue}, T_{red})$ with $T_{blue} \hateq \wedge(\times(\tau, \circlearrowleft(a, \tau)), \times(\tau, \circlearrowleft(d, \tau))$ and $T_{red} \hateq \wedge(\times(\tau, \circlearrowleft(b, \tau)), \times(\tau, \circlearrowleft(c, \tau)))$.

Step III: Given T_i, we can extract and unite all sub event logs by projecting on both subtrees T_{blue} and T_{red} resulting in $\log[blue] = \log[1]\lceil_{T_{blue}} = [\langle\rangle^2, \langle a, d, a, d\rangle^2]$ and $\log[red] = \log[1]\lceil_{T_{red}} = [\langle\rangle, \langle b\rangle, \langle b, c, c, b, c, c\rangle, \langle b, c, c\rangle]$.

Step IV: Given the extracted logs, we rediscover process trees using the Inductive Miner on the logs $\log[blue]$ and $\log[red]$ resulting in $T_{blue}' \hateq \times(\tau, \circlearrowleft(\to(a, d), \tau))$ and $T_{red}' \hateq \times(\tau, \circlearrowleft(\to(b, \times(\tau, \circlearrowleft(c, \tau))), \tau))$ which replace T_{blue} and T_{red} in the process tree T_i resulting in $T_1' \hateq \wedge (T_{blue}', T_{red}')$ shown in Fig. 5.

Here, fitness is preserved as the log log[1] remains replayable, while precision for T_1' is improved since, for example, the trace $\langle c \rangle$ has a running sequence for the process tree T_1 but not for T_1', i.e., $\langle c \rangle \in \mathcal{L}(T_1) \wedge \langle c \rangle \notin \mathcal{L}(T_1')$ holds.

4   Guarantees of the Framework

In this section, we discuss the guarantees of the methods proposed. For this purpose, we show that all steps taken do neither reduce fitness nor precision. We start with Step II where we distinguish two cases. In the first case, we do not have to lower a set of nodes such that the input tree remains unchanged and thus the fitness and precision are preserved. In the second case, we lower a (partitioned) set of children $N_c = \{cn_1', cn_2', \ldots, cn_j'\} \subseteq ch^T(r) = \{cn_1, cn_2, \ldots, cn_n\}$ with $j, n \in \mathbb{N}$ of a (sub-)process tree $T = (V, E, A, l, r)$. Initially, from Definition 2 and 3, we can conclude that the process tree language of the tree T is $\mathcal{L}(T) = \{\mathcal{L}(cn_1) \diamond \mathcal{L}(cn_2) \diamond \ldots \diamond \mathcal{L}(cn_n)\}$. Lowering the set of children N_c results in a node n_{low} being added such that we obtain a process tree $T' = (V', E', A, l', r)$ according to Definition 5. By construction, $\mathcal{L}(T_{n_{low}}) = \{cn_1' \diamond cn_2' \diamond \ldots \diamond cn_j'\}$ and $\mathcal{L}(T') = \{\mathcal{L}(n_{low}) \diamond \mathcal{L}(cn_1) \diamond \mathcal{L}(cn_2) \diamond \ldots \diamond \mathcal{L}(cn_n) \mid \forall_{i \in [1,n]} : cn_i \notin N_c\}$ hold, resulting in $\mathcal{L}(T) = \mathcal{L}(T')$ due to the shuffle operator being associative. Conclusively, lowering a set of children does not change the language of a process tree and in particular does not reduce fitness nor precision.

Next, we want to show that applying Steps III and IV does neither reduce fitness nor precision. Towards fitness, we show that each part of all traces replayed in the replaced process tree remains replayable in the replacing process tree. We follow the following line of argument. For each trace a running sequence (possibly derived from an alignment) can be computed. Given a set of running sequences, we can directly determine their language on the replaced process tree. This corresponds to the traces that result from the occurrences of the leaves of the replaced process tree between the replaced process tree's opening and closing in the running sequence. Taking into account that such a language for only running sequence given, is identical to the sub event log computation, we conclude the language of the replaced process tree to be equal to the extraction and union of all sub event logs as applied in Step III. The resulting log is the basis for the discovery of the replacing process tree and therefore the lower bound of its modeled language (as required in Step IV). Thus, the parts of the running sequences of the event log replayed on the replaced subprocess tree are replayable on the replacing subprocess tree. In conclusion, all traces have an alignment at least as good as before - in particular, fitting traces remain replayable.

Towards precision, we can trivially conclude an overall precision preservation as we do a precision comparison between the replacing and the replaced process tree in Step IV assuring that we do not reduce precision. Such a comparison would be redundant if the discovery algorithm used guarantees that it discovers a process tree whose language is contained in the log obtained by Step III. This is a result of the log obtained by Step III being a subset of the language of the replaced process tree. This property holds as the log obtained by Step III is computed using the running sequences obtained from the input log. Conclusively, the replacing process tree would not allow for more behavior than the replaced process tree resulting in a preservation of precision.

Taking all those arguments into consideration and that further Step I and Step V do not alter the input process tree, there is no step in our framework that reduces either fitness or precision. Thus, both are preserved using our framework.

5   Evaluation

In this section, we evaluate the PtR framework proposed in Sect. 3 with real-life event logs. We implemented a plugin called "Process Tree Projection & Replacement Framework (PtR framework)" in ProM[2] that applies the framework automatically to an input event log and its corresponding process tree.

For our evaluation, we want to quantitatively evaluate precision by using $ETC_{All} - precision$ [7]. We consider pairs of real-life event logs, namely the BPI challenge logs from 2011–2020, the Sepsis event log and the RTFM event

---

[2] Available at https://promtools.org/.

Table 1. Results of our framework for real-life logs, for which our algorithm and ETC$_{All}$-precision are computable in allotted time and space.

Log	ETC$_{All}$-precision			
	Initial	PtR	Difference	Percentage
BPI12 - O events	0.457	0.612	0.155	33.9%
BPI12 - W events	0.431	0.496	0.065	15.1%
BPI13 - closed problems	0.510	0.612	0.102	20.0%
BPI20 - Domestic Declarations	0.216	0.288	0.072	33.3%
BPI20 - Request for Payment	0.236	0.273	0.037	15.7%
Sepsis Cases	0.227	0.234	0.007	3.1%

logs, and their corresponding discovered process trees discovered by the Inductive Miner without noise filtering. Noise filtering is not used, since, this way, imprecise structures are obtained on less complex event logs. Further, $ETC_{All} - precision$ computation becomes more probable to be feasible. As imprecise structures we restrict ourselves to flower and loop constructs. In Table 1, we report the precision before and after the application of the PtR framework for only those pairs, where both the running sequence computation of the input event log (Step III in the framework) and the ETC-precision computation of the evaluation finish in allotted time and space. Further, we report the difference of the precision values and its relative improvement given by the percentage of the increasement.

The other pairs of event logs and their process trees contain three pairs (BPI12 - application, BPI13 - open, RTFM) for which no imprecise structure is identifiable, one pair (BPI13 - open) for which no improvement was achieved, one pair (BPI13 - incidents) for which we improve the input process tree but ETC$_{All}$ precision computation is not feasible within allotted time, and for the process tree of all the other pairs imprecise structures are identified, but running sequence computation is not feasible.

Our results show, that for most real-life event logs an imprecise structure is discovered by the Inductive Miner. For all event logs listed in Table 1 but one, we improve precision significantly by at least 15% compared to the initial precision value. This qualitative improvement clearly shows the applicability and relevance of our approach and motivates further research regarding improvement of running times, which is not the focus of this work.

Given our experiments we suggest to improve the IM by optimizing the way it applies certain fall-throughs. Consider the discovered and replaced structure in Fig. 2. Here, the IM first evaluates two sublogs, one containing only the activity "O_CREATED" and the other containing only the activity "O_SENT". For both sublogs none of the four standard cuts is found and thus fall-throughs (mainly the activity-concurrent fall-through) are applied greedily. Note that the order of fall-through cuts matters and can result in a non-optimal set of subtrees. We propose to re-evaluate sets of such imprecise subtrees based on which we construct one sublog that allows to discover one more precise subprocess tree.

6   Conclusion and Future Work

In this work, we introduce a framework to improve precision by replacing imprecise structures in process trees. It gives guarantees on the preservation of fitness and precision, and therefore never decreases the quality of its input process tree. Further, if we use the IM within our framework, we inherit IM's desirable features such as soundness and fast computation of process models. Our work is supported by experiments on process trees discovered by the well-known Inductive Miner without noise filtering for which we use the IM itself to replace imprecise structures. Our experiments show that imprecise structures occur for most real-life logs available. For six real-life event logs and their corresponding process trees, we improve precision. This indicates the relevance of our work.

However, since running sequences must be computed for all traces before applying the IM, there are inputs for which our implementation did not run within the time and space allotted. Therefore, either efficiency can be improved or could result in being a starting point for adaptations within the IM itself. For the latter, the relevant sub event logs would already exist within the IM and could be used as input for further refinement.

Otherwise, the framework presented in this paper can be evaluated for the IM with noise filtering. Here, the results can be taken as starting point for research on the ranking of desired alignments when computing the sub event log, as the quality of the discovered replacing process tree is strongly related to the sub event log given. Further, heuristics for the identification of promising imprecise structures and for checking how and whether to partition potential imprecise structures are missing.

References

1. Adriansyah, A.: Aligning observed and modeled behavior. Ph.D. thesis, Mathematics and Computer Science (2014). https://doi.org/10.6100/IR770080
2. Augusto, A., Conforti, R., Dumas, M., Rosa, M.L., Polyvyanyy, A.: Split miner: automated discovery of accurate and simple business process models from event logs. Knowl. Inf. Syst. **59**(2), 251–284 (2019). https://doi.org/10.1007/s10115-018-1214-x
3. Bergenthum, R.: Prime miner - process discovery using prime event structures. In: ICPM 2019, Aachen, Germany, pp. 41–48. IEEE (2019). https://doi.org/10.1109/ICPM.2019.00017
4. Li, M., Boehm, B., Osterweil, L.J. (eds.): SPW 2005. LNCS, vol. 3840. Springer, Heidelberg (2006). https://doi.org/10.1007/11608035
5. Leemans, S.J.J., Fahland, D., van der Aalst, W.M.P.: Discovering block-structured process models from event logs - a constructive approach. In: Colom, J.-M., Desel, J. (eds.) PETRI NETS 2013. LNCS, vol. 7927, pp. 311–329. Springer, Heidelberg (2013). https://doi.org/10.1007/978-3-642-38697-8_17
6. de Leoni, M.: Foundations of process enhancement. In: van der Aalst, W.M.P., Carmona, J. (eds.) Process Mining Handbook. LNBIP, vol. 448, pp. 243–273. Springer, Cham (2022). https://doi.org/10.1007/978-3-031-08848-3_8

7. Muñoz-Gama, J., Carmona, J.: A fresh look at precision in process conformance. In: Hull, R., Mendling, J., Tai, S. (eds.) BPM 2010. LNCS, vol. 6336, pp. 211–226. Springer, Heidelberg (2010). https://doi.org/10.1007/978-3-642-15618-2_16
8. Rennert, C., Mannel, L.L., van der Aalst, W.M.P.: Improving the EST-miner models by replacing imprecise structures using place projection. In: ATAED 2023 at Petri Nets 2023. CEUR Workshop Proceedings, vol. 3424. CEUR-WS.org (2023). http://ceur-ws.org/Vol-3424/paper3.pdf
9. Schuster, D., van Zelst, S.J., van der Aalst, W.M.P.: Incremental discovery of hierarchical process models. In: Dalpiaz, F., Zdravkovic, J., Loucopoulos, P. (eds.) RCIS 2020. LNBIP, vol. 385, pp. 417–433. Springer, Cham (2020). https://doi.org/10.1007/978-3-030-50316-1_25
10. van der Werf, J.M.E.M., van Dongen, B.F., Hurkens, C.A.J., Serebrenik, A.: Process discovery using integer linear programming. In: van Hee, K.M., Valk, R. (eds.) PETRI NETS 2008. LNCS, vol. 5062, pp. 368–387. Springer, Heidelberg (2008). https://doi.org/10.1007/978-3-540-68746-7_24

Generating Process Anomalies with Markov Chains: A Pattern-Driven Approach

Jochem Veldman[1], Xixi Lu[1]([✉])[ID], Wouter van der Waal[1][ID], Marcus Dees[2][ID], and Inge van de Weerd[1][ID]

[1] Utrecht University, Utrecht, The Netherlands
x.lu@uu.nl
[2] UWV, Amsterdam, The Netherlands
marcus.dees@uwv.nl

Abstract. Generating anomalies for process executions helps to train anomaly detection methods and evaluate their performance. Anomalous behavior tends to be diverse and very infrequent. Generating process anomalies can help compare detection models and select the suited ones. However, little research has been focused on generating anomalous behavior in a systematic and also stochastic way. In this paper, we built on the idea of training a Markov chain using an event log to capture regular process behavior. We then use a set of predefined *anomaly patterns* to adapt the Markov chain to generate anomalous traces. To evaluate the quality of our generated anomalies, we use them in the downstream task training a detection model. For each pattern, we vary the quantity of injected anomalous traces and their deviation rate. Unsurprisingly, the results show that the models trained with the generated anomalies have a significant improvement in detecting these anomalies. The AUC score increased from 0.63 to reaching a maximum of 0.98 or higher for all three patterns. This confirms our expectation that generating anomalies can help train and evaluate detection models.

1 Introduction

Monitoring business processes and detecting anomalies for early intervention can help prevent compliance issues. Accurate anomaly detection enables the prompt implementation of countermeasures. Anomaly detection is an essential task in data analytics that finds applications across a wide range of industries and is suited for various tasks [1, 2]. In addition to the banking sector, anomaly detection is also applied in intrusion detection, bot detection, fake review detection, identifying terrorist activities, and medical diagnosis [1, 2].

To evaluate the performance of these detection methods, it is necessary to have test data with *labeled anomalies*. However, labeling data instances is expensive and time-consuming, especially in the field of anomaly detection. In domains such as healthcare, banking, or insurance, highly trained experts are needed to manually determine if the instance is an anomaly [3]. Furthermore, anomalies are infrequent, leading to *imbalanced data* issues. For example, in most cases, the

J. De Smedt and P. Soffer (Eds.): ICPM 2023 Workshops, LNBIP 503, pp. 123–135, 2024.
https://doi.org/10.1007/978-3-031-56107-8_10

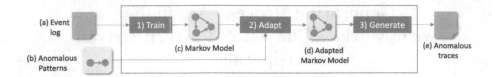

Fig. 1. An overview of the research problem and our proposed approach

majority of individuals are legitimate users rather than fraudsters. Consequently, if labeled anomalies are available, they typically account for only a small percentage, such as 1% of the data [4–6]. The scarcity of labeled data for evaluation is a pervasive challenge within the scientific community.

Generative approaches have emerged as ways to generate additional data sets [7]. A variety of anomalies can be generated and used to evaluate and compare the performance of detection methods.

In this paper, we propose a lightweight generative approach for process anomaly generation using Markov chains and process anomaly patterns. An overview of the approach is shown in Fig. 1. Assuming we have (a) an event log and (b) a set of *anomaly patterns* that denote potentially anomalous behavior of interest. The set of *anomaly patterns* can be obtained by either using (i) domain knowledge, (ii) (interactive) pattern discovery [8], or (iii) some patterns selected from the repository we built based on a systemic literature review [9]. Given these two inputs, we first train a Markov chain on the input event log, which represents the normative behavior (Step 1). We then use (b) the anomaly patterns to adapt the Markov chain (Step 2). Finally, We use (d) the adapted Markov chain to generate anomalous traces (Step 3).

To demonstrate and evaluate this approach, we inject the generated anomalies into the training datasets with varying amounts to investigate their effect on the supervised detection models. However, it is important to note that, in this experiment, the test data remains untouched and contains the true anomalies. The reasoning is that if the generated process anomalies are of high quality and mimic the true anomalies, injecting these generated anomalies should help detection models improve their accuracy. In addition, the objective is not to train a better detection model but to evaluate their performance in diverse settings, for example, when we increase or decrease the ratio of labeled anomalies in the training. Following this setting, we demonstrate the approach using a publicly available BPIC dataset. The results show that injecting the generated anomalous sequences tends to increase the Area Under the Curve (AUC) metric of supervised detection models.

The remainder of this paper is organized as follows. In Sect. 2, we discuss related work. Next, we introduce the preliminaries in Sect. 3, followed by the approach in Sect. 4, the evaluation in Sect. 5, and the results in Sect. 6. Finally, we conclude the paper in Sect. 7.

2   Related Work

In this section, we discuss four different streams of approaches to data and their suitability to generate infrequent process anomalies.

Earlier studies that propose detection methods tend to either use a random approach to add noise or introduce anomalies in an ad-hoc or restricted manner to evaluate the detection performance [10,11]. We argue that our approach complements such random approaches and allows users to have more control and options when generating anomalous traces.

Simulation-based approaches have also been studied and can be adapted to generate accurate anomalies. However, assuming a set of multiple anomalous patterns is of interest, the simulation models have to be manually (re)built or reconfigured. The effort to rebuild such simulation models highly depends on the simulation model/tool used. In this paper, we use the lightweight Markov models and propose (step 2) to adapt the Markov model based on the patterns in an automatic way.

Deep models or AI-based generative approaches, such as GAN [12], have also emerged. In [7], the authors have proposed to integrate Deep models with simulations models to generate traces. However, given our problem setting as shown in Fig. 1, users can train GANs on (a) the event log to generate normal traces, but they will have difficulty using the anomalous patterns to adapt GANs or make GANs to generate anomalous traces. Alternatively, one can train GANs on a small set of anomalous traces if such traces are available. Yet, the GANs trained on anomalies may ignore the normative process, whereas our approach largely maintains the distribution in the normative process (represented by the trained Markov model (c)).

3   Preliminaries

In this section, we briefly recall the preliminary concepts related to event logs and Markov chains.

Event Logs. Let $\mathcal{E}$ be the universe of event identifiers. Let A be a set of activities and $\alpha : \mathcal{E} \rightarrow A$ an event labeling function that returns the activity $\alpha(e)$ of event $e \in \mathcal{E}$. A trace $\sigma = \langle e_1, e_2, \cdots, e_n \rangle \in \mathcal{E}^*$ is a sequence of events. An event log L is a set of traces. An example of an event log is listed in Table 1.

Table 1. Example log for Markov chain explanation

Session ID	CustomerID	Activity	Timestamp
Session 1	1	Start_application	2015-11-06 08:07:22.780
Session 1	1	Input_info	2015-11-06 08:07:40.767
Session 1	1	Send_application	2015-11-06 08:07:51.390
Session 1	1	Accept_offer	2015-11-06 08:08:06.003
Session 2	101	Send_application	2016-02-28 08:17:15.947
Session 2	101	Accept_offer	2016-02-28 08:18:31.454
Session 3	224	Input_info	2016-01-14 08:32:11.511
Session 3	224	Send_application	2016-01-14 08:34:12.123
Session 3	224	Accept_offer	2016-01-14 08:37:23.984
Session 4	7653	Start_application	2016-02-20 20:15:10.321
Session 4	7653	Input_info	2016-02-20 20:16:09.647
Session 5	63	Accept_offer	2016-02-20 20:16:09.647

Markov Chain. We follow the definition of Markov chain in [13]. Let $S = \{s_1, \cdots, s_n\}$ be the set of possible *states* in a Markov chain. For any states s_i, $s_j \in S$, let $\mathbb{P}(s_j \mid s_i) = p_{ij}$ be the *transition probability* from the current state s_i to a subsequent state s_j. A Markov chain is represented by a matrix $T = \{p_{ij}\}$ of transition probabilities, where $p_{ij} = \mathbb{P}(s_j \mid s_i)$, for all $s_i, s_j \in S$. We define a *Markov chain* $M = (S, T)$, where S is the set of states, and T is the transition matrix. For all states $s_i \in S$, $\sum_{s_j \in S} \mathbb{P}(s_j \mid s_i) = 1$. As in [13], we extend the set S with two special states - a start state ($\circ$) and an end state ($\bullet$). For instance,

$\mathbb{P}(s_i \mid \circ)$ is the probability of the Markov chain starting in state s_i; $\mathbb{P}(\bullet \mid s_i)$ is the probability of the Markov chain ending in state s_i. Note that $\sum_{s_i \in S} \mathbb{P}(s_i \mid \circ) = 1$, $\sum_{s_i \in S} \mathbb{P}(\circ \mid s_i) = 0$, and $\sum_{s_i \in S} \mathbb{P}(s_i \mid \bullet) = 0$.

4   Approach

4.1   Log to Markov Chain

Inspired by existing work on training Markov chain using event logs such as [14], the first step of our approach is to train a first-order Markov chain (S, T) from an event log L, where the states S are the set of activities A with the start and end states $\{\circ, \bullet\}$ added. For each trace in the log, we added a dummy "START" at the beginning of the trace and a dummy "END" at the end of the trace, to correspond to the start and end states, respectively.

To compute the transition probabilities T, we first calculate the frequency matrix of any two consecutive activities, i.e., $Freq(a, b) := \sum_{\sigma \in L} \#\{(e_i, e_{i+1}) \mid \alpha(e_i) = a \wedge \alpha(e_{i+1}) = b \wedge e_i, e_{i+1} \in \sigma\}$. For instance, considering the example log listed in Table 1, we obtain the frequency matrix listed in Table 2. Next, for each row, we compute the row total and divide the value in each cell by the row total. The final matrix of transition probabilities is listed in Table 3. In this paper, we only describe the basic algorithm where the last occurred activity is considered as the state; for a more general algorithm, we refer to [14].

4.2   Process Anomaly Patterns

We define process anomaly patterns as directed, labeled graphs $P = (A', \rightarrow)$. The process anomaly patterns of interest can be obtained by using domain knowledge or using interactive pattern explorer [8]. In addition, to support users creating anomaly patterns of interest, a systematic literature review was conducted to establish a repository of anomaly patterns. In total, 24 domain-specific fraudulent patterns and 14 anomaly patterns in process mining were found. A detailed description of each anomaly pattern is presented in [9]. Each of the domain-specific fraudulent characteristics can be used to create a process anomaly pattern $P = (A', \rightarrow)$ and used further by our approach to generate anomalous traces.

In the following, we explain three examples of process anomaly patterns, selected from the repository [9]. We focus on explaining these three patterns because they are used in the evaluation.

Table 2. Frequency matrix resulted from counting of all consecutive events

	Accept_offer	Input_info	Send_application	Start_application	END	sum
START	1	1	1	2	0	5
Accept_offer	0	0	0	0	4	4
Input_info	0	0	2	0	1	3
Send_application	3	0	0	0	0	3
Start_application	0	2	0	0	0	2

Table 3. Transition probabilities discovered using the example event log

	Accept_offer	Input_info	Send_application	Start_application	END
START	0,2	0,2	0,2	0,4	0
Accept_offer	0	0	0	0	1
Input_info	0	0	0,67	0	0,33
Send_application	1	0	0	0	0
Start_application	0	1	0	0	0

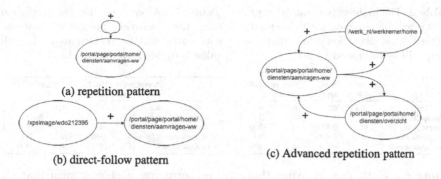

(a) repetition pattern

(b) direct-follow pattern

(c) Advanced repetition pattern

Fig. 2. Examples of the three patterns obtained and used in the evaluation.

Repetition. The repetition pattern is often described in the literature as an anomaly characteristic in process mining [9]. It consists of a single activity that can be performed more or less frequently than expected. This pattern manifests itself as $P = (A', \rightarrow)$ where $A' = \{a\}$ consists of a single activity, and $\rightarrow = \{(a, a)\}$. An example of the repetition pattern can be seen in Fig. 2a, which is a repetition of "../AANVRAGEN-WW".

Direct-follow. The direct-follow relation consists of two consecutively occurring activities in a trace. Note that the directly-follows pattern is directed, i.e., when an activity a is directly followed by another activity b is considered an anomalous pattern, then this does not imply that b directly followed by a is also an anomaly. This pattern manifests itself as $P = (A', \rightarrow)$, where $A' = \{a, b\}$ consists of two activities, and $\rightarrow = \{(a, b)\}$. The direct-follow relation can be seen in Fig. 2b.

Advanced Repetition. The advanced repetition pattern consists of three different activities. Activity a links to activities b and c. Activity b and c link back to activity a. All the links between the activities are direct links. This creates a loop between activity a and b and between activities a and c. We define this pattern as $P = (A', \rightarrow)$, where $A' = \{a, b, c\}$ is the set of three activities, and $\rightarrow = \{(a, b), (b, a), (a, c), (c, a)\}$.

Configured Anomaly Patterns. The reason for these simple anomaly patterns is that they can be easily reused and adapted to different contexts where an event log is available. As we would like to use them to generate anomalous traces, the users should be able to configure the *deviation rate* and *the number of generated traces*. We define a configured anomaly pattern $P_{\delta,k} = (A', \rightarrow, \delta, k)$ where $(A', \rightarrow)$ is the pattern, $\delta : (A' \times A') \rightarrow \mathbb{R}$ is the deviation rate that maps each edge in the pattern to a real number, and $k \geq 1$ is the number of traces to be generated.

4.3   Using Patterns for Adapting Markov Chains

Assuming we have a Markov chain (S, T) trained from the event log L and a configured $P_{\delta,k}$, for each $(a, b) \in \rightarrow$, we update the transition probability T by

Table 4. The highlighted transition probability will be changed for the repetition pattern. If the deviation rate is 10, the cell value will be increased by 10.

	Accept_offer	Input_info	Send_application	Start_ap-plication	END
START	0,2	0,2	0,2	0,4	0
Accept_offer	0	0	0	0	1
Input_info	0	0	0,67	0	0,33
Send_application	1	0	0	0	0
Start_application	0	1	0	0	0

Table 5. After applying the deviation rate, the transition probabilities of the entire row will be recalculated; the cell value is divided by the row total.

	Accept_offer	Input_info	Send_application	Start_ap-plication	END
START	0,2	0,2	0,2	0,4	0
Accept_offer	0	0	0	0	1
Input_info	0	0	0,67	0	0,33
Send_application	0,09	0	0,91	0	0
Start_application	0	1	0	0	0

adding $\delta(a, b)$ to $T(a, b)$. After that, we (re)normalize each row such that the transition probabilities of a row sum up to 1.

For example, let us consider the repetition of "SEND_APPLICATION" as a configured anomaly pattern with a deviation rate of 10. Thus, we change this transition probability to T("SEND_APPLICATION", "SEND_APPLICATION") + 10, see Table 4. We overwrite this value with a new value 10. After that, we (re)normalize the probabilities such that the sum of the probabilities at each row is 1, which resulted in 0.91, see Table 5.

4.4   Generating Anomalies Using Markov Chain

In step (3), we *generate* anomalous traces using the configured anomaly pattern and the adapted Markov chain as our inputs. We briefly sketch the algorithm. It begins with the starting activity. From the "START" row, the activities and their corresponding probabilities are considered. The follow-up activity is chosen randomly based on the given probabilities.

For example, assuming the adapted Markov chain in Table 5, this would mean that there is 20% that "INPUT_INFO" will be selected as the start activity. If this activity is indeed selected as the starting activity, an "INPUT_INFO" event is appended to a new trace. The algorithm then continues with the row "INPUT_INFO" and considers the subsequent activities and their probabilities, i.e., "SEND_APPLICATION" with a 67% probability and "END" with a 33% probability. Let's assume that the function selects "END" as the consecutive activity, then an event of "END" is appended to the trace. The activity "END" signifies that the generated sequence has reached its final state and is considered complete.

To ensure the generated trace is relevant while maintaining the stochastic nature, we check if the trace at least contains the activities of the anomaly pattern. If the trace meets this condition, it is added to the set of generated anomalous traces until the desired *number of generated anomalous traces k* has been reached.

5   Evaluation

We implemented the proposed approach in Python (version 3.9.7). For Python, we used Pandas, Numpy, and Sci-kit learn as our main libraries. The implementa-

Table 6. The three rules for labeling the anomalies and the corresponding patterns.

ID	Rules to label an anomaly	# true anomalies	Pattern
1	A trace has more than fifty direct repetitions of "…/AANVRAGEN-WW"	465	Figure 2a
2	A trace has more than one occurrence of a direct-follows relation from "/XPSIMAGE/WDO212395" to "…/AANVRAGEN-WW"	87	Figure 2b
3	A trace contains more than three non-consecutive executions of activity "…/HOME/SERVICES/REQUESTS-WW"	352	Figure 2c

tion was done in Jupyter Notebook and made publicly available[1]. The objective is to (1) show that our approach can used to generate anomalous traces and (2) investigate the effect on the existing detection methods when injecting the generated anomalous traces into the training set.

5.1 Data Description

We use a public dataset from the BPIC 2016 [15] which is provided by the dutch organization Uitvoeringsinstituut Werknemersverzekeringen (UWV). The UWV is a governmental organization responsible for employee-related social benefits in the Netherlands. In this evaluation, we use the click data of visits to the UWV website for logged-in clients. The original dataset contains no labels.

The event log provided covers the period from 6 November 2015 to 28 February 2016. The data consists of 7,174,934 rows and has a size of 1.06GB. A total of 781 unique activities (i.e., web pages) have occurred in 660,270 sessions (traces). The average number of activities per trace is 10.87, covering 26,647 unique users. The variables that have our interest are CustomerID, SessionID, TIMESTAMP, and URL_FILE. We use the session id as the case id and the URL_FILE as the activity. In addition, we selected a set of 50,000 traces due to the capacity limitation of the laptop used.

Interviews for Labeling Anomalies. For the experiment, two interviews were held with the UWV domain expert who provided the dataset, to obtain anomalies of interest. It is important to note that this step to obtain labels is not a step in our approach (see Fig. 1) but is only a part of the evaluation we designed. During the two interviews, we obtained the three concrete rules to label anomalous traces. Table 6 lists the three rules, the number of anomalies labeled using the rules, and the corresponding pattern used to generate the anomaly. For each rule, we create a separate class label.

5.2 Setup

After obtaining the labeled event log with true anomalies, we use this data set to evaluate our approach to generate anomalies. Assuming we do not have the rules as listed in Table 6 but only the three anomaly patterns as shown in Fig. 2.

---

[1] https://github.com/JochemVeldmanUU/Thesis_anomaly_generation.

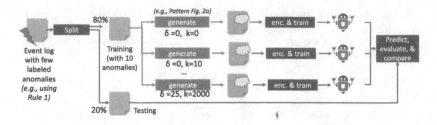

Fig. 3. An overview of the experiment set-up.

We follow a standard pipeline for training and evaluating a supervised model. Figure 3 shows an overview of the setup. In the following, we explain the setup.

Generate Anomalies. We use our approach to generate anomalies. The three patterns are matched to the Markov model and used to manipulate the probability of the corresponding transition probabilities. For the number of anomalous traces injected, we set k to the values of $\{0, 10, 100, 500, 1000, 2000\}$. For the *deviation rate* δ, we use values of $\{0, 0.2, 1, 5, 25\}$ for all relations in δ. For each value, we recalculate the probability such that the total probabilities sum up to one. Using the adjusted Markov model, we apply our approach and generate the anomalous traces. Note that we do not use the rules to generate anomalies but capture the anomalous behavior using the patterns and the deviation rate δ.

Trace Encoding. For encoding the traces to fit the detection technique, we use the simple bag-of-activities encoding, i.e., the activities as the features. For each trace, for each activity, we encode the occurrence frequency of the activity as the feature value.

We split the normal traces randomly into a training set (80% of the original) and a test set (20% of the original). From the true anomaly traces, *10* traces are included in the training data, to mimic the real-life imbalanced data issue with very few anomalous instances labeled. The rest of the true anomaly traces are added to the test data. Next, the generated anomalies are added to the training dataset at different rates. The test set is unchanged.

Training and Evaluating the Detection Models. We use a logistic regression model with default parameters and later a decision tree as the supervised detection method. The max iteration is set to 1000. We evaluate the performance of the detection model using AUC, recall, and precision.

6   Results and Discussion

This section presents the obtained results. As aforementioned, the objective is to show that the approach helps to generate anomalies and to investigate the effect on the downstream anomaly detection techniques. The underlying rationale is that *if the generated process anomalies closely resemble true anomalous behavior*, then injecting these generated anomalies into the training data should lead

Table 7. The AUC scores of the detection model trained with varying settings for the repetition pattern.

Number of anomalous traces injected	AUC score Deviation rate = 0	AUC score Deviation rate = 0.2	AUC score Deviation rate = 1	AUC score Deviation rate = 5	AUC score Deviation rate = 25
0	0.666	0.666	0.666	0.666	0.666
10	0.662	0.649	0.680	0.698	0.670
100	0.796	0.831	0.859	0.832	0.760
500	0.998	0.987	0.984	0.954	0.880
1000	0.995	0.997	0.993	0.978	0.917
2000	0.994	0.994	0.995	0.992	0.953

Table 8. The AUC scores of the model trained with varying settings for the direct-follow pattern.

Number of anomalous traces injected	AUC score deviation rate = 0	AUC score deviation rate = 0.2	AUC score deviation rate = 1	AUC score deviation rate = 5	AUC score deviation rate = 25
0	0.623	0.623	0.623	0.623	0.623
10	0.636	0.636	0.649	0.649	0.688
100	0.630	0.643	0.753	0.773	0.708
500	0.817	0.869	0.914	0.940	0.940
1000	0.907	0.946	0.972	0.998	0.985
2000	0.944	0.976	0.995	0.996	0.996

Table 9. The AUC scores for the advanced repetition pattern.

Number of anomalous traces injected	AUC score deviation rate = 0	AUC score deviation rate = 0.2	AUC score deviation rate = 1	AUC score deviation rate = 5	AUC score deviation rate = 25
0	0.577	0.577	0.577	0.577	0.577
10	0.569	0.572	0.560	0.566	0.556
100	0.621	0.607	0.588	0.577	0.560
500	0.823	0.640	0.612	0.596	0.570
1000	0.936	0.670	0.620	0.597	0.580
2000	0.980	0.710	0.636	0.613	0.572

Table 10. The optimal AUC, precision, and recall scores of our approach (M) compared with the oversampling technique (SO).

Pattern	AUC		Precision		Recall		F1	
	OS	M	OS	M	SO	M	SO	M
Repetition	0.888	**0.995**	**0.99**	0.93	0.78	**0.99**	0.87	**0.96**
Direct-follow	0.870	**0.996**	**0.89**	0.72	0.74	**0.83**	**0.81**	0.77
Advanced repetition	0.757	**0.980**	**0.92**	0.76	0.51	**0.97**	0.66	**0.85**

to *improved detection accuracy* for the detection methods. This improvement is expected since we are to some extent leaking information to the detection methods. In the following, we examine the AUC performance of the detection model under different settings of δ and k.

6.1 AUC Scores

Repetition Pattern. Table 7 lists the attained AUC scores for the repetition pattern. The column names represent the *deviation rate*, while the row names indicate the number of injected anomalous traces. The first row represents the baseline AUC score, thus without injecting the generated anomalies.

As can be seen in Table 7, the AUC score demonstrates a notable increase from 0.666 to 0.995, with an improvement of 0.329. In the setting where the deviation rate is 1 and 2000 anomalous traces are injected, the detection model achieves its highest AUC score. On average, injecting 2000 anomalous traces with different deviation rates yields an AUC improvement of 0.320 compared to the baseline. Interestingly, setting the deviation rate to a high value of 25 yields a less significant improvement.

Direct-follow Pattern. Table 8 shows the AUC scores attained for the direct-follow pattern. The AUC score for this pattern also shows a significant improvement of 0.373, reaching 0.996. This improvement is obtained when the deviation rate is set to 5 or 25. These two settings also achieve the highest AUC score. On average, these settings in the table achieve an increase of 0.358 in the AUC scores.

Advanced Repetition Pattern. Table 9 lists the AUC scores attained for the advanced repetition pattern. The AUC scores for this pattern also show an increase of 0.403 (from 0.577 to 0.980), where the deviation rate is set to 0 and the number of injected anomalous traces to 2000. Interestingly, the performance improvement differs significantly between the deviation rate of 0 and the other deviation rates. In contrast to the previous patterns, the increase in AUC scores diminishes as the deviation rate is set to higher values. For instance, when the deviation rate is set to 25, four out of five obtained AUC scores are even lower than the baseline AUC of 0.577.

Overall, the improvements in AUC are as we expected. In addition, our observations indicate that when the deviation rate is set to a relatively low value, injecting a large number of generated anomalous traces significantly enhances the detection model's AUC performance, compared to not injecting any traces. We also computed the recall and precision, which exhibit similar trends but slightly less significant improvements compared to the AUC scores. The optimal recall and precision scores for each pattern are listed in Table 10.

6.2   Comparative Experiments

We compare our results to a sampling approach. We use the training set that contains the true anomalies but no generated anomalies and the unchanged test set and used an oversampling technique. Additionally, we also use another detection model, i.e., decision tree, to investigate the generalizability of the effects.

Comparing to Oversampling. For the implementation of the oversampling method, we used the RandomOverSampler from the Imbalanced learn library. This function oversamples the minority class by randomly picking samples with replacements. The original training set includes 39,957 normal traces and *10* true anomaly traces. The oversampling function samples these 10 traces and increases the number of anomalous traces to 39,957 to balance the classes. The resulting oversampled training set was used to train a logistic regression model, which was subsequently evaluated using the test set.

Table 10 presents the results attained by the logistic regression trained using the oversampled data. The highest scores are highlighted in bold for comparison with our generative approach. When comparing oversampling with the generative approach, we observe that oversampling achieves a higher precision score but a lower recall score. However, when considering the F1 score, we see that our generative approach achieves a higher score for the repetition and advanced repetition scores. On the other hand, the oversampling technique achieves a better F1 score for the direct-follow pattern.

Considering the AUC scores, it is evident that the generative approach achieves better AUC scores for all three patterns compared to the oversampling technique. Hence, these findings suggest that injecting the anomalous traces helps the detection methods in effectively distinguishing between normal and abnormal behavior, leading to a notable increase in AUC scores. This result is also expected since we are using more complex models (i.e., the Markov chains) to capture the anomalous behavior than just sampling. It is worth noting that the lower precision or F1 score observed may be attributed to the cut-off threshold set for classifying anomalies in the detection methods. Adjusting the anomaly threshold could potentially improve the precision and F1 score.

Using the Decision Tree Model. We conducted a similar experiment using a Decision Tree model instead of a Logistic Regression model. The improvements in the performance of the Decision Tree model were less significant compared to the Logistic Regression model. However, the results still exhibited the same trend observed in the Logistic Regression model. In the AUC curves, we observed that increasing the number of injected anomalous traces led to improved performance. Additionally, increasing the deviation rate also resulted in a slight increase in performance, although this increase differed from that observed in the Logistic Regression model. Notably, the Decision Tree model performed well for the advanced repetition pattern when the deviation rate was increased, which was not the case for the Logistic Regression model.

6.3   Discussion

The evaluation results have shown that generating and injecting the anomalies helps to improve the detection accuracy significantly. For the repetition pattern, our approach helps to achieve an increase of an AUC from 0.666 to 0.995 and an increase in the F1 score from 0.50 to 0.96. For the direct-follow pattern, the AUC increases from 0.623 to 0.996, and the F1 score from 0.39 to 0.77. For the advanced repetition pattern, the injection of anomalies did not help as much as for the other two patterns. It only achieves good results when the deviation rate is 0. For this deviation rate, we achieve an increase in AUC from 0.577 to 0.980 and in F1 score from 0.26 to 0.85.

We observed that injecting more generated anomalies leads to an increase in both the AUC score and recall, while the precision decreases for all three patterns. However, the high AUC scores indicate that the detection model effectively distinguishes anomalies from normal behavior. This suggests that the cutoff threshold could be further optimized, for example, through the use of cross-validation.

Compared to injecting more generated traces, increasing the deviation rate has a less significant impact on the AUC scores obtained by the models for the repetition and direct-follow patterns. The resulting AUC scores related to these two patterns tend to converge to a similar value across different configurations with varying deviation rates. However, for the advanced repetition pattern, we observe a decrease in AUC when the deviation rate is increased. We attribute this to the complexity of the pattern and the simplicity of the features chosen in this experiment. Since the features only consist of the activity frequency, the model may not be able to learn the decision boundary. Adding the directly-follows relations may significantly increase the model performance. In future work, we suggest experimenting with other trace encoding techniques, such as encoding the transitions between activities.

In the experiment, we used three concrete yet relatively simple patterns to demonstrate our approach. Since the patterns are defined as directed graphs, this definition allows our approach to support more complex patterns. For example, and alternatively, when a few traces are manually labeled as anomalies, each trace (or the subsequent events) of interest can be converted to a directed graph as a pattern that can be used by our approach to generating anomalies.

We discuss the following limitations. (1) The anomaly patterns we investigated in the evaluation are rather simplistic. As discussed, our definition of process anomaly patterns is however general and can capture more complex patterns. We consider this study as a first step that confirms the potential of generating stochastic process anomalies. (2) The detection methods and the trace encoding used in the evaluation are rather simplistic, classic machine-learning techniques. Given that the anomaly patterns concern the directly-follows relations, it may be important to include them as features. For future work, we should investigate the effect of injecting generated anomalies on more advanced trace encoding and detection techniques. (3) One may argue that if the anomaly patterns are known, one can use the patterns to detect anomalies, which we agree with. However, our approach aims to generate anomalies, which can also be used to evaluate and compare the detection methods. The experiment performed investigates the performance of the detection models when additional anomalies are injected.

7 Conclusion

In this study, we introduced a lightweight approach for generating stochastic process anomalies using Markov models. Our approach leverages predefined anomaly patterns to adapt the Markov model, subsequently facilitating the generation of anomalous traces. This research contributes a pattern-driven approach for generating anomalies in a stochastic way. The approach is demonstrated in a controlled experiment, allowing for systematic evaluation and comparison of detection methods when an increasing number of labeling anomalies are added to the training set. Our experiment shows that injecting these generated anomalous traces helps increase the AUC of the detection models, achieving a 0.98 or higher, thus affirming our initial expectation. This suggests that the generated anomalies can be used to further evaluate and compare the detection methods.

For future research, we would like to explore the diverse, complex patterns to adapt the Markov chain and perform a systematic evaluation and comparison of existing detection methods using our approach.

References

1. Ahmed, M., Mahmood, A., Islam, M.: A survey of anomaly detection techniques in financial domain. Futur. Gener. Comput. Syst. **55**, 278–288 (2016)
2. Goldstein, M., Uchida, S.: A comparative evaluation of unsupervised anomaly detection algorithms for multivariate data. PLoS ONE **11**(4), e0152173 (2016)
3. Tax, N., et al.: Machine learning for fraud detection in e-commerce: a research agenda, CoRR, vol. abs/2107.01979, 2021
4. Pang, G., Shen, C., Cao, L., van den Hengel, A.: Deep learning for anomaly detection: a review. ACM Comput. Surv. **54**(2), 38:1–38:38 (2021)

5. Adewumi, A., Akinyelu, A.: A survey of machine-learning and nature-inspired based credit card fraud detection techniques. Int. J. Syst. Assur. Eng. Manag. **8**(2s), 937–953 (2017)
6. Achituve, I., Kraus, S., Goldberger, J.: Interpretable online banking fraud detection based on hierarchical attention mechanism. In: 29th IEEE International Workshop on Machine Learning for Signal Processing, MLSP: Pittsburgh, PA, USA, 13–16 October 2019. IEEE 2019, pp. 1–6 (2019)
7. Camargo, M., Dumas, M., Rojas, O.G.: Discovering generative models from event logs: data-driven simulation vs deep learning. PeerJ Comput. Sci. **7**, e577 (2021)
8. Vazifehdoostirani, M., et al.: Interactive multi-interest process pattern discovery. In: Di Francescomarino, C., Burattin, A., Janiesch, C., Sadiq, S. (eds.) Business Process Management. BPM 2023. LNCS, vol. 14159, pp. 303–319. Springer, Cham (2023). https://doi.org/10.1007/978-3-031-41620-0_18
9. Veldman, J.: Generating process anomalies using a taxonomy of fraud characteristics and markov models for accurate detection, Master's thesis, Utrecht University, 2022. https://studenttheses.uu.nl/handle/20.500.12932/42635
10. Alizadeh, M., Lu, X., Fahland, D., Zannone, N., van der Aalst, W.: Linking data and process perspectives for conformance analysis. Comput. Secur. **73**, 172–193 (2018)
11. Lu, X., Fahland, D., van den Biggelaar, F.J.H.M., van der Aalst, W.M.P.: Detecting deviating behaviors without models. In: Reichert, M., Reijers, H.A. (eds.) BPM 2015. LNBIP, vol. 256, pp. 126–139. Springer, Cham (2016). https://doi.org/10.1007/978-3-319-42887-1_11
12. Goodfellow, I.J., et al.: Generative adversarial nets. In: NIPS, pp. 2672–2680 (2014)
13. Ferreira, D.R., Gillblad, D.: Discovering process models from unlabelled event logs. In: Dayal, U., Eder, J., Koehler, J., Reijers, H.A. (eds.) BPM 2009. LNCS, vol. 5701, pp. 143–158. Springer, Heidelberg (2009). https://doi.org/10.1007/978-3-642-03848-8_11
14. van der Aalst, W.M.P., Schonenberg, M.H., Song, M.: Time prediction based on process mining. Inf. Syst. **36**(2), 450–475 (2011)
15. Dees, M., van Dongen, B.B.: BPI Challenge 2016 (2016)

4th International Workshop
on Leveraging Machine Learning
for Process Mining (ML4PM 2023)

4th International Workshop on Leveraging Machine Learning for Process Mining (ML4PM 2023)

Recent academic research and innovative industrial solutions have consistently highlighted the growing need for the integration of Machine Learning (ML) techniques to enhance the effectiveness of Process Mining (PM) methods. ML methods have recently become the cornerstone of a wide range of PM-based applications, ranging from process automation to process simulation. The most recent and striking illustration of the combination of PM and ML can be observed in the area of Predictive Process Monitoring (PPM). In this context, they serve as indispensable components in the development of PPM solutions.

By bringing together practitioners and researchers from both fields, the 4th International Workshop on Leveraging Machine Learning for Process Mining sought to explore recent research advances at the intersection of ML and PM. The broad call for papers invited submissions in various areas, including outcome and time prediction, classification and clustering of business processes, application of deep learning in PM, anomaly detection, natural language processing and text mining for PM, multi-perspective analysis of processes, ML for robotic process automation, automated process modeling and updating, ML-based conformance checking, transfer learning in business processes, ML-enabled IoT business services, multidimensional PM, predictive process monitoring, prescriptive learning in PM, and the convergence of ML and blockchain in process management.

The workshop received fifteen submissions, which underwent a thorough review process involving three to four members of the program committee. Of these, six were accepted for presentation - five as full papers and one as an extended abstract. Papers presented at the workshop were also selected for inclusion in the post-proceedings. A summary of these papers is given below.

The paper by Kim S. et al. explores the impact of design choices on the performance of PPM models, introducing a framework that employs a search space exploration algorithm and explicable AI techniques to analyze different model configurations and their influence on model performance, particularly in the context of outcome-oriented PPM, supported by experimental results from publicly available event logs.

The paper by Li P. et al. introduces a novel approach to automatically identify and interpret influential process-based drivers for case-level outcomes in process mining, aiming to understand the impact of process traces on key performance indicators through a defined optimization problem, addressed using efficient greedy algorithms and validated on real-world datasets, highlighting the effectiveness and efficiency of the proposed method.

The paper by F. Folino et al. proposes a novel approach in process mining research for outcome prediction, introducing a sparse mixture-of-experts trained with logistic regressors, which focuses on interpretability and fast prediction by restricting the input features, offering a promising balance between accuracy and interpretability compared to existing methods, as validated on benchmark logs.

The paper by A. Niro and M. Werner introduces a pioneering framework for anomaly detection in business processes using graph neural networks and object-centric process mining, showing promising performance in detecting anomalies at the activity type and attribute level, although facing challenges in identifying temporal anomalies, by reconstructing event dependencies into attributed graphs and employing a graph convolutional autoencoder architecture.

The paper by M. Vazifehdoostirani et al. introduces a novel post-hoc explainable AI technique inspired by permutation feature importance to evaluate the influence of activity locations in predictive process monitoring models, demonstrating the potential impact of these locations on outcome predictions through experimental validation on real event logs, aiming to improve the interpretability of predictive models by uncovering the significance of activity locations.

The extended abstract by Y. Valero et al. introduces a method that uses process crowding in Generative Adversarial Networks (GANs) to simulate the movement of units in processes by training the GAN using crowding computed from event logs, allowing the model to generate unit movements based on user-defined initial conditions, providing a simplified form of unit-scale simulation in the context of deep learning.

In addition to these papers, the workshop program included a keynote talk titled "Cracking the Nut. Unraveling Challenges in Predictive Process Monitoring" by Jochen De Weerdt and the technical talk "Declarative Process Mining Meets Industry: The Declare4Py Case" by Fabrizio Maria Maggi, Ivan Donadello, and Francesco Riva.

We would like to thank all the authors who submitted papers for publication in this book. We are also grateful to the members of the Program Committee and the external reviewers for their excellent work in reviewing the submitted and revised papers with expertise and patience.

November 2023

Paolo Ceravolo
Sylvio Barbon Junior
Annalisa Appice

Organization

Workshop Chairs

Paolo Ceravolo   Università degli Studi di Milano, Italy
Sylvio Barbon Junior   Università degli Studi di Trieste, Italy
Annalisa Appice   Università degli Studi di Bari Aldo Moro, Italy

Program Committee

Rafael Accorsi   Accenture, Switzerland
Annalisa Appice   University of Bari Aldo Moro, Italy
Sylvio Barbon Junior   Univerity of Trieste, Italy
Mario Luca Bernardi   University of Sannio, Italy
Michelangelo Ceci   University of Bari, Italy
Paolo Ceravolo   University of Milan, Italy
Marco Comuzzi   Ulsan National Institute of Science and Technology, South Korea
Carl Corea   University of Koblenz-Landau, Germany
Jochen De Weerdt   Katholieke Universiteit Leuven, Belgium
Chiara Di Francescomarino   University of Trento, Italy
Matthias Ehrendorfer   University of Vienna, Austria
Maria Teresa Gómez López   University of Seville, Spain
Gabriel Marques Tavares   Università degli Studi di Milano, Italy
Rafael Oyamada   State University of Londrina, Brazil
Emerson Paraiso   Pontifícia Universidade Católica do Paraná, Brazil
Vincenzo Pasquadibisceglie   University of Bari Aldo Moro, Italy
Marco Pegoraro   RWTH Aachen University, Germany
Marcelo Fantinato   University of São Paulo, Brazil
Sarajane M. Peres   University of São Paulo, Brazil
Luigi Pontieri   ICAR, National Research Council of Italy (CNR), Italy
Domenico Potena   Università Politecnica delle Marche, Italy
Flavia Maria Santoro   University of Rio de Janeiro, Brazil
Natalia Sidorova   Eindhoven University of Technology, The Netherlands
Wil van der Aalst   RWTH Aachen University, Germany
Bruno Zarpelao   State University of Londrina, Brazil

Sparse Mixtures of Shallow Linear Experts for Interpretable and Fast Outcome Prediction

Francesco Folino[ID], Luigi Pontieri[✉][ID], and Pietro Sabatino[ID]

Institute for High Performance Computing and Networking (ICAR-CNR), via P. Bucci 8/9C, 87036 Rende, CS, Italy
{francesco.folino,luigi.pontieri,pietro.sabatino}@icar.cnr.it

Abstract. (Process) Outcome Prediction entails predicting a discrete property of an unfinished process instance from its partial trace. Various outcome predictors discovered via Machine Learning (ML) methods, like rule/tree ensembles and (deep) neural networks, have achieved top accuracy performances. However, their opaqueness makes them unsuitable for scenarios necessitating understandable outcome predictors. Aligning with recent efforts to mine inherently interpretable predictors, we suggest training a sparse Mixture-of-Experts, with the "gate" and "expert" sub-nets being Logistic Regressors. This ensemble of specialized predictors is trained in a end-to-end way while restricting the number of input features used in the sub-nets, as an alternative to typical multi-step/objective mining pipelines (including, e.g., a global feature selection step followed by an ML one). This enables different experts to focus on varied input features for predicting the outcomes of instances in their competency regions. Test results on benchmark logs confirmed the ability of this approach to reach a compelling trade-off between accuracy and interpretability compared to existing solutions.

Keywords: Process Mining · Machine Learning · XAI · Green AI

1 Introduction

Predictive Process Monitoring (PPM) methods [7] aim at extending process monitoring mechanisms with the ability to forecast properties of ongoing process instances. This is an active line of research in the area of *Process Mining* (*PM*), owing to the advantages that such methods can bring in terms of run-time decision support and optimization. In this context, we specifically address the *(Process) Outcome Prediction* problem [19], i.e., the problem of predicting the outcome of an unfinished process instance, based on its associated *prefix trace* (i.e., the partial sequence of events available for the instance).

Recently, different supervised learning approaches to this problem were proposed, which allow for discovering an outcome prediction model from labeled traces. Outstanding performances in terms of prediction accuracy have been achieved by two classes of powerful predictors: (i) big ensembles of decision rules/trees discovered with random forest or gradient boosting algorithms [19]; and *Deep Neural Networks* (*DNNs*) (see [10] for a recent survey and benchmark) consisting, for instance, of multiple layers including feed-forward, RNN [18] or CNN [8] sub-nets. In particular, DNNs quickly

© The Author(s), under exclusive license to Springer Nature Switzerland AG 2024
J. De Smedt and P. Soffer (Eds.): ICPM 2023 Workshops, LNBIP 503, pp. 141–152, 2024.
https://doi.org/10.1007/978-3-031-56107-8_11

became popular in this field thanks to their ability to automatically learn hierarchies of abstract features from raw log data without requiring the analyst to preliminary bring the data into a tabular form by using trace encoding schemes [19]. However, the function-approximation power of these models comes at the cost of an opaque internal decision logic, which makes them unfit for real-life settings where decision makers want explainable predictions and interpretable predictors.

The consequent call for transparent outcome prediction first originated a number of proposals relying model-agnostic post-hoc explanation methods (like LIME and SHAP) [2,4,11,13] or explanation-friendly DNN-oriented solutions (e.g., attention modules, gradient/LRP -based feature attribution) [17,20]. More recently, concerns on the reliability of attention/attribution-based explanations [1] and the faithfulness, stability, consistency and efficiency of post-hoc explanations [14,21] pushed PM researchers to face the discovery of inherently-interpretable predictors [9,15,16].

Related work: approaches to discovering inherently interpretable outcome predictors
Two alternative kinds of interpretable models, both leveraging *Logistic Regression* (*LR*) models as a building block, were recently exploited in [16] in the discovery of process outcome predictors from flattened (through aggregation encoding [19]) log traces: (i) *Logit Leaf Model* (*LLM*), a sort of decision tree where each leaf hosts an LR sub-model; and (ii) *Generalized Logistic Rule Model* (*GLRM*) where a single LR model is built upon the original feature and novel features, defined as conjunctive rules over subsets of the former and derived via column generation. LLM and GLRM models were shown to improve plain LR predictors thanks to their ability to capture some non-linear input-output dependencies. An approach leveraging a neural implementation of fuzzy logic, named *FOX*, was instead proposed in [9], which can extract easy-to-interpret IF-THEN rules for outcome prediction, each of which contains a fuzzy set for each input feature of a trace (still encoded propositionally via aggregation encoding [19]) and a membership score for each outcome class. The domain of each data feature is split into three "linguistic" fuzzy sets, so that 3^k rules are learned by training this model over k-dimensional data after selecting the best k features with an MI-based method.

In principle, by learning multiple LRs, an LLM could find an interpretable predictor; however, if using no mechanisms for limiting the number of data features and the size of the decision tree, cumbersome models can be obtained, as noted in [15], which hardly allow the user to grasp a clear and complete understanding of the predictor's behavior. On the other hand, as observed in [15], the GLRM method is very demanding in terms of training data (owing to its sensitiveness to outliers and the sparsity of its transformed space) and computation time (due to column generation). Finally, while the global feature selection and (3-way) feature binning performed in [9] let user control the size of each prediction rule, this may well lead to some information/accuracy loss.

Goal and Contribution. This research work was aimed at seeking a (locally) optimal ensemble of specialized (and complementary) LR models by training a Mixture of Experts (MoE) [6] neural network, which consists of multiple "experts" (the LR models) and a sparse "gate" module responsible for assigning any data instance to one of the experts. The proposed approach shares some features with a method presented in [5]. Specifically, in [5], several MoE variants, differing in the forms of the gate (black-box vs. interpretable) and of the experts (only interpretable vs. also including a DNN), are trained to predict a numerical target, using a combined loss function including many regularization terms (e.g., related to the degree of load balance among the experts).

Our approach to discovering an interpretable MoE-based outcome predictor, called *MoE-OPM*, relies upon several ad hoc design choices and novel technical solutions:

- For the sake of interpretability and scalability, the gate and expert models play as LR classifiers (in fact, all these modules are one-layer neural networks with linear activations and a final softmax/sigmoid link function); this allows for directly learning several local LR-like outcome predictors and an associated interpretable assignment function like in LLM models [15, 16].
- Differently from [5], we let the user control the complexity (and thus the interpretability) of the model by fixing the maximum number $kTop$ of features that the gate and each expert sub-net can use, in addition to specifying the desired number m of experts. However, instead of resorting to a preliminary global feature selection step as in [16] and [9], the model is trained using all the original data features, while using L1-based regularization terms to encourage model sparsity; the parameters of each trained sub-net (i.e., either the gate or an expert) are then pruned in a "feature-based" way, by zeroing all but the $kTop$ most important input features of the sub-net. Each expert can thus use a specific subset of input features when making predictions for the data instances assigned to it.
- We prefer not to enforce expert load balance (e.g., using an ad-hoc loss term as in [5]), to possibly prune redundant experts for the sake of model compactness.

Tests on benchmark logs confirmed that the proposed approach achieves compelling accuracy scores (w.r.t. state-of-the-art interpretable outcome-prediction models [9, 15, 16]), and supports compact and faithful-by-design prediction explanations (in the form of feature-attribution scores) –see Sect. 4.3 for an example concerning a real-life health-care process.

2   Background and Problem Statement

As usual, assume that for every execution instance of the process under analysis (a.k.a. *process instance*), a distinguished *trace* is stored, which consists of a (temporally ordered) sequence of (log) *events*, plus several instance-level attributes that do not vary during the process execution. Each event is a tuple representing a process execution event, which usually stores information on the execution of a process activity (e.g., which activity was executed, the executor, a timestamp, etc.).

At run time, during the unfolding of a process instance, a trace is recorded incrementally which stores the events observed for that instance. Such a trace is called a *prefix trace* and represents pre-mortem log data. Let us denote U the universe of all possible prefix traces produced by the business process under analysis.

Problem OPM *Discovery*. This work aims at discovering a predictive model for (probabilistically) forecasting the outcome class of a running process instance. As mentioned before, for the sake of model interpretability and prediction explainability, we use a propositional representation of all log traces (be them prefix or complete ones) to both train and apply such a model, similarly to [9, 15, 16]. Specifically, we encode each trace into a tuple by using the *aggregation encoding* of [19], which essentially amounts to first turning each categorical attribute into a number of boolean attributes (one for each attribute-value pair) and then replacing all the occurrences of each resulting trace attribute a with a fixed number of aggregate values (namely, the occurrence count of a if it is boolean, or the average and standard deviation of a if it is numerical). The resulting tabular representation of log traces is eventually standardized.

Let us then assume that each trace $\tau \in U$ has been turned into a real-valued vector $x \in \mathbb{R}^d$ (for some suitable $d \in \mathbb{N}$), and its class label is encoded as a one-hot vector $y \in \{0, 1\}^{c-1}$, where c is the number of outcome classes. For the sake of simplicity, and w.l.o.g, let us on the case of two outcome classes (i.e., $c = 2$), as done in [9].

Under this perspective, an *OPM* can be re-defined as a neural network N that encodes a function $f_N : \mathbb{R}^d \to [0, 1]$ mapping the vectorial representation x of any (prefix) trace in U to an estimate of the probability that x belongs to the second class (i.e., the one associated with label 1). Then, the inductive learning problem faced in this work amounts to training a neural net N of this form out of a given collection of class-labeled prefix traces, once turning them into a pair (X, Y) of tensors that store (numerical representations of) the propositional encodings of these traces and their associated outcome labels, respectively.

3   Solution Approach

Similarly, to [5], we rephrase the problem of learning of a *OPM* into discovering a special (extremely sparse) kind of *Mixture of Experts* (*MoE*) ensemble that consists of multiple specialized outcome-oriented classifiers, named "experts", plus a "gate" module that routes each data sample to one of the experts. For the sake of readability, the conceptual architecture of a standard MoE is sketched in Fig. 1.

Definition 1 *(MoE-OPM). A* Mixture-of-Experts-OPM *(MoE-OPM) is a neural net of the form $\mathcal{N} = \langle \mathcal{N}_g, \mathcal{N}_1, \dots, \mathcal{N}_m \rangle$ that assembles two kinds of sub-nets: (i) $\mathcal{N}_1, \dots, \mathcal{N}_m$, called* experts, *which encode different (local) OPM functions $f_1, \dots, f_m \in [0, 1]^{(\mathbb{R}^d)}$, each mapping any trace encoding to an estimate of the probability that the respective process instance belongs to the second outcome class; and (ii) $\mathcal{N}_g$, named* gate, *which encodes a routing function $g : \mathbb{R}^d \to \Delta_m$ (with Δ_m denoting the probability simplex over $\{1, \dots, m\}$) that maps any trace encoding to a discrete probability distribution over the (indexes of the) experts. $\mathcal{N}$ itself is an OPM that encodes a function $f : \mathbb{R}^d \to [0, 1]$ defined as follows: $f(x) \triangleq f_k(x)$ such that $k = \arg\max_{k \in \{1, \dots, m\}} g(x)[k]$ and $g(x)[k]$ is the k-th component of the probability vector returned by g when applied to x.*   □

The experts and the gate sub-nets could be instantiated using different architectures. For the sake of interpretability and memory/computation saving, in this work we assume a *MoE-OPM* to adhere the following design choices: (*a*) expert sub-nets $\mathcal{N}_1, \dots, \mathcal{N}_m$ are all implemented as d-to-1 one-layer feed-forward nets with linear activation functions, followed by a standard sigmoid transformation; (*b*) the gate sub-net $\mathcal{N}_g$ is a one-layer

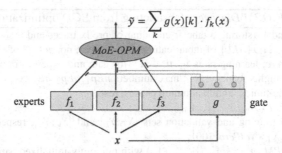

Fig. 1. Standard MoE architecture (for $m = 3$ experts). Each expert sub-net implements a specific classification function f_k, while gate's function g returns per-expert competency scores $g(x)[1], g(x)[2], g(x)[3]$ summing up to 1. In our *MoE-OPM* variant, the gate and experts are LR models, the gate is biased to return sparse competency scores, and x is classified by using only the expert getting the highest score.

d-to-m feed-forward network with linear activation functions followed by softmax normalization. This makes each expert and the gate behave as (standard/multinominal) *LR* models, widely reckoned as interpretable models.

Algorithm MoE-OPM Discovery. Such an ensemble model is discovered through Algorithm 1, named *MoE-OPM Discovery*. This algorithm takes several training instances as input, through tensors X (vectorized prefix traces) and Y (binary class labels), and the percentage *valPerc* of them to use for validation. To control the complexity of both the gate and expert sub-nets in the *MoE-OPM*, the user can set both the desired number m of experts and an upper bound $kTop$ to the number of input features that each of these sub-nets can use at prediction time. This feature-selection-like requisite is fulfilled by zeroing the weights of the connection parameters related to all the input features of a sub-model but the $kTop$ of them that look the most relevant ones for the sub-model (see later on). Further arguments are: the maximum number of SGD-based epochs for training the model (nEp_1), for fine-tuning the gate (nEp_2), and for re-tuning the model again after feature-weight pruning (nEp_3), the learning rates for training the gate (η_g) and each expert (η_e), and the weights λ_R and λ'_R of the loss regularization terms. To support ablation studies, one can set $kTop = ALL$, meaning that no parameters must be pruned and all the input features can be used by both the gate and every expert.

The algorithm consists of four computation phases: (i) train a randomly-initialized *MoE-OPM* end-to-end (Step 4); (ii) fine-tune the gate sub-net while keeping the parameters of the experts frozen (Step 5); (iii) zero all the parameter weights (Steps 7–8), in both the gate and the experts, that do not relate to the $kTop$ input features; (iv) re-train (for nEp_3 epochs) the *MoE-OPM* end-to-end to possibly adapt it to the removal of parameters (Step 19). All the training phases (*i, ii* and *iv*) are performed with the help procedure TRAIN, which implements a standard SGD-based optimization method if called with $freeze = $ **true**; by contrast, when called with $freeze = $ **false**), the optimization is restricted to the gate parameters only, while keeping those of the experts

---

Algorithm 1. *MoE-OPM Discovery* (abstracting from SGD optimization details).

Input: tensors X and Y (storing a tabular encoding of prefix traces and associated outcomes); max. no. $kTop \in \mathbb{N} \cup \{ALL\}$ of input features per sub-net; no. $m \in \mathbb{N}$ of experts; validation percentage *valPerc*; learning rates $\eta_g, \eta_e \in \mathbb{R}^+$ for gate and experts' training, respectively; regularization weights $\lambda_R, \lambda'_R \in \mathbb{R}^+$; max numbers $nEp_1, nEp_2, nEp_3 \in \mathbb{N}$ of epochs for the training, gate fine-tuning, and final tuning phases, resp.

Output: a *MoE-OPM* $\langle \mathcal{N}_g, \mathcal{N}_1, \dots, \mathcal{N}_m \rangle$.

1: split $[X;Y]$ into training and validation sets $[X_T;Y_T]$ and $[X_V;Y_V]$, respectively, such that $|X_V| = |Y_V| = \lfloor |X| \times valPerc/100 \rfloor$;
2: create a *MoE-OPM* $\mathcal{N} = \langle \mathcal{N}_g, \mathcal{N}_1, \dots, \mathcal{N}_m \rangle$ with randomly-initialized parameters Θ;
3: let $\Theta|_g, \Theta|_1, \dots, \Theta|_m$ denote the parameters of $\mathcal{N}_g, \mathcal{N}_1, \dots, \mathcal{N}_m$, respectively;
4:   TRAIN($\mathcal{N}, X_T, Y_T, X_V, Y_V, b, nEp_1, \eta_g, \eta_e, \lambda_R, \lambda'_R, freeze = $ **false**); // *train $\mathcal{N}$ end-to-end*
5:   TRAIN($\mathcal{N}, X_T, Y_T, X_V, Y_V, b, nEp_1, \eta_g, \eta_e, \lambda_R, \lambda'_R, freeze = $ **true**); // *fine-tune the gate only*
6: **if** $kTop \neq ALL$ **then**
7:     zero all $\mathcal{N}_g$'s weights but those linked to its top $kTop$ input features;
8:     zero all $\mathcal{N}_q$'s weights, for $q \in \{1, \dots, m\}$, but those with the top $kTop$ absolute values;
9:     TRAIN($\mathcal{N}, X_T, Y_T, X_V, Y_V, b, nEp_3, \eta_g, \eta_e, \lambda_R, \lambda'_R, freeze = $ **false**); // *re-tune $\mathcal{N}$*
10: **end if**
11: **return** $\mathcal{N}$

---

fixed. Note that all the experts contribute to each ensemble prediction during the training, and the training loss is estimated as in standard MoEs.

Loss and Feature Selection. Let $\mathcal{N} = \langle \mathcal{N}_g, \mathcal{N}_1, \dots, \mathcal{N}_m \rangle$ be a given *MoE-OPM*, $\mathcal{N}_E$ be the sub-net consisting of all its experts $\mathcal{N}_1, \dots, \mathcal{N}_m$, and *wgts(N)* be a function returning the connection-weight parameters of any neural net N. Then, for given paired sub-tensors X and Y, storing n training instances (denoted by $X[1], \dots, X[n]$) and their associated class labels (denoted by $Y[1], \dots, Y[n]$), respectively, the loss $\mathcal{L}(\mathcal{N}, X, Y)$ of $\mathcal{N}$ on X, Y is computed as follows:

$$\mathcal{L}(\mathcal{N}, X, Y) = \mathcal{L}_{acc}(\mathcal{N}, X, Y) + \lambda_R \cdot \mathcal{L}_{reg}(wgts(\mathcal{N}_g)) + \lambda'_R \cdot \mathcal{L}_{reg}(wgts(\mathcal{N}_E)) \quad (1)$$

$$\mathcal{L}_{acc}(\mathcal{N}, X, Y) = \frac{1}{n \cdot m} \sum_{i=1}^{n} \log \left(\sum_{k=1}^{m} g(X[i])[k] \cdot \left(1 + e^{\sigma^{-1}(f_k(X[i])) \cdot (1 - 2 \cdot Y[i])} \right) \right) \quad (2)$$

$$\mathcal{L}_{reg}(W) = \frac{\sum_{\theta \in W} |\theta|}{|W|}, \text{ for any given subset } W \text{ of network parameters} \quad (3)$$

The accuracy loss in Eq. 2, as discussed in both [5] and [6], is expected to favor expert specialization. The loss term in Eq. 3, looking like classic regularization (as in Lasso logistic regression) aims at shrinking less relevant weights, so helping spot the $kTop$ most important input features and eventually retain their associated weights only.

As concerns weight pruning, for each expert $\mathcal{N}_k$, we rank the weights in $wgts(\mathcal{N}_k)$ based on their absolute values, from the highest to the lowest, and zero all but the first $kTop$ of them. A "channel-wise" pruning is performed instead on $\mathcal{N}_g$, based on grouping its weights by the input features they relate to: the group of the i-th input feature gathers the weights of all the connections in $\mathcal{N}_g$ lying on a path starting from the i-th input node of $\mathcal{N}_g$. After ranking these weight groups based on their aggregated magnitude scores (each score is the absolute average value of the weights in a group), we eventually zero the weights of $\mathcal{N}_g$ that do not belong to any of the top $kTop$ groups.

In implementing our approach, each node in the input layer is paired with a multiplicative binary mask. This way, the parameters of each sub-model (i.e., the gate or an expert) can be pruned by setting to 0 all masks but those of its top $kTop$ features.

4 Experiments

For the sake of comparison, the proposed algorithm (implemented in *Python 3.11.4* and *PyTorch 2.0.1*, partly reusing code released in [5]) has been tested against several preprocessed datasets[1], derived from benchmark logs *BPIC 2011* and *Sepsis* that were also used in [9,15,16,19]. All these datasets, in tabular format, were built by making the respective prefix traces undergo the aggregation encoding (see Sect. 2) after extending them all with timestamp-derived temporal features (e.g., weekday, hour, etc.).

Essentially, log *BPIC 2011* stores the clinical history of Gynaecology patients in a Dutch hospital. Its events represent applied treatments and procedures. Four datasets, namely bpic2011_1, bpic2011_2, bpic2011_3, and bpic2011_4, were derived from this log by assigning each trace an outcome label based on the satisfaction of an LTL rule (label '1' for violation and '0' for adherence)—see [19] for details.

Log *Sepsis* stores care-flow data of Sepsis patients in a Dutch hospital, from Emergency Room (ER) registration to final discharge. Three datasets were derived from it by assigning each trace a boolean class label [19] equal to 0 iff the trace concerns an ER revisit within 28 days after discharge (dataset sepsis_1), an ICU admission (dataset sepsis_2), or a discharge type different from 'Release A' (dataset sepsis_3).

Test Procedure, Parameter Setting and Competitors. Each dataset was partitioned into training, validation, and test sets exactly as done in [9,15,19]: after sorting the traces based on their starting time, the first 80% of them were used for training each *OPM* and the remaining 20% for testing it; the last 20% of the training set was used as the validation set. The accuracy of each discovered model was evaluated by computing the AUC score for all test prefixes containing at least two events, as done in [9,15,19].

Algorithm *MoE-OPM Discovery* was run with a fixed configuration of all parameters but λ_R, $kTop$ and b, namely: $nEp_1 = nEp2 = 100$, $nEp3 = 0$, $m = 6$, $\eta_e = 10^{-5}$ and $\eta_g = 10^{-2}$. By the way, the number m of experts was chosen empirically (after trying several values in $[2, \ldots, 16]$), since this choice ensured a good accuracy-vs-simplicity trade-off. The following configurations were used for the regularization weights λ_R and λ_R' in the tests performed on dataset bpic2011_3 while setting $kTop$ equal to 2, 4, 6 and 8: $\lambda_R = \lambda_R' = 0.3$, $\lambda_R = \lambda_R' = 0.4$, $\lambda_R = \lambda_R' = 0.6$ and $\lambda_R = \lambda_R' = 0.8$, respectively. In the other tests, we evaluated the configurations $(kTop = 2; \lambda_R = 0.1)$, $(kTop = 4; \lambda_R = 0.2)$, $(kTop = 6; \lambda_R = 0.4)$ and $(kTop = 8; \lambda_R = 0.6)$, while setting λ_R to either 0.3, 0.4, 0.6, and 1.0, respectively, for datasets sepsis_1, sepsis_2 and sepsis_3, or to the same value as λ_R for the remaining datasets. For each dataset, the batch size was set empirically (using a value in [4..128]), as specified in the following: $b = 4$ for bpic2011_3,

---

[1] https://github.com/vinspdb/FOX.

$b = 4$ for sepsis_2 and sepsis_3 and all the other datasets derived from *BPIC 2011*, and $b = 32$ for sepsis_1.

This experimental analysis encompasses the outcome-predictor discovery methods *FOX* [9] and *GLRM* [15]. For these methods, we here report the results in the respective publications, remarking that they were obtained using exactly the same pre-processed data and test procedure as that described so far. As a further term of comparison, we consider a baseline method, denoted as *1-LR*, that returns one LR model—we simulated this method by running Algorithm *MoE-OPM Discovery* with $m = 1$ and $kTop = ALL$. We are not considering the LLM models discovered in [15], as they were obtained by fixing no bound on the number and size (i.e., the number of non-zero feature coefficients) of LR models appearing in the leaves.

4.1 Prediction Accuracy Analysis

Table 1 reports the AUC scores obtained by the 6-expert *MoE-OPM* models. Notably, *MoE-OPM Discovery* consistently outperforms the baseline *1-LR* in all *kTop* configurations over several datasets, namely bpic2011_1, bpic2011_3, bpic2011_4, sepsis_1 and sepsis_3. For the remaining datasets, there is always at least one *kTop* configuration where *MoE-OPM Discovery* performs better than the baseline. In particular, on average, *MoE-OPM Discovery* achieves an AUC improvement of more than 20% over *1-LR*, with peaks reaching beyond 80%, when combining the latter with feature selection. This confirms that training multiple local LR outcome predictors usually improves the performance of training a single LR model on all the data features (as done by *1-LR*). In addition, *MoE-OPM Discovery* always surpasses state-of-the-art methods FOX and GLRM on all the datasets but bpic2011_2 and bpic2011_3, where some of them perform as well as *MoE-OPM Discovery*.

Notably, *MoE-OPM Discovery* obtains outstanding achievements with different settings of $kTop \neq ALL$, showing that this hyper-parameter helps improve model accuracy (besides reducing model complexity). Precisely, the advantage of exploiting the feature-reduction capability of *MoE-OPM Discovery*, rather than making it just return a *MoE-OPM* trained on all the input features ($kTop = ALL$), is neat on all the datasets but bpic2012_2. Generally, likely owing to information loss, *MoE-OPM Discovery* tends to perform worse when using very few features (namely, $kTop = 2, 4$) than when trained with a slightly larger feature set (namely, $kTop = 6, 8$). However, on dataset bpic2011_1, *MoE-OPM Discovery* manages to achieve outstanding AUC scores even when using just two features.

The fact that the proposed approach achieves compelling AUC results with less than 9 input features per sub-model backs the interpretability of the models that it can discover and their suitability for prediction explanation. A brief discussion on the description and explanation complexities of the models discovered by both this approach and FOX is given in the following subsection. No similar discussion is conducted for GLRM and LLM models, as we did not found detailed information on this regard in the current version of [15]. Anyway, let us remark that all LLM models discovered from (a dataset derived from) logs *BPIC 2011* and *Sepsis* include at least 290 and 84 features per LR model, respectively, and may well contain hundreds of LR models (see [15] for the case

Table 1. AUC scores obtained by: algorithm *MoE-OPM Discovery*, run with a fixed number ($m = 6$) of experts and several values of *kTop* (namely, 2,4,6,8 and *ALL*), the baseline method *1-LR* and three state-of-the-art competitors. For each dataset, the best score is shown in **Bold and underlined**; each score obtained by *MoE-OPM Discovery* is shown in **Bold** if it outperforms all the competitors and in *Italic* otherwise.

Dataset	MoE-OPM Discovery					Competitors		
	kTop					1-LR	FOX [9]	GLRM [15]
	2	4	6	8	ALL			
bpic2011_1	0.97	0.95	0.96	**0.98**	0.88	0.94	0.97	0.92
bpic2011_2	0.85	0.84	0.86	**0.97**	0.87	0.94	0.92	**0.97**
bpic2011_3	0.95	**0.98**	0.96	**0.98**	0.91	0.97	**0.98**	**0.98**
bpic2011_4	0.69	0.81	0.80	0.81	0.80	0.68	**0.89**	0.81
sepsis_1	0.49	0.55	**0.56**	**0.58**	0.49	0.47	**0.58**	0.47
sepsis_2	0.56	0.56	**0.75**	0.73	0.72	0.74	0.73	0.73
sepsis_3	0.56	0.61	**0.72**	**0.72**	0.69	0.70	0.68	0.65

of bpic2011_2). This makes it hard for process stakeholders/analysts to understand and assess the trustworthiness of these LLM models.

4.2 Complexity/Interpretability and Efficiency of the Discovered OPMs

Generally, the lower the description complexity of a prediction model, the easier to interpret (and to trust/debug) the model and explain its predictions. In the cases of *MoE-OPM Discovery* and of baseline *1-LR*, description complexity is computed by counting the non-zero parameters appearing in the respective LR (sub-)models.

In contrast, the complexity of a FOX model can be quantified as the total number of conditions appearing (as conjuncts) in the respective fuzzy rules. Based on [9] if applying FOX to a filtered version of dataset bpic2011_1 (resp., bpic2011_1, ..., bpic2011_4, sepsis_1, ..., sepsis_3) containing only the top 4 (resp., 7, 6, 2, 5, 4 and 6 data features), 81 (resp., 2187, 729, 9, 243, 81, and 729) fuzzy rules are found. This means that the complexities of these models range from 18 to 15309.

To give an idea of the better accuracy-interpretability trade-off achieved by algorithm *MoE-OPM Discovery* on all the datasets (excluding bpic11_4), for each of them, let us focus on the minimal value of *kTop* that allowed the algorithm to match or surpass the AUC achievements of all the competitors, i.e., $kTop = 8$ on bpic2011_1, bpic2011_2, $kTop = 4$ on bpic2011_3 and sepsis_2, and $kTop = 6$ on all the remaining datasets. Since the parameters (including bias vectors) in these *MoE-OPMs* are $2 \times (kTop + 1) \times m$, where $m = 6$ is the desired number of experts, their complexities are bounded by 108. This leads us to believe that *MoE-OPM Discovery* tends to find more compact models than FOX.

On the other hand, when using a *MoE-OPM* to predict a novel trace x, a faithful local explanation of the prediction can be obtained by looking at the *kTop* feature weights of the LR expert that has been exploited to make the prediction. In the case of a FOX

Expert	0	1	2	3	4	5
Activity_CRP	0,00	0,00	0,00	-0,44	0,00	0,35
Activity_IV Liquid	0,85	0,00	-0,47	0,00	0,00	0,00
Activity_Release B	-0,32	-0,40	0,00	0,00	0,00	0,00
DiagnosticArtAstrup	0,00	0,40	0,00	0,00	0,00	0,00
DiagnosticSputum	0,00	0,00	0,00	-0,36	0,00	0,00
Hypotensie	0,00	0,00	0,00	0,00	-0,38	0,00
Oligurie	0,00	0,00	0,00	0,00	0,00	-0,37
SIRSCritHeartRate	0,00	0,00	0,00	0,00	-0,44	0,00
SIRSCritTemperature	0,00	0,00	0,00	0,00	-0,41	0,55
mean_hour	-0,33	0,00	0,00	0,00	0,00	0,00
mean_timesincelastevent	0,00	0,00	0,00	0,00	-0,36	0,00
org:group_A	0,00	0,00	-0,49	0,00	0,00	0,00
org:group_G	0,00	-0,34	0,00	0,00	0,00	0,00
org:group_H	0,00	0,00	0,00	0,52	0,00	0,00
org:group_O	0,00	0,00	0,00	0,00	0,00	0,36
org:group_T	0,00	0,00	-0,46	0,00	0,00	0,00
org:group_V	0,00	0,00	-0,48	0,00	0,00	0,00
org:group_W	0,00	0,34	0,00	0,00	0,00	0,00
org:group_other	-0,34	0,00	0,00	0,00	0,00	0,00
std_timesincemidnight	0,00	0,00	0,00	-0,33	0,00	0,00

Fig. 2. Example *MoE-OPM* discovered by *MoE-OPM Discovery* (with $kTop = 4$) from dataset sepsis_3: parameter weights of the six LR experts. The weights, linking each expert to one input feature, are shown in an orange-to-blue color scale based on their values—the lower (resp., higher) the value, the closer to orange (resp., blue). (Color figure online)

model, though one could focus on a few top-fitting fuzzy rules (or just on the best-fitting one) to explain the prediction returned for x, several other rules may have impacted the forecast substantially. This descends from the fact in a FOX model, the prediction for x is made by fusing (via weighted averaging) those of all of its fuzzy rules (or, at least, of those with non-zero fit) while our *MoE-OPM* uses only one of its experts to this end.

Notably, a *MoE-OPM* can make an outcome prediction in a speedy and compute-efficient way through a forward pass throughout two single-layer linear sub-nets—i.e., the gate and the chosen expert, featuring $m \times (k + 1)$ and $k + 1$ parameters, respectively. This computation entails $(2 \times kTop + 1) \times (m + 1)$ FLOPs (Floating Point Operations)—i.e., less than 120 FLOPs when $m = 6$ and $kTop \leq 8$ as in the tests described above.

4.3 Qualitative Results: An Example of Discovered MoE-OPM

Figure 2 shows the input features and associated weights that are employed by the six LR experts discovered when running algorithm *MoE-OPM Discovery* with $kTop = 4$ on dataset sepsis_3, for which the outcome-prediction task is meant to estimate the probability that an in-treatment patient will leave the hospital with the prevalent release type (i.e., 'Release A'). Only 20 of the 86 data features are used by the experts in total, but the specific feature subset of the experts differ appreciably from one another. In a sense, this means that the experts learned different input-output mappings (capturing different contex-dependent process-outcome use cases).

For instance, Expert 0 attributes a positive influence of 'Activity_IV Liquid' (intra-venous fluid treatment) on predicting class 1 and a negative influence on this class from 'Activity_Release B' (a specific discharge type), 'mean_hour' (certain times of day), and 'org:group_other' (specific hospital groups). On the same class, Expert 1 attributes notable positive influence from 'DiagnosticArtAstrup' (arterial blood gas measurement) and 'org:group_W' (a hospital staff team) and negative influence from 'Activity_Release B' and 'org:group_G' (another hospital group). Expert 2 focuses on scenarios where 'Activity_IV Liquid' and certain hospital groups ('org:group_A', 'org:group_T', 'org:group_V') influence negatively the occurrence of class-1 outcomes. Analogous interpretations can be extracted from the remaining expert models, which also focus on specific activities and hospital groups.

Focusing on such a small number of feature importance scores, a domain expert can quickly inspect and assess the internal decision logic of the model and get simple, faithful explanations for its predictions. However, evaluating the practical relevance of such explanations is left to future work.

5 Conclusion and Future Work

We have proposed an approach to learning an MoE-like interpretable Outcome Prediction Model (OPM) consisting of multiple LR-based expert *OPMs* and an LR-based gate for dynamically selecting one expert to predict the outcome of a new process instance, say x. The discovered model transparently shows the features of x that drove the prediction result and the choice of routing x to a specific expert.

The approach gives the user full control on the size of the discovered *OPM*. Besides favoring interpretability, this feature (combined with the conditional computation scheme implemented by the gate) makes the approach appealing for green AI applications [12]) where compute-efficient ML solutions are needed.

Despite using a lossy encoding of log data, one-layer linear sub-nets, and a rough model pruning strategy, the approach achieved a good trade-off between outcome-prediction accuracy and model/explanation complexity on popular benchmark logs.

As to future work, we will investigate: (i) converting LR-like sub-models returned by our approach into logic rules, which some users may prefer to feature-attribution scores, (ii) tuning hyper-parameters $kTop$ and m automatically; (ii) leveraging prior knowledge and (iv) adapting our framework to predict violations to declarative models [3]. We also plan to expand the empirical study by including more datasets, scalability, and temporal stability analyses [18] and more discussion of qualitative results.

Acknowledgments. This work was partly supported by project FAIR - Future AI Research (PE00000013), under the NRRP MUR program funded by the EU-NGEU, and project PIN-POINT - exPlaInable kNowledge-aware PrOcess INTelligence, under program PRIN, funded by the Italian Ministry of University and Research (grant no. B27G22000160001).

References

1. Bibal, A., et al.: Is attention explanation? An introduction to the debate. In: Proceedings of 60th Meeting of the Association for Computational Linguistics (ACL 2022), pp. 3889–3900 (2022)
2. Elkhawaga, G., Abu-Elkheir, M., Reichert, M.: Explainability of predictive process monitoring results: can you see my data issues? Appl. Sci. **12**(16), 8192 (2022)
3. Fionda, V., Guzzo, A.: Control-flow modeling with declare: behavioral properties, computational complexity, and tools. IEEE Trans. Knowl. Data Eng. **32**(5), 898–911 (2020)
4. Galanti, R., et al.: Explainable predictive process monitoring. In: Proceedings of 2nd International Conference on Process Mining (ICPM 2020), pp. 1–8 (2020)
5. Ismail, A.A., Arik, S.Ö., Yoon, J., Taly, A., Feizi, S., Pfister, T.: Interpretable mixture of experts for structured data. arXiv preprint arXiv:2206.02107 (2022)
6. Jacobs, R.A., Jordan, M.I., Nowlan, S.J., Hinton, G.E.: Adaptive mixtures of local experts. Neural Comput. **3**(1), 79–87 (1991)
7. Márquez-Chamorro, A.E., Resinas, M., Ruiz-Cortés, A.: Predictive monitoring of business processes: a survey. IEEE Trans. Serv. Comput. **11**(6), 962–977 (2017)
8. Pasquadibisceglie, V., et al.: ORANGE: outcome-oriented predictive process monitoring based on image encoding and CNNs. IEEE Access **8**, 184073–184086 (2020)
9. Pasquadibisceglie, V., Castellano, G., Appice, A., Malerba, D.: FOX: a neuro-fuzzy model for process outcome prediction and explanation. In: Proceedings of 3rd International Conference on Process Mining (ICPM 2021), pp. 112–119 (2021)
10. Rama-Maneiro, E., Vidal, J., Lama, M.: Deep learning for predictive business process monitoring: review and benchmark. IEEE Trans. Serv. Comput. (2021)
11. Rizzi, W., Francescomarino, C.D., Maggi, F.M.: Explainability in predictive process monitoring: when understanding helps improving. In: Proceedings of 18th International Conference on Business Process Management (BPM 2020) (2020)
12. Salehi, S., Schmeink, A.: Data-centric green artificial intelligence: a survey. IEEE Trans. Artif. Intell. 1–18 (2023)
13. Sindhgatta, R., Moreira, C., Ouyang, C., Barros, A.: Exploring interpretable predictive models for business processes. In: Fahland, D., Ghidini, C., Becker, J., Dumas, M. (eds.) BPM 2020. LNCS, vol. 12168, pp. 257–272. Springer, Cham (2020). https://doi.org/10.1007/978-3-030-58666-9_15
14. Slack, D., Hilgard, A., Singh, S., Lakkaraju, H.: Reliable post hoc explanations: modeling uncertainty in explainability. Adv. Neural. Inf. Process. Syst. **34**, 9391–9404 (2021)
15. Stevens, A., De Smedt, J.: Explainability in process outcome prediction: guidelines to obtain interpretable and faithful models. arXiv:2203.16073 (2023)
16. Stevens, A., De Smedt, J., Peeperkorn, J.: Quantifying explainability in outcome-oriented predictive process monitoring. In: Process Mining Workshops, pp. 194–206 (2022)
17. Stierle, M., Weinzierl, S., Harl, M., Matzner, M.: A technique for determining relevance scores of process activities using graph-based neural networks. Decis. Support Syst. **144**, 113511 (2021)
18. Teinemaa, I., Dumas, M., Leontjeva, A., Maggi, F.M.: Temporal stability in predictive process monitoring. Data Min. Knowl. Disc. **32**, 1306–1338 (2018)
19. Teinemaa, I., Dumas, M., Rosa, M.L., Maggi, F.M.: Outcome-oriented predictive process monitoring: review and benchmark. ACM Trans. Knowl. Discov. Data **13**(2), 1–57 (2019)
20. Wickramanayake, B., et al.: Building interpretable models for business process prediction using shared and specialised attention mechanisms. Knowl.-Based Syst. **248**, 108773 (2022)
21. Zhou, Y., Booth, S., Ribeiro, M.T., Shah, J.: Do feature attribution methods correctly attribute features? In: Proceedings of AAAI Conference on Artificial Intelligence (AAAI 2022), pp. 9623–9633 (2022)

Understanding the Impact of Design Choices on the Performance of Predictive Process Monitoring

Sungkyu Kim[1] , Marco Comuzzi[1]([✉]) , and Chiara Di Francescomarino[2]

[1] Ulsan National Institute of Science and Technology, Ulsan, Korea
{kimkangf3,mcomuzzi}@unist.ac.kr
[2] University of Trento, Trento, Italy
c.difrancescomarino@unitn.it

Abstract. Predictive process monitoring (PPM) aims at creating models that predict aspects of interest of process execution using historical data available in event logs, mostly using machine learning (ML) techniques. When developing a PPM model, one has several design choices, encompassing both ML-related concerns, such as which classification or regression model to choose, and PPM-specific concerns, such as how to encode the trace prefixes or whether to drop infrequent activities when training a model. While the literature has seen a few attempts to study how these choices impact the performance of a PPM model, no systematic studies on this matter exist. This paper moves towards closing this gap. We propose a framework to interpret the impact of design choices on the performance of a PPM model. The proposed framework uses as building blocks a search space exploration algorithm, which is able to generate different model configurations, and explainable AI techniques, e.g., SHAP, to analyze the impact of design choices on the model performance based on the generated configurations. We show an instantiation of the framework in the use case of outcome-oriented PPM, discussing also the experimental results obtained using publicly available event logs.

Keywords: Business Process · Prediction · Guidelines

1 Introduction

Predictive process monitoring (PPM) aims at creating predictive models of business process execution using the historic data available in event logs, often exploiting machine learning (ML) techniques [8]. PPM historically has considered three aspects to be predicted: the activities that will be executed next in a running case, the timestamps of such activities (including the remaining case duration), and the outcome of running cases, as usually captured by a categorical label.

The development of PPM models requires setting a value for various hyperparameters [1,5]. These include both typical ML hyperparameters of the classification or regression techniques chosen to develop a model, as well as others that

Sponsored by the NRF Korea, Grant Number 2022R1F1A1072843.

J. De Smedt and P. Soffer (Eds.): ICPM 2023 Workshops, LNBIP 503, pp. 153–164, 2024.
https://doi.org/10.1007/978-3-031-56107-8_12

are specific to the PPM task at hand. For instance, one needs to choose how to encode the trace event data to obtain a feature vector and whether to divide the trace prefixes into buckets when training a model, determining if needed the number and types of buckets.

Getting insights into the impact of these design choices on the performance of a PPM model can be crucial for model developers. While a few papers have tried to create benchmarks for different PPM tasks (e.g. [11,13,16]) and few works have focused on searching for the best hyperparameters for a PPM task [1,5], there is no empirical work in the literature specifically aiming at understanding the impact of the hyperparameter values on the performance of a PPM technique. Moreover, since some of these hyperparameters are PPM-specific, we cannot simply adapt insights obtained for other ML scenarios. In this context, this work focuses on the outcome-oriented PPM task, aiming to answer the following research question: "How does the value of PPM-specific hyperparameters impact the performance of outcome-oriented PPM models?"

Answering this question can be crucial for model developers. By knowing in advance which parameter values are more likely to yield a well-performing model, they may save huge amounts of time and computational resources when developing a PPM model. Knowledge about the optimal hyperparameter values can also inform the development of AutoML solutions for PPM, reducing the effort of exploring the space determined by the hyperparameter value combinations.

From a methodological standpoint, this question could be tackled by creating an empirical benchmark testing several configurations of hyperparameter values on different event log datasets. As mentioned earlier, this has been tried in [11, 13,16], even though not systematically, and it requires a massive effort in terms of computational cost and analysis. In this work, we take a novel and more lightweight approach, exploiting the capabilities of explainable AI techniques.

More in detail, we propose a general framework for interpreting the impact of design choices on the PPM model performance that includes three phases. In the first phase, a search space exploration algorithm is used to generate an extensive number of hyperparameter value configurations to configure an outcome-oriented PPM model. In the second phase, these configurations are used as feature vectors associated with a numerical value of the performance of the corresponding PPM model, e.g., model accuracy or AUC, to fit a regression model. Finally, in the third phase, XAI techniques are used to "interpret" the contribution made by each feature, i.e., hyperparameter value, on the model performance, i.e., the predicted numerical label.

We discuss an instantiation of the proposed framework based on the genetic algorithm-based search space exploration techniques proposed in [5], as well as SHAP and Explainable Boosting Machines as XAI techniques, discussing the results obtained on publicly available event logs.

The paper is organised as follows. After a discussion of the related work in Sect. 2, Sect. 3 introduces the general framework. The specific instantiation of the framework that we implemented is discussed in Sect. 4, while the experimental results are reported and discussed in Sect. 5. Conclusions are finally drawn in Sect. 6.

2   Related Work

We can roughly classify the literature related to this paper into two groups: (i) the works related to outcome-oriented Predictive Process Monitoring; (ii) the state-of-the-art concerning AutoML.

Outcome-oriented Predictive Process Monitoring focuses on predicting the outcome (e.g., the satisfaction of a business objective) of a process [13]. In [2,8] the sequence of activities already carried out and the data payload of the last activity are leveraged to make predictions on the fulfilment (or the violation) of a boolean predicate in a running case. In [6], traces are considered as complex symbolic sequences, i.e., sequences of activities each carrying its data payload, and different approaches for feature encoding are considered. In [15], the approach in [6] has been extended by clustering the historical traces before classification. In [13], a comparison of the existing outcome-based predictive monitoring approaches is presented.

AutoML automates the process of developing the best model, e.g., the most accurate one, to address a given machine learning task, or speeding up the model development phase. Different AutoML frameworks, such as Auto-sklearn, Tree-Based Pipeline Optimization Tool (TPOT), or H2O, provide different automated solutions for each different step of the typical machine learning pipeline [4,17], such as data preparation or hyperparameter optimisation. Several approaches in machine learning have been proposed for the selection of a learning algorithm [10], for the tuning of hyperparameters [3], and for the combined optimization of both the algorithm and the hyperparameters [14]. AutoML has been generally neglected by the PPM literature, with the exception of [1,5]. In [1], an approach based on a genetic algorithm has been proposed for the identification of the best configuration, in terms of predictive models, encodings and bucketing methods, for PPM tasks. In [5], besides encoding and bucketing methods, additional parameters, such as the dropping of infrequent activities, as well as a broader set of models have been used.

3   A Framework for Analyzing Design Choices

Figure 1 depicts the proposed framework for the analysis of the design choices in outcome-based PPM. We assume that the design choices are captured by the values of PPM model hyperparameters. As mentioned in the Introduction, these may range from the classification and trace encoding technique adopted, up to the number of buckets in which trace prefixes are divided. The *search space* is constituted by the combination of all the values of such hyperparameters. A *configuration* is a point in the search space, in which one value is assigned to each hyperparameter. For example, a configuration may be determined by choosing to use a decision tree, encoding traces using index-based encoding, and considering only one bucket containing all the encoded trace prefixes when training/testing.

The input of the framework is an event log and, if necessary, an initial hyperparameter configuration. In the first step of the framework, a search-space exploration algorithm is used to generate a set of hyperparameter configurations and

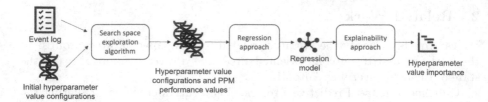

Fig. 1. Framework overview

to compute the corresponding PPM performance values, that is, the PPM performance values obtained by using that configuration. To this aim, we start from an event log and an initial set of hyperparameter configurations and we explore the search space of the PPM model hyperparameter configuration values by generating new configurations. For each configuration, the performance of the PPM model obtained by leveraging it on the event log is computed. Note that different types of algorithms may be chosen, e.g., grid search, optimization-based, or evolutionary-based.

Once the hyperparameter configurations and the performance metrics of the corresponding outcome-oriented PPM model have been generated, in the second step of the framework, they are transformed into numeric feature vectors and used to train a regression model that aims at predicting, given a configuration of hyperparameter values, the performance of the corresponding PPM model, that is, the model built using that particular configuration.

Finally, in the third and last step, a post-hoc explainer for XAI is applied on top of the regression model in order to understand the impact of each feature (i.e., hyperparameter configuration value) on the performance of the model to give users explainability in setting hyperparameter configuration of PPM.

4   Instantiating the Framework in Outcome-Oriented PPM

We instantiate the framework described in Sect. 3 by leveraging for the exploration of the search space an existing GA-based exploration approach (described in [5]). The algorithm aims at optimizing the performance of the outcome-oriented PPM models built leveraging the hyperparameter value configurations. More specifically, for each event log, each individual of the population of the genetic algorithm corresponds to a hyperparameter value configuration as well as to the outcome-oriented PPM model obtained by using that specific configuration. The fitness function, which is defined as:

$$f(i) = [sc(i) + re(i)]/2 \tag{1}$$

aims at optimizing the performance of such a PPM model by maximizing a performance score $sc(i)$, computed as the average AUC and accuracy of the PPM model i, and minimizing the error rate. The latter is captured by the term

$re(i)$, which is defined as $1 - failurerate(i)$, where the failure rate is defined as the percentage of cases in which the outcome predicted by the model i has a class probability lower than 0.7.

The GA-based exploration approach introduced in [5] considers the following design space:

Model: Even though any classification model can be used, the literature highlights that tree-based classifiers show better performance in outcome-based PPM [13]. We consider four tree-based models, including both individual and ensemble classifiers: Decision Tree (DT), Random Forest (RF), XGBoost (XGB), and LightGBM (LGBM).

Drop_act: this configuration parameter captures the process of removing low-frequency activities from an event log, which may reduce the computational cost and improve the model performance [12]. We consider a discrete gap-based scale for this parameter, i.e., dropping the 2, 4, 6, or 8 less frequent activities in an event log.

Bucketing: When pre-processing an event log for outcome-based prediction, the prefixes of each trace are extracted to construct a prefix log. The prefixes then can be grouped into so-called *buckets*. A different classification model is trained for each bucket. In this paper, we consider prefix-length bucketing, in which prefixes are grouped by length, i.e., number of events. A base strategy (zero-bucketing) groups all prefixes in a single bucket, thus training a single classifier. Bucketing allows the grouping of homogeneous prefixes, which may improve the accuracy of the trained models. Given an input event log, this parameter assumes values comprised between 1 (corresponding to zero-bucketing) up to two times the mean length of the traces in an event log. The value n of this parameter signifies that n buckets are created. If for instance, $n = 3$ and the maximum length of trace in a log is six events, then three buckets are created containing the prefixes of length 1 and 2, 3 and 4, 5 and 6, respectively.

Encoding: The prefixes must be numerically encoded to be fed into the model. The problem of encoding prefixes is one of complex symbolic sequence encoding [6] and can be approached in multiple ways. In this paper, we consider the *aggregation* and *index-based* encodings. Aggregation is a lossy encoding, which represents entire event sequence attributes into a single entity, for example, based on frequency. Index-based is a lossless encoding that maintains the order of events in a prefix. In index-based encoding, each event in a prefix is encoded into a fixed number of numerical features.

Table 1 shows an example of a possible set of generated hyperparameter value configurations and the corresponding PPM model performance values.

As a regression model, we consider the Explainable Boosting Machine (EBM), a tree-based cyclic gradient boosting generalized additive model with automatic interaction detection [7]. Despite the simplicity of the prediction task for the regression model in this research, we selected EBM over the simple linear regression model because of its intelligibility, accuracy, and ability to detect pairwise interaction among features. A pairwise interaction refers to how two features in

Table 1. Example of hyperparameter values configurations and corresponding fitness function values

Model	Drop_act	Bucketing	Encoding	Fitness function
DT	2	1	index-based	0.93
XGB	3	3	aggregation	0.97
DT	4	6	aggregation	0.85
...				

a statistical or machine learning model interact with each other to determine the outcome of the model.

Thus, EBM is interpretable and it offers global explanations of the model in terms of both feature contribution and interaction effects. Yet, we also consider the Shapley Additive exPlanations (SHAP) to answer our research question precisely. While EBM provides global explanations with both feature contribution and interaction terms, SHAP is considered to offer more precise feature contribution values by considering marginal contributions. To summarize, the instantiated framework for outcome-oriented PPM provides explanations in the form of feature contribution and feature interaction analysis of the regression model: SHAP is used to calculate the feature contribution, whereas the EBM model is used to analyze the interaction among features towards determining the output of the model.

5　Experimental Results and Discussion

In this section, we first introduce the event log datasets that we considered in the experiment in Sect. 5.1. Then, we aim to answer our research question: "How does the value of PPM-specific hyperparameters impact the performance of outcome-oriented PPM models?". This is done in two steps with XAI techniques. First, we present the results of the design feature contribution analysis using SHAP in Sect. 5.2; then we analyze the results obtained for the design feature contribution interaction analysis using EBM in Sect. 5.3.

5.1　Datasets

We consider four event logs made available by the Business Process Intelligence Challenge (BPIC) that are commonly used in the literature. We followed the same outcome labelling strategy of [13] for a total of 15 datasets. Table 2 shows the characteristics of each dataset.

The BPIC2011 log refers to a diagnosis and treatment process in the gynaecology department of a Dutch academic hospital. Since the treatments do not follow a strict process, it shows relatively high trace length compared to other datasets. The BPIC2012 log refers to a personal loan application process in a Dutch financial institute. There are three outcome labels defined for this log, i.e., whether an application is approved, cancelled, or rejected which yields three datasets in Table 2 (BPIC2012_1, BPIC2012_2, and BPIC2012_3, respectively). The BPIC2015 log refers to a building permit application process in 5

Table 2. Descriptive statistics of the datasets used in the experiments

Datasets	# Traces	Min length	Med length	Max length	# Events	# Activities	# Variants	Class ratio
BPIC2011_1	1058	1	24	1814	57850	193	734	0.77
BPIC2011_2	1058	1	50	1814	138542	251	900	0.36
BPIC2011_3	1045	1	21	1368	69078	190	783	0.91
BPIC2011_4	1058	1	42	1432	84873	231	900	0.76
BPIC2012_1	4685	15	35	175	186693	36	3790	0.46
BPIC2012_2	4685	15	35	175	186693	36	3790	0.70
BPIC2012_3	4685	15	35	175	186693	36	3790	0.84
BPIC2015_1	696	2	42	101	28775	380	677	0.72
BPIC2015_2	753	1	55	132	41202	396	752	0.77
BPIC2015_3	1328	3	42	124	57488	380	1285	0.76
BPIC2015_4	577	1	42	82	24234	319	576	0.82
BPIC2015_5	1051	5	50	134	54562	376	1049	0.64
BPIC2017_20	4982	10	22	148	139232	25	1460	0.71
BPIC2017_30	7473	10	26	148	240537	25	3104	0.63
BPIC2017_40	9964	10	29	148	341953	25	4625	0.60

different Dutch municipalities. The process at each municipality is captured by a different log, hence 5 datasets are considered (BPIC2015_1 to BPIC2015_5). Due to its long recording period (about four years for each municipality), the process has changed over the years, resulting in a significant increase in the number of traces relative to the number of variants compared to other datasets. Finally, the BPIC2017 log is an updated version of the BPIC2012 referring to a more recent period in which a new information system has been used at the Dutch financial institute. It follows the same labelling strategy of BPIC2012. However, since it is a very large event log, we created three versions of it considering only the "accepted" label and sampling 20%, 30%, and 40% of the original datasets, respectively, by removing traces belonging to infrequent variants. The datasets and the code to reproduce the experiments discussed next are available at https://github.com/brucks1217/Understanding-the-impact-of-design-choices.

5.2   Analyzing the Design Choices Using SHAP

Initially, we present the results of the mean absolute SHAP values to analyze the contribution of each configuration feature (that is, design choice) on the performance of the model. Note that the SHAP mean absolute value does not give any insights into the direction of the impact of the feature on the model performance, i.e., whether positive or negative.

Figure 2 shows the results obtained. An initial insight that can be drawn is that the feature bucketing is the most impactful design choice across all datasets. By looking at the differences among the different event logs, it seems that this feature is less impacting for event logs with a high number of activities, such as the BPIC2012 and BPIC 2017 event logs. Apart from bucketing, the choice of the model (in particular choosing RF) and of the index-based

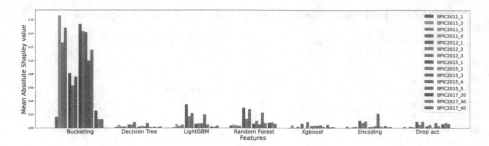

Fig. 2. Mean Absolute SHAP value of design choices

encoding seems to have an impact on the performance, while the impact of
drop-act looks limited. Another interesting remark is that the SHAP values of
model (especially LGBM and RF) for BPIC2012 are relatively higher in respect
of the one of bucketing when compared to other datasets. This implies that,
for BPIC2012, the choice of the model has a more significant impact on the
classification performance compared to other event logs. This is not the case, for
instance, for the BPIC2011_1 and BPIC2017 datasets. For these logs, the SHAP
value of all other features, except for bucketing, appears particularly low.

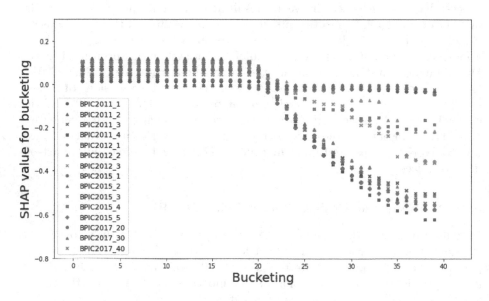

Fig. 3. SHAP values for design dimension bucketing

In contrast to the mean absolute SHAP value, which does not discriminate
between positive and negative feature contributions to the model output, the
SHAP value for each feature reveals how that feature impacts the model prediction according to its variations. We discuss here the results obtained for the

Table 3. SHAP values for the classification model design choice.

	BPIC2011_1	BPIC2011_2	BPIC2011_3	BPIC2011_4	BPIC2012_1
Decision Tree	−0.00669	−0.00969	−0.00879	−0.00664	−0.06741
Random Forest	0.00431	−0.00036	0.003	0.00261	0.02539
LightGBM	0.0001	0.0046	−0.00055	0.00359	0.01108
Xgboost	0.00265	0.00144	0.0028	−0.00307	0.01603
	BPIC2012_2	BPIC2012_3	BPIC2015_1	BPIC2015_2	BPIC2015_3
Decision Tree	−0.04098	−0.06018	−0.01325	−0.02103	−0.02345
Random Forest	0.01206	0.01463	0.00259	0.00308	0.00514
LightGBM	0.00033	0.01789	0.00524	0.0086	0.00312
Xgboost	0.0064	0.022228	0.00535	0.00802	0.0014
	BPIC2015_4	BPIC2015_5	BPIC2017_20	BPIC2017_30	BPIC2017_40
Decision Tree	−0.06446	−0.01537	−0.01542	−0.0169	−0.01391
Random Forest	0.03258	0.00446	-0.00507	−0.00201	−0.00224
LightGBM	−0.00768	0.00294	0.00837	0.00235	0.00288
Xgboost	0.0138	0.0053	0.01198	0.0171	0.01209

bucketing design feature (see Fig. 3), which appears to be the most impactful according to Fig. 2, the type of classification model chosen (see Table 3), and the encoding method (see Table 4). We leave instead out the drop_act feature, which does not seem to have an impact on the performance of the model.

In Fig. 3, we observe that the impact of the design feature **bucketing** is relatively small and positive for low values (below 20) and, at least for some event logs, e.g., the BPIC2011, stronger and negative for higher values. This could be due to the combined effect of the curse of dimensionality and sample size. As the number of buckets considered increases, in fact, while the size of the feature vector remains unchanged, the higher-sized buckets tend to contain a lower number of training observations, from which it becomes harder to learn a high-performing model. To sum up, based on the results shown in Fig. 3, we suggest that choosing a lower number of buckets is generally a good design choice.

From Table 3, we can observe that the decision tree model shows the lowest SHAP value, even negatively contributing to the model performance. The result confirms the trend already observed in existing outcome-oriented predictive process monitoring studies [6]: models based on ensemble principles outperform decision trees. The other models, differently from decision trees, are instead based on ensemble principles and, therefore, are generally more robust against higher dimension input datasets [9]. In the case of bagging (RF), multiple decision trees are built on random subsets of features and data. This randomness helps reducing the dominance of any single feature, thereby reducing the impact of irrelevant or noisy dimensions. On the other hand, the boosting algorithms (LightGBM, XGB) assign higher importance to the most informative features, thus effectively reducing the dimension of the problem. To sum up, our analysis suggests that an ensemble classifier should always be preferred in outcome-oriented PPM.

Regarding **encoding** methods (see Table 4), it appears that the index-based encoding has in most cases a positive, albeit relatively small, impact on the model performance, whereas the aggregation encoding method has a (small) negative impact. Although aggregation encoding leverages information from the events, it still incurs in information loss by disregarding the sequential order of events. Furthermore, event attributes may lose their characteristics as they are

Table 4. SHAP values for the encoding method design choice.

	BPIC2011_1	BPIC2011_2	BPIC2011_3	BPIC2011_4	BPIC2012_1
Index	0.00039	0.00508	−0.00212	0.00406	0.03083
Aggregate	−0.0008	−0.00673	0.00249	−0.00496	−0.03924
	BPIC2012_2	BPIC2012_3	BPIC2015_1	BPIC2015_2	BPIC2015_3
Index	0.02038	0.02012	0.00568	0.00579	0.00646
Aggregate	−0.01476	−0.02269	−0.00592	−0.00652	−0.00596
	BPIC2015_4	BPIC2015_5	BPIC2017_20	BPIC2017_30	BPIC2017_40
Index	0.01876	0.0056	0.00185	0.00117	0.00297
Aggregate	−0.02033	−0.00373	−0.00177	−0.00143	−0.00322

Table 5. Interaction score between design choices `bucketing` and `model`.

Model	Bucket size									
	1	10	20	30	39	1	10	20	30	39
	BPIC2011					BPIC2012				
Decision Tree	0.004257	0.003379	−0.0004314	−0.003761	−0.008527	0.03858	0.03858	0.02379	−0.08415	−0.09621
Random Forest	−0.00005222	−0.0000507	−0.00004967	−0.00148	−0.0009228	−0.005275	−0.006052	−0.000339	0.01191	0.008619
LightGBM	0.000428	0.0007286	0.0006177	−0.002685	−0.007428	−0.02017	−0.008089	−0.007931	0.02883	0.03131
Xgboost	0.0007186	0.000747	0.001203	−0.001244	−0.004534	−0.009792	−0.007307	−0.003472	0.01785	0.01785
	BPIC2015					BPIC2017				
Decision Tree	0.0124	0.01233	0.003992	−0.02707	−0.03202	0.008328	0.000498	−0.003385	−0.003385	−0.004397
Random Forest	−0.005799	−0.005793	−0.005522	0.008644	0.007628	0.004186	0.00001259	−0.001621	−0.001004	−0.0004125
LightGBM	−0.002255	0.002389	0.0002062	−0.006223	−0.006966	−0.001326	−0.0006834	0.0006826	0.0004067	0.0008105
Xgboost	−0.002724	−0.001934	0.001076	0.0009886	0.0102	−0.003683	−0.001349	0.00286	0.00286	0.002662

represented in the form of descriptive statistics rather than in their original state like in index-based encoding. Hence, we conclude that, according to our analysis, index-based should be preferred.

5.3 Analyzing the Feature Interaction Contribution with EBM

Detecting pairwise interactions is one of the key functions of EBM, implemented by a score that captures the combined effect of two features. Briefly, given a pair of features x_i and x_j, the EBM creates a new *interaction* feature $x_{i,j} = (x_i, x_j)$. Then, the interaction score of these two features is the contribution towards the output of the model of $x_{i,j}$.

As an illustration, we discuss here the interaction scores that we obtained between `bucketing` (the most impactful design choice based on the analysis of Sect. 5.2) and `model`, and between `bucketing` and `encoding`. Table 5 reports the mean interaction score across all datasets between the `bucketing` and `model` design choices. We can observe that when the bucketing size is below 20, the DT model shows a higher interaction score than other models. When the bucketing size exceeds 20, the DT interaction score becomes negative. This shows a typical moderation effect that can be highlighted by the EBM analysis: when choosing to use a DT, a lower bucketing size is likely to improve the model performance.

Table 6 shows the mean interaction score across all datasets between `bucketing` and `encoding`. Except for the BPIC2015 case, the table confirms the findings of the SHAP analysis: index-based encoding and low bucketing size are "good" design choices. Index-based encoding, indeed, creates a more positive interaction effect on the model performance than aggregate encoding when the

Table 6. Interaction score between design choices **bucketing** and **encoding**.

Encoding method	Bucket size									
	1	10	20	30	39	1	10	20	30	39
	BPIC2011					BPIC2012				
Index-based	**0.003773**	0.0003773	**0.0008611**	−0.001043	−0.003819	**0.001459**	**0.001459**	−0.0006398	−0.005839	−0.0104
Aggregate	−0.001813	**0.001903**	−0.001327	−0.001677	**−0.001939**	−0.001304	−0.001304	−0.001105	**0.001635**	**0.01911**
	BPIC2015					BPIC2017				
Index-based	−0.005708	**0.001278**	−0.002065	−0.002983	**0.002614**	**0.001155**	**0.001155**	**0.001387**	−0.003359	−0.01516
Aggregate	**0.003296**	0.001943	**0.00259**	**0.002686**	−0.02655	−0.002047	0.0005249	−0.000774	**−0.0002954**	**−0.00003619**

size of buckets is below 20. As mentioned, the only exception to this trend is BPIC2015. This could be due to the fact that the BPIC2015 datasets refer to different municipalities — possibly with different characteristics — so the average scores for these logs may not be reliable.

6 Conclusions

We have presented a framework to understand the impact of design choices on the performance of a PPM model. The framework has been instantiated in the case of outcome-oriented PPM, using an existing GA-based model configuration generator and SHAP/EBM to explain the impact of the model design features on the model performance. We have applied the framework to several publicly available event logs, obtaining a set of general recommendations for developing high-performing outcome-oriented PPM, such as preferring a lower bucketing size, ensemble classifiers, and using index-based trace encoding.

The work presented here can be extended in many ways. New instantiations can be generated and possibly compared. These may refer to other PPM use cases and/or different search space exploration algorithms and explainability approaches. The results presented in this paper suggest that the best design choices may depend on the context, i.e., the type of process generating a log. Event log complexity meta-features can be used to increase the degree of explainability, suggesting design choices for unseen contexts. We are also working on generating synthetic event logs with predefined characteristics to be able to assess more rigorously the insights obtained from the instantiation of the framework.

References

1. Di Francescomarino, C., et al.: Genetic algorithms for hyperparameter optimization in predictive business process monitoring. Inf. Syst. **74**, 67–83 (2018). Information Systems Engineering: selected papers from CAiSE 2016
2. Di Francescomarino, C., Dumas, M., Maggi, F.M., Teinemaa, I.: Clustering-based predictive process monitoring. IEEE Trans. Serv. Comput. **PP**(99), 1 (2017)
3. Hutter, F., Hoos, H.H., Leyton-Brown, K.: Sequential model-based optimization for general algorithm configuration. In: Coello, C.A.C. (ed.) LION 2011. LNCS, vol. 6683, pp. 507–523. Springer, Heidelberg (2011). https://doi.org/10.1007/978-3-642-25566-3_40

4. Karmaker, S.K., Hassan, M.M., Smith, M.J., Xu, L., Zhai, C., Veeramachaneni, K.: AutoML to date and beyond: challenges and opportunities. ACM Comput. Surv. **54**(8). Association for Computing Machinery, New York, NY, USA (2021)

5. Kwon, N., Comuzzi, M.: Genetic algorithms for AutoML in process predictive monitoring. In: Montali, M., Senderovich, A., Weidlich, M. (eds.) Process Mining Workshops. ICPM 2022. LNBIP, vol. 468, pp. 242–254. Springer, Cham (2023). https://doi.org/10.1007/978-3-031-27815-0_18

6. Leontjeva, A., Conforti, R., Di Francescomarino, C., Dumas, M., Maggi, F.M.: Complex symbolic sequence encodings for predictive monitoring of business processes. In: Motahari-Nezhad, H.R., Recker, J., Weidlich, M. (eds.) BPM 2015. LNCS, vol. 9253, pp. 297–313. Springer, Cham (2015). https://doi.org/10.1007/978-3-319-23063-4_21

7. Lou, Y., Caruana, R., Gehrke, J., Hooker, G.: Accurate intelligible models with pairwise interactions. In: Proceedings of the 19th ACM SIGKDD International Conference on Knowledge Discovery and Data Mining, pp. 623–631 (2013)

8. Maggi, F.M., Di Francescomarino, C., Dumas, M., Ghidini, C.: Predictive monitoring of business processes. In: Jarke, M., et al. (eds.) CAiSE 2014. LNCS, vol. 8484, pp. 457–472. Springer, Cham (2014). https://doi.org/10.1007/978-3-319-07881-6_31

9. Mohammed, A., Kora, R.: A comprehensive review on ensemble deep learning: opportunities and challenges. J. King Saud Univ.-Comput. Inf. Sci. (2023)

10. Pfahringer, B., Bensusan, H., Giraud-Carrier, C.: Meta-learning by landmarking various learning algorithms. In: In Proceedings of the 17th International Conference on Machine Learning, pp. 743–750. Morgan Kaufmann (2000)

11. Tama, B.A., Comuzzi, M.: An empirical comparison of classification techniques for next event prediction using business process event logs. Expert Syst. Appl. **129**, 233–245 (2019)

12. Tax, N., Sidorova, N., van der Aalst, W.M.P.: Discovering more precise process models from event logs by filtering out chaotic activities. J. Intell. Inf. Syst. **52**(1), 107–139 (2019)

13. Teinemaa, I., Dumas, M., Rosa, M.L., Maggi, F.M.: Outcome-oriented predictive process monitoring: Review and benchmark. ACM Trans. Knowl. Discov. Data (TKDD) **13**(2), 1–57 (2019)

14. Thornton, C., Hutter, F., Hoos, H.H., Leyton-Brown, K.: Auto-WEKA: combined selection and hyperparameter optimization of classification algorithms. In: Proceedings of the KDD-2013, pp. 847–855 (2013)

15. Verenich, I., Dumas, M., La Rosa, M., Maggi, F.M., Di Francescomarino, C.: Complex symbolic sequence clustering and multiple classifiers for predictive process monitoring. In: BPM Workshops 2015, pp. 218–229 (2015)

16. Verenich, I., Dumas, M., La Rosa, M., Maggi, F.M., Teinemaa, I.: Survey and cross-benchmark comparison of remaining time prediction methods in business process monitoring. ACM Trans. Intell. Syst. Technol. **10**(4), 1–34 (2019)

17. Yao, Q., et al.: Taking human out of learning applications: a survey on automated machine learning (2018). *CoRR*, abs/1810.13306

Discovering Process-Based Drivers
for Case-Level Outcome Explanation

Peng Li[1], Hantian Zhang[1], Xu Chu[2(✉)], Alexander Seeliger[2], and Cong Yu[2]

[1] Georgia Tech, Atlanta, USA
{pengli,hantian.zhang}@gatech.edu
[2] Celonis, New York, USA
{x.chu,a.seeliger,c.yu}@celonis.com

Abstract. Process mining has shown great impact in improving business Key Performance Indicators (KPIs), which are typically measured as aggregations over case-level outcomes. A commonly encountered key question in achieving such impact is understanding the underlying reasons for why a certain outcome appears in some cases (e.g., why certain cases take long to finish). We use the term *drivers* to refer to explanations for case-level outcomes. We hypothesize that how process is run, in other words, process traces, directly influences case-level outcomes, and hence KPIs. In this paper, we propose a new method to automatically and efficiently discover process-based drivers that are effective, significant and interpretable. We formally define the problem of driver discovery as a constrained optimization problem. Given that the problem is NP-hard, we develop efficient greedy algorithms to solve the problem. We evaluate our method on real-world datasets to demonstrate the effectiveness and efficiency of our approach.

Keywords: Process Mining · Explanation · Case outcome

1 Introduction

Process mining is a discipline that aims to discover, monitor, and improve real-world processes. The growing interest in this discipline can be attributed to the increasing availability of recorded process execution data in businesses, as well as the strong desire to improve business outcomes, measured in various Key Performance Indicators (KPIs) [3]. A KPI for process operation is typically measured by taking a historical event log and calculating an aggregation over case-level *outcomes*. For example, on-time delivery rate as a KPI is calculated as the percentage of cases that have an outcome of being delivered on time; and average throughput time is calculated as the average time it takes to complete the execution of cases. Using process mining to discover process inefficiencies, execution gaps have shown significantly impact in terms of improving business KPIs.

H. Zhang—Equal contribution, work done in Celonis.

© The Author(s), under exclusive license to Springer Nature Switzerland AG 2024
J. De Smedt and P. Soffer (Eds.): ICPM 2023 Workshops, LNBIP 503, pp. 165–178, 2024.
https://doi.org/10.1007/978-3-031-56107-8_13

In our experience of delivering process mining solutions to customers for improving their KPIs, there are some important and common questions that are frequently encountered: *Why is a certain KPI so low (or high)? What causes certain cases to have a negative outcome, and hence affecting the overall KPIs?* To answer these real-world questions, we formally define and address the problem of *Driver Discovery* in this paper. *Drivers* refer to the explanations that are most likely to drive a particular case-level outcome, and hence have a direct impact on KPIs. In particular, we want to make use of the event log and discover process-based drivers that contain information about the events or activities in event log traces. The motivation is that process data which describes the execution trace of a case should reveal the fundamental root cause of case-level outcomes. For example, certain cases experiencing long throughput times can be attributed to the involvement of a particular manual activity in their event log traces.

For discovered drivers to be practically useful, they have to be *effective*, *significant*, and *interpretable*. Intuitively, a driver is effective if the probability of observing a certain outcome is highly likely given the driver. A driver should also be significant in that it should cover as many occurrences of a certain outcome as possible. In addition, a driver needs be interpretable so that users can understand the driver, and can then take corresponding actions.

This paper investigates methods to discover drivers on process data that meet those requirements. Concretely, the paper makes the following contributions:

- We formally define the problem of process-based driver discovery as a constrained optimization problem, and propose a discovery workflow (Sect. 2).
- We propose three categories of process-based features as well as efficient methods to enumerate and prune such features (Sect. 3).
- Given that the driver discovery problem is NP-hard, we develop an efficient algorithm based on beam search to solve the problem (Sect. 4).
- We evaluate our method on real-world datasets. The experiment results show the effectiveness and efficiency of our method (Sect. 5).

2   Preliminary

2.1   Input Data and Discovery Workflow

Data Model. We assume a standard case-centric event log data model. In particular, we assume as input a *case table* and an *event log* table. The case table has columns $\{case\_id, X_1, X_1, X_2, ...X_m, Y\}$. $\{X_1, X_2, ...X_m\}$ are case-level attributes, Y is the case-level outcome. We assume in this paper that the target variable Y is a binary outcome variable, while the attributes X_i can be either numerical or categorical. The event log table has three columns $\{case\_id, activity\_name, time\_stamp\}$.

Discovery Workflow. In process mining, the event log records the execution traces of individual cases. The execution trace of a case contains valuable source information and signals that might explain the outcome of a case. How do we leverage the execution traces of cases, together with case-level attributes? Fig. 1 shows the overall workflow: we first flatten the event table by generating multiple process-based features $\{X_{m+1}, X_{m+2}, ...\}$ for each case, which are then joined with the case table on the $\{case\_id\}$ column. For example, for every unique activity A in the event log, we will create a process-based feature X_A to indicate the number of times the activity A appears in each case.

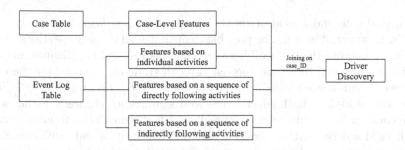

Fig. 1. Driver Discovery Workflow.

2.2 KPI Driver Formal Definition and Goodness

Given a binary outcome $Y = y \in \{0, 1\}$ to explain, we formally define a driver d as a conjunction of constraints on a subset of attribute values:

$$d := (X_1 \odot v_1) \wedge (X_2 \odot v_2)... \wedge (X_k \odot v_k) \tag{1}$$

where $X_j \in \mathbf{X}$ is a feature that could be a case-level feature or a flattened process-based feature, x_j is a feature value and $\odot \in \{=, \neq, <, >, \leq, \geq\}$ is a comparison operator.

Given that there are exponential number of driver with respect to the number of features considered, we define the following goodness metrics for drivers based on various conversations with customers. Let $D = \{t_i | i \in [n]\}$ denote the joined dataset (c.f. Fig. 1) with n cases, where t_i is the ith case. Let $D_d \subseteq D$ denote the subset of cases that fulfill the attribute constraints specified in the driver d:

- **Effectiveness (high precision).** Given a particular outcome $Y = y$, good drivers should effectively drive that outcome rather than preventing the occurrence of that outcome. Therefore, a good driver d should be *effective*, or has high precision, if for cases that satisfy the driver conditions, the probability of the occurrence of the given outcome is high. Formally, this is written as $P_d(D, y) = \frac{\sum_{t_i \in D_d} \mathbb{1}(t_i[Y]=y)}{|D_d|}$.
- **Significance (high recall).** Good drivers are supposed to cover as many cases with the interested outcome as possible. This is especially important if the driver is used to find the underlying reasons for some issues, such as identifying the reasons for low KPI. If the driver only covers a small number (e.g., 1%) of low-KPI cases, it cannot be used to significantly improve the

KPI even if the driver is effective. Hence, a good driver should be *significant*, or has high recall, if it covers as many occurrences of a given outcome as possible. This property can be formally written as $R_d = \frac{\sum_{t_i \in D_d} \mathbb{1}(t_i[Y]=y)}{\sum_{t_i \in D} \mathbb{1}(t_i[Y]=y)}$.

– **Interpretability.** Good drivers should be easily interpretable, and hence users can take actions to fix the problem. Intuitively, the simpler the driver is, the easier it can be understood. Let $|d|$ denote the number of attributes in the driver. Then, we use $|d|$ as the proxy metric for interpretabilty.

Our goal is to find a good driver that is *effective, significant* and easily *interpretable*. However, it may not be possible to optimize all three properties simultaneously. To balance the trade-off between effectiveness and significance, inspired by using F-score [11] to balance precision-recall trade-off, we combine the effectiveness and significance into one metric denoted by F_d: $F_d(D, y) = \frac{2P_d R_d}{P_d + R_d}$. This metric will be high as both effectiveness and significance are high. Either a low effectiveness or low significance will result in a low score. Therefore, optimizing F_d will yield a driver with a good balance on effectiveness and significance. For interpretability, in practice, if the number of attributes involved in the driver is not too large (e.g., $|d| \leq 3$), its interpretability is generally acceptable. Therefore, we only need to ensure $|d|$ under a threshold θ (e.g., $\theta = 3$) to make it easily interpretable rather than optimize it.

Definition 1 (Driver Discovery Problem). *Given a dataset D and an outcome y, we would like to select a driver d that maximizes the metric F_d, while keeping the number of constraints (denoted by $|d|$) smaller than θ. This can be written as a constrained optimization problem as follows.*

$$\arg\max_d \quad F_d(D, y) \quad s.t. \ |d| \leq \theta$$

Problem Complexity. A naive way to solve this constrained optimization problem is to enumerate all drivers with $|d| \leq \theta$ and return the one with the highest score. For datasets with categorical attributes only, the number of possible drivers with at most θ constraints is $O((mc)^\theta)$, where m is the number of attributes, c is the number of possible attribute values. Consider $m = 100$ and $c = 10$. Even for $\theta = 3$, there would be 1 billion possible drivers, let alone that there are infinite drivers for datasets with numerical attributes. Therefore, this naive approach is not feasible in practice. In fact, we can prove the problem is NP-hard (formal proof omitted due to space).

3   Process-Based Feature Engineering

We include three categories of process-based features: (1) features based on individual activities; (2) features based on a sequence of activities that directly follow one another; and (3) features based on a sequence of activities that indirectly follows one another.

Feature Selection. Given the exponential number of sequence-based features, we perform feature selection based on their effectiveness (precision) and significance (recall). As we will see, our sequence-based (directly follow and indirectly follow) features are binary features. We define the precision and recall of a binary feature X with respect to a target outcome y as follows:

$$P_X = \frac{\sum_{t_i \in D} \mathbb{1}(t_i[Y] = y) \ \& \ t_i[X] = 1}{\sum_{t_i \in D} t_i[X] = 1} \qquad R_X = \frac{\sum_{t_i \in D} \mathbb{1}(t_i[Y] = y) \ \& \ t_i[X] = 1}{\sum_{t_i \in D} \mathbb{1}(t_i[Y] = y)}$$

We keep a process-based sequence feature X if its precision and recall are greater than some thresholds $P_X \geq \theta_p$ and $P_X \geq \theta_r$. Note that we set θ_p and θ_r to low numbers ($\theta_p = 0.5$ and $\theta_r = 0.2$ in our experiments) so as not to lose any features might contribute to useful drivers when combined with other features.

Features Based on Individual Activities. Let $\mathcal{A}$ denote all unique activities. We will create a feature X_A for each unique activity $A \in \mathcal{A}$ that appears in the event log of all cases. For each case t_i, the feature value $t_i[A]$ is the number of times the activity A appears in the trace of the case t_i. The complexity for generating these features is $O(|\mathcal{A}|)$.

Features Based on a Sequence of Directly Following Activities. A feature in this category consists of a sequence of directly following activities, such as $X^D_{\{A_1, A_2\}}$ or $X^D_{\{A_2, A_4, A_5, A_1\}}$, where the superscript D means directly following and the subscript is the activity sequence of the feature. For each case t_i, a directly following sequence-based feature value is 1 if the feature's sequence appears at least once as a sub-sequence in the case's event log, and 0 otherwise.

We have two potential ways to generate features in this category. First, we could enumerate all possible sequences using $\mathcal{A}$, which is exponential $O(2^{|\mathcal{A}|})$. However, a feature is only useful if at least one case's feature value is 1. Therefore, we can alternatively generate candidate features by enumerating all cases. For each case t_i, we enumerate the start index s and the end index e of the case's trace, and the sub-sequence between s and e would be a candidate feature. The number of features generated this way is $O(L^2 * n)$, where n is the number of cases and L is the maximum trace length of any case. We first compare the two numbers $2^{|\mathcal{A}|}$ and $L^2 * n$, and pick the enumeration method with the lower complexity. In practice, we took the second enumeration option for all datasets we experimented with. We then prune features that do not meet the minimum precision and recall thresholds.

Features Based on a Sequence of Indirectly Following Activities. A feature here consists of a sequence of indirectly following activities, such as $X^I_{\{A_1, A_2\}}$ or $X^I_{\{A_2, A_4, A_5, A_1\}}$, where the superscript I means indirectly following and the subscript is the activity sequence of the feature. For each case t_i, in indirectly following sequence-based feature value is 1 if the feature's sequence's activities appear in the right order at least once in the case's trace, and 0 otherwise.

Example 1. Let us consider two features $X^D_{\{A_1,A_2\}}$ and $X^I_{\{A_1,A_2\}}$. For a case t_i with trace $\{A1, A4, A2, A5\}$, $t_i[X^D_{\{A_1,A_2\}}] = 0$ and $t_i[X^I_{\{A_1,A_2\}}] = 1$.

For this category of features, we will have to enumerate all possible sequences using $\mathcal{A}$, which is exponential $O(2^{|\mathcal{A}|})$. This is because, the enumeration method starting from cases would have a similar, and sometimes even higher given big n, exponential complexity of $O(n \times 2^{|L|})$.

We followed the famous *Apriori* algorithm [1] for enumerating and pruning features in this category using a lattice data structure. For the ith level of the lattice, we generate and prune all candidate sequences of length i. The candidates in level i are generated using frequent candidates in the previous level $i - 1$. Specifically, a candidate of length i can only be frequent if all of its sub-sequences of length $i - 1$ are frequent. For example, the indirectly following sequence A_1, A_2, A_3 can only be frequent if A_1, A_2, A_1, A_3, and A_2, A_3 are frequent. Given that we only want to retain candidate features that are above a certain recall threshold θ_r, the minimum support, i.e., number of cases where the feature is 1, for a candidate to be frequent is $|\mathbb{1}(t_i[Y] = y)| \times \theta_r$. Concretely, we generate the indirectly following sequence features in the following steps:

1. Generate $|\mathcal{A}|$ length 1 candidate using $\mathcal{A}$. Calculate the support for them and retain only those with support bigger than or equal to $|\mathbb{1}(t_i[Y] = y)| \times \theta_r$.
2. Generate length i candidate using the frequent length $i - 1$ candidates. Note that a length i candidate is generated only if all its sub-sequences of length $i - 1$ are frequent.
3. Calculate the support for length i candidates, and retain only the frequent ones. Iterate step (2) and step (3) until we have no more frequent candidates.
4. Calculate the precision of all frequent candidates from all levels and retain those meeting the precision threshold θ_p.

4   Driver Discovery Algorithm

Given the hardness of the problem, this section introduces our greedy algorithm to solve the aforementioned issue. Specifically, we present an efficient greedy searching algorithm based on beam search.

A straightforward greedy algorithm starts from a driver with no constraint and iteratively adds one constraint with the highest benefit into the driver until the number of constraints in the driver exceeds the given limit. The benefit of a constraint can be computed as the F_d score after adding the constraint into the current driver. Note that it is possible that the F_d score decreases with any additional constraint. Therefore, we keep track of the driver with the highest F_d score during exploration and return it as the final result.

However, this greedy algorithm has a drawback: adding one optimal constraint at each step may not lead to the global optimal driver. For example, assume the global optimal driver is $X_1 = a \wedge X_2 = b$. However, for drivers with one constraint, the optimal driver is $X_3 = c$. Then the greedy algorithm will select $X_3 = c$ at the first step and it is no longer possible to reach global optimal driver by adding more constraints.

To increase the probability of finding the best driver, we use beam search [12], which is a heuristic search algorithm. Instead of only keeping and developing one best driver at each step, we keep the top K (e.g, K = 10) drivers with the highest F_d scores in a "beam". At each step, we will extend each driver in the beam with one additional constraint, and keep the top K resulting drivers for the next step. We will still keep track of the best driver that we have seen during beam search and return it as the final result. The term "beam search" refers to the way the algorithm explores the search space by considering a limited number of candidates at each step, forming a "beam" of possible solutions.

Algorithm. The pseudocode of the beam search algorithm is shown in Algorithm 1. We start from an empty driver (Line 1 - 2). At each iteration, we extend each driver in the beam by one additional constraint (Line 4 - 7). The candidate set of constraints can be generated by enumerating all possible combination of attributes, operators, and attributes values. For numerical attributes, we can choose c splitting points (e.g., 10-percentile, 20-percentile, etc.) and for each splitting point v, we can generate two candidate constraints as $X \leq v$ and $X > v$. We compute the F_d score of each driver (Line 8), and we keep the top K drivers with the highest score for the next step (Line 12 - 13). This process will be repeated for θ iterations such that the number of constraints in the driver will not be greater than θ (Line 3). We keep track of the best driver d^* that we have seen (Line 10–11) and return it at the end (Line 14).

Algorithm 1: Beam Search Algorithm

    input   : Input dataset D, an outcome y, threshold θ, beam width K
    output : A driver d
1 $d^* \leftarrow d_{empty}$
2 $B_{cur} \leftarrow [d_{empty}]$
3 **for** $i = 1, 2, \ldots \theta$ **do**
4     $B_{next} \leftarrow []$
5   **foreach** d in B_{cur} **do**
6   **foreach** $(X_j \odot v_j)$ in candidates **do**
7             $d' \leftarrow d \wedge (X_j \odot v_j)$
8             $d'.score = F_{d'}(D, y)$
9             $B_{next}.append(d_{next})$
10   **if** $d'.score > d^*.score$ **then**
11               $d^* \leftarrow d'$
12   sort B_{next} by $d.score$
13     $B_{cur} \leftarrow B_{next}[: K]$
14 **return** d^*

Complexity. Consider a dataset with n examples and m features, and each attribute can take c values (assuming numerical attributes are split into c intervals). The number of candidate constraint will be $O(mc)$. Let K be the beam size. For each iteration, we compute the F_d score $O(Kmc)$ times, which takes $O(nmc)$ time. Therefore, the total time complexity for our algorithm is $O(Knmc\theta)$.

5   Experiment

We evaluate the effectiveness and efficiency of both the process-based feature engineering and the beam search algorithm for driver discovery.

5.1   Experimental Setup

Datasets. We use three popular datasets from BPI Challenge, which are widely used in the literature, and a synthetic dataset to test the scalability of the driver discovery algorithm. The stats of the datasets are listed in Table 1. BPIC 2017 [7] contains 31,509 loan application cases of a Dutch financial institute; BPIC 2018 [9] contains 43,809 applications for EU direct payments for German farmers from the European Agricultural Guarantee Fund; and BPIC 2019 [8] contains 251,734 purchase orders for a dutch company. For all three real datasets, our target is a binary outcome that indicates whether each case is taking long to finish or not. For a given dataset, we consider a case to have long throughput time if it takes longer than 75 percentile throughput time of all cases.

Table 1. Dataset Statistics (AAPC: average activities per case; DF: directly follows features; IDF: indirectly follows features)

Dataset	#Cases	#Case Features	#Activities	AAPC	DF	IDF
BPIC 2017	31,509	4	26	38.2	7	20
BPIC 2018	43,809	61	41	57.4	111	404
BPIC 2019	251,734	16	42	6.3	112	258
Synthetic	1,000,000	100	N/A	N/A	N/A	N/A

Methods Compared. We compare the following driver discovery methods. Note that, all methods use the same feature set generated by Sect. 3. We will evaluate the effectiveness of process-based feature engineering in Sect. 5.2 and compare driver discovery algorithms in Sect. 5.3.

- Beam Search (Beam): This is our proposed algorithm in Sect. 4. By default we set the maximum number of constraints in a driver θ to be 3, and we set the beam search width K to bc 8.
- Decision Tree (DT): We run the decision tree algorithm to find the drivers. The decision tree is trained to classify the KPI. Then we down the tree from root to leaf, each path would be a driver and all the points in the leaf would be the cases that satisfies the given driver.
- Exhaustive Search (ES): This approach enumerates all possible drivers and find the best one with the highest score.

Evaluation Metrics. We use F1 score to measure the quality of the drivers, as defined in Sect. 2.2. We use running time to evaluate algorithm efficiency.

Table 2. Top 1 driver with different set of features on three datasets.

Features	Top 1 Driver
BPIC 2017 A	"Application Type==New credit" & "Requested Amount > 0"
BPIC 2017 B	"Count of A_Cancelled > 0" & "Count of A_Submitted > 0" & "Count of W_Call after offers > 4"
BPIC 2017 C	"A_Cancelled directly followed by O_Cancelled" & "A_Concept directly followed by W_Complete application" & "Count of W_Call after offers > 4"
BPIC 2017 D	"A_Submitted indirectly followed by A_Cancelled" & "A_Cancelled directly followed by O_Cancelled" & "Count of W_Call after offers > 4"
BPIC 2018 A	"Year==2015" & "number parcels > 3" & "amount applied0 > 1135.24"
BPIC 2018 B	"Count of initialize > 4" & " Count of begin preparations <= 0 " & "Count of save > 0"
BPIC 2018 C	"Count of initialize > 4" & " amount applied0 > 4025.81 " & "finish payment directly followed by save"
BPIC 2018 D	"finish payment indirectly followed by save" & "case year != 2017"
BPIC 2019 A	"Item Category != Consignment" & "Item Type != Third-party"
BPIC 2019 B	"Count of Record Invoice Receipt > 0" & "Item Type != Third-party"
BPIC 2019 C	"Clear Invoice directly followed by Record Invoice Receipt" & "Item Type != Third-party" & "Count of Record Invoice Receipt>=2"
BPIC 2019 D	"Change Quantity indirectly followed by Record Goods Receipt" & "Item Type != Third-party" & "Count of Record Invoice Receipt>=2"

5.2 Evaluating Process-Based Feature Engineering

We evaluate the effectiveness of the process-based feature engineering described in Sect. 3. The number of each type of features is shown in Table 1. Specifically, we compare the following feature set in a cumulative manner:

- Feature Set A: case-level features only
- Feature Set B: features based on activity counts and features in A
- Feature Set C: directly following activities and all features in B
- Feature Set D: indirectly following activities and all features in C

Qualitative Assessment. We show the Top-1 driver discovered by each feature set in Table 2. For example, for the BPIC 2017 dataset, an important driver is "Count of W_Call after offers > 4", the repetition is likely to be the cause of long throughput time, and is highlighted by the driver discovery algorithm. The directly following feature "A_Cancelled directly followed by O_Cancelled" and the indirectly following feature "A_Submitted indirectly followed by A_Cancelled" show that cancelled cases takes longer than normal cases, which is counter-intuitive. After we looked at the data more deeply, we noticed that this is caused by automatic cancellation, which takes 30 days and

Table 3. F1 Score of the driver with feature set.

Dataset and Feature Set	Top 1	Top 5	Top 10
BPIC 2017 A	0.429	0.429	0.428
BPIC 2017 B	0.650	0.648	0.643
BPIC 2017 C	0.653	0.652	0.649
BPIC 2017 D	0.655	0.653	0.650
BPIC 2018 A	0.647	0.646	0.646
BPIC 2018 B	0.714	0.713	0.708
BPIC 2018 C	0.718	0.716	0.710
BPIC 2018 D	0.906	0.905	0.903
BPIC 2019 A	0.506	0.506	0.505
BPIC 2019 B	0.522	0.521	0.521
BPIC 2019 C	0.532	0.530	0.523
BPIC 2019 D	0.535	0.532	0.527

Table 4. F1 Score of the Top 1 driver with driver discovery algorithm, NA means that the algorithm cannot finish in 1 day.

Dataset	Beam	DT	ES
BPIC 2017 D	0.655	0.608	0.664
BPIC 2018 D	0.906	0.904	NA
BPIC 2019 D	0.535	0.493	NA

causes long throughput time. For BPIC 2018 dataset, we find that the indirectly following feature "finish payment indirectly followed by save" has a high relevance with long throughput time Overall, our feature generation algorithm can generate features related to the process and provide insightful patterns that are worth looking into more carefully.

Quantitative Assessment. Table 3 shows the F1 score of top drivers found by our algorithm. Here top 5 is the average F1 score of top 5 drivers and Top 10 is the average F1 score of the top 10 drivers. We observe that adding the count features can already increase the F1 score significantly compared with only using case-level features, because we are focusing on long throughput time as the target and usually long throughput time is closely related to rework, which is captured by the count features. After adding the directly following and indirectly following features, the F1 score also increases, indicating that new features are used in the top drivers, revealing more causes that are related to the processes. Especially, we see that after adding the indirectly following features, the F1 score of the top-1 driver for the BPIC 2018 dataset (BPIC 2018 D) becomes 0.906, which shows that the driver has very high relevance with the long throughput time.

Feature Selection Knob Analysis. We evaluate the how tuning the precision and recall threshold would have an impact on the number of features generated, and the F1 score of the drivers found using the BPIC 2017 dataset. In Fig. 2(a), we fix the recall threshold, $\theta_r = 0.2$ and tune the precision threshold θ_p, we see that as θ_p becomes higher, there are less features, but the impact on the top 1 F1 is pretty insignificant. Similarly, In Fig. 2(b), we fix the precision threshold, $\theta_p = 0.5$ and tune the recall threshold θ_r, we see that the top 1 F1 does not change at all. The reason is that after the features are generated, we still need to run the driver discovery algorithm, which would select the high quality features.

The selected features in the top drivers usually have high precision and recall, which means that the result is not sensitive on the knob for feature selection.

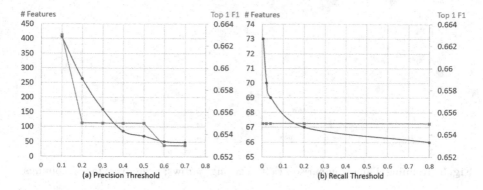

Fig. 2. Knob Analysis.

5.3   Evaluating the Driver Discovery Algorithm

Quality of the Driver. We evaluate the F1 score of the found driver using the three algorithms: beam search, decision tree (DT) and exhaustive search (ES), and the result is shown in Table 4. For exhaustive search, it takes a long time to run and cannot finish in 1 day for the BPIC 2018 and BPIC 2019 dataset. For BPIC 2017, exhaustive search achieved the highest F1 score at 0.664, which is understandable because it searches the entire search space. However, our beam search achieved a F1 score of 0.655, and the difference is less than one percentage point. Compared to the decision tree algorithms, our beam search can consistently outperform the decision tree algorithm significantly, by up to 4.7 percentage points.

Running Time Comparison. We use the synthetic dataset to verify the scalability of driver discovery algorithm. Figure 3 shows the running time comparison of different methods with varying size of datasets. As we can see, in Fig. 3 (a), as the number of rows increases, all three grows linearly, and decision tree and beam search have similar running time, and they are 4x faster than exhaustive search. In Fig. 3 (b), as the number of columns grows, the running of the exhaustive search method grows polynomial and takes over 1 h to finish when the number of columns is greater than 100. However, both decision tree and beam search algorithm grow almost linearly and thus have a better scalability, and decision tree and beam search have similar running times.

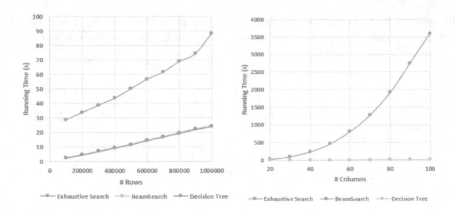

Fig. 3. Running Time Comparison (left: Varying # rows; right: Varying # columns)

6   Related Work

Feature Importance. Our work is related to estimating feature importance in ML, which estimates the impact of each feature on model predictions [10]. Some interpretable ML models provides feature importance by themselves. For example, in logistic regression [6], the weight of a feature indicates its importance. In tree-based methods, such as decision tree [15] and random forest [4], the feature importance is computed as the reduction of the prediction error brought by that feature. Permutation importance [2] defines the importance of feature by the decrease of the model performance when that feature value is randomly shuffled. Chung et al. [5] propose an automated data slicing method to validate ML models to find potential performance issues. Also, SHAP values [17] are used to determine the importance of a feature in ML models to explain KPI changes.

Drivers discovered by our method also refer the most important features in a dataset, but different from feature importance in ML based on model predictions, our method does not tie to a specific ML model and focuses on the impact of features on outcomes.

Decision Mining in Process Mining. In process mining, decision mining is first introduced in [18] to identify the set of features as rules that define the choices made in a process. An extension to support conditions with disjunctions and inequalities is introduced by de Leoni et al. [14]. A typical limitation of decision tree learning is the assumption of full deterministic process executions and, therefore, non-overlapping rules. Mannhardt et al. [16] introduce an additional step to learn new decision trees for each leaf node in the first iteration for wrongly classified instances. An alignment based approach was introduced in [13] which additionally allows to discover rules associated with XOR-splits/joins and certain types of loops. Our work focuses on the factors that influenced the outcome and not only a particular choice. Consequently, our approach aims to find factors on a case-level end to end instead of a local decision point.

7   Conclusion

We formally define the problem of driver discovery, which is a technique to explain case-level outcomes in process mining. We form three categories of process-based features, and we propose a beam search method to automatically and efficiently discover effective, significant and interpretable drivers. We show the effectiveness and efficiency of our approach.

References

1. Agrawal, R., Srikant, R., et al.: Fast algorithms for mining association rules. In: Proceedings of the 20th International Conference on Very Large Data Bases, VLDB, vol. 1215, pp. 487–499. Santiago, Chile (1994)
2. Altmann, A., Toloşi, L., Sander, O., Lengauer, T.: Permutation importance: a corrected feature importance measure. Bioinformatics **26**(10), 1340–1347 (2010)
3. Badakhshan, P., Wurm, B., Grisold, T., Geyer-Klingeberg, J., Mendling, J., vom Brocke, J.: Creating business value with process mining. J. Strateg. Inf. Syst. **31**(4) (2022)
4. Breiman, L.: Random forests. Mach. Learn. **45**, 5–32 (2001)
5. Chung, Y., Kraska, T., Polyzotis, N., Tae, K.H., Whang, S.E.: Slice finder: automated data slicing for model validation. In: IEEE 35th International Conference on Data Engineering (ICDE), pp. 1550–1553. IEEE (2019)
6. Cox, D.R.: The regression analysis of binary sequences. J. R. Stat. Soc.: Ser. B (Methodol.) **20**(2), 215–232 (1958)
7. van Dongen, B.: Bpi challenge 2017 (2017). https://doi.org/10.4121/uuid:5f3067df-f10b-45da-b98b-86ae4c7a310b
8. van Dongen, B.: Bpi challenge 2019 (2019). https://doi.org/10.4121/uuid:d06aff4b-79f0-45e6-8ec8-e19730c248f1
9. van Dongen, B., Borchert, F.F.: Bpi challenge 2018 (2018). https://doi.org/10.4121/uuid:3301445f-95e8-4ff0-98a4-901f1f204972
10. Hooker, S., Erhan, D., Kindermans, P.J., Kim, B.: Evaluating Feature Importance Estimates (2018). arXiv https://arxiv.org/pdf/1806.10758.pdf
11. Hossin, M., Sulaiman, M.N.: A review on evaluation metrics for data classification evaluations. Int. J. Data Min. Knowl. Manag. Process **5**(2), 1 (2015)
12. Kumar, A., Vembu, S., Menon, A.K., Elkan, C.: Beam search algorithms for multilabel learning. Mach. Learn. **92**, 65–89 (2013)
13. de Leoni, M., van der Aalst, W.M.P.: Data-aware process mining: discovering decisions in processes using alignments. In: Proceedings of the 28th Annual ACM Symposium on Applied Computing, pp. 1454–1461. SAC '13, Association for Computing Machinery, New York, NY, USA (2013)
14. de Leoni, M., Dumas, M., García-Bañuelos, L.: Discovering branching conditions from business process execution logs. In: Cortellessa, V., Varró, D. (eds.) FASE 2013. LNCS, vol. 7793, pp. 114–129. Springer, Heidelberg (2013). https://doi.org/10.1007/978-3-642-37057-1_9

15. Lewis, R.J.: An introduction to classification and regression tree (CART) analysis. In: Annual Meeting of the Society for Academic Emergency Medicine in San Francisco, California, vol. 14. Citeseer (2000)
16. Mannhardt, F., de Leoni, M., Reijers, H.A., van der Aalst, W.M.P.: Decision mining revisited - discovering overlapping rules. In: Nurcan, S., Soffer, P., Bajec, M., Eder, J. (eds.) CAiSE 2016. LNCS, vol. 9694, pp. 377–392. Springer, Cham (2016). https://doi.org/10.1007/978-3-319-39696-5_23
17. Padella, A., de Leoni, M., Dogan, O., Galanti, R.: Explainable process prescriptive analytics. In: 2022 4th International Conference on Process Mining (ICPM). IEEE (oct 2022)
18. Rozinat, A., van der Aalst, W.M.P.: Decision mining in ProM. In: Dustdar, S., Fiadeiro, J.L., Sheth, A.P. (eds.) BPM 2006. LNCS, vol. 4102, pp. 420–425. Springer, Heidelberg (2006). https://doi.org/10.1007/11841760_33

Detecting Anomalous Events
in Object-Centric Business Processes
via Graph Neural Networks

Alessandro Niro[✉][iD] and Michael Werner[iD]

University of Amsterdam, Amsterdam, The Netherlands
{a.niro,m.werner}@uva.nl

Abstract. Detecting anomalies is important for identifying inefficiencies, errors, or fraud in business processes. Traditional process mining approaches focus on analyzing 'flattened', sequential, event logs based on a single case notion. However, many real-world process executions exhibit a graph-like structure, where events can be associated with multiple cases. Flattening event logs requires selecting a single case identifier which creates a gap with the real event data and artificially introduces anomalies in the event logs. Object-centric process mining avoids these limitations by allowing events to be related to different cases. This study proposes a novel framework for anomaly detection in business processes that exploits graph neural networks and the enhanced information offered by object-centric process mining. We first reconstruct and represent the process dependencies of the object-centric event logs as attributed graphs and then employ a graph convolutional autoencoder architecture to detect anomalous events. Our results show that our approach provides promising performance in detecting anomalies at the activity type and attributes level, although it struggles to detect anomalies in the temporal order of events.

Keywords: Object-centric Process Mining · Graph Neural Networks · Anomaly Detection

1 Introduction

Process mining aims to discover, monitor, and enhance existing business processes by leveraging data traces generated by their execution and stored into event logs [2]. Business processes can be defined as a set of activities that enable the organization to achieve a specified goal. They are seldom friction-less. Errors, inefficiencies, and fraud during process executions can lead to significant losses for the organizations. The ability to detect and mitigate harmful anomalies is crucial for maintaining the effectiveness and efficiency of business operations.

Traditional approaches to process mining rely on 'flattened' event logs. Events are characterized by a single case identifier [1] and process instances are assumed to be strictly ordered sequences of events. Anomaly detection techniques have primarily centered on approaches applied to flattened event logs.

J. De Smedt and P. Soffer (Eds.): ICPM 2023 Workshops, LNBIP 503, pp. 179–190, 2024.
https://doi.org/10.1007/978-3-031-56107-8_14

Conformance checking approaches [9,10,12] have focused on identifying deviations of sequential process instances, as captured by the event logs, from an *a priori* process model, which is a necessary input for this type of techniques. Machine learning approaches, based on distance measures [21,30] or reconstruction errors [20,26–28], have focused on detecting anomalies directly from event logs, adopting methods suited for strictly ordered sequences of events.

However, in real-world processes there usually exist multiple potential identifiers. A single case notion leads to a loss of information (i.e. *deficiency*, *convergence* and *divergence* issues [2]). Object-centric process mining [18] is an emerging paradigm that drops the single case assumption and instead assumes events can be associated to any number of objects (cases) of different types, with the aim to overcome the limitations of traditional approaches and provide a more accurate depiction of the actual process. Compared to the strictly ordered linear structure of process instances resulting from the single case notion, object-centric process instances can be naturally represented as directed graphs [6].

This study introduces an approach for anomaly detection in business process that is natively designed for object-centric event logs. We propose an unsupervised machine learning approach based on Graph Neural Networks (GNNs), and specifically on a graph convolutional autoencoder (GCNAE) [25,33] architecture.

The approach is illustrated in Fig. 1. It first reconstructs the dependencies between events within an object-centric event log as a set of attributed graphs, then it uses the GCNAE to compute the events' anomaly scores. We employ a simple heuristic based on the inter-quartile range (IQR) to automatically set the threshold and label the anomalies without the need of prior knowledge of the contamination rate of the data.

The main contribution of this study is the introduction of a novel unsupervised anomaly detection approach for business processes, leveraging GNNs and the enriched event data structure offered by object-centric process mining. We are not aware of any other studies that employ GNN on object-centric events logs for anomaly detection. Our approach does not rely on prior information about the process model, contamination rate, or a clean training set, making it suitable for real-world applications.

We evaluated the performance of our approach on two different publicly available[1] object-centric event logs: one a synthetic dataset and the other a real-life dataset. We measured the performance of the approach across different metrics by injecting various types of anomalies in the event logs. The evaluation results demonstrate that our approach performs well in regard to events activity type and attributes anomalies. They also showed limitations regarding the detection of anomalies in the temporal order of events, which requires further exploration of GNN architectures that can better detect such anomalies.

2   Preliminaries and Background

Object-Centric Process Mining. Traditional approaches to process mining involve 'flattened' event logs that are based on the assumptions of a single case

---

[1] Event logs and source code are available at: github.com/niro-a/DAEiOcBPvGNN.

notion and of each event to be associated to exactly one case [1]. This leads to a gap between the real event data and the event log, and specifically to the issues of *deficiency* (deletion of events), *convergence* (duplication of events) and *divergence* (ordering unrelated events) [1]. An object-centric event log [18] is a collection of events where each event is associated with one or more objects, which may be of different types. Similarly to traditional event logs, each event is also associated to an activity, timestamp, and additional attributes.

Definition 1 (Object-centric Event Log). *Let T be the universe of timestamps. An object-centric event log $L = (E, O, OT, A, AV, \pi_{type}, \pi_{time}, \pi_{trace}, \pi_{act}, \pi_{attr})$ is a tuple where:*

- *E is a set of events, O is a set of objects, OT is a set of object types, A is a set of activities and AV is a set of attribute values,*
- *$\pi_{type}: O \to OT$ maps each object to an object type,*
- *$\pi_{time}: E \to T$ maps each event to a timestamp,*
- *$\pi_{trace}: O \to E^*$ maps each object to a temporally ordered sequence of events,*
- *$\pi_{act} : E \to A$ maps each event to its activity,*
- *$\pi_{attr} : E \nrightarrow AV$ maps each event onto attributes values.*

By modeling the relationship between events and multiple objects of different types, object-centric event logs exhibit a graph structure [8] and also the traditional concepts of cases (i.e. process instances) and variants have been extended, in the object-centric setting, from sequences to graphs [6].

Definition 2 (Object-centric Process Instance). *Let L be an object-centric event log. Given all the temporally ordered traces of events $\pi_{trace}(o_i) = \langle e_1, \ldots, e_n \rangle$ associated to each object $o_i \in L$, an object-centric process instance $P = (E', D)$ is a directed graph with nodes E' (representing events), edges D (representing the events temporal dependencies) for a set of traces joined directly or transitively by one or more common events.*

Given this definition, an object-centric event log can be reconstructed as a set of one or more process instances, where process instances are made by set of traces that are connected by common bridge events. This representation is free of convergence, deficiency, or divergence issues [4] and is equivalent to the *connected component process execution* found in [6]. It represents a generalization of the traditional case concept to object-centric event logs.

Problem Statement. While most of the traditional process mining literature has focused on detecting anomalous process instances (i.e. cases), we move our focus to detecting anomalous events since, in the context of object-centric process mining, process instances can be overly complex and large, to the extreme of comprising one single instance for the whole event log [6].

Unlike some of the previous machine learning approaches that characterized anomaly detection as a semi-supervised task [21,24,26] which assumes the availability of a suitable labeled dataset of normal behavior, we characterize anomaly detection as an unsupervised task. We further impose the requirement for the algorithms to explicitly discriminate the anomalous events from the normal ones.

Definition 3 (Event Anomaly Detection). *Event anomaly detection is the task of identifying events that deviate significantly from normal behavior in an object-centric event log. Formally, given an object-centric event log L, let $E_n \subseteq E$ be the set of normal events and $E_a \subset E$ be the set of anomalous events. The goal of event anomaly detection is to learn a function $f : E \rightarrow \{0, 1\}$ that assigns a binary label to each event $e_i \in E$ indicating whether it is anomalous or not, based only on the knowledge of L.*

3   Related Work

Anomaly Detection in Business Processes. The task of anomaly detection involves identifying observations that do not follow a pattern of normal behavior [14], or more specifically in the context of business processes and of process mining, of normal process behavior [23]. The exact notion of normal behavior and conversely of anomalous behavior are heavily dependent on the application domain [14] and on the level of analysis of the specific detection approach [23]. A possible categorization of process anomalies is between event-level and process instance-level anomalies [23], where the first refers to anomalies in one or more attributes of an event, while the latter to anomalies in the order or attribute dependencies of events belonging to the same process instance. Following the more general taxonomy found in [13,14] classifies process anomalies into three categories based on their nature: *point anomalies, contextual anomalies*, and *collective anomalies*. Point (or global) anomalies refer to individual observations that are anomalous compared to the rest of the data, while contextual (or local) anomalies are observations that are only anomalous in specific contexts. Collective anomalies are sets of related observations that are anomalous compared to the entire dataset, even if the individual observations may not be anomalies on their own.

In regard to existing approaches, [3] have proposed a generalization of the traditional conformance checking concepts of precision and fitness to object-centric process mining, but otherwise approaches to anomaly detection in object-centric event logs are, to the best of our knowledge, currently unexplored. More research has been done in the context of traditional process mining, which has mostly focused on detecting anomalous cases (i.e. process instances) [23].

Conformance checking based approaches revolve around detecting anomalous behavior in an event log compared to a reference process model or a discovered process model. These approaches can either focus on a control-flow perspective [9,10] or consider also additional event attributes [7,12].

Distance-based approaches group traces based on distance measures, either via clustering [21] or classification [30] algorithms, while reconstruction-based approaches employ autoencoder neural networks to compute the reconstruction errors for the case encodings, which are used as anomaly scores. Approaches applying standard autoencoders [26,27] involve representing each case as an ordered vector of event activity types and events attributes, eventually padding shorter cases to the maximum length found in the event log. Similarly, approaches based on recurrent neural networks leverage the sequential nature of the traditional case concept to train autoencoders based on gated-recurrent units (GRUs) [28] or long-short term memory (LSTM) neural networks [24, 26]. [20] proposed an approach based on graph autoencoders that represented cases as loops and self-loops between activity types.

A common characteristic of the aforementioned approaches is that they require the definition of a threshold to discriminate between anomalous and normal cases [23] derived from domain knowledge or some heuristic.

Graph Neural Networks. GNNs are a class of neural networks designed to operate on graphs. They have been applied successfully to various tasks, including anomaly detection [25]. In general terms, GNNs are based on learning representations of the nodes of graphs and of their neighborhood (a k-hop of connected nodes) via a local function that is invariant to permutation of the neighboring nodes ordering [31]. [11] categorizes most GNNs into three classes based on their local function: convolutional, attentional, and generic message-passing. We are not aware of GNNs applications to object-centric process mining, but, in the context of traditional process mining, they have been employed in approaches to process discovery [29], predictive process mining [15, 19, 32] and anomaly detection [20]. These approaches have relied on encodings of process instances as ordered sequences of connected nodes, with the exception of [15], who employed a technique proposed in [16] to embed some temporal loops and events parallelism in the process instances, and of [20] who, as mentioned, encoded process instances as loops and self-loops between activity types (instead of events).

4 Method

Approach Overview. Our approach, as illustrated in Fig. 1, relies on a GCNAE [33] trained on object-centric event logs containing both normal and anomalous events. We first reconstruct the object-centric process instances from the event logs as a single (disconnected) graph that serves as input for the GCNAE. The GCNAE is trained to reconstruct the nodes attributes of the input graph. The nodes' reconstruction errors serve as the anomaly scores. We finally apply a simple heuristic based on the IQR to automatically assign a binary label

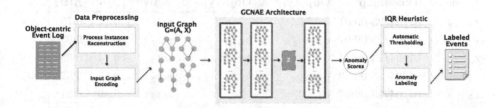

Fig. 1. An overview of our proposed approach.

to each event indicating whether it is anomalous or not, without the need to manually set an anomaly score threshold. The following sub-sections explain the different steps in detail.

4.1 Data Preprocessing

Process Instances Reconstruction. We reconstruct the object-centric process instances via the *ocpa* Python library [5] to represent the dependencies between events in the object-centric event log.

As an example, given the simple object-centric event log L in Table 1, the resulting process instances P_1 and P_2 can be visualized in Fig. 2, where P_1 is composed by the set of traces $\pi_{\text{trace}}(a_1) \cup \pi_{\text{trace}}(a_3) \cup \pi_{\text{trace}}(b_3) = \langle e_1, e_4, e_7 \rangle \cup \langle e_4, e_7 \rangle \cup \langle e_4, e_8 \rangle$ which are bridged by events e_4 and e_7 and where P_2 is composed by the set of traces $\pi_{\text{trace}}(a_2) \cup \pi_{\text{trace}}(b_1) \cup \pi_{\text{trace}}(b_2) = \langle e_2, e_5, e_6 \rangle \cup \langle e_2, e_3 \rangle \cup \langle e_2, e_3, e_6 \rangle$ which are bridged by events e_2, e_3 and e_6.

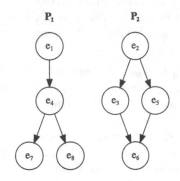

Fig. 2. The reconstructed process instances for the object-centric event log in Table 1.

Input Graph Encoding. We combine the process instances into a single graph $\mathcal{G}$, composed of a set of disconnected subgraphs (i.e., the process instances). This way, we do not need to apply padding or other transformations to the instance graphs. For the example in Fig. 2, therefore the input graph would correspond to the set of the two subgraphs P_1 and P_2, $\mathcal{G}_L = \{P_1, P_2\}$.

Definition 4 (Adjacency Matrix, A). *Given the input graph $\mathcal{G}$ for the event log L, where $\mathcal{G} = (\mathcal{V}, \mathcal{E})$ is a directed graph with nodes $\mathcal{V} = E_L$ and edges $\mathcal{E} \subseteq \mathcal{V} \times \mathcal{V}$, we represent it with an adjacency matrix $\mathbf{A} \in \mathbb{R}^{|\mathcal{V}| \times |\mathcal{V}|}$ where, for an ordered pair of nodes (u, v), $a_{u,v}$ is equal to 1 if $(u, v) \in \mathcal{E}$ and 0 otherwise.*

Table 1. An object-centric event log with two object types (A, B).

Event ID	Timestamp	Obj. Type A	Obj. Type B	Activity	Attr$_1$	Attr$_2$	...
e_1	01/04/23 09:01	a_1		act$_1$	0.12	0.75	...
e_2	01/04/23 09:07	a_2	b_1, b_2	act$_1$	0.33	0.98	...
e_3	01/04/23 09:14		b_1, b_2	act$_2$	0.24	0.39	...
e_4	01/04/23 09:22	a_1, a_3	b_3	act$_3$	0.15	0.67	...
e_5	01/04/23 09:37	a_2		act$_3$	0.89	0.21	...
e_6	01/04/23 09:44	a_2	b_2	act$_4$	0.58	0.46	...
e_7	01/04/23 10:02	a_1, a_3		act$_5$	0.73	0.81	...
e_8	01/04/23 10:09		b_3	act$_4$	0.42	0.34	...

Definition 5 (Feature Matrix, X). *Given an object-centric event log L and its input graph $\mathcal{G} = (\mathcal{V}, \mathcal{E})$, we map to each node $u \in \mathcal{V}$ a feature vector, $\mathbf{x}_u \in \mathbb{R}^k$ corresponding to the event activity type $\pi_{act}(u)$ and original attributes $\pi_{attr}(u)$, where categorical features are one-hot encoded, and thus k is equal to the sum of unique activity types in A_L, unique categorical values in AV_L and numerical attributes in AV_L. Then, we stack all the feature vectors into a feature matrix $\mathbf{X} \in \mathbb{R}^{|\mathcal{V}| \times k}$, where $\mathbf{X} = [\mathbf{x}_1, \mathbf{x}_2, \ldots, \mathbf{x}_{|\mathcal{V}|}]^\top$.*

Accordingly, the input graph $\mathcal{G}$ for the GCNAE is encoded as $\mathcal{G} = (\mathbf{A}, \mathbf{X})$. For the running example of the object-centric event log L in Table 1, the adjacency matrix $\mathbf{A}_L$ and the feature matrix $\mathbf{X}_L$ would look as:

$$
\mathbf{A}_L = \begin{bmatrix} 0\,0\,0\,1\,0\,0\,0\,0 \\ 0\,0\,1\,0\,1\,0\,0\,0 \\ 0\,0\,0\,0\,0\,1\,0\,0 \\ 0\,0\,0\,0\,0\,0\,1\,1 \\ 0\,0\,0\,0\,0\,1\,0\,0 \\ 0\,0\,0\,0\,0\,0\,0\,0 \\ 0\,0\,0\,0\,0\,0\,0\,0 \\ 0\,0\,0\,0\,0\,0\,0\,0 \end{bmatrix} \quad
\mathbf{X}_L = \begin{bmatrix} 1\,0\,0\,0\,0\,0.12\,0.75 \cdots \\ 1\,0\,0\,0\,0\,0.33\,0.98 \cdots \\ 0\,1\,0\,0\,0\,0.24\,0.39 \cdots \\ 0\,0\,1\,0\,0\,0.15\,0.67 \cdots \\ 0\,0\,1\,0\,0\,0.89\,0.21 \cdots \\ 0\,0\,0\,1\,0\,0.58\,0.46 \cdots \\ 0\,0\,0\,0\,1\,0.73\,0.81 \cdots \\ 0\,0\,0\,1\,0\,0.42\,0.34 \cdots \end{bmatrix}
$$

4.2 GCNAE Architecture

The GCNAE uses a graph convolutional network (GCN) [22] component both for the the encoder and for the decoder. Graph convolution aggregates the information from neighboring nodes and updates node representations based on their local graph structure.

The encoder component of the GCNAE learns a latent representation of the input graph while the decoder learns to reconstruct the nodes features from this latent representation. The GCNAE is trained by minimizing the reconstruction error between the original nodes features and the reconstructed ones.

Adapted from [33], our encoder consists of a two-layer GCN:

$$
\mathbf{Z} = GCN(\mathbf{X}, \mathbf{A}) = \mathrm{ReLU}(\tilde{\mathbf{A}}\,\mathrm{ReLU}(\tilde{\mathbf{A}}\mathbf{X}\mathbf{W}_{(0)})\mathbf{W}_{(1)}) \tag{1}
$$

where the output $\mathbf{Z}$ is a matrix of node embeddings, $\mathbf{X}$ is the feature matrix, $\mathbf{A}$ is the adjacency matrix of the graph. ReLU is the rectified linear unit activation function with $\mathrm{ReLU}(x) = \max(0,x)$. $\tilde{\mathbf{A}}$ is the symmetrically normalized adjacency matrix with $\tilde{\mathbf{A}} = \mathbf{D}^{-\frac{1}{2}}(\mathbf{A} + \mathbf{I})\mathbf{D}^{-\frac{1}{2}}$ (where $\mathbf{I}$ is the identity matrix and $\mathbf{D}$ is the diagonal degree matrix), used to add self-loops and normalize nodes features aggregation. $\mathbf{W}_{(l)}$ denotes a learnable weight matrix for each l-th layer.

The decoder's reconstructed node attributes $\hat{\mathbf{X}}$ are computed with a third GCN layer that maps the node embeddings back to the original input space:

$$
\hat{\mathbf{X}} = \mathrm{ReLU}(\tilde{\mathbf{A}}\mathbf{Z}\mathbf{W}_{(2)}) \tag{2}
$$

As the loss function to optimize the GCNAE we take the average row-wise mean squared error (MSE) between $\mathbf{X}$ and $\hat{\mathbf{X}}$, while, to account for different shapes in the features encoding, we compute the events anomaly scores by taking the average MSE for each event original feature which are then averaged again.

4.3   IQR Heuristic: Automatic Thresholding and Anomaly Labeling

The IQR is is often used to detect outliers and is defined as the difference between the first quartile (Q_1) and the third quartile (Q_3) of a dataset, $IQR = Q_3 - Q_1$.

To determine a threshold to label anomalies, we compute the Q_3 and the IQR for the set of anomaly scores generated by the GCNAE and set the threshold τ as:

$$\tau = Q_3 + k \cdot \text{IQR} \tag{3}$$

Once the threshold is set, we can automatically label the events in the event log as normal or anomalous based on whether their anomaly score is respectively below or above the threshold. In this study, we set $k = 1.5$ based on convention, but this value can be adjusted to tailor the sensitivity of the threshold to specific uses.

5   Experiments

We evaluate our proposed approach on both synthetic and real object-centric event logs, since real event logs can help prove the feasibility of the approach but at the same can also contain unlabeled real-life anomalies which can impact the reliability of the results [26,28]. Like in previous work [24,26–28], we introduce artificial anomalies into the event logs to simulate various types of irregularities that can occur in real-world processes. Summary statistics for the datasets and the reconstructed process instances can be found in Table 2.

We use an object-centric version of the *BPIC 2017* dataset [17] as a representative of a real event log. It contains almost 400.000 events for the loan application process of a Dutch financial institution between 2016 and 2017. The event log has two types of objects (the application and the offer) and thirteen attributes.

The second event log is the synthetic *DS2* dataset found in [6]. It simulates an order management process with an especially high amount of connected objects and variability. The event log has three types of objects (items, orders, and packages) and four attributes.

Table 2. Summary statistics for the datasets, the reconstructed process instances and the injected anomalies.

Dataset	Original Events	Final Events	Injected Anomalies	Process Instances	Events per P. Instance (max, min, avg)
BPIC 2017	393931	407499	40704	31509	(45, 6, 12.9)
DS2	22367	23137	2310	83	(1434, 8, 278.8)

5.1   Anomalies Injection

Before reconstructing the process instances, we directly manipulate the object-centric event logs by introducing three types of anomalies in equal parts, amounting in total to circa 10% of the final number of events in each event log.

Attributes Swap: these anomalies are created by altering the attributes of an event, introducing inconsistencies when compared to events in the same process instance. Given the candidate event i, we select the event j whose attributes deviate the most from the attributes of event i by maximizing the euclidean distance $||x_i - x_j||$ and replace the original attributes of i with those of j.

Timestamp Shift: these anomalies are introduced by sampling an existing event in the event log and shifting its timestamp within the time-frame ($\pm 5\%$) of all other events that share a common object with the candidate event. This leads to discrepancies in the temporal order of the events in the process instance.

Random Activities: similarly to [28], we inject events into the process instances with an activity type that does not come from the original process, while the attributes are sampled from the target process instance.

5.2   Baselines

We compare the performance of our graph-based approach to existing approaches for traditional event logs. To be able to do so, we 'flatten' the object-centric process instances to temporally ordered sequences composed by the set of events belonging to each process instance. While this flattening strategy still leads to divergence issues, it does not lead to the deletion or duplication of events [4].

As baselines, we implement a standard autoencoder (AE) similar to the one in [26,27] and a LSTM autoencoder (LSTMAE) similar to the recurrent neural network approaches found in [24,26,28]. For both, we used the hyperparameters found in previous implementations [26,28] in the literature.

5.3   Results

Table 3 shows the experiments results. We ran our experiments five times with different random seeds. To compute the F1 Scores we applied the IQR heuristic to all models, while the other metrics are computed on the raw anomaly scores.

Table 3. Performance comparison of the different models. Results reported as mean ± standard deviation. Best model in bold.

Dataset	Model	F1 Score	AUC ROC	AUC PR	Recall @ 10
BPIC 2017	AE	52.4 ± 0.2	**85.6 ± 0.1**	43.5 ± 0.3	52.1 ± 0.2
	LSTMAE	44.6 ± 0.3	82.9 ± 0.1	34.3 ± 0.2	43.9 ± 0.2
	GCNAE	**61.2 ± 0.2**	82.4 ± 0.1	**60.3 ± 0.2**	**64.8 ± 0.3**
DS2	AE	OOM	OOM	OOM	OOM
	LSTMAE	31.1 ± 0.6	68.4 ± 0.4	23.5 ± 0.8	30.6 ± 0.7
	GCNAE	**59.2 ± 0.3**	**82.5 ± 0.3**	**64.9 ± 0.4**	**66.6 ± 0.1**

The GCNAE generally outperforms the baselines, which could be attributed to the inherent ability of GNNs to reason over graphs and account for dependencies between events. We also note how the AE goes out-of-memory on the *DS2* dataset since the high number of events in the process instances of this dataset result in long vector encodings.

Furthermore, in Table 4 we present the *Recall@10* for each type of anomaly and model. Since in this specific instance of the *Recall@k* metric we set k equal to the amount of ground truth anomalies in the datasets, it can be used to measure how well the models rank the different anomalous events over the normal ones.

Table 4. Recall@10 for the different type of anomalies. Results reported as mean ± standard deviation. Best model in bold.

Dataset	Model	Attr. Swap	Timestamp Shift	Random Act.
BPIC 2017	AE	89.1 ± 0.5	**25.5 ± 0.1**	41.8 ± 0.4
	LSTMAE	81.8 ± 0.4	18.8 ± 0.2	30.9 ± 0.6
	GCNAE	**96.9 ± 0.4**	4.0 ± 0.1	**93.4 ± 0.6**
DS2	AE	OOM	OOM	OOM
	LSTMAE	76.3 ± 2.8	**7.4 ± 0.6**	8.0 ± 1.3
	GCNAE	**96.4 ± 0.1**	3.6 ± 0.4	**100.0 ± 0.0**

The GCNAE struggles detecting the *Timestamp Shift* anomalies. A possible explanation is that GCNs learn nodes representations by aggregating local neighborhood information. Shifting an event within a process instance time-frame might create very subtle changes in the event neighborhood, which therefore would limit the performance of the GCNAE for this specific anomaly.

6 Conclusion

Detecting anomalies is important for identifying inefficiencies, errors, or fraud in business processes. Object-centric event logs provide benefits over traditional event log representations. We have presented a novel approach for anomaly detection in business processes that can leverage the joint capabilities of GNNs and object-centric process mining. Our approach has displayed promising performance, while also not requiring a process model, knowledge of the contamination rate, or the availability of a clean training set.

Future work could explore the use of GNNs architectures that are better suited to learn the temporal and structural dependencies of business process instances and address the limitations displayed by the GCNAE. Future work could also extend the focus to additional anomaly types and object-centric perspectives, for example moving the level of analysis to anomalous process instances and sub-process instances, or investigating anomalies arising in the relationships between and within multiple objects.

References

1. Aalst, W.M.P.: Object-centric process mining: dealing with divergence and convergence in event data. In: Ölveczky, P.C., Salaün, G. (eds.) SEFM 2019. LNCS, vol. 11724, pp. 3–25. Springer, Cham (2019). https://doi.org/10.1007/978-3-030-30446-1_1
2. van der Aalst, W.M.P.: Process mining: a 360 degree overview. In: van der Aalst, W.M.P., Carmona, J. (eds.) Process Mining Handbook. LNBIP, vol. 448, pp. 3–34. Springer, Cham (2022). https://doi.org/10.1007/978-3-031-08848-3_1
3. Adams, J.N., van der Aalst, W.M.P.: Precision and fitness in object-centric process mining. In: 2021 3rd International Conference on Process Mining (ICPM), pp. 128–135. IEEE, Eindhoven, Netherlands (2021)
4. Adams, J.N., van der Aalst, W.M.P.: Addressing convergence, divergence, and deficiency issues. In: De Weerdt, J., Pufahl, L. (eds.) BPM 2023. LNBIP, vol. 492, pp. 496–507. Springer, Cham (2024). https://doi.org/10.1007/978-3-031-50974-2_37
5. Adams, J.N., Park, G., van der Aalst, W.M.P.: Ocpa: a python library for object-centric process analysis. Software Impacts, p. 100438 (2022)
6. Adams, J.N., Schuster, D., Schmitz, S., Schuh, G., van der Aalst, W.M.P.: Defining cases and variants for object-centric event data. In: 2022 4th International Conference on Process Mining (ICPM), pp. 128–135 (2022)
7. Bergami, G., Maggi, F.M., Marrella, A., Montali, M.: Aligning data-aware declarative process models and event logs. In: Polyvyanyy, A., Wynn, M.T., Van Looy, A., Reichert, M. (eds.) BPM 2021. LNCS, vol. 12875, pp. 235–251. Springer, Cham (2021). https://doi.org/10.1007/978-3-030-85469-0_16
8. Berti, A., Herforth, J., Qafari, M., van der Aalst, W.M.P.: Graph-Based Feature Extraction on Object-Centric Event Logs. preprint, In Review (2022)
9. Bezerra, F., Wainer, J.: Algorithms for anomaly detection of traces in logs of process aware information systems. Inf. Syst. **38**(1), 33–44 (2013)
10. Bezerra, F., Wainer, J., van der Aalst, W.M.P.: Anomaly detection using process mining. In: Halpin, T., et al. (eds.) BPMDS/EMMSAD -2009. LNBIP, vol. 29, pp. 149–161. Springer, Heidelberg (2009). https://doi.org/10.1007/978-3-642-01862-6_13
11. Bronstein, M.M., Bruna, J., Cohen, T., Veličković, P.: Geometric Deep Learning: Grids, Groups, Graphs, Geodesics, and Gauges (2021). arXiv:2104.13478 [cs, stat]
12. Böhmer, K., Rinderle-Ma, S.: Multi-perspective Anomaly Detection in Business Process Execution Events, pp. 80–98 (2016). mAG ID: 2538859255
13. Böhmer, K., Rinderle-Ma, S.: Anomaly Detection in Business Process Runtime Behavior – Challenges and Limitations (2017). arXiv:1705.06659 [cs]
14. Chandola, V., Banerjee, A., Kumar, V.: Anomaly detection: a survey. ACM Comput. Surv. **41**(3), 1–58 (2009)
15. Chiorrini, A., Diamantini, C., Mircoli, A., Potena, D.: Exploiting instance graphs and graph neural networks for next activity prediction. In: Munoz-Gama, J., Lu, X. (eds.) ICPM 2021. LNBIP, vol. 433, pp. 115–126. Springer, Cham (2022). https://doi.org/10.1007/978-3-030-98581-3_9
16. Diamantini, C., Genga, L., Potena, D., van der Aalst, W.M.P.: Building instance graphs for highly variable processes. Expert Syst. Appl. **59**, 101–118 (2016)
17. van Dongen, B.F.: BPI Challenge 2017 (2017). publisher: 4TU.ResearchData
18. Ghahfarokhi, A.F., Park, G., Berti, A., van der Aalst, W.M.P.: OCEL: a standard for object-centric event logs. In: Bellatreche, L., et al. (eds.) ADBIS 2021. CCIS, vol. 1450, pp. 169–175. Springer, Cham (2021). https://doi.org/10.1007/978-3-030-85082-1_16

19. Harl, M., Weinzierl, S., Stierle, M., Matzner, M.: Explainable predictive business process monitoring using gated graph neural networks. J. Decis. Syst. **29**(sup1), 312–327 (2020)
20. Huo, S., Völzer, H., Reddy, P., Agarwal, P., Isahagian, V., Muthusamy, V.: Graph autoencoders for business process anomaly detection. In: Polyvyanyy, A., Wynn, M.T., Van Looy, A., Reichert, M. (eds.) BPM 2021. LNCS, vol. 12875, pp. 417–433. Springer, Cham (2021). https://doi.org/10.1007/978-3-030-85469-0_26
21. Junior, S.B., Ceravolo, P., Damiani, E., Omori, N.J., Tavares, G.M.: Anomaly detection on event logs with a scarcity of labels. In: 2020 2nd International Conference on Process Mining (ICPM), pp. 161–168 (2020)
22. Kipf, T.N., Welling, M.: Semi-Supervised Classification with Graph Convolutional Networks (2017). arXiv:1609.02907 [cs, stat]
23. Ko, J., Comuzzi, M.: A Systematic Review of Anomaly Detection for Business Process Event Logs. Business & Information Systems Engineering (2023)
24. Lahann, J., Pfeiffer, P., Fettke, P.: LSTM-based anomaly detection of process instances: benchmark and tweaks. In: Montali, M., Senderovich, A., Weidlich, M. (eds.) Process Mining Workshops. ICPM 2022. LNBIP, vol. 468, pp. 229–241. Springer, Cham (2023). https://doi.org/10.1007/978-3-031-27815-0_17
25. Liu, K., et al.: BOND: Benchmarking Unsupervised Outlier Node Detection on Static Attributed Graphs (2022). arXiv:2206.10071 [cs]
26. Nguyen, H.T.C., Lee, S., Kim, J., Ko, J., Comuzzi, M.: Autoencoders for improving quality of process event logs. Expert Syst. Appl. **131**, 132–147 (2019)
27. Nolle, T., Luettgen, S., Seeliger, A., Mühlhäuser, M.: Analyzing business process anomalies using autoencoders. Mach. Learn. **107**(11), 1875–1893 (2018)
28. Nolle, T., Luettgen, S., Seeliger, A., Mühlhäuser, M.: BINet: multi-perspective business process anomaly classification. Inf. Syst. **103**, 101458 (2022)
29. Sommers, D., Menkovski, V., Fahland, D.: Process discovery using graph neural networks. In: 2021 3rd International Conference on Process Mining (ICPM), pp. 40–47 (2021)
30. Tavares, G.M., Barbon, S.: Analysis of language inspired trace representation for anomaly detection. In: Bellatreche, L., et al. (eds.) TPDL/ADBIS -2020. CCIS, vol. 1260, pp. 296–308. Springer, Cham (2020). https://doi.org/10.1007/978-3-030-55814-7_25
31. Veličković, P.: Everything is Connected: Graph Neural Networks (2023). arXiv:2301.08210 [cs, stat]
32. Weinzierl, S.: Exploring gated graph sequence neural networks for predicting next process activities. In: Marrella, A., Weber, B. (eds.) BPM 2021. LNBIP, vol. 436, pp. 30–42. Springer, Cham (2022). https://doi.org/10.1007/978-3-030-94343-1_3
33. Yuan, X., Zhou, N., Yu, S., Huang, H., Chen, Z., Xia, F.: Higher-order structure based anomaly detection on attributed networks. In: 2021 IEEE International Conference on Big Data (Big Data), pp. 2691–2700 (2021)

Uncovering the Hidden Significance of Activities Location in Predictive Process Monitoring

Mozhgan Vazifehdoostirani[✉], Mohsen Abbaspour Onari, Isel Grau,
Laura Genga, and Remco Dijkman

Eindhoven University of Technology, Eindhoven, The Netherlands
{m.vazifehdoostirani,m.abbaspour.onari,i.d.c.grau.garcia,
l.genga,r.m.dijkman}@tue.nl

Abstract. Predictive process monitoring methods predict ongoing case outcomes by analyzing historical process data. Recent studies highlighted the increasing need to enhance the interpretability of these prediction models. This is often achieved by exploiting post-hoc explainable methodologies to assess the importance of different process features on the predicted outcome. However, the significance of the *location* of process activities on prediction models remains unexplored. In several real-life contexts, there might be potential meaningful relations between the location of the activities and process outcome. This information facilitates insights into process management optimization and decision-making. This paper introduces a novel post-hoc explainable artificial intelligence technique inspired by permutation feature importance to assess the impact of activity locations in predictive models. The experimental results on real-life event logs validate the feasibility of the proposed method, showcasing the influence of the location of (group of) activities on outcome predictions.

Keywords: Predictive Process Monitoring · Explainbale AI · Feature Permutation Importance

1   Introduction

Predictive Process Monitoring (PPM) methods aim to predict the future status of ongoing cases by analyzing historical process data. In recent years, a plethora of Machine Learning (ML) approaches have been proposed to support PPM. Extensive studies and benchmarks have indicated the effectiveness of black-box models, such as XGBoost and Random Forest [18], in accurately predicting process outcomes across diverse domains. Recently, the adoption of Deep Learning approaches in PPM has been on the rise [7]. Although these black-box models demonstrate impressive predictive capabilities, they also bring complexity and limited interpretability as trade-offs.

eXplainable Artificial Intelligence (XAI) aims to address the lack of interpretability of black-box models by supporting process analysts in investigating

J. De Smedt and P. Soffer (Eds.): ICPM 2023 Workshops, LNBIP 503, pp. 191–203, 2024.
https://doi.org/10.1007/978-3-031-56107-8_15

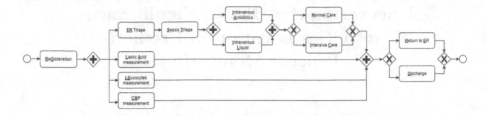

Fig. 1. A simplified version of the sepsis patient trajectory [14]

Table 1. An example of a training event log from Sepsis.

ID	Trace	Label
1	RG, *LA*, LE, CR, ER, ST, IL, IA, NC, ER, CR, LE, CR	Negative
2	RG, ER, ST, IL, LE, CR, IA, *LA*, IC, DI	Positive
3	RG, *LA*, ER, ST, LE, CR, IA, NC, CR, LE, CR, LE, CR	Negative
4	RG, LE, LE, *LA*, ER, ST, CR, IA, IC, LE, *LA*, NC, DI	Positive
5	RG, ER, ST, LE, CR, IL, IA, *LA*, NC, CR, LE	Positive
6	RG, *LA*, CR, ER, ST, LE, IL, IA, NC, DI	Negative

how a given classifier made its decisions. A popular class of XAI methods is *post-hoc* methods, which explain decisions made by black-box models after they are built. Earlier research in PPM has utilized techniques like SHAP [4,23], LIME [16], and Permutation Feature Importance (PFI) [5] to obtain the importance of different process features at both local and global levels. Utilizing these existing XAI methods, prior research has addressed the impact of executing each activity on process outcome [4]; however, the importance of the location of executing activities through the process has not been discussed.

As an example, let us consider the process model in Fig. 1, which is a simplified version of the *Sepsis* patient pathways presented in [14]. Table 1 shows an excerpt of an *event log* used to train a model to predict patients returning to the emergency room within 28 days of discharge. Let us consider the activity *Lactic Acid measurement* (*LA*). This activity can be executed at different moments (locations) in the process. From the table, no relation can be detected between the occurrence of this activity and the process outcome. However, the situation is different when its location is considered. The execution of activity *LA* in position 2 corresponds to negative process outcomes, whereas its occurrence in other locations correlates with positive outcomes. This intriguing observation might encourage a process analyst to assess the importance of the location of *LA* and compare this importance with other activities.

To assess the importance of activity locations with post-hoc methods, one needs to employ a trace encoding technique able to represent activity locations explicitly. To incorporate the location information in training an ML classifier, index-based encoding has been used in several studies [13,18]. Existing post-hoc XAI approaches usually return two kinds of explanations using index-based encoding. The first one only measures the importance of each *index (location)* in the process. For example, we might understand that the third activity is more important than the second activity executed in the process, regardless of the type of activity. The second one, instead, considers both the kind of the activity and its location, generating explanations in the form "*Occurrence of activity $\mathcal{A}$ at index 3 in case 10 impacts the prediction.*" While providing useful insights, this form of explanation combines the effect of *executing* activity $\mathcal{A}$ and the *location* of its execution in the process. Therefore, the lingering question is whether executing activity $\mathcal{A}$ impacts the process outcome regardless of its occurrence in a particular location. As a result, uncertainties arise regarding the potential impact of relocating activities, like shifting activity $\mathcal{A}$ from timestamp 3 to timestamp 8, on the predictive model. This query can be extended to encompass *multiple* activities that occur collectively (e.g., activities belonging to the same *subprocess*). Prior research has unveiled distinct outcomes when activities are considered in groups as opposed to their individual effects [19]. However, the impact of their location on the outcome remains unexplored.

We argue that being able to provide explanations on which activities may affect the classifier's performance and whether their impact depends on their position provides the process manager with valuable insights about the process. In flexible processes, there is often little or no prior knowledge of how the decision to execute a (group of) activity(ies) at a given moment may affect the outcome. Furthermore, the extracted relations can support process managers in different tasks. For instance, insights on the importance of activity location in determining the process performance can be used in selecting suitable redesign heuristics [6] to explore alternative control-flow constraints during business process re-engineering efforts.

In this paper, we seek to address the following research question: "Given a predictive model trained on a set of process executions, how can we assess the importance of the location of a group of process activities on the classifier performance?" Our main contribution is a novel post-hoc model-agnostic method, inspired by the PFI method, designed to assess the importance of the location of executing activities on outcome prediction. Our experimental results on real-life event logs show the feasibility of the method and provide evidence of the importance of the location of activities for trained outcome prediction models.

The remainder of this paper is organized as follows. In Sect. 2, we present a review of the relevant related work. Next, in Sect. 3, we introduce our proposal. The experimental settings and results are discussed in Sect. 4. Finally, Sect. 5 concludes the research and outlines potential directions for the future.

2   Related Work

XAI approaches proposed within the PPM domain can be broadly categorized into *factual* and *counterfactual* explanations [3]. The former aims to reveal the reasoning behind specific predictions, emphasizing the most influential features. On the other hand, counterfactual explanations provide insights into what changes are necessary for an input sample to achieve a desired prediction [3].

Significant efforts have been made to generate realistic counterfactual explanations for process prediction such as DiCE4EL [9], LORELEY [10], and CREATED [11]. While counterfactual explanations offer valuable insights into hypothetical scenarios, this paper's primary focus remains on factual explanations to gain a deeper understanding of the functionality of black-box models in the context of PPM. Regarding factual explanations, two groups of methods have been exploited in PPM: *intrinsically interpretable* and *post-hoc* methods. Intrinsically interpretable methods seek to build interpretable models from scratch, such as rule-based classifiers [12], neuro-fuzzy networks [15], and linear regression [5]. However, intrinsically interpretable models often underperform compared to their black-box counterparts [1].

Post-hoc methods can be classified into two groups: *model-specific* and *model-agnostic* [1]. Model-specific methods are designed to work with specific prediction models, such as Gated Graph Neural Network [8], LSTM with Layer-wise Relevance Propagation [20], and LSTM with attention layers [21]. In contrast, model-agnostic methods compute explanations based on the inputs and their associated outputs, allowing the process analyzer to use various prediction models.

Regarding the model-agnostic post-hoc techniques, several studies employed LIME to address the problem of low accuracy by identifying the features that cause wrong predictions [16] and providing an explanation for various feature representations of the event log [17]. Various model-agnostic post-hoc methods, such as SHAP and FPI, are widely used in the literature to provide a local and global explanation [5,23]. A recent study introduced an ML-based approach for generating multi-level explanations, employing logistic regression, attention-based LSTM, and the eXplainable Dual-learning Deep network [22]. However, it is notable that none of these studies have tackled the global importance of activity locations within a process. Hence, we are filling the mentioned gap by proposing a model-agnostic post-hoc explanation method.

3   Methodology

Figure 2 illustrates our proposed method for measuring the global importance of the location of one or a group of activities on the process outcome prediction. The steps depicted with hatched patterns represent this research's primary focus and contribution. Drawing inspiration from the PFI technique designed for tabular data, our method quantifies the reduction in model performance resulting from the random shuffling of a single feature value [2]. In our analysis, we are interested in analyzing the effect of changing activity locations in process executions. However, the direct application of conventional PFI to a tabular-encoded event log is not suitable for our analysis. Let us assume to encode the event log using index-based encoding. In this encoded log, the location of an activity does not

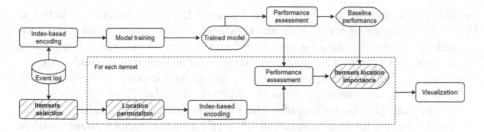

Fig. 2. Overview of the location permutation importance method.

map to a single column; instead, it encompasses all the columns related to the same activity. Therefore, the shuffling implemented by standard PFI techniques, which shuffles one column independently from the others, is inadequate for our analysis due to intricate interdependencies among features. Indeed, relocating an activity necessitates coordinated shuffling of all associated location-related columns to maintain distinct activity locations in generated traces. Furthermore, shifting the location of an activity inevitably impacts also the location of other activities in the trace. Therefore, we introduced a tailored method that accommodates the sequential nature of processes.

The method takes as an input an *event log*, that is, a multiset of *traces*, each tracking the execution of a given process *instance* (or *case*). Each trace involves a sequence of *events* representing the execution of a given process *activity* at a given timestamp. Within the context of this work, we consider only the activity names as event attributes, assuming that their order in the trace is based on their execution timestamps. Table 1 shows an excerpt of an event log, where each execution corresponds to the treatment administered to a sepsis patient.

First, we *train* a black-box model using index-based encoding and evaluate its performance through k-fold cross-validation on the event log. This provides us with the *baseline performance*. Then, we identify a group of activities (aka. itemsets) whose location importance we want to measure. For each itemset, first, we use the location permutation module to shuffle the location of each item in the itemset across the existing traces. Then, we apply index-based encoding to the shuffled event traces. Next, we assess the model's performance on the permuted event logs using the original trained model through k-fold cross-validation. The difference between the baseline performance and the performance on the permuted event log indicates the importance of the itemset in question. These iterative steps are repeated for each individual itemset. Finally, we plot the importance of each itemset in one plot to facilitate the location importance comparison. In the remainder of this section, we delve into the itemsets selection (Sect. 3.1) and location permutation (Sect. 3.2) modules.

3.1   Itemsets Selection

Depending on the purpose of the analysis, a process analyst might be interested in exploring the significance of the location of different groups of activities. To

facilitate this exploration, we utilize an **I**temsets **E**xtractor function denoted as
$IE(\mathcal{L})$. Given an event log $\mathcal{L}$, this function generates itemsets of activities considered of interest for the analysis. This function can be customized according to the analyst's notion of interest and may encompass diverse methods. A common and straightforward approach is measuring an itemset's interest through frequency, often accomplished using the Apriori algorithm [24].

As an example, let us consider the event log depicted in Table 1 and let us assume to use an implementation of $IE(\mathcal{L})$ which returns itemsets with a minimum frequency of 80%. An excerpt of the output of the itemset selection step would then be $IE(\mathcal{L}) = \{\{RG\}, \{ER, CR\}, \{RG, LE, CR\}, \dots\}$.

3.2 Location Permutation

We perform the location permutation module for each discovered itemset to shuffle the location of activities in that itemset within all traces. However, randomly shuffling activities' locations has important drawbacks. First, it is likely to result in unrealistic traces . Second, when permuting itemsets involving more than one activity, a completely random shuffle may result in a permuted trace where the relative order of activities in the itemset has also been changed, thus introducing noise in assessing the importance of the itemset location. To mitigate these issues, we introduce the following two constraints:

- **Feasibility Constraint**: We restrict the location permutation of an activity to the observed locations of the occurrences of that activity throughout the event log.
- **Preserving Ordering Relation**: When shuffling itemset activities, we preserve their relative order within each trace.

These constraints allow us to balance between maintaining meaningful process behaviors in generated traces and introducing enough randomness and variability in itemset locations within the event log.

Keeping these constraints in mind, given an itemset $\mathcal{I}$ extracted by an event log $\mathcal{L}$, we permute the location of $\mathcal{I}$ in each trace in which it occurs by implementing the following steps. We first extract a set of **O**bserved **L**ocations for $\mathcal{I}$ throughout the event log. To uphold the sequential order of activities within an itemset, we define tuples encompassing the itemset activities. For instance, the **O**bserved **L**ocations for the itemset $\{ER, CR\}$ in the event log $\mathcal{L}$ shown in Table 1 can be defined as $OL(\mathcal{L}, (ER, CR)) = \{(5,4), (10, 11), (2,6), (3,6), (5,7), (2,5), (4,3)\}$. In certain locations, activity CR follows activity ER, whereas, in other instances, CR precedes ER. It's important to note that if a single activity from the itemset appears multiple times in a trace and results in an overlapped occurrence of the itemset, only the first complete occurrence is considered for collecting observed locations and subsequent permutation. For instance, in case number 1 in Table 1 we observe the occurrence of $\{CR, ER\}$ twice, along with an additional CR. Since the final occurrence of CR lacks a distinct accompanying ER to form the itemset, its location is not included in the function's output.

Next, we randomly rearrange the positions of itemsets in traces using the pool of observed locations. We extract a random location from the set of observed locations for every activity of the itemset within a trace. If the chosen location conforms to the existing sequential order of activities of the itemset instance, it is retained. Otherwise, an alternative location is drawn to ensure that the activity relations remain consistent within that specific itemset instance. This operation is repeated for each occurrence of the itemset in the trace.

As an example, let us consider case number 1 from the running example: $\sigma_1 = \langle RG, LA, LE, \mathbf{CR}, \mathbf{ER}, ST, IL, IA, NC, \mathbf{ER}, \mathbf{CR}, LE, CR \rangle$. A possible permutation for itemset {ER, CR} generates the permuted trace $\sigma_1^? = \langle RG, LA, \mathbf{CR}, \mathbf{ER}, \mathbf{ER}, LE, \mathbf{CR}, ST, IL, IA, NC, LE, CR \rangle$.

4   Implementation and Experiments

4.1   Settings

We utilized XGBoost, a top-performing ensemble model in outcome prediction according to [18], and evaluated it using a 5-fold cross-validation. To account for the variability introduced by the permutation process, we repeated the location permutation 10 times and utilized box plots to visualize the results. A decrease in the f1-score indicates the importance of each itemset under consideration.

We considered two analysis goals, i.e., deriving the location importance for the single and frequent group of activities. For the latter, we extracted the top 10 frequent itemsets of size greater than one using the Apriori algorithm [24].

In addition to assessing the importance of itemset locations, we have also employed the conventional PFI technique to assess the importance associated with the existence of itemsets. To achieve this, we utilized binary encoding, where each feature represented a distinct itemset. We trained an XGBoost model on the binary-encoded event log. It is worth mentioning that the difference between the importance of the location and the existence of the selected itemsets is also due to using different encoding methods. Our aim is not to establish an absolute comparison between the obtained values but, instead, to shed light on the insights gained from examining the location of activities as opposed to their existence. The implementation of the proposed method is available at GitHub[1].

We used public event logs widely used in the literature, such as *bpic2011*, *bpic2012*, and *Sepsis* event logs with the same labeling strategy as in [18].

4.2   Results and Discussion

Single-activity Itemsets. Figure 3 represents the top 20 most important single activities regarding their location in the process (in green) and their corresponding existence importance values (in blue). Activities that hold the greatest positional significance do not necessarily maintain equivalent existence importance. For instance, in the *bpic2012 accepted* event log, the location of the activity

---

[1] https://github.com/MozhganVD/PermutationLocationImportance.

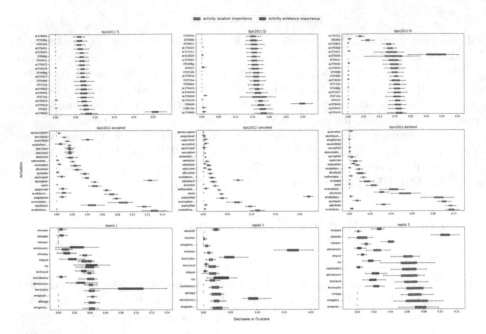

Fig. 3. Single activities location importance vs. their existence importance. (Color figure online)

"W Nabellen Offer" stands out as an influential factor, leading to a decrease in performance between 12% and 14%. However, its existence does not yield substantial explanatory power for the predictive model. To delve more into this activity, since we lack expert access to validate explanations from the black box model, we have explored the event log to assess whether the data aligns with our findings. In particular, we have plotted the distribution of process outcomes associated with different locations of this activity in Fig. 4a. According to the event log, the occurrence of this activity leads to the process being accepted in 61% of the cases; however, we observe variations in the acceptance percentage from 50% to 70% in different locations. While these observations cannot serve as direct validation for the presented results, they suggest that our findings in terms of location and existence importance are meaningful in the log under analysis.

Likewise, across all three labeled event logs extracted from the *bpic2011* dataset, most activities demonstrate high significance based on their location, while their existence is insignificant for the model. Conversely, we encounter activities showing a relatively strong influence due to their sheer presence. Take the activity "ac370000" within the *bpic2011 f1* event log; for instance, it demonstrates notably high importance in relation to its existence. A similar trend is observable across all event logs extracted from the *sepsis* dataset, where multiple activities such as "leucocytes" in *sepsis 1* (see Fig. 4b), "release A" in *sepsis 2*, and "release B" in *sepsis 3* showcase the same behavioral patterns. As depicted in

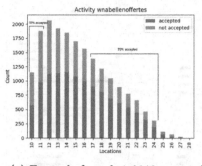
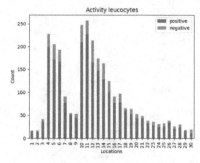

(a) Example from *bpic2012 accepted*.   (b) Example from *sepsis 1*.

Fig. 4. Distribution of the locations of activities over different outcomes.

Fig. 4b, the presence of the "leukocytes" activity strongly correlates with positive outcomes, only with minor variations in location.

Multiple-activities Itemsets. Figure 5 represents the location and existence importance of the extracted itemsets. A first observation is that, in general, the existence of the frequent itemsets does not exhibit much importance for the prediction model. This observation could potentially stem from our selection of the most frequent itemsets, which might not necessarily be the most predictive ones. However, permuting their location could still affect the prediction model. Notably, within the *bpic2011 f1* log, except for the itemset {ac370000, ac370419} whose existence demonstrates a noticeable effect on the prediction model, the remainder of the frequent itemsets are primarily influential due to their location.

We have plotted the distribution of outcomes across diverse locations for itemset with the highest *existence* importance in *bpic2011 f1* (Fig. 6b) and with the highest *location* importance in *bpic2011 f2* (Fig. 6a). Note that when plotting itemset locations, we can easily have a lot of locations with low-frequency values. This would lead to many locations in the X-axis with many small bars, resulting in a very cluttered figure. To simplify the visualization, we aggregated all locations with the same starting point. For example, all locations of (1,3), (1,5), and (1,10) are shown in index 1 in the plot. While this representation is less accurate since only the starting position of each itemset is considered, it still provides a reasonable estimate of how the output distribution varies in relation to different locations. Notably, the itemset {ac379999, ac370000} exhibits significant variation in positive and negative class proportions across varying locations. There are also more possible locations for this itemset in general. In contrast, the itemset {ac370000, ac370419} maintains an almost consistent positive and negative fraction across different locations.

Discussion. The obtained results confirm the feasibility and practicality of the proposed methods in measuring the importance of the location of activities. They also underscore the need to delve further into the significance of locations within

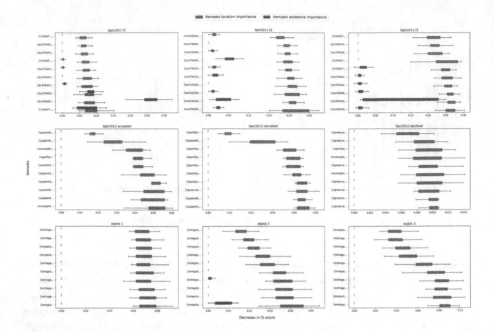

Fig. 5. Location vs. existence importance for 10 most frequent itemsets.

process analysis, given the meaningful relationships between activity location and associated outcomes detected in real-life event logs.

Nonetheless, our approach presents some limitations. First, our method's focus is on classifier performance, which might not fully reveal the underlying relationships between activities and outcomes in the dataset. This prompts the need for expert validation of the insights gathered. Moreover, an activity location's importance is inherently intertwined with other activity locations. While we have addressed this issue by implementing repeated permutations, quantifying the exact impact of these permutations remains a complex challenge. Also, despite imposing feasibility constraints, the risk of placing activities in prohibited locations due to dependencies persists, and more sophisticated methods are needed. Additionally, the effectiveness of our method is influenced by the design choices made during various methodological steps. This acknowledges the potential for refining strategies, such as employing predictive pattern detection methods, as previous studies discussed that frequent patterns are not necessarily the most predictive ones [19].

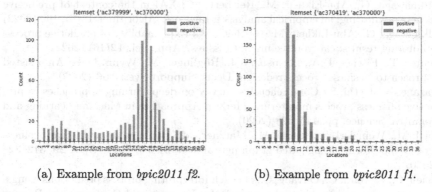

(a) Example from *bpic2011 f2*.   (b) Example from *bpic2011 f1*.

Fig. 6. Distribution of the locations of itemsets over different outcomes.

5 Conclusion and Future Work

Our exploration into XAI within PPM has shed light on the importance of understanding activities' location-based significance. Our novel post-hoc method, inspired by the Permutation Feature Importance, endeavors to address this gap by quantifying the impact of activities locations on predictive process outcomes. We performed several experiments on real-life event logs widely used in the PPM domain. Our experiments underscore the method's feasibility, as demonstrated through its successful application to real-life event logs. The results provide clear evidence regarding the latent importance of activities' location. This insight into the significance of location adds a new dimension to our understanding, one that is frequently overlooked by existing XAI techniques.

These considerations highlight the potential for further extension of this research, prompting us to investigate different approaches for itemset selection, seeking more meaningful itemsets rather than just being frequent. For instance, we intend to construct outcome-oriented patterns introduced in [19] rather than relying on frequent itemsets. Additionally, we are working on a methodology to evaluate the importance of the order of activities within each itemset, besides their location importance. Furthermore, our future research endeavors to develop more sophisticated approaches to ensure the feasibility of permuted traces.

References

1. Arrieta, A.B., et al.: Explainable artificial intelligence: concepts, taxonomies, opportunities and challenges toward responsible AI. Inf. Fusion **58**, 82–115 (2020)
2. Breiman, L.: Random forests. Mach. Learn. **45**, 5–32 (2001)
3. Buliga, A., Di Francescomarino, C., Ghidini, C., Maggi, F.M.: Counterfactuals and ways to build them: evaluating approaches in predictive process monitoring. In: Indulska, M., Reinhartz-Berger, I., Cetina, C., Pastor, O. (eds.) Advanced Information Systems Engineering. CAiSE 2023. LNCS, vol. 13901, pp. 558–574. Springer, Cham (2023). https://doi.org/10.1007/978-3-031-34560-9_33

4. El-khawaga, G., Abu-Elkheir, M., Reichert, M.: XAI in the context of predictive process monitoring: an empirical analysis framework. Algorithms **15**(6), 199 (2022)
5. Elkhawaga, G., Abu-Elkheir, M., Reichert, M.: Explainability of predictive process monitoring results: can you see my data issues? Appl. Sci. **12**(16) (2022)
6. Fehrer, T., Fischer, D.A., Leemans, S.J., Röglinger, M., Wynn, M.T.: An assisted approach to business process redesign. Decis. Support Syst. **156** (2022)
7. Harane, N., Rathi, S.: Comprehensive survey on deep learning approaches in predictive business process monitoring. Modern Approaches in Machine Learning and Cognitive Science, pp. 115–128 (2020)
8. Harl, M., Weinzierl, S., Stierle, M., Matzner, M.: Explainable predictive business process monitoring using gated graph neural networks. J. Decis. Syst. **29**, 312–327 (2020)
9. Hsieh, C., Moreira, C., Ouyang, C.: Dice4el: interpreting process predictions using a milestone-aware counterfactual approach. In: International Conference on Process Mining, pp. 88–95. IEEE (2021)
10. Huang, T.H., Metzger, A., Pohl, K.: Counterfactual explanations for predictive business process monitoring. In: Themistocleous, M., Papadaki, M. (eds.) Information Systems. EMCIS 2021. LNBIP, vol. 437, pp. 399–413. Springer, Cham (2021). https://doi.org/10.1007/978-3-030-95947-0_28
11. Hundogan, O., Lu, X., Du, Y., Reijers, H.A.: CREATED: generating viable counterfactual sequences for predictive process analytics. In: Indulska, M., Reinhartz-Berger, I., Cetina, C., Pastor, O. (eds.) Advanced Information Systems Engineering. CAiSE 2023. LNCS, vol. 13901, pp. 541–557. Springer, Cham (2023). https://doi.org/10.1007/978-3-031-34560-9_32
12. Lee, S., Comuzzi, M., Kwon, N.: Exploring the suitability of rule-based classification to provide interpretability in outcome-based process predictive monitoring. Algorithms **15**(6), 187 (2022)
13. Leontjeva, A., Conforti, R., Di Francescomarino, C., Dumas, M., Maggi, F.M.: Complex symbolic sequence encodings for predictive monitoring of business processes. In: Motahari-Nezhad, H.R., Recker, J., Weidlich, M. (eds.) BPM 2015. LNCS, vol. 9253, pp. 297–313. Springer, Cham (2015). https://doi.org/10.1007/978-3-319-23063-4_21
14. Munoz-Gama, J., et al.: Process mining for healthcare: characteristics and challenges. J. Biomed. Inform. **127**, 103994 (2022)
15. Pasquadibisceglie, V., Castellano, G., Appice, A., Malerba, D.: Fox: a neuro-fuzzy model for process outcome prediction and explanation. In: International Conference on Process Mining, pp. 112–119. IEEE (2021)
16. Rizzi, W., Di Francescomarino, C., Maggi, F.M.: Explainability in predictive process monitoring: when understanding helps improving. In: Fahland, D., Ghidini, C., Becker, J., Dumas, M. (eds.) BPM 2020. LNBIP, vol. 392, pp. 141–158. Springer, Cham (2020). https://doi.org/10.1007/978-3-030-58638-6_9
17. Sindhgatta, R., Moreira, C., Ouyang, C., Barros, A.: Exploring interpretable predictive models for business processes. In: Fahland, D., Ghidini, C., Becker, J., Dumas, M. (eds.) BPM 2020. LNCS, vol. 12168, pp. 257–272. Springer, Cham (2020). https://doi.org/10.1007/978-3-030-58666-9_15
18. Teinemaa, I., Dumas, M., Rosa, M.L., Maggi, F.M.: Outcome-oriented predictive process monitoring: review and benchmark. ACM Trans. Knowl. Discov. Data **13**(2) (2019)
19. Vazifehdoostirani, M., Genga, L., Lu, X., Verhoeven, R., van Laarhoven, H., Dijkman, R.: Interactive multi-interest process pattern discovery. In: Di Francesco-

marino, C., Burattin, A., Janiesch, C., Sadiq, S. (eds.) Business Process Management. BPM 2023. LNCS, vol. 14159, pp. 303–319. Springer, Cham (2023). https://doi.org/10.1007/978-3-031-41620-0_18

20. Weinzierl, S., Zilker, S., Brunk, J., Revoredo, K., Matzner, M., Becker, J.: XNAP: making LSTM-based next activity predictions explainable by using LRP. In: Del Río Ortega, A., Leopold, H., Santoro, F.M. (eds.) BPM 2020. LNBIP, vol. 397, pp. 129–141. Springer, Cham (2020). https://doi.org/10.1007/978-3-030-66498-5_10

21. Wickramanayake, B., He, Z., Ouyang, C., Moreira, C., Xu, Y., Sindhgatta, R.: Building interpretable models for business process prediction using shared and specialised attention mechanisms. Knowl.-Based Syst. **248**, 108773 (2022)

22. Wickramanayake, B., Ouyang, C., Xu, Y., Moreira, C.: Generating multi-level explanations for process outcome predictions. Eng. Appl. Artif. Intell. **125**, 106678 (2023)

23. Yang, M., et al.: Design and implementation of an explainable bidirectional LSTM model based on transition system approach for cooperative AI-workers. Appl. Sci. **12**(13), 6390 (2022)

24. Yuan, X.: An improved apriori algorithm for mining association rules. In: AIP Conference Proceedings, vol. 1820. AIP Publishing (2017)

6th International Workshop
on Process-Oriented Data Science
for Healthcare (PODS4H 2023)

6th International Workshop on Process-Oriented Data Science for Healthcare (PODS4H 2023)

Data has become a highly valuable resource in today's world. The ultimate goal of data science techniques is not to collect more data, but to extract knowledge and valuable insights from existing data. To analyze and improve processes, event data is a key source of information. In recent years, a new discipline has emerged that combines traditional process analysis and data-centric analysis: Process-Oriented Data Science (PODS). The interdisciplinary nature of this new research area has resulted in its application to analyze processes in a wide variety of domains. This workshop has an explicit focus on healthcare.

The International Workshop on Process-Oriented Data Science for Healthcare 2023 (PODS4H 2023) provided a high-quality forum for interdisciplinary researchers and practitioners to exchange research findings and ideas on data-driven process analysis techniques and practices in healthcare. PODS4H research includes a variety of topics ranging from process mining techniques adapted for healthcare processes to practical issues related to the implementation of PODS methodologies in healthcare organizations.

The 6th edition of the workshop was organized in conjunction with the 5th International Conference on Process Mining in Rome (Italy). Similarly to last year, we allowed full papers to be either research papers or case studies. While research papers had to focus on extending the state of the art of PODS4H research, case studies had to focus on a practical application of PODS4H in a real-life context.

In total, we received 22 full paper submissions, which were thoroughly reviewed by experts from our Program Committee such that each submission got three reviews. After the review process, 9 full papers were accepted. The distinction between research papers and case studies was also reflected in the accepted papers, which consisted of 5 research papers and 4 case studies. The research papers focused on a wide range of topics: generating an event log in a healthcare context using logical reasoning over ontologies, building a clinical event knowledge graph to enrich healthcare event data with entities and clinical concepts, using Directly Follows Graphs and hypergraphs to conduct frailty analysis, discovering BPMN processes with duplicated activities in a healthcare context, and visualizing knowledge-intensive and context-sensitive process instances in healthcare by incorporating external information sources such as taxonomies or ontologies. The case studies also considered a variety of healthcare-related problems and contexts: exploring the impact of socio-economic status on the treatment of musculoskeletal disorders in a Dutch care network, conducting an ontology-based multi-perspective process mining analysis in a German laboratory, using error-correcting techniques in conformance checking to highlight the degree of deviation from the clinical guidelines for rectal cancer patients, and identifying variations in a person's daily routines using process mining. Besides the presentation of the full papers included in these proceedings, the workshop program also contained an interactive poster session where 12 posters were presented.

This year's edition of the workshop featured two awards: a Best Paper Award and a Best Student Paper Award. Based on the assessment by the reviewers, the Best Paper Award was given to Carlos Fernandez-Llatas and Andrea Burattin for their paper "I-PALIA: Discovering BPMN Processes with Duplicated Activities for Healthcare Domains". The Best Student Paper Award was awarded to Owen P. Dwyer, Lara Chammas, Emanuel Sallinger, and Jim Davies for their paper "Investigating an Ontology-Informed Approach to Event Log Generation in Healthcare".

The PODS4H workshop is an initiative of the Process-Oriented Data Science for Healthcare Alliance (PODS4H Alliance) within the IEEE Task Force on Process Mining. The goal of the PODS4H Alliance is to promote awareness, research, development, and education regarding process-oriented data science in healthcare. For more information, we would like to refer the reader to our website, http://www.pods4h.com/.

The organizers would like to sincerely thank all authors for their contributions to the workshop, all Program Committee members for their valuable work in reviewing the papers, and the ICPM 2023 workshop chairs and local organizers for supporting this successful event.

November 2023

Niels Martin
Carlos Fernandez-Llatas
Owen Johnson
Marcos Sepúlveda
Jorge Munoz-Gama

Organization

Workshop Chairs

Niels Martin   Hasselt University, Belgium
Carlos Fernandez-Llatas   Universitat Politècnica de València, Spain
Owen Johnson   University of Leeds, UK
Marcos Sepúlveda   Pontificia Universidad Católica de Chile, Chile

Jorge Munoz-Gama   Pontificia Universidad Católica de Chile, Chile

Program Committee

Davide Aloini   University of Pisa, Italy
Robert Andrews   Queensland University of Technology, Australia
Iris Beerepoot   Utrecht University, The Netherlands
Elisabetta Benevento   University of Pisa, Italy
Andrea Burattin   Technical University of Denmark, Denmark
Daniel Capurro   University of Melbourne, Australia
Marco Comuzzi   Ulsan National Institute of Science and Technology, South Korea
Jonas Cremerius   HPI – University of Potsdam, Germany
Benjamin Dalmas   Computer Research Institute of Montreal, Canada
René de la Fuente   Pontificia Universidad Católica de Chile, Chile
Onur Dogan   İzmir Bakırçay University, Turkey
Carlos Fernandez-Llatas   Universitat Politècnica de València, Spain
Roberto Gatta   Università Cattolica del Sacro Cuore, Italy
Joscha Grüger   Universität Trier, Germany
Emmanuel Helm   University of Applied Sciences Upper Austria, Austria
Owen Johnson   University of Leeds, UK
Felix Mannhardt   Eindhoven University of Technology, The Netherlands
Ronny Mans   Philips Research, The Netherlands
Niels Martin   Hasselt University, Belgium

Renata Medeiros de Carvalho	Eindhoven University of Technology, The Netherlands
Jorge Munoz-Gama	Pontificia Universidad Católica de Chile, Chile
Marco Pegoraro	RWTH Aachen University, Germany
Simon Poon	University of Sydney, Australia
Luise Pufahl	Technical University of Munich, Germany
Ricardo Quintano	Philips, The Netherlands
Hajo A. Reijers	Utrecht University, The Netherlands
Eric Rojas	Pontificia Universidad Católica de Chile, Chile
Gema Ibañez Sanchez	Universitat Politècnica de València, Spain
Fernando Seoane	Karolinska Institutet, Sweden
Marcos Sepúlveda	Pontificia Universidad Católica de Chile, Chile
Minseok Song	Pohang University of Science and Technology, South Korea
Alessandro Stefanini	University of Pisa, Italy
Emilio Sulis	University of Turin, Italy
Pieter Toussaint	Norwegian University of Science and Technology, Norway
Vicente Traver	Universitat Politècnica de València, Spain
Zoe Valero Ramón	Universitat Politècnica de València, Spain
Wil van der Aalst	RWTH Aachen University, Germany
Mathias Weske	HPI – University of Potsdam, Germany

Using Process Mining to Explore the Impact of Socio-economic Status on the Treatment of Musculoskeletal Disorders – A Case Study

Ruben Claus[1], Niels Martin[1,3]([✉]), Esther R. C. Janssen[2],
Gert Janssenswillen[1,3], Tim A. E. J. Boymans[2], and Rob J. B. Vanwersch[2]

[1] Research group Business Informatics, Hasselt University,
Martelarenlaan 42, 3500 Hasselt, Belgium
ruben.claus@student.uhasselt.be,
{niels.martin,gert.janssenswillen}@uhasselt.be
[2] Maastricht University Medical Center, P. Debyelaan 25,
6229 HX Maastricht, The Netherlands
{esther.janssen,t.boymans,rob.vanwersch}@mumc.nl
[3] Expertise Centre for Digital Media, Hasselt University, Wetenschapspark 2, 3590
Diepenbeek, Belgium

Abstract. Musculoskeletal disorders (MSDs) reduce a person's mobility and are a worldwide problem. The optimal care for MSDs implies that various healthcare providers, such as hospitals and physiotherapists, collaborate. Moreover, in order to shape the optimal care for MSD patients, their medical and personal background should be considered. Research has shown that care consumption can differ among patients depending on their socio-economic status. In order to explore the influence of the socio-economic status of patients on their MSD treatment trajectory, data from the *Beweeghuis* care network for MSDs is analyzed using process mining. The exploratory process mining analysis only highlights minor differences between socio-economic status groups. The findings need to be reflected against the prevailing data-related limitations, showing the clear need for follow-up research.

Keywords: Musculoskeletal disorders · Process mining ·
Socio-economic status

1 Introduction

Musculoskeletal disorders (MSDs) encompass conditions inflicting pain in the muscles, joints, bones and nerves causing people to lose part of their dexterity and mobility [7]. Examples of common MSDs are osteoarthritis [3], rheumatoid [11] and back issues [10], all conditions that lead to a reduced quality of life and persist to be a worldwide problem [2,11]. Common treatments include physical therapy practices, physical exercise, pharmacological treatments and surgeries [2]. Often, a combination of treatments is desirable for optimal care [17].

© The Author(s), under exclusive license to Springer Nature Switzerland AG 2024
J. De Smedt and P. Soffer (Eds.): ICPM 2023 Workshops, LNBIP 503, pp. 211–222, 2024.
https://doi.org/10.1007/978-3-031-56107-8_16

As optimal care for MSDs typically consists of a combination of various treatments [17], different healthcare providers such as hospitals, general practitioners and physiotherapists will need to collaborate in the patient's treatment trajectory [2]. To streamline this collaboration, *Beweeghuis* has been set up in the Maastricht-Heuvelland region (the Netherlands), which is a care network of general practitioners, medical specialists, physiotherapists and movement coaches. This network aims to offer patients optimal care by creating an individualized treatment trajectory across different healthcare providers [24].

In this effort to provide optimal care to each individual, it is key to consider not only the medical background of a patient, but also their personal background. In this respect, an important factor is their socio-economic status (SES), i.e. the social and economic well-being of a person [18]. Prior research has shown that care consumption can differ depending on the SES of a patient [13,25]. As the service region of *Beweeghuis* consists of areas with inhabitants with varying SES, it is considered highly relevant to gain insights into the impact of the SES of patients on their treatment trajectories. To analyze the treatment trajectories, process execution data will be leveraged.

Against this background, this paper uses process mining to conduct an exploratory study on the impact of the SES on the treatment trajectory of MSDs at *Beweeghuis*. Until now, the SES of patients has not been given consideration in the process mining in healthcare literature, despite its demonstrated impact on care consumption. In this way, the paper contributes to challenge "C8: Look at the process through the patient's eyes" coined by Munoz-Gama et al. [16], as it explicitly takes the perspective of the patient instead of a healthcare organization or department. Moreover, by considering the context of a care network, the case study also follows the recommendation by Martin et al. [14] to look beyond the hospital walls when studying healthcare processes.

The remainder of this paper is structured as follows. Section 2 provides pointers to related work on both process mining and the impact of SES on care consumption. Section 3 describes the research questions and methodology. Section 4 presents the results, which are discussed in Sect. 5. Section 6 concludes the paper.

2   Related Work

This exploratory study touches upon two key streams of literature: process mining in healthcare and the impact of SES on care consumption. While a full review of these topics is beyond the scope of this paper, some valuable pointers are provided.

Process Mining in Healthcare. Process mining has intensively been studied in a healthcare setting as it serves as a facilitator for care process improvement by translating process execution data into useful process-related insights [6]. A variety of use cases can be distinguished such as discovering how a care process is performed in reality and assessing the adherence of the care process to clinical guidelines and protocols [15]. Given the focus of this paper on comparing patients from different SES groups, this paper relates to prior research on comparative process mining [1]. In a healthcare context, comparative process mining can relate, for instance, to comparing patient groups, time periods and care organizations [15]. For example: Rojas and Capurro [19] compare three patient groups based on the used medication category to study the medication use process for sepsis patients. For a more extensive review on process mining in healthcare, the reader is referred to Rojas et al. [20] and De Roock and Martin [6].

Impact of SES on Care Consumption. Research has shown that people with a lower SES persist to be in worse health than those at the other end of the spectrum [5,13]. The worse health state among people of lower SES can be explained by the higher occurrence of smoking, poor diets and physical inactivity [25]. For instance, Wang et al. [26] showed that people with a low SES are four times as likely to initiate physical inactivity, and twice as likely to continue physical inactivity and smoking after the diagnosis of a non-communicable disease (e.g. heart diseases, cancer, diabetes and MSDs [27]) compared to their high SES counterparts. Such behavior can be partly explained by lower health literacy in low SES groups [26], referring to the ability of a person to obtain and interpret health-related information and act accordingly [9].

The poorer health status of people with a lower SES is also reflected in their care consumption. Veugelers et al. [25], for instance, report more visits to the general practitioner and hospital by people with a low SES. However, this higher consumption rate is not reflected in the usage of specialist services [25]. A recent study by Loef et al. [13] confirms these findings.

Besides curative care, preventive care, such as vaccinations, also has an important influence on the health status of a person [21,23]. The use of preventive care is found to be linked to the health literacy of an individual. Consistent with the finding that a low SES is generally associated with a lower health literacy [23], it has been shown that the use of preventive care is lower among people with a low SES [22,23].

3   Research Questions and Methodology

From Sect. 2, it follows that existing research has shown that the SES of individuals impacts their care consumption. While SES can also impact the treatment trajectory, it has not been taken into consideration in process mining in healthcare research. This paper extends the knowledge base by using process mining to explore the impact of SES on the treatment trajectory for MSDs within the *Beweeghuis* care network. In particular, the following research questions are considered:

- Q1: Do patients with a different SES tend to start their MSD treatment trajectory at a different healthcare provider from the network?
- Q2: Do patients with a different SES tend to show differences in their treatment trajectory?

To answer these questions, the PM^2 methodology by van Eck et al. [8] is adopted, which distinguishes six key stages in a process mining project: planning, extraction, data processing, mining & analysis, evaluation, and process improvement & support. As a full outline of the operationalization of PM^2 is infeasible out of space considerations, the remainder of this section provides some key pointers on the extracted data, the data wrangling that took place, the tools used and the evaluation with domain experts.

Available Datasets. Data relating to degenerative and non-specific disease patterns of the back and knee was extracted from the health information systems from two entities in the *Beweeghuis* network: the Maastricht University Medical Center (MUMC+) and the outpatient city clinic. While MUMC+ is the hospital within the network, the outpatient city clinic acts as an intermediary actor between the general practitioner and hospital to improve patient routing. This data covers MSD treatment activities that took place in one of two periods: a first period running from 01-01-2017 until 31-12-2019 and a second period running from 01-01-2021 until 30-06-2022. Data from the period in between was not considered to omit any disruptive impact due to the initial stage of the COVID-19 pandemic. Data recording the SES of patients was sourced from the Central Bureau of Statistics. This organization publishes SES scores by zip-code [4], which were used as a proxy for the SES of patients in this exploratory analysis. The SES scores take on values between -0.875 and $+0.625$, with 0 serving as a breaking point. As a result, values above 0 are linked to people with a high SES, while values below 0 are linked to people with a low SES. However, as the SES score is only a rough approximation of an individual's SES, since it is computed by zip-code, SES scores between -0.125 and 0.125 were considered neutral.

Data Wrangling. The original data contained 1 296 distinct activities for knee patients and 1 346 for patients with back disorders. The very fine-grained nature of these activities highlighted the need to perform event aggregation. Overarching categories of activities were created to remove unnecessary details in the data, while also guaranteeing its usability, e.g. all lab-related activities were combined into a single lab activity. The mapping from low-level to high-level activities took place together with domain experts from *Beweeghuis* and resulted in 43 distinct activities for knee patients and 41 for back patients. Besides event aggregation, filters were applied to the data, removing patients younger than 18 years old due to the specific nature of the treatment trajectories of minors. Furthermore, only patients living within the allocated care region of the hospital and outpatient city clinic were considered. Patients living outside of this region, e.g. patients forwarded from other areas for specialist care, could distort the analysis as they immediately visit the hospital, regardless of their SES.

Tools. The tools used for this case study comprise of R, and bupaR specifically, the process mining ecosystem in R [12]. The required data wrangling happened in R, after which the analysis of the data could start. To that end, bupaR was used.

Evaluation with Domain Experts. The analysis was performed in an iterative way by organizing interim feedback sessions with domain experts from *Beweeghuis*. During these meetings, research results were presented and thoroughly discussed. These discussions led to a further refinement of the research questions and analysis.

4 Results

This section presents the key results of the conducted analysis. Section 4.1 focuses on the first research question, related to differences in starting points of treatment trajectories. The second research question, related to differences in the overall treatment trajectories, is analyzed in Sect. 4.2.

4.1 Q1: Starting Point of Trajectory versus SES of Patients

Period 1. Table 1 presents an overview of the distribution of patients starting their treatment trajectory at either the outpatient city clinic or hospital. This overview is given for the two groups of musculoskeletal problems considered: degenerative and non-specific disease patterns of the knee, as well as of the back.

Table 1. Patient summary statistics - Period 1.

Problem	SES	Patients		Inhabitants		Started at			
		Total	%	Total	%	City clinic	%	Hospital	%
Knee	Low	1 365	39.73%	64 550	2.11%	333	24.40%	1 032	75.60%
	Neutral	975	28.38%	52 345	1.86%	217	22.26%	758	77.74%
	High	1 096	31.90%	58 250	1.88%	249	22.72%	847	77.28%
Back	Low	1 479	42.62%	64 550	2.29%	210	14.20%	1 269	85.80%
	Neutral	1 003	28.90%	52 345	1.92%	136	13.56%	867	86.44%
	High	988	28.47%	58 250	1.70%	120	12.15%	868	87.85%
		(a)	(b)	(c)	(d)	(e)	(f)	(g)	(h)

Patients with a low SES make up the largest group in this dataset (column a b). This is to be expected as relatively more of the inhabitants within the region under review are considered to have a SES below average (column c). However, even taking into account the number of inhabitants in each SES group (column d), it can be seen that patients in the low SES group are slightly over-represented for both knee (2.11% for the low SES group vs 1.86% and 1.88% for the neutral and high SES group, respectively), and back problems (2.29% for the low SES group vs 1.92% and 1.70% for the neutral and high SES group, respectively).

The relative percentages of patients starting at the outpatient city clinic show that patients with knee problems tend to start their trajectory more often at the city clinic compared to patients with back problems, independently of their SES (column e). Looking at both groups of problems separately, numbers show that differences between people with a low and high SES are negligible in this period. The percentage point difference between both equals 2.05pp for problems related to the back and 1.62pp for problems related to the knee (column f, h).

Period 2. Table 2 presents an overview considering the second period under review. At the start of this second period, an online reference module was introduced, making it easier for general practitioners to refer patients to the outpatient city clinic. As a result, an increase in the relative percentages of patients starting at the outpatient city clinic is expected. Table 2 shows indeed that considerably more trajectories were started at the outpatient city clinic (column e), on average 60.06% for knee problems (versus on average 23.11% in period 1), and on average 30.21% for back problems (versus on average 13.30% in period 1). The higher percentage of patients with back problems starting at the hospital, compared to knee problems, is in line with the findings in period 1.

Whereas patients with a low SES were the most represented in the first period, this is no longer generally true in the second period. Here, patients with a high SES are the most represented for problems related to the knee (column d). However, the difference between both is very small (0.02pp).

While the difference in starting points between people with a low and high SES remained negligible in this second period for patients with back problems, this is not the case for patients with knee problems (column e). For this last group, the difference between both groups grew by 9.31pp, which is more outspoken. Some caution is needed in drawing conclusions as the second period covers a significantly smaller amount of patients.

Table 2. Patient summary statistics - Period 2.

Problem	SES	Patients		Inhabitants		Started at			
		Total	Rel.	Total	Rel.	City clinic	Rel.	Hospital	Rel.
Knee	Low	697	37.21%	64 550	1.08%	398	57.10%	299	42.90%
	Neutral	533	28.46%	52 345	1.02%	302	56.66%	231	43.34%
	High	643	34.33%	58 250	1.10%	427	66.41%	216	33.59%
Back	Low	735	40.41%	64 550	1.14%	224	30.48%	511	69.52%
	Neutral	542	29.80%	52 345	1.04%	155	28.60%	387	71.40%
	High	542	29.80%	58 250	0.93%	171	31.55%	371	68.45%
		(a)	(b)	(c)	(d)	(e)	(f)	(g)	(h)

4.2   Q2: Trajectory Differences for Patients with a Different SES

This subsection approaches the second research question from three angles. Firstly, the treatment trajectories will be analyzed by looking at the relative occurrence of treatment activities for each of the SES groups defined. Secondly, the average amount of consultations will be compared for each SES group within the respective period. Finally, differences in activity sequences among SES groups will be assessed.

Period 1. The first period involves 6 905 cases, i.e. 3 435 related to knee issues and 3 470 related to back issues. For these cases, respectively 1 247 and 952 traces were identified. A trace is defined as a unique sequence of activities. These high numbers of traces are due to the variability in the treatment trajectories, which is common in a healthcare setting [14, 16]. In order to elaborate on the treatment trajectories and the possible differences between SES categories, an overview of the most important treatment activities is provided in Table 3.

Table 3. Relative use of MSD treatment activities - Period 1.

Problem	Treatment activity	SES		
		Low	Neutral	High
Knee	Surgeries	12.04%	13.13%	12.50%
	Consultation	99.19%	99.38%	99.91%
	Medical-imaging	60.57%	59.79%	60.49%
Back	Surgeries	7.84%	9.37%	8.20%
	Consultation	98.51%	97.61%	97.17%
	Medical-imaging	53.35%	57.03%	54.55%

The overview in Table 3 shows the relative amount of patients from each SES category for which each listed activity has been executed. In general, no real differences between patients from different SES categories can be observed, showing their similar presence in the treatment trajectories for each group of patients. Note that a similar observation holds for the other treatment activities, of which the numeric results are not included out of space considerations.

As consultations can take place at the outpatient city clinic or hospital, differences between SES categories might be found after further subdividing them. This is done in Table 4. Here, the average number of each consultation type is shown per SES category. Numbers show that hospital consultations happen, on average, more irrespective of the SES category of the patient. No remarkable differences between SES categories were observed.

Table 4. Average amount of consultations - Period 1.

Problem	Consultation type	SES		
		Low	Neutral	High
Knee	Hospital	2.56	2.60	2.67
	Outpatient city clinic	1.08	1.06	1.10
Back	Hospital	2.07	2.18	1.99
	Outpatient city clinic	1.13	1.08	1.12

In order to compare the actual order of activities in more detail, directly-follows process maps were created, focusing on the major activities as listed in Table 3. Figure 1 shows the resulting process for knee problems in period 1, both for patients in the low and high SES groups. Percentages show the relative number of patients connected to a specific flow or activity. It can be seen that no differences are present in the flows, except for relatively minor fluctuations in the relative frequencies of patients. The same conclusion was reached concerning the neutral SES group, as well as concerning the back problems.

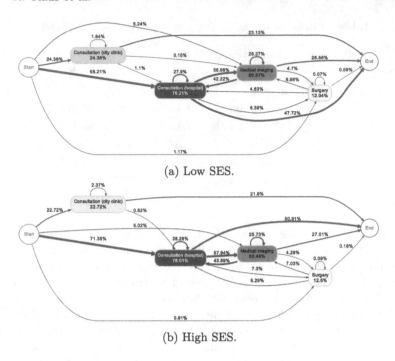

(a) Low SES.

(b) High SES.

Fig. 1. Patient trajectories - Knee Problems - Period 1.

Period 2. The same analyses were performed for the second period, encompassing trajectories that started after the introduction of the online reference module. Table 5 shows the same statistics as Table 3, yet for 3 692 cases, i.e. 1 873 related to knee issues and 1 819 related to back issues. For those cases, respectively 457 and 458 traces were identified.

As the statistics in Table 5 show, no remarkable differences become apparent between patients from different SES categories. However, the relative percentages related to medical imaging for patients with knee issues appear to show larger differences. Domain experts were not able to give an explanation for this observation. For other treatment activities not included in the table, no noticeable differences were identified.

Table 6 shows the average amount of consultations per SES category for the second period. Again, differences appear to be minimal, pointing at similar treatment behavior among patients belonging to a different SES category. The higher number of consultations in the city clinic can be seen as a result of the online reference module, which significantly increased the number of trajectories starting at the city clinic. Also for the second period, process maps for different SES groups were created. As before, no differences in the overall trajectories could be observed.

Table 5. Relative use of MSD treatment activities - Period 2.

Problem	Treatment activity	SES		
		Low	Neutral	High
Knee	Surgeries	3.44%	4.88%	3.58%
	Consultation	99.71%	98.87%	99.38%
	Medical-imaging	35.29%	34.71%	27.53%
Back	Surgeries	2.86%	4.80%	3.69%
	Consultation	99.46%	98.15%	98.34%
	Medical-imaging	42.31%	43.91%	41.70%

Table 6. Average amount of consultations - Period 2.

Problem	Consultation type	SES		
		Low	Neutral	High
Knee	Hospital	2.37	2.34	2.54
	Outpatient city clinic	1.31	1.39	1.30
Back	Hospital	2.11	2.12	2.20
	Outpatient city clinic	1.42	1.41	1.40

5   Discussion

Literature has shown that people with a lower SES have a worse health status, which also impacts their care consumption [13,25]. This case study explored whether the SES of a patient impacts the treatment trajectory of MSDs at *Beweeghuis*. To this end, data of patients suffering from back and knee disorders have been considered in two time periods (01-01-2017 - 31-12-2019 and 01-01-2021 - 30/06/2022), where the second period is characterized by the presence of an online reference module, which makes it easier for general practitioners to refer patients to the outpatient city clinic.

Consistent with the results reported by Loef et al. [13] and Veugelers et al. [25], patients with a low SES are the most strongly represented in the *Beweeghuis* data. However, differences in representation do not imply differences in the treatment trajectory as well.

When assessing the differences between SES groups in terms of their treatment trajectory, only minor differences have been detected. The first research question specifically focused on the start of the treatment trajectory, i.e. whether the starting point is the hospital or the outpatient city clinic. Results generally show small differences in terms of starting point between patients with a low SES and a high SES. The only exception is situated in the second period for patients with knee conditions, where the difference between patients with a low SES and a high SES increased from 1.62pp to 9.31pp. Domain experts considered this difference highly relevant, but could not provide a clear explanation, showing the need for further investigation.

The second research question targets the entire treatment trajectory, but also did not surface substantial differences between SES groups. When looking at the use of treatment activities, limited differences have been detected. The only noteworthy difference relates to the use of medical imaging for knee patients in the second period, where a difference of 7.76pp is present between low and high SES groups. This indicates that low SES patients receive more medical imaging than high SES patients. Domain experts indicated that, in order to assess the relevance of this difference, its effect on the quality of the provided treatment should be assessed. This effect is currently unknown and marks an area for follow-up research.

From the previous, it follows that the results of the exploratory analysis did not surface a substantial impact of a patient's SES on the treatment trajectory of MSDs at *Beweeghuis*. However, these results need to be reflected against two key limitations of the conducted analyses. Firstly, to determine the SES of a patient, the SES scores published by the Central Bureau of Statistics [4] have been used as a proxy. These SES scores are based on the financial wealth, education level and employment history of private households and were computed per zip-code. As a result, the same SES score will be assigned to all inhabitants of an area with the same zip-code. While this SES score is appropriate for the population of that area in general, it might not be an accurate reflection of the SES for individual patients. Therefore, the accuracy of the results reported in this paper depends on the quality of this proxy. Future research could focus on assessing the quality of the SES proxy and its refinement, also taking into account privacy considerations.

Secondly, this exploratory analysis has only been based on data from the hospital and the outpatient city clinic. To get a full view on the treatment trajectory, data from the other partners of the *Beweeghuis* network such as general practitioners, physiotherapists and movement coaches should also be taken into consideration. As data connections between partners have not yet been established, data from these other partners was not available. Hence, differences in the MSD treatment trajectory of patients with a different SES might have remained hidden due to data unavailability. For instance, differences might arise when physiotherapeutic care is taken into consideration as this type of care is not included in the basic health insurance package [13].

6   Conclusion

This paper reports on the results of a case study at *Beweeghuis*, a care network for the treatment of MSDs in the Maastricht-Heuvelland region. In particular, an exploratory process mining analysis has been conducted on the effect of the SES of patients on their treatment trajectory. In general, the analysis results only highlight minor differences between the treatment trajectories of patients from different SES groups. Some specific differences have been discovered, requiring more in-depth analyses. While this paper clearly demonstrates the potential of process mining to tackle the considered research questions, data-related limitations stress the need to interpret the findings with great care.

Several avenues for future research are promising to address the limitations of the current paper. Firstly, a more individualized proxy for the SES of a patient would enable more accurate analyses compared to the use of a SES score by zip-code. This would imply the analysis of sensitive data related to topics such as a patient's educational background or income, which are subject to ethical and privacy considerations. Secondly, a more complete view on the treatment trajectory of *Beweeghuis* patients is warranted, necessitating the integration of data along all involved parties in the care network. Finally, a toolkit can be developed to perform these analyses on a regular basis. This would enable *Beweeghuis* to follow up on the impact of policy measures taken when undesirable discrepancies between SES groups would appear. In that respect, it is also important to connect findings regarding differences in the treatment trajectory to outcomes for a particular patient group.

References

1. van der Aalst, W.M.P.: Process mining: a 360 degree overview. In: van der Aalst, W.M.P., Carmona, J. (eds.) Process Mining Handbook. LNBIP, vol. 448, pp. 3–34. Springer, Cham (2022). https://doi.org/10.1007/978-3-031-08848-3_1
2. Bergman, S.: Management of musculoskeletal pain. Best Pract. Res. Clin. Rheumatol. **21**(1), 153–166 (2007)
3. Canjels, K.F., Imkamp, M.S., Boymans, T.A., Vanwersch, R.J.: Unraveling and improving the interorganizational arthrosis care process at maastricht UMC+: an illustration of an innovative, combined application of data and process mining. In: Proceedings of the BPM Industry Forum, pp. 178–189 (2019)
4. CBS: Sociaal-economische status per postcode, 2019 (2022). https://www.cbs.nl/nl-nl/maatwerk/2022/26/sociaal-economische-status-per-postcode-2019. Accessed 23 Mar 2023
5. Davis, K., Gold, M., Makuc, D.: Access to health care for the poor: does the gap remain? Annu. Rev. Public Health **2**(1), 159–182 (1981)
6. De Roock, E., Martin, N.: Process mining in healthcare - an updated perspective on the state of the art. J. Biomed. Inform. **127**, paper 103995 (2022)
7. Du, S., Yuan, C., Xiao, X., Chu, J., Qiu, Y., Qian, H.: Self-management programs for chronic musculoskeletal pain conditions: a systematic review and meta-analysis. Patient Educ. Couns. **85**(3), e299–e310 (2011)
8. van Eck, M.L., Lu, X., Leemans, S.J.J., van der Aalst, W.M.P.: PM^2: a process mining project methodology. In: Zdravkovic, J., Kirikova, M., Johannesson, P. (eds.) CAiSE 2015. LNCS, vol. 9097, pp. 297–313. Springer, Cham (2015). https://doi.org/10.1007/978-3-319-19069-3_19
9. Furuya, Y., Kondo, N., Yamagata, Z., Hashimoto, H.: Health literacy, socioeconomic status and self-rated health in japan. Health Promot. Int. **30**(3), 505–513 (2015)
10. Gatchel, R.J.: Musculoskeletal disorders: primary and secondary interventions. J. Electromyogr. Kinesiol. **14**(1), 161–170 (2004)

11. Hutting, N., et al.: Physical therapists and importance of work participation in patients with musculoskeletal disorders: a focus group study. BMC Musculoskelet. Disord. **18**, 1–16 (2017)
12. Janssenswillen, G., Depaire, B., Swennen, M., Jans, M., Vanhoof, K.: bupaR: enabling reproducible business process analysis (2019)
13. Loef, B., et al.: Socioeconomic differences in healthcare expenditure and utilization in The Netherlands. BMC Health Serv. Res. **21**(1), 1–17 (2021)
14. Martin, N., et al.: Recommendations for enhancing the usability and understandability of process mining in healthcare. Artif. Intell. Med. **109**, paper 101962 (2020)
15. Martin, N., Wittig, N., Munoz-Gama, J.: Using process mining in healthcare. In: van der Aalst, W.M.P., Carmona, J. (eds.) Process Mining Handbook. LNBIP, vol. 448, pp. 416–444. Springer, Cham (2022). https://doi.org/10.1007/978-3-031-08848-3_14
16. Munoz-Gama, J., et al.: Process mining for healthcare: characteristics and challenges. J. Biomed. Inform. **127**, paper 103994 (2022)
17. Nielson, W.R., Weir, R.: Biopsychosocial approaches to the treatment of chronic pain. Clin. J. Pain **17**(4), S114–S127 (2001)
18. Nyame, Y.A., et al.: Deconstructing, addressing, and eliminating racial and ethnic inequities in prostate cancer care. Eur. Urol. **82**(4), 341–351 (2022)
19. Rojas, E., Capurro, D.: Characterization of drug use patterns using process mining and temporal abstraction digital phenotyping. In: Daniel, F., Sheng, Q.Z., Motahari, H. (eds.) BPM 2018. LNBIP, vol. 342, pp. 187–198. Springer, Cham (2019). https://doi.org/10.1007/978-3-030-11641-5_15
20. Rojas, E., Munoz-Gama, J., Sepulveda, M., Capurro, D.: Process mining in healthcare: a literature review. J. Biomed. Inform. **61**, 224–236 (2016)
21. Scott, T.L., Gazmararian, J.A., Williams, M.V., Baker, D.W.: Health literacy and preventive health care use among medicare enrollees in a managed care organization. Med. Care **40**(5), 395–404 (2002)
22. Stormacq, C., Van den Broucke, S., Wosinski, J.: Does health literacy mediate the relationship between socioeconomic status and health disparities? Integrative review. Health Promot. Int. **34**(5), e1–e17 (2019)
23. Svendsen, M.T., et al.: Associations of health literacy with socioeconomic position, health risk behavior, and health status: a large national population-based survey among Danish adults. BMC Public Health **20**(1), paper 565 (2020)
24. UMC+, M.: Het beweeghuis (2023). https://beweeghuis.mumc.nl/het-beweeghuis. Accessed 20 Feb 2023
25. Veugelers, P.J., Yip, A.M.: Socioeconomic disparities in health care use: does universal coverage reduce inequalities in health? J. Epidemiol. Community Health **57**(6), 424–428 (2003)
26. Wang, D., et al.: Association between socioeconomic status and health behaviour change before and after non-communicable disease diagnoses: a multicohort study. Lancet Public Health **7**(8), e670–e682 (2022)
27. World Health Organization: Noncommunicable diseases (2023). https://www.who.int/health-topics/noncommunicable-diseases. Accessed 22 Aug 2023

Identifying Variation in Personal Daily Routine Through Process Mining: A Case Study

Gemma Di Federico[1]($\boxtimes$) (ID), Carlos Fernández-Llatas[2] (ID), Zahra Ahmadi[3] (ID),
Mohsen Shirali[4] (ID), and Andrea Burattin[1] (ID)

[1] Technical University of Denmark, Kgs. Lyngby, Denmark
gdfe@dtu.dk
[2] Universitat Politècnica de València, Valencia, Spain
[3] LIRIS, KU Leuven, Brussels, Belgium
[4] Shahid Beheshti University, Tehran, Iran

Abstract. The study of daily routines has gained substantial attention, especially in healthcare. Understanding the activities and behaviors of individuals, particularly older adults, has the potential to play a crucial role in providing effective care and support, for example, when it comes to spotting deviations from it automatically.

Process mining is a valuable tool for analyzing routine dynamics and identifying variations. However, human behavior is unstructured and characterized by variability, making it difficult to derive a process model representing only the control flow.

In this paper, we employ a multi-dimensional process discovery and conformance checking methodology to a real-world dataset representing a person's behavior in a smart environment. The derived model combines control flow and statistics on the data. The results, on the real-world data, highlight that the approach can identify variations in the inhabitant's behavior.

1 Introduction

The study of daily routines has gained substantial attention, especially within the healthcare field. Understanding the activities and behavior of individuals, particularly older adults, has the potential to play a crucial role in providing effective care and support [6]. There is evidence in the literature demonstrating the importance of deriving individual behavioral models that contribute to personalized healthcare [6,13]. For example, an early diagnosis of dementia can be made through the detection of alterations in daily habits [5].

Process mining is a powerful methodology to analyze and extract information from event logs, allowing experts to gain insight into the dynamics of daily routines. In healthcare, process mining can contribute to a deeper comprehension of patients' activities, their patterns, and potential deviations from expected routines [11]. The study is made possible by the use of smart environments [23] in which sensors collect information about the activities carried out by the inhabitants. By applying process mining techniques to event data captured through

J. De Smedt and P. Soffer (Eds.): ICPM 2023 Workshops, LNBIP 503, pp. 223–234, 2024.
https://doi.org/10.1007/978-3-031-56107-8_17

sensor networks or wearable devices [3], a model representing the daily routine of the patient can be derived. The continuous monitoring of the behavior throughout the day can help identify variations and provide medical support to the patient.

The derivation of a model that faithfully represents and abstracts the individual daily behavior is a challenging task [9]. In fact, routines are not fixed as they are dependent on the context, and result in the variability of the behaviors. Variations can be an alternative way to accomplish a task or the introduction of a new behavior. Furthermore, although it might be possible to predict the set of activities that compose a routine, we cannot define with certainty their order of execution. All of these factors make it inadequate to derive a process model that represents only the control flow.

For this reason, Di Federico et al. [8] implemented an algorithm able to derive a multi-dimensional model composed not only by the control flow but also embedding the data dimension in the form of various statistics. The approach derives multiple process models, both declarative and imperative, together with statistics on the activities. The approach can also be used to identify variations in the execution of the routine itself by proposing a conformance checking algorithm that balances control-flow alignment and data.

In this paper, we demonstrate the capability of this approach in recognizing variations of behaviors through its application to a real-world dataset [12]. The dataset collects information regarding the daily routine of a person living in a smart environment. Differently from other publicly available datasets, in this case, we have evidence of events that impacted the routine of the inhabitant (i.e., the ground truth of the routine variation), and we are able to identify these changes.

The paper is structured as follows. Section 2 presents the state of the art of the analysis of routines. The algorithm used in the work is explained in Sect. 3, and its application is further elaborated in Sect. 4, i.e. the use case of this paper. The results are discussed in Sect. 5. Section 6 concludes the paper.

2   State of the Art

Human behavior can be defined as a combination of intentions, perceptions and states. The execution of a behavior, and its purpose, is influenced by all of these factors [9]. Human beings establish routines and perform them repetitively [2]. However, routines are not static; rather, they exhibit variations over time and are greatly influenced by situational factors, reflecting the unpredictable nature of human behavior. The main challenge when analyzing human behavior is whether the behavior is structured enough to be represented using a process model. In fact, behavioral models usually result in spaghetti-like models [17]. As a consequence, the identification of variations becomes even more challenging. A variation in the daily behavior can be defined as an unexpected but significant irregularity in otherwise normal data, which could be indicative of an adverse condition [23].

Several approaches in the literature tried to discover a behavioral model for daily routines. Palermo et al. [21] propose an approach to analyze the risk of agitation in people living with Dementia. Unusual patterns of activities could be an indication of an agitation episode. The authors construct a Long-Short Term Memory (LSTM) network from the behavior of 46 patients to characterize their daily routine. The approach predicts whether the behavior of an individual is classified as agitated or not agitated. Nevertheless, the behavioral model is neither personalized nor easily interpretable. Specifically, it only returns the predicted class, and no additional information can be provided.

Dogan et al. [11] apply process mining techniques to discover and classify human behavior patterns. The authors use a discovery algorithm to identify trajectories in the smart environment, then a clustering technique is applied to identify behavioral patterns, subsequently represented using a calendar view. It is noteworthy that the resulting models are not individual, but they represent groups of people, and then each participant is assigned to a group. The approach classifies deviations as a difference between the participant's behavior and the modeled one. However, the reference model is a generalization and doesn't take into account the specific person in detail. What is more, the approach only considers the process flow perspective. When representing human behaviors, other dimensions should be considered, e.g., the excessive repetition of an activity cannot be captured by the control flow alone.

Di Federico et al. [8] propose an approach to derive a personalized behavioral model which combines control flow and data dimensions. The authors argue the importance of considering statistics on the data while deriving a model. What is more, they propose both imperative and declarative modeling languages to represent the control flow, as there is not yet a conclusive solution capable of dealing with routine behavior. However, so far, the approach has only been tested on simulated data [10].

In the context of this paper, we apply the algorithm proposed by Di Federico et al. [8] on a real dataset. Before delving into the use case description, we describe the approach in the following background section.

3   Background

The approach used in this paper is a multi-dimension algorithm described in [8]. The algorithm proposes the discovery of both control flow models and the computation of statistics and it also verifies the conformance between such multi-dimensional model and new instances of the process. In the following sections, the two stages are explained in detail.

3.1   Process Discovery

The discovery consists of deriving both the control flow and the data perspectives. Observing the process from different points of view allows us to consider all the aspects characterizing human behaviors. The control flow is composed of the discovery of three models, i.e., a Petri Net [19], a Declare model [22], and a DCR graph [15]. The Inductive Miner [16] is used to obtain the Petri Net, while for the declarative models the discovery algorithms of the corresponding languages are used [14,18,20]. On one hand, a declarative language represents the process in the form of constraints, therefore more suitable to abstract from the problem of variability. On the other hand, imperative languages have a more structured and clear representation of the process.

The data dimension focuses on deriving significant statistics related to the activities' frequency, duration, and occurrence time. These aspects are deemed relevant as they allow the monitoring of the repetition of activities and position them on a timeline. The activity frequency is determined by counting the occurrence of each unique activity identifier in each trace. Then, the values are aggregated to the entire event log, and mean, standard deviation, median, minimum, and maximum are computed. The activity duration is assessed through the average duration per activity identifier, with statistics like mean, median, minimum, and maximum duration computed across traces. The absolute time dimension is derived by using histograms to depict activity occurrence frequency within specific time intervals. The last dimension is the trace length, and min, max, mean, and standard deviation are derived. All these insights offer a comprehensive understanding of process behavior, unveiling recurring patterns, timing delays, and variations in activity execution.

3.2   Conformance Checking

The model derived in the discovery phase can be used as a reference model in the conformance checking. The conformance algorithm presented includes the verification of all the mentioned perspectives, and returns an enriched fitness value which is an aggregation of all of them. In particular, the conformance checking between the Petri Net and new instances of the process is computed using alignments [1] (we'll refer to this value as CCInd). Additionally, the precision value computed using the alignments is also considered. For the Declare model, the algorithm implemented by Burattin et al. [4] is used. In this case, the algorithm returns the number of activations, fulfillment, and violations of each constraint in the input model and for each trace in the log, and we computed the fitness value (CCDeclare). For the conformance of the DCR graph (CCDcr), a rule checker algorithm is deployed [7]. For the verification of the data flow dimensions, comparison functions are used. For the frequency of the activities (CCFreq), the assumption is that the average value serves as a benchmark. The probability density function lets us measure how likely it is that the mean frequency value for each activity identifier in the trace is close to this reference. The same approach is adopted to obtain a fitness value for the duration (CCDur) of the activities and for the trace length (CCLen).

For the absolute time dimension (CCTime), the reference is the histogram of the frequencies of each activity over time intervals. The conformance of a new absolute time is then computed as the normalized frequency for the time interval the new absolute time belongs to.

The resulting enriched fitness value is an aggregation of the four values obtained from the conformance of the control flow dimension and the four values obtained from the conformance of the data flow dimension.

4   Application

The objective of the paper is to demonstrate that the daily routine can be modeled using a multi-dimension model and that behavioral changes can be identified. In particular, the model is personalized for an individual, therefore it is highly representative of the habits and characteristics of that person. It is important to mention that the daily routine evolves over time; hence the reference model should be updated consequently. The case study presented in this paper is the daily routine of a person living in a smart environment.

4.1   Dataset Description

The dataset used in this case study refers to the behavior of a 60-year-old woman living in her private house [12]. The components of the setting are a smart home, a smartphone, and a smart wristband. The smart home is equipped with sensors used to perceive the environment and the activities performed by the resident during the day. The installed devices are 15 binary sensors positioned on furnishing elements, appliances, and doors.

With the aid of a mobile application, smartphone usage information is collected. The wristband is instead used to obtain sleeping data and to collect the number of daily steps. The data were collected in the timeframe 08/01/2020 - 02/06/2020. During the collection period, various events happened that influenced the behavior of the resident. From the 40th day from the beginning of the collection process, the Covid-19 pandemic was prevalent in the region, affecting the habits of the participant. From the 109th day to the 137th day was the Ramadan month; therefore, the resident changed their habits such as meal times, praying time and duration, and sleeping intervals.

4.2   Pre-processing

Since the objective is to monitor the behavior of the subject at the level of activities executed during the day, the dataset requires some abstraction. In fact, the dataset includes sensors' raw readings at a low level of abstraction representing the presence of the subject near the appliances, the open or closed state of doors and the use of the stove. We pre-process the raw data to extract information about the subject's presence in different locations of the house (e.g. bedroom, kitchen) by looking at the locations in which sensors are mounted. In this way, we are able to detect events related to the visited home locations for the entire dataset period. In addition, the executed activities at a higher level (for instance, sleeping, eating, watching TV) are also determined based on the sensor states. Then, for each detected location or activity, a record is added to the event log with the labels in the form of location-activity (e.g., *LivingRoom-Mobile-Cooking*, meaning that the person was in the living room, they were using the mobile phone, and something was left cooking on the stove). However, we decided to simplify the labels and rename them with the location only (e.g., the previous label is replaced by *LivingRoom*). This choice is driven by the presence of activities that occur without direct involvement from the participant, as seen in the cooking activity from the previous instance. If the person is in the living room at that moment, we are interested in that specific event. What is more, all the mobile events have an additional corresponding entry *Mobile*. All events related to the *corridor* location are removed, as the corridor can be considered a hub and not a place that actually contributes to the execution of an activity. We also removed all the events in the *bathroom* location, referring to the usage of the toilet to ensure the privacy of the resident, while we considered only those events located in the anteroom. To divide the log in cases, we group them by day. At this point, we obtained 43 278 events organized in 146 cases. What is more, it is good practice to focus on a specific routine, therefore we decided to investigate the day routine without considering the evening and the night routine. Hence, we filter the event log to preserve only events in the timeframe 10am to 6pm. Last, because of the renaming of the labels, we could observe a lot of consecutive events with the same event name, thus we merged them considering the start time as the timestamp of the first event, and the end time as the timestamp of the last consecutive event. To sum up, we obtain an event log with 146 cases, 9237 events, and 14 unique activity identifiers.

4.3   Method

For the analysis of the dataset we use the approach reported in Sect. 3. An important factor to consider while analyzing human behavior is that the routine evolves over time. For this reason, we have applied a sequential approach, in which we consider two weeks to derive the reference model, and one week for the conformance, with a sliding of 1 week for the subsequent training/testing. We decided on this strategy to accommodate the natural evolution of routines that might naturally happen over the course of time. In total, we obtained 18 logs for training and 18 for testing. Once we applied the algorithm, we obtained results for 18 data points, i.e., a result every other week. In the rest of the paper, we will refer to the discovery phase as *training*, while to the conformance checking phase as *testing*.

5   Results

In this section, we present the results obtained by the application of the multi-dimension discovery and conformance approach to the dataset under examination. In all the graphs, we'll highlight the two events that probably affect the routine (i.e., Covid-19, Ramadan) as horizontal bars in blue shades.

Prior to delving into the specifics of how to balance the different dimensions, it's important to grasp the overall direction of the analysis. For this reason, the

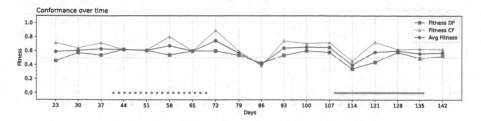

Fig. 1. Fitness value given by the average between the control flow perspective (CCInd, CCDcr and CCDeclare) and the data flow perspective (all)

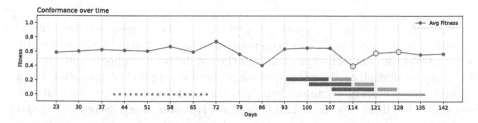

Fig. 2. Propagation of the variations on the results. The red/orange bars refer to training/test sets, while the yellow dots the corresponding fitness result (Color figure online)

first result we analyze is a fitness value obtained by averaging the control flow and the data flow perspectives. The values considered are the average between CCInd, CCDcr, and CCDeclare for the control flow, and the average between CCFreq, CCDur, CCTime, and CCLen for the data flow. The result is plotted in Fig. 1. The plot highlights two negative trends: from day 72 to 86 and from day 107 to 114. In general, control flow and data flow follow the same trend, especially in the second half of the graph.

In order to understand these downward spikes, we have to understand the propagation of events, specifically the time required for the reference model to incorporate the new routine. Let's consider as an example Fig. 2 and the Ramadan event, starting from day 109. In the figure we indicate the training period using a red bar, and the testing period using a orange bar. Taking the interval of days 94 to 106 for model training (prior to Ramadan), and days 107 to 113 for testing (the initial week of Ramadan), a divergence emerges between the expected behavior and the observed one. In fact, the Fitness value drops below 0.5 on the 114th day. Progressing to the subsequent application (the second set of red/orange horizontal bars), we note that the new routine is gradually integrated into the training set, hence it is becoming more representative of the Ramadan behavior, and this is the reason why the fitness value starts increasing again. In the following iteration, marked by the final pair of red/orange horizontal bars, the training set fully incorporates the Ramadan routine. As a result, the observed behavior aligns perfectly, causing the fitness value to rise and stabilize.

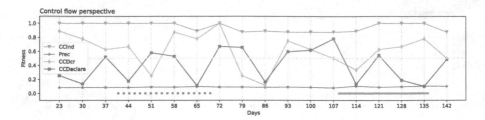

Fig. 3. All the control flow dimensions: fitness values obtained by CCInd, CCDcr, CCDeclare, and the Precision value

Before analyzing the motivations behind the negative spikes, we have to investigate how to balance the different components of the approach. In fact, especially in the case of the control flow, we consider three different modeling languages and discovery/conformance algorithms, which all have different characteristics. For a faithful representation of human behavior, the modeling language must allow a certain level of flexibility in the execution flow. However, when deriving the Petri Nets by using the Inductive Miner, the models exhibit low precision and have a propensity to underfit the behavior. On the declarative side, Declare has demonstrated a higher degree of strictness by deriving notably more constraints when compared to DCR. The Fitness values and the precision are plotted in Fig. 3. The graph illustrates a significant difference between the CCInd Fitness values and the Precision. The Fitness values are consistently high, indicating a strong match between the model and the observed behavior. However, Precision values remain close to zero throughout the graph. The divergence between the two metrics underscores a potential gap between overall alignment with the observed behavior and the model's capacity to generalize the behavior. Yet, as previously mentioned, relying solely on the control flow is insufficient for comprehending human behavior; hence, the viewpoint of data flow also demands consideration. Figure 4 plots the Fitness values of the data flow. It can be noticed that CCDur, CCFreq, and CCTime roughly follow the same trend, whereas CCLen shows two negative spikes, followed by a higher positive one, on day 86 and on day 114.

To find a balance between all the dimensions, we make use of the moving average so that we can identify peaks more accurately. We compute different configurations to obtain the total fitness value, which is then used to compute the moving average and the corresponding signal for the spike. If the difference in the signal between two data points is greater than 0.1, it is labeled as a spike.

Figure 5 illustrates the spike detector across three distinct configurations. In the first run, a balanced configuration was employed, allocating equal weight to all dimensions, that is the same weight we gave to the dimensions to compute the average fitness values plotted in Fig. 1. The calculation highlights a spike on day 114, as expected. Contrary to what was observed before, the downward trend on day 86 is not identified as a peak. This is due to the gradual nature of the decrease, which spans over more than a week. As a result, the difference between the moving averages of consecutive data points does not satisfy the

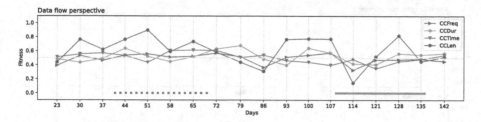

Fig. 4. All the data flow dimensions: fitness values obtained by CCFreq, CCDur, CCTime, CCLen

minimum threshold employed to confirm the occurrence of a spike. In the second and third configurations, we only consider Precision and CCDcr in the control flow, while for the data flow all the dimensions are considered. In the case of the second configuration, when calculating the average fitness value between the control flow and data flow, greater emphasis is given to the control flow dimension. Specifically, a higher significance is attributed to control flow by assigning it a weight of $4/5$, whereas data flow contributes with a weight of $1/5$. The resulting signal is plotted on the second graph in Fig. 5. In this case, two spikes are identified, meaning that the control flow identifies a variation in the behavior on the data point at day 51.

The signal function depicted in the third graph adopts an inverse weighting compared to the prior setup. Here, the data flow has more importance, contributing for $4/5$ to the average fitness, while the control flow $1/5$. In this case, the spike at day 51 is not identified, meaning that the variation is not reflected in the data flow.

As the last result, we compare the behavior of the inhabitant at two different moments in time. In particular, we examine the behavior during Ramadan and the behavior preceding that period. When selecting the time frames, we consider the signal function in the first graph of Fig. 5, opting for a date when the fitness fluctuation is low. The pre-Ramadan behavior is selected from day 44 to 64, while the period during Ramadan is from day 107 to 127. We use the same setup as before: two weeks for training and one for testing. Firstly we train and test a model for each timeframe independently to verify if the behavior is constant. The fitness value is set up according to the balanced configuration explained above. The result shows that the tested behaviors are actually the ones depicted by the corresponding training log, with a fitness value of 0.7 and 0.62 respectively. Delving into the differences, we notice that the *Eating* activity is not present in the log during Ramadan, in fact the mean value of the frequency statistic for this activity is 0.8 before Ramadan and 0.1 during Ramadan. The reason is that during Ramadan the *eating* activity is performed early in the morning or late in evening, so it is not executed during the timeframe we are considering. To conclude, we check if the behavior during Ramadan (days 121–128) can be represented by the model pre-Ramadan. In this case, the obtained fitness value is 0.4, indicating a difference between the behaviors.

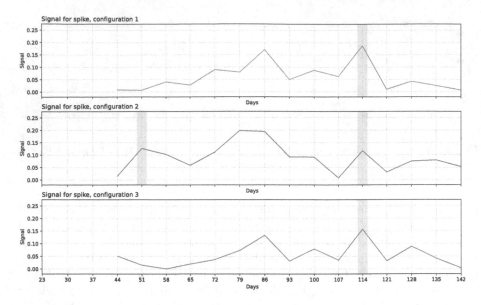

Fig. 5. Spike detection applied on three different configurations of the signal. A spike is identified when there is an increase of 0.1 in two subsequent points.

Finally, we link the identified variation to the events which probably impacted the behavior of the participant. The first event is Covid-19 (from day 40). In the spike detector in Fig. 5 the signal function starts at day 44, as 4 weeks are used as a subset to compute the first moving average value. Therefore, we cannot characterize the difference between the behavior before and during Covid-19 as we don't have enough data to analyze before this event. In addition, there is no end to the Covid-19 behavior in the recorded period, hence the only difference that can be identified is the beginning of the pandemic. The second event is the Ramadan period (from day 109 to 137). In this case, we have both the start and end of the event, but the recording period terminates only one week after, hence we do not have the time to propagate and recognize the end of Ramadan. However, the beginning of Ramadan is recognized by the approach across all configurations of the signal function, as well as by both the control flow and data flow independently.

6   Conclusions

In conclusion, the presented case study has demonstrated the effectiveness of the employed methodology in identifying significant variations within an individual's daily routine. By using an algorithm that integrates both the control flow and the data flow, the work derived a reference behavioral model representing the daily routine of the participant. Then, a conformance checking algorithm is applied to verify the discrepancies between the expected and the actual behavior. The model is updated every 7 days, to reflect changes in the routine. The findings demonstrated the effectiveness of the approach in identifying significant events that signify variations in the participant's behavior.

To sum up, this paper shows the capability of the approach presented in [8] which can automatically detect variations in the behavior of a subject during their time in a smart home. Proving the capability of such a system on real data paves the way to its application in contexts where the actual change in behavior is not known in advance and which could result in impactful in new disciplines (e.g., Dementia worsening, as discussed before). This also represents the main endeavor for the future: deploying the technique on new domains, where no information is known.

References

1. Van der Aalst, W., Adriansyah, A., Van Dongen, B.: Replaying history on process models for conformance checking and performance analysis. Wiley Interdisc. Rev.: Data Min. Knowl. Discov. **2**(2), 182–192 (2012)
2. Banovic, N., Buzali, T., Chevalier, F., Mankoff, J., Dey, A.K.: Modeling and understanding human routine behavior. In: Proceedings of the 2016 CHI Conference on Human Factors in Computing Systems, pp. 248–260 (2016)
3. Bertrand, Y., Van den Abbeele, B., Veneruso, S., Leotta, F., Mecella, M., Serral, E.: A survey on the application of process discovery techniques to smart spaces data. Eng. Appl. Artif. Intell. **126**, 106748 (2023)
4. Burattin, A., Maggi, F.M., Sperduti, A.: Conformance checking based on multi-perspective declarative process models. Expert Syst. Appl. **65**, 194–211 (2016)
5. Chalmers, C., Fergus, P., Montanez, C.A.C., Sikdar, S., Ball, F., Kendall, B.: Detecting activities of daily living and routine behaviours in dementia patients living alone using smart meter load disaggregation. IEEE Trans. Emerg. Top. Comput. **10**(1), 157–169 (2020)
6. Chimamiwa, G., Giaretta, A., Alirezaie, M., Pecora, F., Loutfi, A.: Are smart homes adequate for older adults with dementia? Sensors **22**(11), 4254 (2022)
7. Debois, S., Hildebrandt, T.T., Laursen, P.H., Ulrik, K.R.: Declarative process mining for DCR graphs. In: Proceedings of the Symposium on Applied Computing, pp. 759–764 (2017)
8. Di Federico, G., Burattin, A.: Do you behave always the same? A process mining approach. In: Montali, M., Senderovich, A., Weidlich, M. (eds.) ICPM 2022. LNBIP, vol. 468, pp. 5–17. Springer, Cham (2022). https://doi.org/10.1007/978-3-031-27815-0_1
9. Di Federico, G., Burattin, A., Montali, M.: Human behavior as a process model: which language to use? In: ITBPM@ BPM, pp. 18–25 (2021)
10. Di Federico, G., Nikolajsen, E.R., Azam, M., Burattin, A.: Linac: a smart environment simulator of human activities. In: Munoz-Gama, J., Lu, X. (eds.) ICPM 2021. LNBIP, vol. 433, pp. 60–72. Springer, Cham (2022). https://doi.org/10.1007/978-3-030-98581-3_5
11. Dogan, O., et al.: Individual behavior modeling with sensors using process mining. Electronics **8**(7), 766 (2019)
12. Falah Rad, M., Shakeri, M., Khoshhal Roudposhti, K., Shakerinia, I.: Probabilistic elderly person's mood analysis based on its activities of daily living using smart facilities. Pattern Anal. Appl. 1–14 (2022)

13. Fernández-Llatas, C., Benedi, J.M., García-Gómez, J.M., Traver, V.: Process mining for individualized behavior modeling using wireless tracking in nursing homes. Sensors **13**(11), 15434–15451 (2013)
14. Hildebrandt, T., Mukkamala, R.R.: Declarative event-based workflow as distributed dynamic condition response graphs. PLACES **69** (2011). https://doi.org/10.4204/EPTCS.69.5
15. Hildebrandt, T.T., Mukkamala, R.R.: Declarative event-based workflow as distributed dynamic condition response graphs. In: Electronic Proceedings in Theoretical Computer Science, vol. 69, pp. 59–73 (2011)
16. Leemans, S.J.J., Fahland, D., van der Aalst, W.M.P.: Discovering block-structured process models from event logs - a constructive approach. In: Colom, J.-M., Desel, J. (eds.) PETRI NETS 2013. LNCS, vol. 7927, pp. 311–329. Springer, Heidelberg (2013). https://doi.org/10.1007/978-3-642-38697-8_17
17. Leotta, F., Mecella, M., Mendling, J.: Applying process mining to smart spaces: perspectives and research challenges. In: Persson, A., Stirna, J. (eds.) CAiSE 2015. LNBIP, vol. 215, pp. 298–304. Springer, Cham (2015). https://doi.org/10.1007/978-3-319-19243-7_28
18. Maggi, F.M., Mooij, A.J., Van der Aalst, W.M.: User-guided discovery of declarative process models. In: 2011 IEEE Symposium on Computational Intelligence and Data Mining (CIDM), pp. 192–199. IEEE (2011)
19. Murata, T.: Petri nets: properties, analysis and applications. Proc. IEEE **77**(4), 541–580 (1989)
20. Nekrasaite, V., Parli, A.T., Back, C.O., Slaats, T.: Discovering responsibilities with dynamic condition response graphs. In: Giorgini, P., Weber, B. (eds.) CAiSE 2019. LNCS, vol. 11483, pp. 595–610. Springer, Cham (2019). https://doi.org/10.1007/978-3-030-21290-2_37
21. Palermo, F., et al.: Designing a clinically applicable deep recurrent model to identify neuropsychiatric symptoms in people living with dementia using in-home monitoring data. In: 35th Conference on Neural Information Processing Systems (NeurIPS 2021) (2021)
22. Pesic, M., Schonenberg, H., Van der Aalst, W.M.: DECLARE: full support for loosely-structured processes. In: 11th IEEE International Enterprise Distributed Object Computing Conference (EDOC 2007), p. 287. IEEE (2007)
23. Rashidi, P., Mihailidis, A.: A survey on ambient-assisted living tools for older adults. IEEE J. Biomed. Health Inform. **17**(3), 579–590 (2012)

Investigating an Ontology-Informed Approach to Event Log Generation in Healthcare

Owen P. Dwyer[1]([✉]) [iD], Lara Chammas[1] [iD], Emanuel Sallinger[1,2],
and Jim Davies[1]

[1] University of Oxford, Oxford, UK
owen.dwyer@gtc.ox.ac.uk
[2] TU Wien, Vienna, Austria

Abstract. Process mining methods have the potential to reveal useful patterns in hospital data and provide insights into patterns of treatment, but healthcare has proven an exceptionally challenging domain due to the significant heterogeneity of possible events and the diversity of individual patients. When studying a patient's pathway, their history might contain hundreds of events unrelated to the disease of interest; determining which to include or exclude in an event log is difficult, and highly dependent on the situation. Typically, researchers only include the most common or correlated events (risking missing rare but significant exceptions), or hand-curate a list of events (slow and difficult, especially where there might be thousands of possible events). We discuss an alternative approach that uses logical reasoning over ontologies to deduce plausibly related events, which might have implications in terms of time savings, the facilitation of reproducible research, and the enabling of comparisons across datasets and healthcare systems. We investigate the practical feasibility of such an approach by demonstrating it on real data, finding that the discovered processes approximate those produced through established approaches, with some caveats. The approach is a promising way to support conversations with domain experts and expedite human processes, and highlights the potential of structured domain knowledge to inform and enhance the event log generation process.

Keywords: preprocessing · filtering · ontologies

1 Introduction

Clinical pathways describe the sequences of events that patients are expected to experience over the course of their journey through the healthcare system. The relationship between these ideal pathways and the real journeys experienced by patients, as observed in data from electronic health records (EHR), is an area of significant research interest, and process mining (PM) is a popular set of methods often proposed as a solution [19]. However, PM can struggle to produce useful insights from healthcare processes because they present several

J. De Smedt and P. Soffer (Eds.): ICPM 2023 Workshops, LNBIP 503, pp. 235–246, 2024.
https://doi.org/10.1007/978-3-031-56107-8_18

challenges: they are highly dynamic, changing as new interventions and technologies are introduced; they are highly complex, relying on large amounts of data and unpredictable events; they are increasingly multidisciplinary, requiring communication and coordination between multiple specialists; and they are ad hoc, modified and interpreted according to individual preferences and professional judgement [20]. These challenges create data that is characterised by incomplete and noisy signals, high levels of process variation, and multitudes of exceptional behaviours that should ideally be captured rather than disregarded.

Given the complex state of raw healthcare data, preparing it for analysis is an intensive and time-consuming step, where modelling decisions and assumptions can have a significant impact on results; this is most evident when determining which clinical events to include in an event log. Human curation of events ensures a high degree of reliability, especially when domain experts are involved, but it is time-consuming and becomes increasingly challenging in a healthcare scenario where the possible events can easily number in the thousands. Statistical approaches, such as only considering the most common events, can be an easy way to simplify data for analysis. However, they risk overlooking rare but significant exceptions, or conversely including very common events that are wholly unrelated to the disease of interest.

In this paper, we describe a third approach to preprocessing for healthcare process mining: an ontological approach. Given that healthcare data is typically encoded in standardised terminologies, and that these terminologies are mappable to ontologies rich with semantics, we propose to use these ontologies to facilitate event log generation. By specifying domain-informed constraints, plausibly related events can be deduced, helping to reduce a large log of events to a smaller subset of more informative and pertinent ones.

Exploiting structured domain knowledge from ontologies has the potential to bring a number of improvements to the process of event log generation, such as:

- expediting the slow and labour-intensive process of codelist curation
- allowing codelists to be expressed as a set of intuitive, explainable rules
- providing rules that can be translated into dataset-specific terminologies, enabling reproducibility across healthcare systems and datasets
- promoting reproducibility and code sharing within the research community
- providing an approach available irrespective of a dataset's sample size

This paper therefore aims to investigate the extent to which event log generation can be automated through the use of ontologies. We first review previous work on preprocessing healthcare data, and the use of semantic reasoning in PM (Sect. 2). We outline an approach to event log generation (Sect. 3), and demonstrate it on real-world healthcare datasets, presenting our initial results (Sect. 4). Finally, we discuss the implications of these results and consider whether it effectively resolves the challenges identified, as well as explore the potential for future research (Sect. 5).

The approach presented here is inspired by, and aims to address, a number of the current challenges in healthcare PM, as established by Munoz-Gama et al. [19]. In particular, we address the ideas that there naturally exists high variability between patients; that infrequent behaviour should be valued; and that transparent approaches should be prioritised. Additionally, we also target two of the current key challenges: *designing dedicated methodologies* by describing a healthcare-specific PM framework that leverages domain knowledge and facilitates comparison across healthcare providers; and *dealing with reality*, by demonstrating our approach on two different real-world datasets.

2   Background

In this section, we consider established approaches to preprocessing healthcare data for process mining, and introduce some of the sources of structured knowledge available in the healthcare domain.

2.1   Preprocessing in Healthcare Process Mining

A 2021 literature review of preprocessing in PM [17] highlights event- and trace-level filtering as one of the most common preprocessing techniques used in the PM literature. However, this framework defines a filtering technique as one that determines the likelihood of the occurrence of events based on its surrounding behaviour, meaning it effectively focuses on the removal of logging mistakes. Determining whether a recorded event actually happened is a question of interest in healthcare PM, but given the very large size of a patient's record and the number of possible events, a more important question to answer first is whether a particular event—whether it happened or not—is even relevant to the particular disease or pathway being studied.

The obvious answer is to consider only the most common events in the study population. However, Tax et al. [22] demonstrate that filtering activities based on frequency alone does not fix problems of chaotic activities, and affects the quality of the final process model. It has been observed that "researchers and practitioners must go beyond simply filtering out infrequent behaviour from the event log" [19].

An alternative to this approach is human curation. In healthcare research, researchers studying health records typically create a *codelist*, a list of concepts in the dataset's terminology that are to be included for study, in order to rigorously define which exposures and outcomes are being investigated. The development of such a list requires three steps: a clear definition of the clinical feature of interest, a shortlist of the potential codes to include, and an iterative process of expert review [23]. This process is therefore naturally very time-consuming, and must be repeated for different datasets using different terminologies. Many researchers that hand-curate codelists in this way have created shared repositories of codes, in an attempt to establish standard and reproducible phenotypes for particular diseases. However, these libraries are focused around the phenotyping of diagnoses rather than procedures, with codelists largely consisting of ICD diagnostic codes [1,4]. Given that PM involves a similar process of deciding which procedural codes to extract from a healthcare record, the field of PM might benefit from an equivalent repository of procedure and event codelists, to similarly establish common phenotypes of disease pathways and facilitate reproducible research.

More recently, a standard approach to generating event logs from healthcare datasets has been proposed [9]: here, activity filtering involves a human identifying a codelist of procedures from those described in relevant medical guidelines. However, this approach is limited by the fact that the language of medical guidelines is typically vague. For example, the UK's guidance on colorectal cancer simply recommends that "surgery" be offered to patients: this does not represent a clear rule for which specific events should be included in a study, and will be interpreted differently by different healthcare systems and individuals [6]. Guidelines will also differ by location, making comparing results difficult. There is therefore a need to explore this activity selection stage in deeper detail, and establish clear and consistent rules for what is and is not included.

2.2   Ontologies, Terminologies, and Clinical Coding

Healthcare procedures are represented in the electronic health record by clinical codes, which can follow one of many possible coding standards [11]. These standards allow for the conversion of medical records into terms that can then be statistically analysed, and provide a framework for standardisation between hospitals and countries. In this work, we encounter two major coding standards.

ICD is an international disease classification standard maintained by the World Health Organization. Its usage world-wide allows for comparability on rates of morbidity, including causes of death. ICD version 9 codes represent both diagnoses and procedures; ICD version 10 does not directly support procedure coding, but the USA maintains a local extension, the ICD-10 Procedure Coding System (ICD-10 PCS), which does.

OPCS is the procedure coding system used by hospitals within the UK's National Health Service. OPCS codes consist of one alphabetical character denoting one of 23 "chapters" organised by anatomical site, followed by two numeric digits representing a subcategory, and an optional third digit for further sub-types. Strictly speaking, OPCS and ICD are *statistical classifications*, a subset of terminologies in which concepts are mutually exclusive and monohierarchical (every concept having exactly one parent), which aid in statistical reporting [11].

In comparison, **SNOMED-CT**—an international standard containing over 350,000 medical terms—describes semantic relationships and polyhierarchies amongst over 350,000 entities, making it closer to a true ontology. These can be reasoned over using logical languages such as the SNOMED Expression Constraint Language (ECL) [7]. This means that SNOMED-based logical reasoning can be a valuable source of knowledge, but real datasets still encode data in terminologies, meaning that terms need to be translated into their SNOMED equivalents for the benefits of a semantically rich ontology to be realised.

The combination of semantics and ontological reasoning with PM has been explored in the past. Alves de Medeiros and van der Aalst [18] describe the core idea of *semantic process mining* as the explicit relation or annotation of elements in a log with the concepts they represent, thereby making it possible to automatically reason or infer other relationships between them. They suggest that such ontologies might be useful in the log cleaning process. Other approaches have used ontological structure to abstract events into less granular categories for analysis, or even to aggregate sequences of events into single events based on rules [16,21]. The difference between fine-grained events in EHR data and more abstract events in treatment guidelines has also been highlighted, with ontology-based abstraction proposed as a way to bridge this gap [15]. The use of ontologies in online systems has also been proposed, as a way of continuously verifying the plausibility of new events [12].

In summary, the preprocessing stages are a key part of the PM framework. Modelling assumptions and decisions, such as which events in a raw health record are included and which are discarded, will inevitably have an impact on the outcome of any analysis. The exact codelists and preprocessing steps used in studies are not always elaborated upon in detail in publications, which limits their reproducibility and usefulness. Cremerius et al. [9] have made some progress in rectifying this with a standard framework for preprocessing the popular MIMIC dataset. The remainder of this paper dives deeper into the event selection stages of this framework, considering how researchers might arrive at a rationale for the inclusion of individual events, and how ontologies might assist in this process.

3   Methods

Given that healthcare data is typically encoded in standardised terminologies, and that these terminologies are mappable to ontologies rich with semantics, we propose leveraging these properties and using domain knowledge to facilitate elements of the event log generation process. In our approach, a candidate list of procedure codes for analysis can be quickly generated by the execution of semantic rules over a domain ontology.

This paper aims to investigate the extent to which event log generation can be automated through the use of ontologies. To answer this question, we define several different possible sets of constraints that might be used to generate a list of candidate SNOMED concepts, we evaluate the resulting codelists in terms of their agreement with an established expert-curated codelist, using colon cancer as a case study, and we analyse the resulting processes in a real EHR dataset.

3.1   Logical Constraints

Through an iterative process, we consider four candidate ECL queries for identifying concepts of interest in SNOMED, listed in Table 1. Firstly, to retrieve all concepts that might be plausibly related to colon cancer, we formalise the question "which concepts are chemotherapy, radiotherapy, or are procedures that occur on the colon or part of the colon?" into a set of rules (Query 1).

This initial query retrieved many codes which were only tangentially colon-related: for example, G02.4, *total oesophagectomy and interposition of microvascularly attached colon* is unlikely to be related to colorectal cancer as the oesophagus is the primary site, and the colon is of secondary concern. Therefore, we

Table 1. SNOMED ECL queries 1–4

```
1   (< 71388002|Procedure| :
        405813007|Procedure site - Direct|
        = << (* : R 363698007|Finding site| = <<363406005))
    OR << 367336001 | Chemotherapy (procedure) |
    OR << 108290001 | Radiation oncology AND/OR
        radiotherapy (procedure) |
```

```
2   (< 71388002|Procedure| :
        ( 405813007|Procedure site - Direct|
        = << (* : R 363698007|Finding site| = <<363406005) )
        AND ([1..1] 405813007|Procedure site - Direct| = *))
    OR << 367336001 | Chemotherapy (procedure) |
    OR << 108290001 | Radiation oncology AND/OR
        radiotherapy (procedure) |
```

```
3   (< 71388002|Procedure| :
        405813007|Procedure site - Direct| = <<71854001)
    OR << 367336001 | Chemotherapy (procedure) |
    OR << 108290001 | Radiation oncology AND/OR
        radiotherapy (procedure) |
```

```
4   (< 71388002|Procedure| :
        ( 405813007|Procedure site - Direct| = <<71854001 )
        AND ([1..1] 405813007|Procedure site - Direct| = *))
    OR << 367336001 | Chemotherapy (procedure) |
    OR << 108290001 | Radiation oncology AND/OR
        radiotherapy (procedure) |
```

introduced an additional constraint that procedures must have one and only one site (Query 2).

Query 1 also retrieved some procedures not related to the colon at all, for example H34.3, *open cryotherapy to lesion of rectum*. These arise because the SNOMED concept representing *malignant neoplasm of colon* has child concepts including *overlapping malignant neoplasm of colon and rectum*, so the rectum is introduced as a procedure site of interest. Therefore, we created a more specific query: instead of any possible site for any colon cancer concept, we consider only the procedures on the colon, or a descendant thereof (Query 3).

Finally, we combine the additions from Queries 2 and 3 to constrain our output to those procedures with exactly one procedure site and a procedure site that is a descendant of the colon, or the colon itself (Query 4).

3.2   Analysis

To benchmark the usability of logic reasoning for clinical activity selection, and to evaluate the retrieval performance of Queries 1–4, we compare their result sets to a reference list of colorectal cancer treatments, as curated by domain experts. Specifically, we use a codelist from the COloRECTal cancer Repository (CORECT-R) project [10]. The project's codelist [5] maps 197 different OPCS codes to five different treatment categories: major resection, minor resection, stoma, stent, and bypass. Furthermore, to investigate the entire patient journey for colorectal cancer, we extended this code list, in consultation with subject matter experts, to include additional codes for diagnostic tests, chemotherapy, radiotherapy, and surgical procedures related to the maintenance of treatments, amounting to a total of 497 OPCS codes[1]. Each ECL query is evaluated according to precision (the proportion of retrieved codes that were in the reference list) and recall (the proportion of codes in the reference list successfully retrieved). Following this, we examine the resulting process model from our derived codelist, and compare it to one generated from our benchmark list.

---

[1] available at https://github.com/larachammas/EventLists.

Table 2. Query precision and recall against original and extended CORECT codelists

Query	Precision		Recall	
	original	*extended*	*original*	*extended*
1	25.78	40.06	**84.69**	**57.59**
2	34.26	52.13	82.14	54.69
3	35.37	52.16	35.37	45.76
4	**50.62**	**73.44**	50.62	39.51

3.3 Data

We demonstrate this methodology by applying it to two separate real-world datasets. Firstly, we use data collected by Oxford University Hospitals (OUH) NHS Foundation Trust, which operates four hospitals in Oxfordshire, southeast England. In this dataset, procedures are coded using OPCS. We also make use of the MIMIC-IV dataset [13,14], a freely accessible EHR dataset from Massachusetts, USA which has been widely used in previous PM studies. This dataset uses a mixture of ICD-9 and ICD-10-PCS procedure codes.

We use the official NHS maps for converting SNOMED codes to their corresponding OPCS codes [8], which are intended to assist clinical coders in converting codes for billing purposes. Most SNOMED concepts actually map to multiple OPCS codes—either a choice of multiple codes, or a mandatory set of multiple codes. Given that the aim of this study is to establish plausibility rather than to guarantee causality, we assume that any OPCS code that is mapped in any way to a SNOMED concept could plausibly be related to it.

4 Results

In this section, we present the initial results of our proposed approach. Firstly, we compare the quality of the generated codelists against our reference list. We then compare the process models generated using these lists, and discuss differences and similarities. Finally, we examine the distribution of codes in an additional dataset to see how a statistical element might add value to our approach.

4.1 Codelist Quality

Table 2 compares each of the four queries in terms of their precision and their recall, against both the original and extended CORECT-R lists. OPCS codes in chapters Y and Z—supplementary codes that describe additional information such as sites or approaches—are excluded since as a rule they never appear in the primary position in records, and therefore have little bearing on PM results.

Query 1 exhibits high recall, retrieving 85% of the original CORECT-R codes, but a low precision (26%), meaning that many extra codes were retrieved. Conversely, Query 4, the most restrictive, has the highest proportion of CORECT-R codes amongst its results (51%), but captures a much smaller set of the whole list (51%). In the extended codelist, precision is naturally higher and recall lower than in the original list, since more of the retrieved codes are in the reference list, but a smaller proportion of the entire list is retrieved. A consistent pattern is that increasing the constraints on the original ECL query can significantly increase precision, but at a cost of much lower recall.

Figure 1 shows the recall of each query, further broken down by the concepts' categories. Concepts representing blood tests, diagnostic testing and patient assessment were never retrieved, presumably because they are not disease specific and therefore do not have a clear site; similarly, endoscopy of the upper gastrointestinal tract was not retrieved as it does not have a relevant procedure site, but it is commonly included in colon cancer analyses as a common route to diagnosis. Recall was highest in surgical topics, since they were well annotated with procedure sites in the ontology. The differences in constraints between queries 1–4 only had a noticeable affect on the *resection* and *other operations* codes.

4.2   Processes

To investigate the usefulness of these codelists in PM, we generate two directly follows graphs (DFGs), one using the extended CORECT-R codelist and one using the Query 1 codelist, chosen as it was the list with the highest overlap with CORECT-R. In these graphs (Fig. 2), node labels represent relative case frequency, i.e. the number of patients experiencing that event, whilst edge labels represent the relative antecedent frequency, i.e. the proportion of instances of the source event that are followed by the destination event. The codes in our new codelist were grouped onto a smaller number of categories for visualisation based on the OPCS codes' text descriptions (e.g. 'resection' encompasses all codes mentioning 'resection', 'excision', 'lesion' or 'exentoration'). For clarity and simplicity, *minor* and *major* resection were grouped into one *resection* category, as were *lower GI* and *upper GI endoscope*. Activities that only occured in a very small proportion of patients (stoma, stent, bypass, other, imaging, assessment) were excluded.

The two processes resemble each other in many ways. A similar proportion of patients underwent resections (58.51% in our codelist, 53.89% according to the CORECT codelist), indicating that the derived codelist arrived on a broader

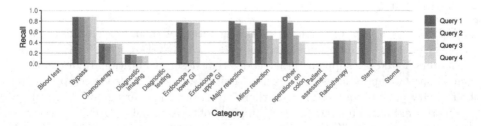

Fig. 1. Recall of queries by category compared to the extended CORECT reference set

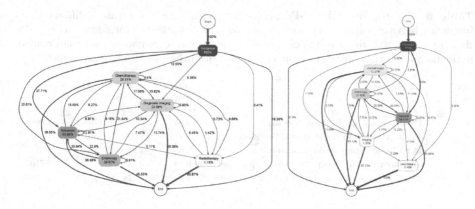

Fig. 2. Directly-follows graphs for CORECT-R codelists (left) and Query 1 (right)

definition of what constitutes a resection. Both processes share similarities: the most common first event was resection; imaging and radiotherapy were typically the last event in a pathway; and radiotherapy very rarely follows a resection. However, there are also some significant differences: the proportion of patients experiencing chemotherapy, imaging and endoscopies were all markedly lower in our model than the CORECT model. These differences will in turn affect the entire process model. In particular, this potentially explains why chemotherapy, endoscopy, resection and imaging were so often the last event in a pathway: in actuality, 21% of chemotherapies are followed by endoscopies, 15% by imaging, and 20% by resection, but an extra 17% of patients had chemotherapy, and an extra 20% had imaging, which were never properly identified in the first place. Therefore, whilst our generated codelist does in some aspects provide a rough sketch of patient journeys, it is certainly far from complete.

4.3   Statistics and the MIMIC Dataset

A limitation of the OUH dataset used here is that the data available at this point only consists of patients with colorectal cancer. An ontological approach could potentially be enhanced by combining both logical and statistical knowledge, enabling the identification of codes that do not have a clear logical link, but are nonetheless correlated with colon cancer. To test this, we examined the MIMIC dataset, which contains data on an entire cohort of patients regardless of disease history.

We divided the MIMIC patients into a control cohort (those without a colon cancer (ICD-10 C18) diagnosis, $n = 120,906$) and a case cohort (those with the diagnosis, $n = 1,046$), and calculated how frequently each code appeared in each group. The codes with the greatest difference in frequency between the two patient groups that did not have a known counterpart in Query 1's codelist [2,3] are listed in Table 3. This immediately raises some interesting results: *large-to-large intestinal anastomosis* and *other small-to-large intestinal anastomosis*

Table 3. The top five MIMIC-IV procedure codes with the greatest differences in frequency between colon cancer and non-colon cancer patients. Considered were codes that appeared >20 times in the case cohort, were more common in case than control patients, and statistically significant ($P < 0.05$) according to Fisher's exact test.

ICD version	ICD concept	control frequency (%)	case frequency (%)	odds ratio	P
9	**17.35** Laparoscopic left hemicolectomy	0.04	2.49	70.02	$1.06e^{-35}$
9	**45.93** Other small-to-large intestinal anastomosis	0.15	7.65	55.54	$1.39e^{-99}$
9	**45.94** Large-to-large intestinal anastomosis	0.08	2.87	34.97	$1.27e^{-33}$
10	**0D1B0Z4** Bypass Ileum to Cutaneous, Open Approach	0.18	2.58	15.08	$6.71e^{-22}$
9	**45.25** Closed [endoscopic] biopsy of large intestine	1.14	11.28	11.05	$2.71e^{-74}$

are highly correlated with colorectal cancer diagnosis, and are obviously colon related, but are not in our codelist. More suprisingly, *laparoscopic right hemicolectomy* does appear in our codelist, but *laparoscopic left hemicolectomy* does not. An examination of the mapping files reveals that left hemicolectomy has no mapping to any SNOMED concept, so regardless of whether its SNOMED counterpart was identified in our search, it would not be detected in an ICD-9 encoded dataset.

5   Discussion and Conclusions

These results establish that a logical query over SNOMED's domain knowledge is capable of approximating a human-prepared codelist with some accuracy, but there exists a clear trade-off between precision and recall: either a relatively complete codelist is retrieved with a large number of extra codes, or an incomplete codelist is retrieved in which every code has as high chance of being known to be relevant. The differences between process models produced via this approach and from a traditional curated codelist support this. Additionally, challenges appeared in the form of grouping codes into categories. The original approach considered was to group codes according to relationships in the SNOMED ontology - for example, all codes that were a descendent of "imaging" could safely be considered imaging. However, in a high proportion of cases, many possible SNOMED concepts mapped onto one OPCS code creating multiple possible categories. An additional problem is the need for these categories to be aligned with the ones from the benchmark codelist to allow for a useful comparison. Hence, the solution of grouping codes by text was arrived upon.

The supplementary analysis of the MIMIC dataset indicated that many codes existed that were clearly correlated with colon cancer, but not identified by our proposed approach. In addition, some unusual results highlighted gaps in the mappings' coverage. Overall, these results suggest that the approach proposed here is, whilst an interesting experiment, far from a replacement for discussion and input from domain experts, and in fact underline their importance.

There are some potential advantages to the presented approach. It does provide a reasonably accurate list on which to begin discussions, speeding up the initial stages of the development process. It allows the majority of concepts in a codelist to be described simply, as a set of intuitive, explainable rules. It in principle allows the description of codelists in terms of a well-known ontology that can be translated into the specific languages used by individual datasets, although this is highly dependent on both the completeness of the original ontology and the quality of mappings available. It also provides a viable approach for applications where datasets are very small, rendering statistical examinations of the most common codes unhelpful. Finally, the specification of desired process events in terms of their relationship to a particular target disease keeps PM focused on a concrete health issue, ensuring clinical meaningfulness and alignment between PM studies and research questions around healthcare delivery.

It also highlights several avenues for future research; in particular, further work is required to establish the extent to which this approach is generalisable to other diseases, and whether it might also work in other application areas outside of healthcare with their own ontologies.

In summary, we have found that domain knowledge, even in the form of established ontologies, is far from perfect and cannot instantly automate the process of event log preparation. However, it can provide a meaningful framework to generate initial ideas to be iterated upon. This study highlights that no single approach—whether reliant on ontologies, conversation with domain experts, or pure statistics—can fully capture the complex nature of healthcare processes, and that a combination of all are required to fully explore health processes and answer questions around modern healthcare delivery.

Acknowledgements. OPD and LC are supported by the EPSRC Centre for Doctoral Training in Health Data Science (EP/S02428X/1). OPD is supported by Elsevier. ES is supported by the Vienna Science and Technology Fund (WWTF) (10.47379/ICT2201, 10.47379/VRG18013, 10.47379/NXT22018); and the Christian Doppler Research Association (CDG) JRC LIVE. Access to anonymised healthcare data was facilitated by the NIHR Health Informatics Collaborative Colorectal Cancer Programme, with ethical approval from the East Midlands and Derby Research Ethics Committee (21/EM/0028).

References

1. HDRUK Phenotype Library. https://phenotypes.healthdatagateway.org/
2. ICD-9-CM Diagnostic Codes to SNOMED CT Map. https://www.nlm.nih.gov/research/umls/mapping_projects/icd9cm_to_snomedct.html
3. ICD-9-CM to and from ICD-10-CM and ICD-10-PCS General Equivalence Mappings. https://www.nber.org/research/data/icd-9-cm-and-icd-10-cm-and-icd-10-pcs-crosswalk-or-general-equivalence-mappings
4. OpenCodelists. https://www.opencodelists.org/
5. CORECT-R Data Coding v1.0 (2020). https://www.ndph.ox.ac.uk/corectr/files/corect-r-data-coding-v1-0-oct20.pdf

6. Colorectal cancer (NICE guideline NG151) (2021). https://www.nice.org.uk/guidance/ng151/resources/colorectal-cancer-pdf-66141835244485
7. Expression Constraint Language - Specification and Guide Version 2.1 (2022). http://snomed.org/ecl
8. SNOMED CT to ICD-10 and OPCS-4 Map Table Technical Specification and Implementation Guidance (UK Edition) (2023). https://nhsengland.kahootz.com/gf2.ti/f/762498/159916325.1/PDF/-/doc_SnomedCTICD10OPCS4MapTableTechnicalSpecificationImplementationGuidance_UK%20Edition_Current-e.pdf
9. Cremerius, J., Pufahl, L., Klessascheck, F., Weske, M.: Event log generation in MIMIC-IV research paper. In: Montali, M., Senderovich, A., Weidlich, M. (eds.) ICPM 2022. LNBIP, vol. 468, pp. 302–314. Springer, Cham (2023). https://doi.org/10.1007/978-3-031-27815-0_22
10. Downing, A., et al.: Data resource profile: the COloRECTal cancer data repository (CORECT-R). Int. J. Epidemiol. **50**(5), 1418–1418k (2021)
11. Haendel, M.A., Chute, C.G., Robinson, P.N.: Classification, ontology, and precision medicine. N. Engl. J. Med. **379**(15), 1452–1462 (2018)
12. Helm, E., Buchgeher, G., Ehrlinger, L.: Online plausibility checks for patient pathways with medical ontologies. In: PODS4H at ICPM (Posters) (2022)
13. Johnson, A., Bulgarelli, L., Pollard, T., Horng, S., Celi, L., Mark, R.: MIMIC-IV (version 1.0) (2020). https://doi.org/10.13026/s6n6-xd98
14. Johnson, A.E.W., et al.: MIMIC-IV, a freely accessible electronic health record dataset. Sci. Data **10**(1), 1 (2023)
15. Klessascheck, F., et al.: Domain-specific event abstraction. In: Business Information Systems, pp. 117–126 (2021)
16. Leonardi, G., Striani, M., Quaglini, S., Cavallini, A., Montani, S.: Towards semantic process mining through knowledge-based trace abstraction. In: Ceravolo, P., van Keulen, M., Stoffel, K. (eds.) SIMPDA 2017. LNBIP, vol. 340, pp. 45–64. Springer, Cham (2019). https://doi.org/10.1007/978-3-030-11638-5_3
17. Marin-Castro, H.M., Tello-Leal, E.: Event log preprocessing for process mining: a review. Appl. Sci. **11**(22), 10556 (2021)
18. Alves de Medeiros, A.K., van der Aalst, W.M.P.: Process mining towards semantics. In: Dillon, T.S., Chang, E., Meersman, R., Sycara, K. (eds.) Advances in Web Semantics I. LNCS, vol. 4891, pp. 35–80. Springer, Heidelberg (2008). https://doi.org/10.1007/978-3-540-89784-2_3
19. Munoz-Gama, J., et al.: Process mining for healthcare: characteristics and challenges. J. Biomed. Inform. **127**, 103994 (2022)
20. Rebuge, Á., Ferreira, D.R.: Business process analysis in healthcare environments: a methodology based on process mining. Inf. Syst. **37**(2), 99–116 (2012)
21. Remy, S., Pufahl, L., Sachs, J.P., Böttinger, E., Weske, M.: Event log generation in a health system: a case study. In: Fahland, D., Ghidini, C., Becker, J., Dumas, M. (eds.) BPM 2020. LNCS, vol. 12168, pp. 505–522. Springer, Cham (2020). https://doi.org/10.1007/978-3-030-58666-9_29
22. Tax, N., Sidorova, N., van der Aalst, W.M.P.: Discovering more precise process models from event logs by filtering out chaotic activities. J. Intell. Inf. Syst. **52**(1), 107–139 (2019)
23. Watson, J., Nicholson, B.D., Hamilton, W., Price, S.: Identifying clinical features in primary care electronic health record studies: methods for codelist development. BMJ Open **7**(11), e019637 (2017)

I-PALIA: Discovering BPMN Processes with Duplicated Activities for Healthcare Domains

Carlos Fernandez-Llatas[1,3]([✉]) and Andrea Burattin[2]

[1] Universitat Politecnica de Valencia, Valencia, Spain
cfllatas@itaca.upv.es
[2] Technical University of Denmark, Kongens Lyngby, Denmark
[3] Karolinska Institutet, Solna, Sweden

Abstract. Process mining encompasses a range of methods designed to analyze event logs. Among these methods, control-flow discovery algorithms are particularly significant, as they enable the identification of real-world process models, known as *in-vivo* processes, in contrast to anticipated models. An obstacle faced by control-flow discovery algorithms is their limited ability to recognize duplicated activities, which are activities that occur in multiple locations within a process. This issue is particularly relevant in the healthcare sector, where numerous instances of duplicated activities exist in processes but remain undetected by conventional algorithms. This article introduces a novel concept for a control-flow discovery algorithm capable of effectively revealing duplicated activities. The effectiveness of this technique is demonstrated through experimentation on a synthetic dataset. Moreover, the algorithm has been implemented and its source code is available as open-source software, accessible both as a ProM plugin and a Java Maven dependency.

Keywords: Process mining · Control-flow discovery · BPMN · Duplicated activities

1 Introduction

Process mining is the scientific discipline aiming at connecting process models and recordings of activity executions [17]. In particular, *control-flow discovery* techniques pertain to the synthesis of models which are capable of explaining in a compact way all (or most of) the executions reported in an event log.

The ultimate goal of process mining techniques is to improve processes and how these are actually deployed in the real world. Since these models are supposed to improve actual processes it is essential that the models identified are as reliable and *good* as possible.

When considering the control-flow discovery techniques, the main challenge they need to face consists of extracting a model which is the most suitable representation possible. Defining "most suitable representation" is a challenge in itself

J. De Smedt and P. Soffer (Eds.): ICPM 2023 Workshops, LNBIP 503, pp. 247–258, 2024.
https://doi.org/10.1007/978-3-031-56107-8_19

and, in the literature, numerical approaches to quantify this dimension have been proposed, in particular *fitness, precision, generalisation* and *simplicity* [17]. Fitness indicates that a model should be able to replicate the log it has been generated from; precision quantifies how much more behavior (w.r.t. the starting log) the mined model permits; generalization tries to capture to what extent behavior not observed in the log is present in the model; and, finally, simplicity verifies that the model should be as simple as possible, to foster understandability. All these metrics should be maximized in order to obtain good results.

While many algorithms for control-flow discovery have put a lot of focus on optimizing fitness and precision [1,11,19], less emphasis has been put on the simplicity dimension, in particular regarding the type of supported behavior. Specifically, as mentioned in the Process Mining Manifesto [10] (as guiding principle GP3), control-flow discovery algorithms should be able to identify basic control-flow constructs [15,18], such as concurrency and choice. In many situations, a limiting factor towards better simplicity is the problem of *duplicated activities*. This problem stems from the fact that most control-flow discovery algorithms are not able to produce process models where the same activity occurs more than once.

Within the healthcare sector, it's common to encounter activities that occur repeatedly. Instances such as revisiting medical appointments, undergoing assessment procedures like laboratory tests and medical imaging, or undergoing cyclic treatments like dialysis or chemotherapy are recurrent events throughout a patient's journey within the care process. These activities carry significant importance in representing the overall process. To illustrate, the sequencing of treatments can vary significantly based on the timing of assessments. For instance, in the context of cancer treatments, administering chemotherapy before and/or after surgery can yield distinct results. The initial treatment aims to shrink the tumor size and streamline the surgical procedure, while the subsequent treatment focuses on preventing the proliferation of harmful cells, introducing differing objectives and complexities that impact process delineation.

When applying conventional process discovery algorithms to this scenario, the ability to differentiate between these distinct behaviors becomes compromised. In this example, as well as in numerous other cases within the healthcare sphere, the utilization of duplicated nodes becomes imperative. Not only do they contribute to a lucid depiction of the process, but they also facilitate comprehension of the preparatory and follow-up stages surrounding these recurrent activities.

In this paper we present a new algorithm capable of extracting process models, represented as BPMN [12]. The algorithm can identify all the basic workflow patterns (i.e., sequence, parallel split, synchronization, exclusive choice, and simple merge) with the addition of duplicated activities.

The rest of the paper is structured as follows: Sect. 2 introduces the background and the state of the art of the proposed technique; Sect. 3 presents the actual algorithm proposed in the paper; Sect. 4 describes the implementation of the technique; Sect. 5 presents some performance results of the algorithm against some extreme scenarios; and finally Sect. 6 concludes the paper.

2 Background and State of the Art

In the literature on control-flow discovery [1] many algorithms have been developed able to identify all the basic workflow patterns. Among these, the Alpha miner is typically recalled as one of the first algorithms explicitly tackling the control-flow discovery problem. More advanced algorithms, such as the Heuristics Miner, the Fuzzy Miner, the Split Miner, and the Inductive Miner, have gained a lot of popularity due to the quality of the output they produce and their performance. However, none of these is actually capable of producing duplicated activities. The algorithms which are able to achieve this are very few, including the $\alpha*$-algorithm [5] which nonetheless have very restrictive assumptions on the event log. Fodina [5] can discover duplicated activities by pre-processing the event log only based on some heuristics. Genetic Process Mining [6], ETM [2], AGNES [9] are evolutionary algorithms that, in principle, can discover duplicated activities at the expense of extreme computational complexity. Other algorithms that exploit region theory are also capable of mining duplicated activities which however SLAD [20] is another approach that post-processes the mined model for duplicated activities. Also in this case, however, the algorithm exploits some heuristics for simplifying the model by duplicating some behavior.

As a basis for the paper we should provide some definitions. Classic PALIA algorithm [8,14] uses as a representation model, a Timed Parallel Automaton [7]. This model has an expressiveness equivalent to a safe Petri Net [13] and has a Regular complexity [7] based on the concept of Parallel Finite Automaton [16]. For this paper a TPA is defined as follows:

Definition 1. *A Timed Parallel Automaton(TPA) [7] is a tuple $T = \{N, Q, \gamma, \delta, S, F\}$ where:*

- *N is a finite set of Nodes, where a Node n is a graphical representation of the action a,*
- *Q is a finite set of states where $q \subseteq N^+ \forall q \in Q$,*
- *$\gamma : N^+ \to N^+$ is the Node Transition function, where $\gamma = \{(n_0^s, .., n_i^s), (n_0^e, .., n_j^e)\}$. Γ is the set of γ functions;*
- *$\delta : Q \to Q$ is the State transition function where $\delta = \{q^s, q^e\}$. Δ is the set of δ functions where $(\forall \delta \in \Delta \; \exists \; \gamma \in \Gamma \; / \; (n_0^s, \ldots, n_i^s) = q^s \wedge (n_0^e, \ldots, n_i^e) = q^e)$ where γ is the associated transition of δ;*
- *$S \subseteq N$ is the set of Starting Nodes;*
- *$F \subseteq N$ is the set of Final Nodes.*

A TPA has a double transition function, defining Nodes (N) and States (Q). The transitions between nodes can be n to n multiple for defining parallelism. For example, a transition $\gamma_1 = \{(n_1), (n_2, n_3)\}$ represents a parallel split from the node n_1 to the nodes n_2 and n_3. In the same way, a transition $\gamma_2 = \{(n_1, n_2), (n_3)\}$ represent a parallel synchronization from the nodes n_1 and n_2 to the node n_3. Exclusive Choice can be represented using several γ transitions. For example, having $\gamma_1 = \{(n_1), (n_2)\}$ and $\gamma_2 = \{(n_1), (n_3)\}$ we can represent that, from n_1 is possible to go to n_2 or n_3.

The view of States provides a regular language view over the interpretation of the automaton. In the states view (Δ set), the parallelism is represented at the state level, A State q is a set of Nodes that represents the actions that are active in the state q in an analogous way to a Petri-Net marking. Δ and Γ are complementary. The state transitions (δ) keep the regular complexity due to their simplicity (N to N) where the Node Transitions (Γ) represent parallel situations (N^+ to N^+). In practice, there is only one state active in a moment in time, which supposes that it could be several nodes active. Node transitions represent the single pass from one node to another. This double transition function allows representing complex workflow patterns, like milestones or interleaved parallel routines [7]. There is an algorithm that given a Γ set it is possible to construct a basic Δ set of states [7]. The objective of the discovery algorithm of this paper is to construct a TPA with a Γ set assuming that Δ can be automatically inferred.

Following, we present the definitions of Event and Event Log:

Definition 2. *An Event is a pair $e = \{a, \pi\}$ where $a \in \mathcal{A}$ is the set of possible actions in a process, π is the timestamp execution of the action.*

Definition 3. *An Event Log ($\mathcal{L}$) is a set of traces $\mathcal{L} = \{t_0, \ldots, t_i\}$, where a trace is a sequence of events $t = \{e_0, \ldots, e_j\}$*

An *Event* is the digital representation of an action in a moment in time. A set of events referenced to the same user or the same execution instance is called *Trace*.

3   Inductive PALIA (I-PALIA): The Algorithm

Within this document, we introduce an upgraded iteration of the PALIA algorithm, specifically devised to uncover activity logs through the application of Grammar Inference methods. Subsequently, the algorithm undertakes the task of detecting parallel configurations within the inferred model. To facilitate this process, we have established certain foundational definitions:

Definition 4. *Given events $e_0 = \{a_0, \pi_0\}, e_1 = \{a_1, \pi_1\}, e_0$ is equivalent to e_1 ($e_0 \equiv e_1$) where $a_0 = a_1$.*

Given event $e = \{a_0, \pi\}$ and a Node n representing the action a_1, e_0 is equivalent to n ($e_0 \equiv n$) where $a_0 = a_1$.

Given two Nodes n_0, n_1, they are equivalents ($n_0 \equiv n_1$) if they have the same representing action.

Definition 5. *Given two sets of nodes N_0, N_1 they are equivalent ($N_0 \equiv N_1$) if $|N_0| = |N_1|$ and $\exists n_i \equiv n_j | \forall n_i \in N_0, n_j \in N_1$*

Colloquially, Nodes and Events are equivalent when they refer to the same action, and two sets of nodes are equivalent if each one of the nodes of each set is equivalent to a node of the other set.

Definition 6. *Given two Node Transitions $\gamma_0 = \{D_0, R_0\}, \gamma_1 = \{D_1, R_1\}$, they are equivalents ($\gamma_0 \equiv \gamma_1$) if their Domains ($D_0$, D_1) and Ranges (R_0, R_1) are equivalent*

In an analogous way, two Node Transitions are equivalent if their domains and ranges are equivalent.

Definition 7. *Given a TPA, and $n_0, n_1 \in N$, n_0 is directly followed by n_1 ($n_0 \to n_1$) if $\exists$ a node transition $\gamma_0 \in \gamma | n_0 \to n_1$.*
  γ_0 is directly followed by γ_1 ($\gamma_0 \to \gamma_1$) if $n^e \in \gamma_0 = n^s \gamma_1$

Definition 8. *Given a TPA, and $n_0, n_1 \in N$, n_0 is eventually followed by n_1, ($n_0 \Rightarrow n_1$) where $\exists$ a sequence of node transition $\{\gamma_0 .. \gamma_j\}$ $\forall_{0<i<j} | \gamma_i \to \gamma_{i+1} \wedge n^s \in \gamma_0 = n_0 \wedge n^e \in \gamma_j = n_1$*
  γ_0 is eventually followed by γ_1, ($\gamma_0 \Rightarrow \gamma_1$) if $n^e \in \gamma_0 \Rightarrow n^s \in \gamma_1$

The next definitions define when two node transitions are directly followed ($\to$) when the second transition can be immediately accessed from the first one and eventually followed ($\Rightarrow$) when the second transition can be eventually accessed from the first one.

Definition 9. *A Prefix Acceptor Tree (PAT) is a tree-like TPA built from the learning Log by taking all the prefixes in the sample as states and constructing the smallest TPA which is a tree, strongly consistent with the Log.*

The Prefix Acceptor Tree creates a TPA that represents a tree from left to right with the events of the samples. The head of the tree is formed by the nodes representing the starting events of the traces, and the leaves represent the last events of the traces. Figure 1 shows an example of how this tree is created. Should be noticed that although TPA is able to represent parallel situations, the Prefix Acceptor Tree creates only non-parallel δ functions so this algorithm is not able to represent parallelism.

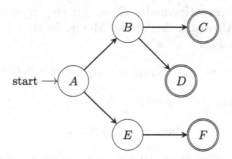

Fig. 1. Prefix Acceptor Tree of Log = {ABC, ABD, AEF}

Algorithm 1 shows the pseudocode of the presented algorithm. The first action is to compute the Prefix Acceptor Tree that represents the Log. Using the Prefix Acceptor Tree as a basis, Inductive PALIA will perform some generalizations over the algorithm using Grammar Inference techniques. First, the algorithm merges equivalent consecutive nodes, generalizing all the transitions

Algorithm 1. Inductive PALIA Algorithm

Require: $\mathcal{L}$
Ensure: $\mathcal{T}$
1: $\mathcal{T} \leftarrow PrefixAceptorTree(\mathcal{L})$
2: **for all** $\gamma : (n^s, n^e) \in \Gamma)$ **do**
3:      **if** $n^s \equiv n^e$ **then** Merge(n^s, n^e)
4:      **end if**
5: **end for**
6: **for all** $n_0, n_1 \in F | n_0 \equiv n_1$ **do** $Merge(n_0, n_1)$
7: **end for**
8: **while** $\mathcal{T}$ has changes **do**
9:      **for all** $\gamma_x \Rightarrow \gamma_y \mid \gamma_x = \{d_x, r_x\}, \gamma_y = \{d_y, r_y\} \in \Gamma$ **do**
10:          **if** $\gamma_x \equiv \gamma_y$ **then**
11:              $Merge(d_x, d_y)$
12:              $Merge(r_x, r_y)$
13:          **end if**
14:      **end for**
15: **end while**
16: $\mathcal{T} \leftarrow ParallelMerge(\mathcal{T})$ ▷ See Algorithm 2

---

from one node to itself. Second the algorithm merges all the final nodes that are equivalent. Finally, the algorithm Merge the domains (d_x, d_y) and ranges (r_x, r_y) of each couple of γ in Γ that are eventually followed ($\gamma_x \Rightarrow \gamma_y$) and are equivalent ($\gamma_x \equiv \gamma_y$). This action is performed until the TPA $\mathcal{T}$ has no new merges. This algorithm allows an ordered merging of the nodes that prevent their massive merging like in other basic algorithms such as Directly Follows Graphs (DFG).

Until this moment, the algorithm has discovered a process structure Discovering with sequences, splits, and loops, assuming no parallelism, but differentiating repeated non-consecutive nodes. The next step is to identify the parallel sequences with the Algorithm 2: Parallel Merge. In this algorithm, the parallelism has been defined as:

Definition 10. *Given $n_0, n_1 \in N$, n_0 and n_1 are parallel ($n_0 \| n_1$) where:*

$$n_0 \Rightarrow n_1 \wedge n_1 \Rightarrow n_0 \tag{1}$$

$$!n_0 \Leftrightarrow n_1 \wedge !n_1 \Leftrightarrow n_0 \tag{2}$$

Colloquially, two nodes are parallel ($n_0 \| n_1$) if both are eventually followed between themselves and these nodes are not acting as a loop, that means, not exist a path of transitions that contains $n_0 \Rightarrow n_1$ and $n_1 \Rightarrow n_0$ in the same path ($n_0 \Leftrightarrow n_1$), and vice-versa. With that definition, the Parallel Merge (Algorithm 2) defines the Parallel Regions for discovering the parallel situations:

Definition 11. *Given a TPA $\mathcal{T}$ and node n_{Split}, A Parallel Region is a set of nodes R where $n_{Split} \Rightarrow n_x \wedge \exists n_y : n_x \| n_y | \forall n_x, n_y \in R$*

A Parallel Region is a set of nodes that occurs after a split node n_{Split} and have parallelisms between themselves.

Definition 12. *Given a TPA $\mathcal{T}$, a node n_{Split}, and a Parallel Region R, a Syncronization Node is a node n_{Syncro} where $n_i \Rightarrow n_{Syncro}|\forall n_i \in R$ and $\forall n_x|n_{Split} \Rightarrow n_x \wedge n_x \Rightarrow n_{Syncro}|n_x \in R$*

A Synchronization Node n_{Syncro} is a node that occurs immediately after the Parallel region. n_{Split} and n_{Syncro} delimits the Parallel Region and are the nodes that will define the start and the end of parallelism. According to that, the Algorithm 2 Discover and create the Parallel structures.

Algorithm 2. Parallel Merge

Require: $\mathcal{T}$
Ensure: $\mathcal{T}$
1: **for all** $n_{Split} \in N$ **do**
2:     $R \leftarrow GetParallelRegions(\mathcal{T}, n_{Split})$
3:     **for all** $p \in R$ **do**
4:         $n_{Syncro} \leftarrow GetSyncroNode(\mathcal{T}, n_{Split}, R)$
5:         $seq \leftarrow$ IdentifyParallelSequences($\mathcal{T}, R$)   ▷ See Algorithm 3
6:         $\mathcal{T} \leftarrow$ CreateParallelTransitions($\mathcal{T}, n_{Split}, n_{Syncro}, R, seq$)
7:     **end for**
8: **end for**

The *Parallel Merge* Algorithm tries to discover parallel regions after each node on the TPA (representing this node the n_{split} of the Parallel Region). Once a Parallel Region is detected, the subsequent task involves pinpointing the synchronization node that marks the boundaries of said Parallel Region. Subsequently, the algorithm proceeds to determine the parallel sequences within the identified Parallel Region. This specific process is detailed in Algorithm 3.

Algorithm 3. Identify Parallel Sequences

Require: $\mathcal{T}, R$
Ensure: $SeqMap$
1: **for all** $r \in R$ **do**
2:     $SeqMap(r) \leftarrow (r, S)$ where $S \subset R \wedge s_i \nparallel r|\forall s_i \in S$
3: **end for**

The algorithm *Identify Parallel Sequences* segregates the nodes within the Parallel Region into distinct groups, classifying those that do not exhibit parallelism in relation to the rest. This methodology serves to discern the parallel sequences contained within the defined Parallel Region.

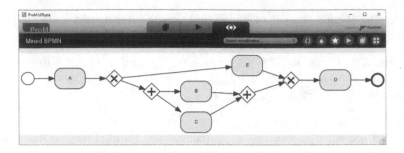

Fig. 2. The PaliaProM plugin showing the result of a mining session.

Upon successful identification of the parallel sequences, the Parallel Merge Algorithm (Algorithm 2) allows the creation of the ascertained parallel structure. This involves establishing connections between each parallel sequence and the Split node at the beginning, as well as the Synchronization node at the conclusion of the respective sequences.

4   Implementation

I-PALIA has been implemented in Java and as a Maven project as well as a ProM plugin[1]. Having the code available as stand-alone Java project simplifies its embedding into new projects (the code can easily be imported into any Maven/Gradle/Ivy project[2]). The PaliaProM package, which imports the Maven dependency, allows us to easily benefit from the algorithm leveraging the infrastructure made available by ProM. The package contains two plugins, one called "Palia Miner" which takes an XES log object as input and produces a standard BPMN object as result. The second plugin made available in the PaliaProM package is a visualizer for BPMN called "Graphviz BPMN visualisation" which exploits Graphviz to display any BPMN process model. A graphical representation of the latter is reported in Fig. 2.

5   Evaluation and Discussion

In order to evaluate the effectiveness of the algorithm, we decided to compare the models resulting from the mining of the process using the state of the art algorithms and tools for control-flow discovery. We designed a process (available in Fig. 3) specifically expressing the challenges of duplicated activities, in the case of the process it is activity A. In addition to that, we incorporated behavior coming from the most common workflow patterns [18]: sequences, parallel split, synchronization, exclusive choice, and simple merge.

---

[1] The Maven project is available at https://github.com/delas/palia. The ProM package, called PaliaProM, is available at https://github.com/delas/PaliaProM.

[2] See https://jitpack.io/#delas/palia.

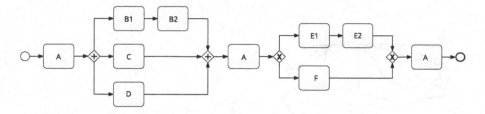

Fig. 3. The reference process we used for our simulation

We simulated the process using the tool Purple [4][3], configuring the tool for the rediscoverability purpose, which led to an event log with 990 traces and 8415 events. We mined this log with I-PALIA as well as with Fluxicon Disco[4], Celonis[5], Apromore[6] and the Inductive Miner [11]. The results are available in Fig. 4. While the model mined with I-PALIA matches perfectly the expected one, all other mining tools and algorithms fail at extracting a model that resembles the original one. The main issue, as expected, is the duplication of activity A which is observed at the beginning, in the middle, and at the end of the process. This causes all models to show unstructured behavior, quite similar for each mining algorithm: the process can start with activity A and finish immediately, or can have repetitions of the combinations of the other activities (the part before and after the A in the middle).

In another battery of tests we aimed at learning something about the computational performance of the I-PALIA implementation. For this purpose, we generated a random process model using PLG2 [3] (cf. Fig. 5). With this model, we generated 6 event logs with 100, 500, 1000, 2000, 5000, and 10000 traces. These logs were mined with I-PALIA and we monitored the execution time. The tests were performed on a standard laptop, equipped with Java 1.15(TM) SE Runtime Environment on Windows 10 Enterprise 64bit, an Intel Core i7-7500U 2.70 GHz CPU and 16 GB of RAM. Results are reported in Fig. 6. As the plot shows, the time required to process is not negligible and could grow quite quickly. Considering the biggest log we had 10000 traces, 58713 events, and our implementation of I-PALIA took almost 7 s for the actual mining.

While the algorithm shows very promising results, it still suffers from important issues. The most important ones are the current lack of robustness to noise and its computational complexity. Regarding the lack of robustness to noise, this is certainly a problem that makes the algorithm not mature enough for many industrial settings, however, we believe this is an issue that can easily be addressed by considering frequencies of the direct following relations and applying some threshold on those before applying the rest of the computation. A more fundamental challenge regards the complexity of the algorithm. Right now, sev-

---

[3] See http://pros.unicam.it:4300/.
[4] See https://fluxicon.com/disco/.
[5] See https://www.celonis.com/.
[6] See https://apromore.com/.

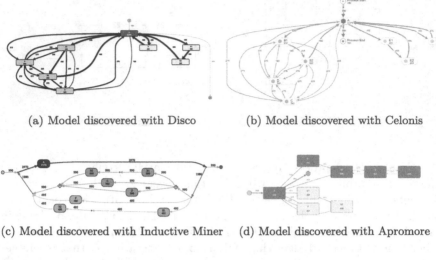

(a) Model discovered with Disco   (b) Model discovered with Celonis

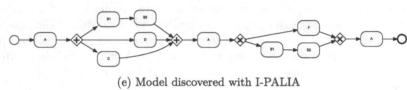

(c) Model discovered with Inductive Miner   (d) Model discovered with Apromore

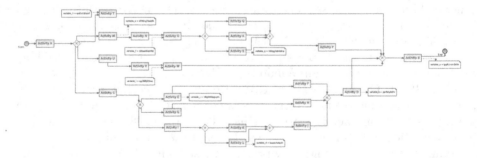

(e) Model discovered with I-PALIA

Fig. 4. Results of the mining of the log using different techniques

Fig. 5. Random model generated for the stress test

eral steps and needed in order to reach the goal, and each of these contribute substantially to the complexity. For small logs the mining time is acceptable, but it grows quickly as the numbers of traces and events grow. Optimizations can be employed also in this case, both in terms of implementation (e.g., multi-threading) as well as more conceptual ones.

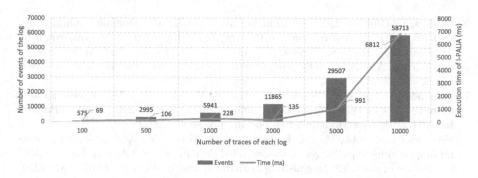

Fig. 6. Stress test on the algorithm against log with different sizes

6   Conclusion and Future Work

In this paper we presented I-PALIA, a process mining algorithm for control-flow discovery. The algorithm is capable of synthesising BPMN process models containing all basic workflow patterns (i.e., sequence, parallel split, synchronization, exclusive choice, and simple merge) as well as duplicated activities. The algorithm, which has a publicly available implementation as both ProM package as well as a Java Maven dependency has been tested and evaluated both qualitatively (against state of the art tools) as well as quantitatively on logs of different sizes.

Future work for I-PALIA certainly includes the extension of the algorithm to become noise tolerant, for example employing frequencies. Additionally improving the performance and the computational complexity of the approach certainly represents a fundamental step towards wider adoption.

Acknowledgements. This research has been supported through projects MINE-GUIDE(PID2020-113723RB-C21) funded by MCIN/AEI/10.13039/501100011033 and LIFECHAMPS(Grant Agreement No 875329) under European Union's Horizon 2020 research and innovation program.

References

1. Augusto, A., et al.: Automated discovery of process models from event logs: review and benchmark. IEEE Trans. Knowl. Data Eng. **31**(4), 686–705 (2019)
2. Buijs, J.C.A.M., van Dongen, B.F., van der Aalst, W.M.P.: Quality dimensions in process discovery: the importance of fitness, precision, generalization and simplicity. Int. J. Coop. Inf. Syst. **23**(01), 1440001 (2014)
3. Burattin, A.: PLG2: multiperspective process randomization with online and offline simulations. In: Online Proceedings of the BPM Demo Track 2016. CEUR-WS.org (2016)
4. Burattin, A., Re, B., Rossi, L., Tiezzi, F.: A purpose-guided log generation framework. In: Di Ciccio, C., Dijkman, R., del Río Ortega, A., Rinderle-Ma, S. (eds.) BPM 2022. LNCS, vol. 13420, pp. 181–198. Springer, Cham (2022). https://doi.org/10.1007/978-3-031-16103-2_14

5. Calders, T., Günther, C.W., Pechenizkiy, M., Rozinat, A.: Using minimum description length for process mining. In: Proceedings of the 2009 ACM symposium on Applied Computing - SAC 2009, pp. 1451–1455. ACM Press, New York (2009)
6. de Medeiros, A.K.A.: Genetic process mining. Ph.D. thesis, Technische Universiteit Eindhoven (2006)
7. Fernandez-Llatas, C., Pileggi, S.F., Traver, V., Benedi, J.M.: Timed parallel automaton: a mathematical tool for defining highly expressive formal workflows. In: 2011 Fifth Asia Modelling Symposium, pp. 56–61 (2011)
8. Fernández-Llatas, C., Meneu, T., Benedí, J.M., Traver, V.: Activity-based process mining for clinical pathways computer aided design. In: 2010 Annual International Conference of the IEEE Engineering in Medicine and Biology, pp. 6178–6181 (2010)
9. Goedertier, S., Martens, D., Vanthienen, J., Baesens, B.: Robust process discovery with artificial negative events. J. Mach. Learn. Res. **10**, 1305–1340 (2009)
10. van der Aalst, W., et al.: Process mining manifesto. In: Daniel, F., Barkaoui, K., Dustdar, S. (eds.) BPM 2011. LNBIP, vol. 99, pp. 169–194. Springer, Heidelberg (2012). https://doi.org/10.1007/978-3-642-28108-2_19
11. Leemans, Sander J. J.., Fahland, Dirk, van der Aalst, Wil M. P..: Discovering block-structured process models from event logs containing infrequent behaviour. In: Lohmann, Niels, Song, Minseok, Wohed, Petia (eds.) BPM 2013. LNBIP, vol. 171, pp. 66–78. Springer, Cham (2014). https://doi.org/10.1007/978-3-319-06257-0_6
12. OMG. Business Process Model and Notation (BPMN) - Version 2.0, Beta 1 (2009)
13. Peterson, J.L.: Petri nets. ACM Comput. Surv. (CSUR) **9**(3), 223–252 (1977)
14. Rojas, E., et al.: PALIA-ER: bringing question-driven process mining closer to the emergency room. In: 15th International Conference on Business Process Management (BPM 2017) (2017)
15. Russell, N., ter Hofstede, A.H.M., van der Aalst, W.M.P., Mulyar, N.: Workflow control-flow patterns: a revised view. BPM Center Report BPM-06-22, BPMcenter.org (2006)
16. Stotts, P.D., Pugh, W.: Parallel finite automata for modeling concurrent software systems. J. Syst. Softw. **27**(1), 27–43 (1994)
17. van der Aalst, W.M.P.: Process Mining, 2nd edn. Springer, Heidelberg (2016)
18. van der Aalst, W.M.P., ter Hofstede, A.H.M., Kiepuszewski, B., Barros, A.P.: Workflow patterns. Distrib. Parallel Databases **14**(1), 5–51 (2003)
19. van der Aalst, W.M.P., Weijters, T.A.J.M.M., de Medeiros, A.K.A.: Process mining with the heuristics miner-algorithm. BETA Working Paper Series, WP 166 (2006)
20. Vázquez-Barreiros, B., Mucientes, M., Lama, M.: Enhancing discovered processes with duplicate tasks. Inf. Sci. **373**, 369–387 (2016)

Enhancing Clinical Insights: Knowledge-Intensive and Context-Sensitive Process Instance Visualization in Health Care

Joscha Grüger[1,2]([✉]) and Ralph Bergmann[1,2]

[1] Business Information Systems II, University of Trier, Trier, Germany
grueger@uni-trier.de
[2] SDS Branch Trier, German Research Center for Artificial Intelligence (DFKI),
Trier, Germany

Abstract. The paper focuses on enhancing the understanding of treatment processes, particularly in healthcare, through process visualization. Healthcare processes are complex and data-rich due to Electronic Health Records (EHRs). Existing visualization approaches often overlook the crucial data perspective alongside the control-flow perspective. To address this, the paper introduces the Knowledge-Intensive and Context-sensitive Process Instance Visualization approach, incorporating external sources like taxonomies and ontologies. A descriptive language enables flexible visualizations, and the enriched XES format supports tailored representations. Thus, the paper emphasizes the importance of context-sensitive visualizations for efficient interpretation by healthcare professionals. By addressing the challenges in healthcare process mining, the approach seeks to improve patient care through comprehensive and meaningful process visualization.

Keywords: Process Visualization · Process Mining for Healthcare · Information Visualization

1 Introduction

The understanding of treatment processes quickly and effectively is crucial [1]. To overcome the challenge of understanding processes, the subfield of Information Visualization known as Process Visualization is employed [2]. Its focus primarily lies in visualizing process models and generating specific insights through visual representations, such as for process revision or for monitoring multiple process instances simultaneously. Nevertheless, healthcare processes pose distinct challenges owing to their elevated complexity, dynamic nature, multidisciplinary aspects, and the vast volume of data in Electronic Health Records (EHRs) [3].

Nevertheless, for individual patients, healthcare providers need a concise process instance overview within a limited timeframe. They need to quickly grasp

© The Author(s), under exclusive license to Springer Nature Switzerland AG 2024
J. De Smedt and P. Soffer (Eds.): ICPM 2023 Workshops, LNBIP 503, pp. 259–270, 2024.
https://doi.org/10.1007/978-3-031-56107-8_20

the essential details relevant to a particular patient's case without getting overwhelmed by an excessive amount of data [4]. Additionally, the interest in understanding treatment processes goes beyond the control-flow perspective. The data perspective provides many crucial insights for comprehending and tracing treatment cases effectively. It contains vital information such as patient demographics, lab results, medication history, and other relevant clinical data, which are essential for a comprehensive understanding of the patient's journey. Furthermore, the importance of different aspects of the data can vary depending on the specific context. For example, in emergency situations, certain critical information may take precedence over other details. As a result, not every visualization is universally suitable for every healthcare context. Tailoring visualizations to the specific needs of each scenario becomes imperative to ensure that healthcare professionals can efficiently interpret and act upon the information presented.

To address this need, approaches for visualizing process instances with specific views were developed [5]. Yet, most existing approaches fail to consider the data perspective, combined with the control flow perspective [2,5]. Furthermore, incorporating the data perspective presents the challenge of interpreting and evaluating the data. For instance, in the case of laboratory values, it is important to highlight any exceedance or deficiency of threshold values, provide potential explanations, and minimize the path to further relevant information [4]. While the necessary knowledge, such as taxonomies, ontologies, and classifications, partially exists, current systems do not effectively leverage it.

In this paper, we present an approach called Knowledge-Intensive and Context-sensitive Process Instance Visualization. The approach enables context-sensitive visualization of treatment processes by incorporating external information sources, such as taxonomies, ontologies or knowledge provided by web services, e.g., information extraction, external databases or analysis of events or traces. We have developed a descriptive language for process instance visualization, allowing for flexible specification of the visualization. Additionally, we enrich the eXtensible Event Stream (XES) format with context-sensitive visualization information, empowering various visualization techniques to create flexible and tailored visual representations. By doing so, we address challenge *C9 Complement HISs* from the Process mining for healthcare challenges [6].

The remainder of the paper is organized as follows. Section 2 provides related works and existing approaches. In Sect. 3 we introduce our approach and describe in Sect. 4 the implementation. In Sect. 5 we evaluate the approach in a clinical setting. Following the evaluation, we discuss the results, provide a summary, and outline potential future research directions.

2   Related Work

Process visualization, also known as event sequence visualization [7] is an emerging research area, with process views being a specific subfield of interest [5]. Previous works have predominantly concentrated on public and internal (private) process views [8,9].

Within the Proviado project [10], a process visualization and process monitoring component was developed to enable configurable and personalized visualization of business processes. One key aspect of the project is the personalized visualization of processes for specific target audiences. To achieve this, the authors devised an approach for parameterizable views to visualize process models and process instances [2,5,11]. At the core of this approach lies the ability to adapt and configure the complexity within the views through reduction and aggregation, tailored to specific usage contexts. The authors primarily focused on the control flow perspective.

On the other hand, the field of patient data visualization addresses the increasing need for representations of the growing volume of digital data per patient in a manner that is both rapid and easily comprehensible. Rind et al. [12] provide an extensive survey of information visualization systems utilized for visualizing, exploring, and querying Electronic Health Records (EHRs). These approaches, pertaining to EHRs, can be broadly classified into two categories: those that concentrate on an individual patient record and those that focus on a collection of patient records. Approaches in the first category center on delivering comprehensive information concerning an individual patient, encompassing factors such as patient history, notable events, prescribed medications, and treatment protocols. Conversely, the second category endeavors to present a holistic overview derived from multiple patients.

In the scientific study [13], a novel visualization method employing vertical lines or boxes is proposed for representing the temporal aspect of data in an Electronic Health Record (EHR) system. By incorporating this visual element, the temporal dimension of the data is effectively conveyed, enabling healthcare professionals to discern and analyze the timing of various events or data points within the EHR. Another notable example in the realm of medical data visualization is Patient History in Pocket (PHiP) as introduced by Belden et al. in their work [14]. In PHiP, horizontal lines are employed as a medication timeline visualization to depict the duration and timing of medication.

In contrast to the existing works, this paper presents an approach that focuses on the visualization of process instances, with a particular emphasis on the medical domain. The primary objective is to achieve flexible visualization that incorporates all perspectives, integrates with other knowledge sources, and adapts to specific contextual requirements. The proposed approach is demonstrated through examples within the medical domain.

3   Context-Sensitive Knowledge-Intensive Process Instance Visualization

The fundamental idea of the framework is based on the assumption that there are numerous ways to visualize a trace for a specific context. Each type of visualization highlights important information differently, utilizing distinct markers to indicate event aggregation or the removal of events for complexity reduction. Therefore, the approach of knowledge-intensive and context-sensitive process instance visualization aims to generate XES files enriched with visualization information specific to contexts. XES is the prevailing standard event log model, relying on XML and finds extensive application in both industrial and academic domains [15,16]. These extended XES files can then be read by various visualization engines. To achieve this, the XES file is extended with visualization attributes through a rule-based and context-sensitive knowledge-intensive process instance visualization engine.

3.1   Visualization-Engine

The framework facilitates configuring visualizations for various contexts, each represented by unique identifiers and a set of visualization rules. Thus, a context can be seen as a mapping to a collection of visualization rules. Medical domain examples of contexts include, e.g., the *tumor board, follow-up* or *operating room*.

Definition 1 (Universes). *We define the following universes to be used in this paper:*

- *$\mathcal{C}$ is the universe of all possible context identifiers.*
- *$\mathcal{U}$ is the universe of all values*
- *$\mathcal{R}$ is the universe of all rules*
- *$\mathcal{A}$ is the universe of all actions*

Definition 2 (Context). *A context is a distinct mapping context : $\mathcal{C} \to \mathcal{R}^*$ that associates a context identifier with a set of rules.*

The visualization rules (rules) describe conditions and actions. Conditions are evaluated on the given trace; if met, associated actions (like highlighting an attribute) are executed sequentially.

Definition 3 (Rules). *Let $r \in \mathcal{R}$ be a rule. Then, r is a tuple consisting of a condition and an ordered list of actions. Thus, for a given set of variables V, we denote all possible rules by $\mathcal{R}_V = EXPR(V) \times \mathcal{A}^*$, where $EXPR(V)$ represents the set of expressions involving the variables in V, and $\mathcal{A}^*$ denotes the set of all possible lists of actions.*

The conditions are logical statements that can be evaluated as *True* or *False*. They involve querying and comparing properties of the scope on which they are executed, utilizing operations such as *AND, OR, GREATER THAN*, and others.

Definition 4 (Condition). *Let V be a set of variables. We define $EXPR(V)$ as the universe of all boolean expressions over the variables in V. A condition is a boolean formula $c \in EXPR(V)$ that can be evaluated to either true or false. Conditions can be formally described using a Context-Free Grammar (CFG) as:*

```
<condition>  ::= <logical-expr>
<logical-expr> ::= '(' <condition> ' AND ' <condition> ')'
     | '(' <condition> ' OR ' <condition> ')'
     | 'NOT ' <condition>
```

```
           |  <comp-expr>
<comp-expr>  ::=  '('  <variable>  <comp-op>  <value>  ')'
<variable>   ::=  <variable-name>
<comp-op>    ::=  '>'|  '>='|  '<'|  '=='|  '<='|  '!='
<value>      ::=  <constant>|  <variable>
```

Definition 5 (Condition evaluation). *Let U be the universe of all variable values and σ a given trace. Let V be a set of variables. Let U_V be a set of variable value assignments for all $v \in V$. Let $c \in EXPR(V)$ be a condition. The truth of a condition is evaluated by a function:*

$$eval : EXPR(V) \times U_V^* \rightarrow \{true, false\}$$

In the context of traces and attributes, variables are assessed based on attributes and their corresponding attribute values. These attributes can either be event attributes or trace attributes.

Visualization operations (operations) can relate to control flow, data perspective, or edges. However, not every operation is defined for every scope. The operations are derived from requirements for context-aware visualization, which were collected through semi-structured interviews with two doctors. The interviews focused on medical decision-making scenarios and providing an overview of the patients, as well as direct access to the information required in the given situation. The situations were discussed in detail, and examples were considered to figure out how to procedurally represent the vast amount of patient data and quickly grasp the necessary information in the given contexts. Every mentioned idea was integrated into the approach. Three subdomains were identified: complexity reduction, highlighting, and enrichment.

Complexity reduction operations aim to distill relevant information within a context by eliminating irrelevant data, abstracting to context-appropriate levels, and summarizing details. Highlighting operations visually emphasizes information, including vital values or domain-specific associations using symbols/colors. Apart from highlighting and complexity reduction, accessing external or analyzed data for process instances was suggested to enhance trace examination. These operations fall under the category enrichment. Examples include incorporating ontologies and taxonomies, for instance, to provide explanations for encoded information, or linking to the current surgical operation plan.

Definition 6 (Operations). *Let O be the set of all operations with $O = HO \cup CO \cup EO$, while*

– *Let HO denote the set of all highlighting operations, defined as*

$$HO = \{highlight, iconization, importance, colorization\}$$

– *Let CO denote the set of all complexity reducing operations, defined as*

$$CO = \{reduction, aggregation, abstraction\}$$

– *Let EO denote the set of all enriching operations, defined as*

$$EO = \{tooltip, information\}$$

In concluding the framework, actions include execution context and necessary parameters. Regarding traces, operations can target three scopes: control flow (events), data (event and trace attributes), and edges (event edges). Parameters encompass values like icons, colors, criticality levels, and additional information used during execution.

Definition 7 (Action). *Let O be the set of all possible operations, let $S = \{controllflow, data, edges\}$ be the set of scopes, $\mathcal{U}$ the universe of values and I the set of identifiers, while I can be an attribute identifier, an event identifier or the identifier of an edge, formalized as a tuple of event identifiers. If $s \in S$, then I_s describes all identifiers for scope s. Then the set of all possible actions is defined as $\mathcal{A} = O \times I_s^* \times \mathcal{U}^*$.*

Not every identified operation can be mapped to control flow, data perspective, and edges (see Table 1). Complexity reductions can only be applied at the control flow and data levels, while the edge level is indirectly addressed through control flow rules (when hiding events, the edges are also removed). The same applies to the application of abstraction to events algorithms for computing new information for the control flow perspective, as no case was identified in the interviews that directly pertains to the control flow perspective.

Table 1. Operations defined for the different scopes in the categorized *Complexity Reduction (CO)*, *Highlighting (HO)* and *Enrichment (EO)*

	Operations	Scopes		
		Control flow	Data	Edge
CO	**Reduction:** hiding events or attributes	x	x	–
	Aggregation: Aggregating events to new event or attributes to new attribute	x	x	–
	Abstraction: Replace attribute by more abstract information	–	x	–
HO	**Highlight:** highlighting events, attributes, or edges	x	x	x
	Status: marking events, attributes or edges to have a specific status, i.e. critical	x	x	x
	Iconization: Add icon to event or replacing attribute by icon	x	x	x
	Colorization: giving specific events, attributes or edges a defined color	x	x	x
EO	**Tooltip:** adding information for mouse over	x	x	x
	Information: adding additional information (visualization dependent)	x	x	x

3.2   Visualization XES-Extension

The objective of this approach is twofold: enabling knowledge-intensive and context-sensitive visualization and providing a basis for future visualization

```
1   <trace> ...
2     <event>
3       <string key="visualization:color" value="#F3FD2d"/>
4       <string key="concept:name" value="radio_MRI">
5         <string key="visualization:abstract" value="MRI"/>
6       </string>
7       <string key="ICD10-CM" value="C43.30">
8         <string key="visualization:information"
9         value="Malignant melanoma of unspecified part of face"/>
10      </string>
11      <string key="org:resource" value="Hospital Trier">
12        <boolean key="visualization:hide" value="true"/>
13      </string>
14      ...
```

Listing 1. Example of visualization elements in XES, coloring the event, abstracting the attribute *radio_MRI* to *MRI*, adding the textual descritpion to the ICD-code and hiding the resource.

developments that can leverage the defined rule set and engine. Hence, results from the Visualization Engine and applied trace rules must be converted into an adaptable format for other visualization methods.

A widely adopted format for event logs is XES. Numerous tools and applications support the XES format, such as ProM, RapidMiner, and Apromore. It standardizes event data representation and supports seamless extensions. Hence, the choice was to extend the current XES format with visualization properties, offering targeted details to the visualization approach, including attributes to hide, highlight, and additional relevant contextual data. The visualization engine records these details into an XES file for a given context and trace, while the visualization approach handles their implementation in its distinct format. The decision to integrate directly into XES, as opposed to outsourcing visualization information, was made because XES does not prescribe unique identifiers for events. Therefore, an extension would be necessary in either case to establish a relationship between outsourced visualization properties and the events.

To facilitate this, a new namespace, namely "visualization" is introduced. Within this namespace, the visualization information is encoded. Specifically, for events and attributes, they are encoded in the respective underlying hierarchical levels. In the case of events, they are encoded as event attributes, while for attributes, they are nested attributes (refer to Listing 1). As for edges, they are encoded as trace attributes in the XES format.

4   Implementation

For evaluation, the approach was implemented. On one hand, the visualization engine was developed, and on the other hand, a visualization approach was designed and implemented. Both components form the basis for the evaluation.

4.1 Visualization-Engine

The visualization engine is implemented in Python and is structured into three components (see Fig. 1). The rule engine is responsible for evaluating the predefined rules. The action engine interprets and executes the actions and operations specified in the configuration, while seamlessly integrating external resources such as taxonomies and web services. The integration of web services (e.g., for getting knowledge from external database, information extraction or generation) and taxonomies (e.g., ICD-10-CM) occurs through actions, where the corresponding taxonomy or web service can be provided as a value. Web services are registered in the knowledge registry and can be invoked with a given value (e.g., value of the attribute for which the rule is being executed). To achieve interoperability and conform to the XES standard, the XES engine is employed to transform and implement the operations in the XES format.

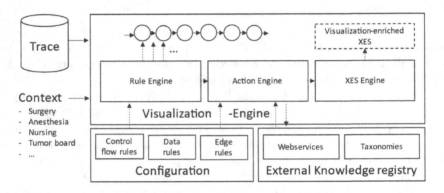

Fig. 1. Visualization Engine's architecture, the Inputs and Knowledge Registry, offering access to external knowledge as ICD-10-CM, SNOMED CT, calculations.

The rule engine evaluates the rules defined in the rule set for a given trace and context. Following the order specified in the configuration, each rule is executed on the trace either as a whole or event by event. The conditions in the rules refer to variables, which can be trace or event attributes. To ensure successful evaluation of the conditions, logical expressions are automatically added, verifying in each conjunction if the used variable is defined in the given context. If not, the conjunction is set to the logical value "False". When the conditions are satisfied by a trace or event, the action engine evaluates the configured actions and operations. This process utilizes the Python library "fpyparsing" (see Listing 2). The operation registry identifies the specific operation to be executed, including whether it is composed of other operations.

4.2 Visualization

The visualization is realized as a timeline visualization [7]. It is based on the concept of representing events as nodes, enabling the integration of extensive

```
    ...
"controlflow":[
    {"condition":"(LDH > 248) OR (S100B_martial == 'Liquor' AND
    ((sex == 'm' AND  S100B > 3.4) OR (sex == 'f' AND S100B
    > 2.5))) OR S100B_martial == 'Serum' AND S100B > 0.1),
    "operation":"highlight current event critical" } ... ] ...
```

Listing 2. Example medical domain rule: evaluates TRUE if defined tumor markers exceed reference values, highlighting the event as critical.

information while facilitating the representation of easily comprehensible knowledge on multiple levels. To implement this, the framework *Graphly D3*[1] was employed, leveraging the computational capabilities of the *d3.js*[2] force simulation and data administration.

The visualization approach introduces innovative functionalities by presenting events in a hexagonal structure, divided into several areas. The areas include: (1) the utilization of color highlighting, such as uniformly coloring events of a specific type, (2) the display of event names, and (3) the aggregation of attributes, which can be visually emphasized, replaced by an icon, or enriched with additional information through tooltips (see Fig. 2).

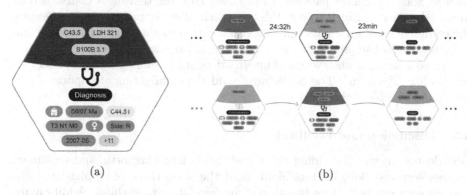

(a)   (b)

Fig. 2. (a) Visualizing a single *Diagnosis* event with data perspective. Signifying significance of high LDH and S100B tumor markers, primary diagnosis C43.5. Attributes are highlighted and iconized. *TNM* classification *T3 N1 M0* aggregated from three attributes. (b) Example of the visualization of a part of a trace

5   Evaluation

The knowledge-intensive process visualization was evaluated in the Dermatological Oncology domain with the participation of two medical doctors. The evaluation was divided into two phases: context definition and generation of rules for those scenarios, followed by a qualitative analysis of the outcomes.

---

[1] https://docs.graphly.dev/.
[2] https://d3js.org/.

5.1   Context and Rules Definition

During the initial phase, two contextual scenarios, *Tumor Conference* and *Follow-up Examination*, were chosen. For each context, objectives were identified along with the key data points necessary to achieve them. Context-specific and generic rules were established, leveraging domain knowledge encompassing ICD10-CM[3], OPS codes[4], residual tumor classifications, general performance status, and a TNM classification[5] web service, explaining the components of the code. The visualization highlighted important data and data exceeding thresholds and emphasizes missing critical information, such as home medication and allergies. Similar activities were color-coded consistently, and attributes like gender and tumor location were depicted using symbols. Tooltips provided additional insights into treatment events and attributes.

5.2   Individual Assessment by Medical Practitioners

In the evaluation phase, the visualization of real patients was presented to each doctor individually. Their task was to assess its usefulness qualitatively, comparing it to their existing HIS. The doctors emphasized the value of procedural representation, particularly for cases deviating from standard treatment paths, such as Stage IV cancer patients. In the used HIS, the treatment course is documented in text form; however, this approach offers improved clarity. Despite the comprehensive information in the visualization, the doctors felt that certain granular details like precise procedure codes and titles were less important. They suggested a stronger abstraction of information, such as mapping to broader categories like "Excision". The physicians found the highlighting of important and missing attributes highly beneficial.

5.3   Discussion and Feedback

One doctor suggested dividing the visualization into diagnostic and treatment process sections. Both doctors highlighted the importance of emphasizing disease progression indicators like tumor markers and stage shifts. Additionally, they noted the absence of a summary of the patient's current medical status. Furthermore, it was suggested to establish direct links from the events to the documents within the HIS, taxonomies or guidelines. Moreover, it was emphasized that the visualization should be continuously adapted to meet evolving needs and current developments, which could vary significantly based on the specific medical specialty.

The evaluation underscored the effectiveness of the visualization in delivering contextual insights. Feedback from the medical practitioners illuminated the need for a balance between comprehensive data representation and meaningful abstraction, especially in the context of non-standard cases. The insights

---

[3] International Classification of Diseases, 10th Revision, Clinical Modification.

[4] Operation and Procedure Classification System.

[5] Tumor, Node, Metastasis Classification System.

provided valuable guidance for further refining the tool to better meet clinical needs. Subsequent iterations will incorporate these recommendations to create an improved and more user-friendly solution.

6   Conclusion

In conclusion, the knowledge-intensive context-sensitive process instance visualization approach presented in this paper offers a valuable method for visualizing traces from multiple perspectives, enriched with pertinent knowledge tailored to specific contexts. Our research has showcased the utilization of contextual information and knowledge within the procedural perspective, specifically in the evaluation use case of the medical domain. This approach holds promise for enhancing information capture, comprehending treatment status, and the overall data. Integrating contextual information and knowledge into a procedural perspective on patients is a valuable way to assist in clinical practice.

By bringing procedural views, augmented with relevant data, into information systems, such as hospital information systems, we take a significant step towards enhancing the decision-making process in complex domains. Another advantage of the approach lies in its adaptability and the capability to apply visualization annotations across various alternative visualization methodologies. The approach's limitations involve the complex rule definition, demanding domain and IT expertise, as well as the inability to generate summaries or monitor the progress of specific variables.

The field's future research holds promise. One avenue is automatic configuration via usage tracking and documentation, streamlining implementation. Additionally, integrating taxonomies and ontologies into constraints can unveil novel applications and opportunities. Moreover, incorporating a patient's current status summary, tracking individual value progression, and integrating directly with FHIR (Fast Healthcare Interoperability Resources) would be valuable. Additionally, exploring the visualization of process models and guideline deviations can deepen process understanding, open up new fields of application, and incorporate results of various analysis methods. Furthermore, extending the evaluation to a larger number of participants and investigating its application in other domains will provide more comprehensive insights into its effectiveness and adaptability.

In conclusion, the knowledge-intensive context-sensitive process instance visualization approach shows great promise as a powerful tool for understanding and leveraging data within specific contexts. By addressing the current limitations and pursuing further research, we can unlock its full potential and foster its integration into various information systems, thus empowering professionals to make more informed decisions in their respective domains.

References

1. Aigner, W., Miksch, S.: CareVis: integrated visualization of computerized protocols and temporal patient data. Artif. Intell. Med. **37**(3), 203–218 (2006)
2. Bobrik, R., Bauer, T.: Towards configurable process visualizations with proviado. In: 16th IEEE International Workshops on Enabling Technologies: Infrastructure for Collaborative Enterprises (WETICE 2007), pp. 367–369 (2007)
3. Rebuge, Á., Ferreira, D.R.: Business process analysis in healthcare environments: a methodology based on process mining. Manage. Eng. Process-Aware Inf. Syst. (2012)
4. West, V.L., Borland, D., Hammond, W.E.: Innovative information visualization of electronic health record data: a systematic review. J. Am. Med. Inform. Assoc. **22**(2), 330–339 (2015)
5. Bobrik, R., Reichert, M., Bauer, T.: View-based process visualization. In: Alonso, G., Dadam, P., Rosemann, M. (eds.) BPM 2007. LNCS, vol. 4714, pp. 88–95. Springer, Heidelberg (2007). https://doi.org/10.1007/978-3-540-75183-0_7
6. Munoz-Gama, J., et al.: Process mining for healthcare: characteristics and challenges. J. Biomed. Inform. **127**, 103994 (2022)
7. Yeshchenko, A., Mendling, J.: A survey of approaches for event sequence analysis and visualization. Inf. Syst. 102283 (2023)
8. Chiu, D.K.W., Cheung, S.C., Till, S., Karlapalem, K., Li, Q., Kafeza, E.: Workflow view driven cross-organizational interoperability in a web service environment. Inf. Technol. Manage. **5**(3), 221–250 (2004)
9. Chebbi, I., Dustdar, S., Tata, S.: The view-based approach to dynamic inter-organizational workflow cooperation. Data Knowl. Eng. **56**(2), 139–173 (2006)
10. Bobrik, R., Reichert, M., Bauer, T.: Requirements for the visualization of system-spanning business processes. In: 16th International Workshop on Database and Expert Systems Applications (DEXA 2005), pp. 948–954. IEEE (2005)
11. Bassil, S., Reichert, M., Bobrik, R., Bauer, T.: Access control for monitoring system-spanning business processes. Microsystem technologies-micro-and nanosystems-information storage and processing systems (2007)
12. Rind, A., et al.: Interactive information visualization to explore and query electronic health records. Found. Trends Hum.-Comput. Interact. **5**(3), 207–298 (2013)
13. Zhang, Z., et al.: A visual analytics framework for emergency room clinical encounters. In: IEEE Workshop on Visual Analytics in Health Care (2012)
14. Belden, J.L., et al.: Designing a medication timeline for patients and physicians. J. Am. Med. Inform. Assoc.: JAMIA **26**(2), 95 (2019)
15. Günther, C.W., Verbeek, E.: XEX standard definition - version 2.0 (2014)
16. van Dongen, B.F., Shabani, S.: Relational XES: data management for process mining. In: CAiSE Forum (2015)

Hypergraphs for Frailty Analysis
Research Paper

Zoe Hancox[1]([⊠]) [iD], Samuel D. Relton[1] [iD], Andrew Clegg[1] [iD],
Philip G. Conaghan[1] [iD], and Dan Schofield[2] [iD]

[1] University of Leeds, Leeds LS2 9JT, UK
{z.l.hancox,s.d.relton}@leeds.ac.uk
[2] NHS England, Quarry House, Leeds LS2 7UE, UK

Abstract. Frailty and multimorbidity becomes more prevalent as the
population continues to age. We employ directed hypergraphs to represent the complex interactions among multiple health conditions and
capture the inter-dependencies within multimorbidity sets. We introduce
the inclusion of 'Mortality' nodes into directed hypergraphs. Through
the analysis of ResearchOne data, we aim to identify the most prevalent combinations of frailty conditions alongside their co-occurrence with
mortality, providing valuable knowledge for healthcare professionals to
improve patient care and develop targeted interventions. We demonstrate
that hypergraphs enable us to determine the probability of acquiring
another electronic frailty index (eFI) condition, understand condition
connectivity and sequentiality, and identify the most influential hyperarcs. The findings from this study suggest that hypergraphs enable us
to retain progression information compared to holistic views, facilitating
the implementation of more effective healthcare strategies.

Keywords: Frailty · Multimorbidity · Process Mining · Hypergraphs

1 Introduction

As the population ages, multimorbidity (the coexistence of two or more long-term
conditions in an individual) increases, negatively impacting people's health [10].
Frailty is a condition closely related to multimorbidity that is characterised by
loss of biological reserves, failure of physiological mechanisms and resulting vul-
nerability to a range of adverse outcomes [5]. The presence of multimorbidity can
potentially exacerbate frailty, leading to increased risk of disability and extended
hospital stays [9]. In 2015, 54% of people over 65 years old had multimorbidity,
projected to rise to 67.8% by 2035 [10]. About 12% of individuals aged over 50
experience frailty, while 24% have an eFI condition [13]. Some population-based
clinical pathways have been established to provide standard treatment routes for
frailty patients[1]. However, healthcare cannot always follow a uniform approach

---

[1] https://www.england.nhs.uk/rightcare/wp-content/uploads/sites/40/2019/07/
frailty-toolkit-june-2019-v1.pdf.

J. De Smedt and P. Soffer (Eds.): ICPM 2023 Workshops, LNBIP 503, pp. 271–282, 2024.
https://doi.org/10.1007/978-3-031-56107-8_21

due to the individual needs and preferences of individuals, and their responses to treatment. Categorising patients as having frailty offers a practical concept for managing older people, moving away from inappropriate care decisions based solely on chronological age. By shifting the emphasis from specific organ diagnoses, frailty encourages a more holistic understanding of the patient and their unique circumstances rather than one-size-fits-all approaches. Early detection of frailty, understanding health trajectories and proper planning of care is crucial to enhance quality of life and for improved resource utilisation.

Frailty is complicated and has many underlying causes [5]. More research is required to identify risk factors and early indicators linked to various frailty trajectories. To distinguish between different frailty sub-types that require different management strategies, we must better understand the heterogeneity of frailty trajectories and the effect factors have on individuals.

The eFI is an extensively validated measure of frailty derived from routinely available healthcare data [4]. The eFI calculates an index from 36 health condition groupings, which is constructed using 2,133 electronic health record (EHR) Read codes, providing a standardised measure of frailty through condition accumulation [4]. Healthcare providers can use the eFI score to optimise treatment plans, care pathways, and resources allocations. To analyse frailty trajectories and common pathways we use the eFI to assess the prevalence of frailty condition sets. Socioeconomic status is gauged by Index of Multiple Deprivation (IMD) scores, this is vital as lower status correlates with poorer health and multimorbidity [3]. Frailty and multimorbidity are more common among females and older patients compared to males and younger patients [3,8]. We use process mining to find the prevalence of pairwise conditions. We build directed hypergraphs with demographic groups to observe the affect of age, gender and IMD on multimorbidity sets.

The contributions from this paper can be summarised as follows:

1) We apply a novel hypergraph technique to augment traditional Directly Follows Graphs (DFGs) with sequential information.
2) We stratify patients to analyse directed hypergraphs with diverse demographic sets, observing the effects of age, sex, and IMD on frailty patterns.

2   Process Mining Background

Process mining is an analytical approach used to map time-stamped events to graphs. In healthcare, process mining plays a crucial role in analysing process data to uncover patterns and insights that can be harnessed for predictive analytics [12]. In the healthcare context, the analysis of historical process data can be used to reveal predictable patterns that can be utilised to identify patients at risk of adverse events, anticipate resource requirements, and enable proactive interventions for preventing complications and optimising care delivery [7].

DFGs can be used for the visualisation and analysis of event sequencing. DFGs are directed graphs that capture the relationships between events and help in visualising the flow of activities in a process. These visual representations can

aid in identifying bottlenecks or inefficiencies in healthcare processes, ultimately
leading to better patient care and resource management. In this paper, we use
DFGs to identify common eFI pathways and compare them to hypergraphs.

3   Hypergraphs Background

A hypergraph is defined as $\mathcal{H}(V, E)$, where V represents the set of vertices
and E the set of hyperedges. In this report we use directed B-Hypergraphs.
B-Hypergraphs have hyperarcs (directional edges) with ≥ 1 tail node and a single head node each, where the tail nodes are the node(s) from which the hyperarc
begins and the head node(s) are where the hyperarc terminates.

Hypergraphs are advantageous over standard graphs for healthcare applications due to their ability to represent complex relationships between two or
more entities [1], for example, that Hypertension (HTN) followed by Myocardial
Infarction can lead to Heart Failure (HF) [11].

Previous hypergraph work has been carried out on the Charlson Comorbidity and Elixhauser Indexes using the SAIL DataBank [2,15]. Rafferty et al. used
eigenvector centrality within undirected hypergraphs to measure the influence
diseases have on each other [15]. Directionality was introduced within hypergraphs. Various hyperedge calculations were explored to observe sequential transitions between disease sets [2]. Random walk Markov chains were used to find
the probability of transitioning between conditions. PageRank centrality was
used to find node importance based on node inter-connectivity in the directed
hypergraphs by retrieving the eigenvalues from the transition matrices [2].

The Modified Sørensen-Dice coefficient is used to calculate the hyperedge
weights $W(e_i)$ as shown in Eq. 1. We direct readers to our Streamlit applet[2] for
a interactive walkthrough of how to calculate the hyperedge weights, hyperarc
weights, transition probability, and node centrality for directed hypergraphs. We
expand the research to include frailty to gain insights into potential pathways,
because of the interconnected development of eFI conditions over time.

$$W(e_i) = \frac{C(e_i)}{C(e_i) + \sum_{e_j \in L(e_i)} C(e_j) + \sum_{e_k \in U(e_i)} C(e_k)}, \quad (1)$$

where

$$L(e_i) = \{e_j \in E : e_j \subset e_i\}, \quad (2)$$
$$U(e_i) = \{e_k \in E : e_i \subset e_k\} \quad (3)$$

are all proper subsets and supersets of e_i (related to the power and super-
power set, respectively). In particular, $L(e_i)$ contains all disease sets which are
a proper subset of the diseases in e_i (with $C(\emptyset) = 0$ for the empty set). The set
$U(e_i)$ contains all disease sets which already contain all diseases in e_i, and other
diseases. $C(e_i)$ is the raw prevalence count for disease set e_i.

---

[2] https://nhsx-hypergraphical-streamlit-hypergraphs-hklixt.streamlit.app/.

Hyperarc weightings incorporate disease prevalence among children hyper-arcs, their parent hyperedge, and the hyperedge itself. We use Eq. 4 to calculate hyperarc h_i weights.

$$w(h_i) = W(p(h_i)) \frac{C(h_i)}{\sum_{h_j \in \mathcal{K}(h_i)} C(h_j)}, \quad \text{where} \quad \mathcal{K}(h_i) = \{h_j \; : \; p(h_j) = p(h_i)\}$$

(4)

where $\mathcal{K}(h_i)$ are the siblings of hyperarc h_i. And $W(p(h_i))$ is the hyperedge weight of the parent hyperedge of h_i.

We use an adaptation of the work of [6], as shown in the Streamlit applet, to find the probability of there being a transition between diseases. PageRank scores are derived from transition matrix eigenvalues [14].

4   Dataset

We analyse a real-world EHR dataset with 151,565 patients who had joint pain, sourced from routine NHS data via ResearchOne (not publicly available). The de-identified dataset includes timestamped clinical and administrative data for patients registered at participating ResearchOne general practices using Syst-mOne in England, who have not opted-out of data sharing at a patient-level.

The study included patients aged 40 to 75 at the start date (April 1st, 1999) who experienced joint pain between 1st April 1999 and 31st March 2014. Follow-up continued until censorship due to loss to follow-up or the observation period's end. This age range was chosen for its relevance to musculoskeletal diseases.

4.1   Baseline Characteristics

Prior to excluding patients without an eFI condition, the dataset comprised 151,565 patients. 2,133 distinct CTV3 codes were used to establish the 36 frailty conditions based on eFI. Baseline characteristics are detailed in Table 1, while Fig. 1 illustrates the distribution of diseases, highlighting arthritis as the most common eFI condition and Activity Limitation (AL) as the least common.

Patients without mortality recorded have a mean of 2.1 ± 1.26 conditions, while the mortality group showed a higher average of 3.11 ± 1.63 conditions. Suggesting increased frailty and age, raises mortality chance [4].

HTN (61.5%), Ischaemic Heart Disease (IHD) (59.4%), Respiratory Disease (RD) (57.0%), and Thyroid Disease (TD) (55.4%) predominantly appear as start conditions, while the other 11 conditions are commonly end conditions. Fragility Fracture (FF) (84.5%), memory and cognitive problems (81.3%), and Chronic Kidney Disease (CKD) (81.2%) have the highest occurrence as end conditions.

4.2   Inclusion Criteria and Pre-processing

Data is included only for individuals with any of the 36 eFI conditions. 118,323 patients have at least one eFI condition from our code list, encompassing 379

Table 1. Baseline characteristics of the dataset. [a]Electronic frailty index (eFI) scores. IMD quintiles [b] from least (1) to most deprived (5).

		ResearchOne Data	
Patient age range		40–75	
Average age ± SD		55.22 ± 9.29	
Female		60.38%	
Total # of patients		151,565	
Total # of patients meeting inclusion criteria		118,308	
Total deaths in study period		0.81%	
Frailty category[a]	Population (%)	IMD quintile[b] (score)	Population (%)
Fit (0–0.12)	93.86%	1 (≤8.49)	22.10%
Mild (0.13–0.24)	6.10%	2 (8.5–13.79)	21.51%
Moderate (0.25–0.36)	0.04%	3 (13.8–21.35)	20.90%
Severe (>0.36)	0.00%	4 (21.36–34.17)	17.23%
		5 (≥34.18)	18.26%

out of the 2,133 eFI codes and 15 of the 36 conditions. The 15 diseases are: Atrial Fibrillation (AF), Arthritis, AL, CKD, Cerebrovascular Disease (CVD), Diabetes (DM), FF, HF, HTN, IHD, Memory and Cognitive Problems (M&C), Osteoporosis (OP), Peripheral Vascular Disease (PVD), RD, and TD.

IMD was determined at inception. 15 patients (0.01%) did not have an IMD score recorded so we excluded these patients for simplicity. We split IMD scores into quintiles (Table 1). We also split the patients based on sex and three age groups: 40–55, 55–65 and 65+.

5   Methodology

5.1   Process Mining Methodology

Using eFI conditions as events, we employ the PM4PY Python package[3] to construct DFGs, capturing condition prevalence from initial occurrence to last or mortality. A variant is defined as a unique pathway from a start condition to an end condition or mortality. In this study, DFG nodes represent eFI conditions, and edges signify their sequence and frequencies (edge labels). The 'Alive' node is excluded from the DFG, but a condition node connected to the finish node implies equivalence to the 'Alive' node.

5.2   Hypergraph Methodology

We introduce 'Mortality' into the B-hypergraphs as an end-state node. Patients with a single condition will be represented as a hyperarc where the tail node

---

[3] https://github.com/pm4py/pm4py-core.

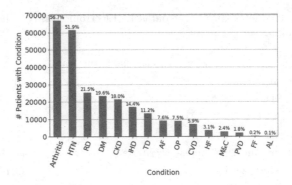

Fig. 1. Count of how many patients have each of the eFI conditions. Where AF = Atrial Fibrillation, AL = Activity Limitation, CKD = Chronic Kidney Disease, CVD = Cerebrovascular Disease, DM = Diabetes, FF = Fragility Fracture, HF = Heart Failure, HTN = hypertension, IHD = Ischaemic Heart Disease, M&C = Memory and Cognitive Problems, OP = Osteoporosis, PVD = Peripheral Vascular Disease, RD = Respiratory Disease, and TD = Thyroid Disease.

of the hyperarc is the condition and the head node will be either 'Mortality' or 'Alive'. We choose to have a single 'Mortality' node and an 'Alive' node to enforce symmetry. Alternatively, we could have x 'Mortality' nodes for the number of conditions present when mortality occurs (e.g., $HTN, CKD \rightarrow M_2$ or $AL \rightarrow M_1$), but this inflates computational expense as the number of nodes increase.

When calculating hyperedge weights, if an end state node is in the current set, its super set should be empty. This ensures that we only consider a final state as 'Alive' if no mortality is recorded during the analysis period. Consequently, 'Mortality' and 'Alive' nodes become dominant successors in PageRank scores, converging to a successor PageRank of zero. To address this, we applied three PageRank corrections: 'loop', 'loop-all', and 'replace'.

The 'loop' correction adds self-loops only to the end-state nodes, removing their end-state status. The 'loop-all' correction adds self-loops to all nodes, equalising node importance across all instead of just end-state nodes, improving centralisation. The 'replace' correction calculates PageRank for each disease, excluding end-state nodes. Then, it incorporates the end-state nodes by summing the non-mortality and mortality PageRank for each disease and end-state node and normalises the combined values as given in Eq. 5.

$$PR_{replace} = \frac{PR_{d,nomort} + PR_{d,mort}}{\sum_d (PR_{d,nomort} + PR_{d,mort})} \tag{5}$$

where $PR_{replace}$ is the replace corrected PageRank, $PR_{d,nomort}$ is the PageRank of disease d for the non-mortality hypergraph and $PR_{d,mort}$ is the PageRank of disease d for the hypergraph which includes mortality.

The 'replace' correction is chosen as it is the only method preventing the successor condition PageRanks from iterating to zero. We plot the predecessor and successor PageRank scores to identify diseases likely to be predecessors or successors based on their ratio. Then, we compare the raw occurrence of eFI conditions as first or last conditions and match them with our hypergraph's predecessors and successors to demonstrate consistency.

Finally, we compare the top 10 pathways of the DFG with the top 10 hyperarc weights for the entire population.

5.3 Statistical Analysis

We perform Chi-square goodness of fit tests to compare proportions across 15 conditions in various demographic groups (sex, IMD, age) independently with the entire population. The null hypothesis assumes that the proportions in all demographic groups are similar to the whole population ($\alpha = 0.05$).

Spearman's rank correlation was performed on all (9,094) hyperarc weights between demographic groups to assess their correlations. In cases where a hyperarc was absent in a stratified group, we assigned a hyperarc weight of 0.

6 Results

The whole population's DFG exhibits dense connectivity among the 15 nodes, with 11,259 variants. Figure 2 shows the top 10 DFG variants in descending order of occurrence: 1) Arthritis, 2) HTN, 3) HTN $\rightarrow$ Arthritis, 4) RD, 5) Arthritis $\rightarrow$ HTN, 6) TD, 7) DM, 8) RD $\rightarrow$ Arthritis, 9) HTN $\rightarrow$ DM, 10) IHD. Figure 3 depicts a visualisation of the top hyperarc weights associated with HTN, encompassing both inbound and outbound connections for the entire population.

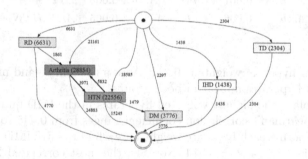

Fig. 2. Top 10 variants visualised using a DFG.

The Chi-Square value was 23.68, and the test statistics ranged from 36.75 to 802.28 with an average of 471.81 $\pm$ 263.18. The Chi-square goodness of fit test leads to null hypothesis rejection, indicating that the different demographic groups showed dissimilar proportions compared to the entire population dataset.

Table 2 displays the top 10 hyperarc weights for the entire population and separately for the male and female populations. The Spearman's rank correlation

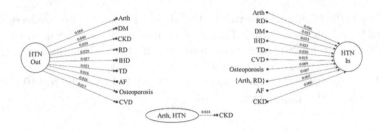

Fig. 3. Visualisation of hyperarc weights surrounding hypertension: top 10 hyperarcs inbound and outbound. Relevant tail nodes which contain more than one disease are represented as collective sets e.g. Arth, RD and Arth, HTN in the figure.

Table 2. Top 10 hyperarc weights in the whole population vs the female and male cohorts. A = Alive, M = Mortality, Arth = Arthritis.

Top	Whole Population		Female Only		Male Only	
	Hyperarc	Weight	Hyperarc	Weight	Hyperarc	Weight
1	$Arth \rightarrow A$	0.171	$Arth \rightarrow A$	0.170	$Arth \rightarrow A$	0.173
2	$RD \rightarrow A$	0.122	$RD \rightarrow A$	0.121	$RD \rightarrow A$	0.125
3	$TD \rightarrow A$	0.118	$TD \rightarrow A$	0.121	$HTN \rightarrow A$	0.121
4	$HTN \rightarrow A$	0.116	$OP \rightarrow A$	0.116	$M\&C \rightarrow A$	0.104
5	$OP \rightarrow A$	0.114	$HTN \rightarrow A$	0.113	$TD \rightarrow A$	0.100
6	$M\&C \rightarrow A$	0.097	$AL \rightarrow A$	0.109	$OP \rightarrow A$	0.090
7	$AL \rightarrow A$	0.076	$M\&C \rightarrow A$	0.094	$DM \rightarrow A$	0.080
8	$DM \rightarrow A$	0.072	$AL \rightarrow M$	0.068	$FF \rightarrow A$	0.080
9	$Arth, HTN \rightarrow A$	0.067	$HTN \rightarrow Arth$	0.065	$IHD \rightarrow A$	0.073
10	$HTN \rightarrow Arth$	0.066	$DM \rightarrow A$	0.065	$Arth, HTN \rightarrow A$	0.070

among all 9,094 hyperarc weights is 0.311. Across the female and male cohorts, 3,527 (38.78%) hyperarcs appear in both groups.

Table 3 displays the highest weighted hyperarcs in the IMD quintile 1 and 5 groups. The Spearman's correlation coefficient ranges from 0.445 to 0.492 when iteratively comparing each hyperarc weight for each of the five IMD groups. The average coefficient is 0.462 ± 0.014. Notably, the most correlated IMD groups (0.492) are IMD 1 and IMD 2, while the least correlated (0.445) are IMD 3 and IMD 4. In all five IMD cohorts, a total of 1,770 hyperarcs (19.46%) are present, and the hyperarc pairs from the IMD quintiles exhibits around 25% similarity.

Table 4 compares the top 10 hyperarcs and their weights for three age groups. The 55−64 and 65+ age groups show the highest correlation with a Spearman's coefficient of 0.729. The 40−54 and 55−64 age groups have a correlation of 0.510, while the 40−54 and 65+ age groups have a coefficient of 0.459. Across all three age groups, 2,560 (28.15%) hyperarcs appear.

Table 3. Top 10 hyperarc weights across IMD quintiles 1 and 5.

Top	Hyperarc IMD 1	Weight	Hyperarc IMD 5	Weight
1	$Arth \rightarrow A$	0.192	$Arth \rightarrow A$	0.143
2	$AL \rightarrow M$	0.191	$RD \rightarrow A$	0.108
3	$TD \rightarrow A$	0.138	$HTN \rightarrow A$	0.096
4	$OP \rightarrow A$	0.138	$TD \rightarrow A$	0.092
5	$RD \rightarrow A$	0.136	$M\&C \rightarrow A$	0.085
6	$HTN \rightarrow A$	0.133	$OP \rightarrow A$	0.069
7	$M\&C \rightarrow A$	0.116	$DM \rightarrow A$	0.067
8	$DM \rightarrow A$	0.083	$Arth, HTN \rightarrow A$	0.062
9	$HTN \rightarrow Arth$	0.070	$HTN \rightarrow Arth$	0.059
10	$IHD \rightarrow A$	0.070	$PVD \rightarrow A$	0.058

Table 4. Top 10 hyperarc weights across the different age groups.

Top	Hyperarc 40–54	Weight	Hyperarc 55–64	Weight	Hyperarc 65+	Weight
1	$Arth \rightarrow A$	0.231	$Arth \rightarrow A$	0.133	$Arth \rightarrow A$	0.112
2	$OP \rightarrow A$	0.186	$M\&C \rightarrow A$	0.105	$M\&C \rightarrow A$	0.090
3	$M\&C \rightarrow A$	0.175	$OP \rightarrow A$	0.099	$OP \rightarrow A$	0.077
4	$RD \rightarrow A$	0.167	$HTN \rightarrow A$	0.090	$HTN \rightarrow A$	0.076
5	$TD \rightarrow A$	0.166	$AL \rightarrow A$	0.089	$HTN \rightarrow Arth$	0.066
6	$HTN \rightarrow A$	0.164	$RD \rightarrow A$	0.076	$Arth, HTN \rightarrow A$	0.065
7	$DM \rightarrow A$	0.106	$Arth, HTN \rightarrow A$	0.073	$AL \rightarrow A$	0.064
8	$IHD \rightarrow A$	0.102	$TD \rightarrow A$	0.069	$RD \rightarrow A$	0.063
9	$AF \rightarrow A$	0.098	$HTN \rightarrow Arth$	0.068	$TD \rightarrow A$	0.055
10	$AL \rightarrow M$	0.093	$AL \rightarrow M$	0.067	$Arth \rightarrow HTN$	0.046

The $AL \rightarrow Mortality$ hyperarc, which only appears in the female and 40−54 age groups, is the sole hyperarc associated with mortality among the top 10 hyperarcs. Irrespective of demographic, the hyperarc $Arthritis \rightarrow Alive$ consistently ranks as the top hyperarc. The following hyperarcs appear in the top 10 hyperarcs in all groups: $RD \rightarrow Alive$, $TD \rightarrow Alive$, $HTN \rightarrow Alive$, $OP \rightarrow Alive$.

We show the successor and predecessor PageRank of the eFI conditions in this dataset in Fig. 4, the conditions to the left of the transitive line are more likely to be predecessors and those to the right are more likely to be successors.

In Fig. 4 we can see that CKD and M&C are more often successor conditions. Whilst, HTN, DM, TD, and IHD are clearer predecessors. The rest of the

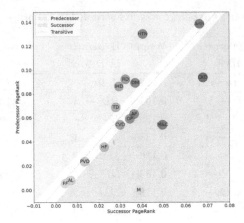

Fig. 4. The whole population's PageRank successor and predecessor scores.

conditions lie close to the transitive line, suggesting that they are no more likely to come before or after another condition.

The highest probability transition is from AL to 'Mortality' (99%). The next six largest probabilities are: OP → FF (34%), HF → AL (32%), HTN → Arthritis (29%), AF → HF (23%), Arthritis → HTN (23%), and HTN → RD (23%).

7   Discussion

The population hypergraph contains 9,094 hyperarcs, while the DFG comprises 11,259 variants. This difference is due to the hypergraph's representation, where individuals with conditions contribute to the tail set instead of being represented as sequentially ordered chains, reducing the number of potential pathways.

When comparing the top 10 pathways generated from the DFG and the hypergraph, we observe a 60% similarity. The matching pathways include: *Arthritis → Alive, HTN → Alive, RD → Alive, Arthritis → HTN → Alive, TD → Alive,* and *DM → Alive.* The process mining model relies solely on disease prevalence, while our hypergraphs model considers the prevalence of neighbouring condition nodes. In Fig. 3, we observe that the top 10 hyperarc weights stemming from HTN are greater in sum than those going in. We can also make observations such as that CVD is more likely to follow HTN, whilst RD is more likely to precede it. Notably, the substantial weight from HTN to Arth contributes significantly to the weight of {Arth, HTN} → CKD.

DFGs focus on pairs of connections, while hypergraphs consider a wider network of related conditions. In the DFG (Fig. 2), we observe additional pathways like *RD → Arthritis → HTN* beyond the top 10 variants. Hyperarcs excel by representing sets of over two conditions in a single entity, while DFGs are confined to pairs. Consequently, DFG edge weights only account for prior conditions, ignoring the complete patient history. However, the B-Hypergraphs we employ do not retain the chronological order of past conditions.

The Chi-square goodness of fit results indicate the importance of incorporating demographics when creating population-based models. The Spearman's correlation is relatively weak between males and females. The correlation between IMD quintiles and age groups is fair, but 55−64 year-olds and 65+ year-olds show a higher correlation. Disaggregating the population into smaller groups allows for more nuanced insights rather than holistic, highlighting the necessity of stratifying groups when evaluating disease trajectories in a population. Less than 40% of hyperarcs match across the different demographic groups. None of the IMD hyperarcs were over 30% similar between quintile groups, suggesting that the disparity between the lowest and highest deprivations is not significantly different from any other deprivation quintile pair.

The PageRank scores obtained from our hypergraph model currently align with the frequency of occurrence of each condition as a starting or ending point. In this regard, conditions such as IHD and HTN are frequently identified as predecessors, while CKD, FFs, and M&C tend to occur following other conditions.

Other research has looked into grouping multimorbidities for example social network analysis identified frailty sub-groups [8], forming 4 clusters based on living environment, age, and recent hospitalisation. Violan et al. employed Hidden Markov Models to observe multimorbidity patterns by identifying health event sequences using dynamic Bayesian networks [16]. Throughout the analysis period, 59% stayed within one of ten multimorbidity clusters. However, instances of movement were mainly towards the mortality or drop-out clusters [16].

To the best of our knowledge this is the first paper using hypergraphs to analyse eFI trajectories. Unlike standard graphs, hypergraphs provide a more intuitive representation of complex relationships between events, making it easier to understand intricate connections and patterns within the data. This leads to more meaningful analyses, offering insights for clinical decision-making, care strategies, and resource allocation, with the ultimate goal of improving patient outcomes and healthcare delivery.

8   Conclusion

Using DFGs and hypergraphs, we analyse the pathways of individuals with eFI. Stratifying the population by age, sex, and IMD reveals a weak positive correlation among most groups, emphasising the importance of stratification to avoid excessive generalisations. A strong correlation exists between AL and mortality, underscoring the need to prioritise AL patients. This can lower mortality by improving their quality of life and health through effective treatment strategies. Our analysis demonstrates that hypergraphs enable us to determine the probability of transitioning between eFI conditions, understand condition connectivity, identify the occurrence sequence of conditions, and identify influential multimorbidity sets. Hypergraphs offer advantages over standard graphs due to retaining progressive information.

Acknowledgements. This work uses data provided by patients and collected by the NHS as part of their care and support. The methodological hypergraphs work was conducted during a PhD internship at NHS England. Zoe Hancox receives support through EPSRC funding (Grant No. EP/S024336/1).

References

1. Berge, C.: Graphs and Hypergraphs. Mathematical Studies. North-Holland Publishing Company (1976)
2. Burke, J., et al.: Representing multimorbid disease progressions using directed hypergraphs. medRxiv (2023). https://doi.org/10.1101/2023.08.31.23294903
3. Cassell, A., et al.: The epidemiology of multimorbidity in primary care: a retrospective cohort study. Br. J. Gen. Pract. **68**(669), e245–e251 (2018)
4. Clegg, A., Bates, C., Young, J., et al.: Development and validation of an electronic frailty index using routine primary care electronic health record data. Age Ageing **45**(3), 353–360 (2016)
5. Clegg, A., Young, J., Iliffe, S., Rikkert, M.O., Rockwood, K.: Frailty in elderly people. Lancet **381**(9868), 752–762 (2013)
6. Ducournau, A., Bretto, A.: Random walks in directed hypergraphs and application to semi-supervised image segmentation. Comput. Vis. Image Underst. **120**, 91–102 (2014)
7. Farid, N.F., De Kamps, M., Johnson, O.A.: Process mining in frail elderly care: a literature review. In: Proceedings of the 12th International Joint Conference on Biomedical Engineering Systems and Technologies-Volume 5: HEALTHINF, vol. 5, pp. 332–339. SciTePress, Science and Technology Publications (2019)
8. Franchini, M., Pieroni, S., Fortunato, L., Knezevic, T., Liebman, M., Molinaro, S.: Integrated information for integrated care in the general practice setting in Italy: using social network analysis to go beyond the diagnosis of frailty in the elderly. Clin. Transl. Med. **5**(1), 1–13 (2016)
9. Han, L., Clegg, A., Doran, T., Fraser, L.: The impact of frailty on healthcare resource use: a longitudinal analysis using the clinical practice research datalink in england. Age Ageing **48**(5), 665–671 (2019)
10. Kingston, A., Robinson, L., Booth, H., Knapp, M., Jagger, C.: for the MODEM project: projections of multi-morbidity in the older population in England to 2035: estimates from the Population Ageing and Care Simulation (PACSim) model. Age Ageing **47**(3), 374–380 (2018). https://doi.org/10.1093/ageing/afx201
11. Kuan, V., Denaxas, S., Patalay, P., et al.: Identifying and visualising multimorbidity and comorbidity patterns in patients in the English national health service: a population-based study. Lancet Digit. Health **5**(1), e16–e27 (2023)
12. Munoz-Gama, J., Martin, N., Fernandez-Llatas, C., Johnson, O.A., Sepúlveda, M., Helm, E., Galvez-Yanjari, V., et al.: Process mining for healthcare: characteristics and challenges. J. Biomed. Inform. **127**, 103994 (2022)
13. O'Caoimh, R., Sezgin, D., O'Donovan, M.R., Molloy, D.W., Clegg, A., et al.: Prevalence of frailty in 62 countries across the world: a systematic review and meta-analysis of population-level studies. Age Ageing **50**(1), 96–104 (2021)
14. Page, L., Brin, S., Motwani, R., Winograd, T.: The PageRank citation ranking: bring order to the web. Technical report, Stanford University (1998)
15. Rafferty, J., Watkins, A., Lyons, J., et al.: Ranking sets of morbidities using hypergraph centrality. J. Biomed. Inform. **122**, 103916 (2021)
16. Violán, C., Fernández-Bertolín, S., Guisado-Clavero, M., et al.: Five-year trajectories of multimorbidity patterns in an elderly Mediterranean population using hidden Markov models. Sci. Rep. **10**(1), 16879 (2020)

Ontology-Based Multi-perspective Process Mining in Laboratories: A Case Study

Elisabeth Mayrhuber[1]([✉]) [iD], Emmanuel Helm[1] [iD], and Lisa Ehrlinger[2] [iD]

[1] Advanced Information Systems and Technology,
University of Applied Sciences Upper Austria, Hagenberg im Mühlkreis, Austria
{elisabeth.mayrhuber,emmanuel.helm}@fh-hagenberg.at

[2] Software Competence Center Hagenberg GmbH, Hagenberg im Mühlkreis, Austria
lisa.ehrlinger@scch.at

Abstract. In real-world process mining scenarios, event logs are extracted from relational databases. The de-facto standard for event log exchange, XES (eXtensible Event Stream), has the limitation that it is restricted to a single case notion and hence viewpoint. Although recent trends towards object-centric process mining propose new standards, they are not yet widely adopted by the tool industry. In this paper, we show how to enable multi-perspective process mining based on the established XES standard by means of a case study from the laboratory domain. Inspired by an existing approach, we use semantic technology to enable the mapping between a domain ontology and a relational database. This allows to dynamically switch the perspective with every new query. In addition, we employ the semantic extension of XES to enrich the resulting event log with semantic information from the domain ontology. Our prototype has been evaluated on real-world data from a German laboratory and therefore specifically addresses the challenge on how to process protected health information.

Keywords: Process Mining · Ontologies · Semantic Header · Laboratory

1 Introduction

Healthcare institutions, in their continuous pursuit of enhanced operational efficiency and quality patient care, face challenges in managing and optimizing complex processes [12]. Process mining has emerged as a promising approach to address these challenges by harnessing event log data to gain valuable insights into process execution and bottlenecks [12]. In this paper, we present an approach on how to seamlessly switch perspectives on different aspects of event logs from the laboratory domain. To achieve this, the approach utilizes semantic web technology.

© The Author(s), under exclusive license to Springer Nature Switzerland AG 2024
J. De Smedt and P. Soffer (Eds.): ICPM 2023 Workshops, LNBIP 503, pp. 283–295, 2024.
https://doi.org/10.1007/978-3-031-56107-8_22

1.1 Problem Statement

Analyzing different perspectives to the data is considered crucial for process mining in healthcare and thus, also in the laboratory domain [12]. However, a problem arises concerning the representation and exchange of event log data because the widely used standard data exchange format in process mining, XES (eXtensible Event Stream) [18], exhibits certain limitations.

The most important limitation pertains to the single-case notion prevalent in XES. At the time the XES is created, the case notion is hard-wired in the data. By adopting a single-case approach, event logs are structured around a singular perspective, typically focusing on individual patient cases or isolated laboratory processes. This rigid perspective limits the ability to analyze processes from different viewpoints, hindering the comprehensive understanding of the interconnections between patients, workplaces, and samples within the laboratory ecosystem. The lack of diversity in perspectives impedes the ability to uncover hidden bottlenecks and inefficiencies that may vary across different contexts. This limitation hinders a laboratory's potential to achieve a granular and detailed analysis of process performance, and the identification of critical areas for optimization.

1.2 Related Work

In a recent paper, Wynn et al. [20] conducted a survey that identifies limitations inherent in the XES standard. The primary shortcoming is its single-case perspective, restricting process analysis to a single viewpoint. This restriction contrasts with contemporary process mining trends, such as object-centric process mining, which underscore the need for a multi-case notion. Additionally, they identified that the flexibility of XES, achieved through numerous extensions, contributes to increased complexity.

Semantic process mining seeks to amalgamate process mining methodologies with semantic web technologies to enable deeper business process analysis. This involves leveraging ontologies to model semantic information, enhancing process mining techniques [11]. Multiple approaches for achieving this synthesis have been explored in the literature, e.g., [3,7–10,13]. These studies illustrate diverse methodologies. One approach involves creating event logs from instantiated ontologies, as demonstrated by Nykänen et al. [13]. Additionally, Calvanese et al. [3] propose an ontology-driven method for extracting event logs from relational data, while Knoll et al. [9] extend this approach to the logistics domain. Research by Leonardi et al. [10] utilize the concept of semantic process mining, enabling analysis across different abstraction levels. Their framework facilitates process discovery on varying levels of an ontology. In a related vein, Kingsley et al. [8] concentrate on semantically annotating event logs and process models, enhancing process analysis through the infusion of semantics and adaptable perspectives. Further Soltani et al. [16] propose an ontology-based representation of OCEL (Object-Centric Event Log) to enable filtering and flattening event logs using SPARQL.

Domain ontologies can also be used to enrich the event logs with information for other use cases. In prior work [7], we discuss the use of open ontologies like SNOMED-CT and the W3C standard SHACL (Shapes Constraint Language)[1] to validate patient pathways.

1.3 Proposed Solution

Following the notion of Dirk Fahland [5], we develop a *semantic header* for event data. A semantic header specifies *"how the stored data maps to the domain data model of the process"* [5]. Hence, our approach is similar to the one of Calvanese et al. [3], in that it utilizes semantic web technologies to guide the extraction of different XES event logs from a relational database. In our case study, we want to highlight two major opportunities that arise from this approach: (1) multi-perspective analysis, and (2) tailored event logs, e.g., anonymization for protected health information (PHI).

Regarding (1), laboratories can shift from the single-case notion to a more interconnected and holistic representation of event log data. This transformation enables a multifaceted view of processes, offering novel angles to analyze and interpret laboratory workflows. Consequently, stakeholders can gain more detailed insights into bottlenecks, resource utilization, and interdependencies across different process dimensions, such as patients, workplaces, or samples.

Moreover, the introduction of semantic web technologies creates another promising opportunity (2), i.e., dynamically creating tailored datasets through SPARQL queries. By employing SPARQL queries, laboratories can filter event log data based on specific criteria, tailoring datasets to meet the unique needs of analysts and decision-makers. It also allows to extract anonymized event logs where the privacy of patients, doctors, and employees is protected. This dynamic event log extraction facilitates fine-grained analysis, allowing researchers to focus on relevant subsets of data, identify patterns, and draw actionable conclusions that can drive targeted process optimization strategies.

2   Method

In this section, we present the pipeline that we implemented. Following, we discuss the components of the pipeline in more detail: the domain ontology in Sect. 2.1, the SPARQL query parsing in Sect. 2.3, the semantic header in Sect. 2.2, data filtering in Sect. 2.4, and the custom XES creation in Sect. 2.5.

To alter the analytical perspective, several steps need to be executed. Figure 1 shows the ideal scenario for executing our pipeline, where a user queries the data and receives a perspective-adjusted XES file as result. Prior to initiation, an ontology must be established and mapped to the relational database (i.e., the *semantic header* is created). Users analyzing the dataset need only understand the ontology structure, alleviating complexities inherent in the actual data

---

[1] https://www.w3.org/TR/shacl.

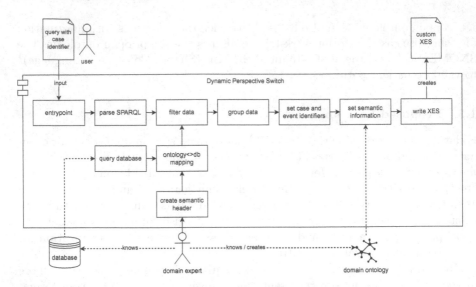

Fig. 1. Module to perform a dynamic perspective switch by utilizing an ontology and a semantic header to create custom event logs based on a SPARQL query.

structure. This process can safeguard sensitive data access, as different privacy-preserving or more comprehensive ontology variants can be selected. This work implements a simplified approach, where the ontology mapping is confined to data properties and the semantic header is embedded within the SQL query. The ideal version involves expanding this to also accommodate object properties. The XES creation module is domain-independent, since only the SQL query, including the ontology mapping, needs to be updated in case of changes of the domain ontology.

2.1 Domain Ontology

The domain ontology has a lightweight nature since it is not instantiated at any point. The purpose of the ontology is to provide a shared domain representation which is readable by humans as well as machines. One major advantage of using the semantic header is that a user does not need to know the underlying database structure but only needs to be familiar with the ontology.

In the semantic web context, an ontology serves as a structured portrayal of knowledge, encompassing concepts, relationships, and properties within a designated domain. Its primary role involves enhancing data integration, interoperability, and automated reasoning [4,17]. Basic ontologies in RDF and RDFS are appropriate for fundamental knowledge representation and modest inferencing [14], enabling class, property, and basic relationship definitions. In contrast, OWL offers a more powerful language with advanced features like constraints, cardinality limits, and sophisticated inference abilities, making it suitable for intricate domains with comprehensive semantics [14]. Therefore in this work, OWL has been used to create the ontology, which serves as a semantic header.

2.2   Semantic Header and Database Mapping

The semantic header describes how concepts of the domain ontology are represented in the database. There are different ways to implement this. In our case study, the domain ontology-database mapping is implemented within the SQL query where the identifier in the ontology serves as an alias in the SQL query. The main advantage of including the mapping in the SQL query is that the prototype stays independent of the underlying database management system.

2.3   SPARQL Query Parsing

SPARQL [19] is a language for querying RDF graphs. Its queries use triple patterns mirroring the subject-predicate-object format of RDF. These patterns pinpoint specific elements within a graph, like an ontology. Analogous to SQL [1], SPARQL provides operators, including filters and sorting, to refine search results. The process of parsing SPARQL queries involved the utilization of RDFlib [15]. This library assesses the query's syntax and generates an AST (Abstract Syntax Tree) that embodies the query's structural composition. Subsequently, this AST is traversed by adopting the visitor pattern [6]. As the traversal progresses, a specialized structure is generated, as depicted in Listing 1.3, for the purpose of extracting pertinent components from the query to facilitate data filtering.

2.4   Data Filtering

The data filtering process in the context of the parsed SPARQL query occurs along two dimensions: column-wise and row-wise. Column filtering hinges on the contents of the SELECT segment of the query. Consequently, only the columns explicitly designated in the SELECT section are utilized for constructing the XES file. Notably, certain columns such as event type, timestamp, and case identifier are omitted from this selection. These particular columns are retained even if they aren't explicitly listed in the SELECT attributes, given their indispensability in the XES creation process. Furthermore, columns that contain exclusively null values across all rows are excluded. If the SELECT block does not specify any attributes (SELECT *), then all columns contribute to the XES file generation.

Turning to row filtering, two factors are taken into consideration: the WHERE conditions and the FILTER conditions. Initially, attention is directed towards the WHERE condition. For each attribute outlined in the WHERE section, rows are sifted through the removal of those containing null values for any of the specified attributes. Subsequently, the previously parsed FILTER conditions are employed to winnow the dataset based on the provided values and operations. Within this prototype's implementation, the subsequent operations are viable for data filtering: $<$, $>$, $<=$, $>=$, $==$, and $!=$. In situations where multiple filters need application, SPARQL permits their combination solely with the OR operator. Worth noting is that the use of RegEx [2] within filters, as supported by SPARQL, is not compatible with this prototype. Similarly, constructs like LIMIT and OFFSET lack support. The viability of this prototype is contingent upon a PREFIX clause, while functions like AVG and COUNT, along with the usage of DISTINCT, are incompatible within the SELECT clause.

2.5   Custom XES Creation

For accurate identification of event, case, and time attributes within the XES, it is imperative to establish a correspondence between the respective columns and then assign appropriate names to them. The event and case identifier are referred to as "concept:name", and the ordering attribute is represented by "time:timestamp".

The remaining columns retain their original names in accordance with the ontology. To ensure the seamless creation of a valid XES file, it is crucial that none of the aforementioned event, case, or time attributes contain null values. Thus, prior to generating the XES file, any rows containing null values in these three attribute types are systematically excluded. Additionally, any columns that solely consist of null values are likewise removed.

A strategy to enhance the semantic context embedded within the XES involves augmenting each bottom-level tag with an accompanying child tag. This supplementary child tag is linked to a semantic model, manifesting as a URI that interacts with the ontology based on the associated concept's name. This approach enriches the representation of XES data by incorporating pertinent semantic context.

3   Results and Evaluation

The prototype has been evaluated on a real-world dataset provided by a German laboratory. The evaluation of these results includes a comparison of different directly-follows graphs (DFGs), as well as the XES files. It has been evaluated with different case identifiers, filter criteria, and the use of both the full and the privacy-preserving ontology. This evaluation gave meaningful insights into the laboratory workflow and showed the feasibility of this prototype. Unfortunately, for reasons of non-disclosure, we can only present the results for a small part of the work, i.e., the domain ontology. We developed a minimal dataset as a proof of concept for the rest of the pipeline.

3.1   Domain Ontology

The implemented ontology consists of two modules as shown in Fig. 2. The core module shows the laboratory domain in a privacy-preserving form. The non-privacy-preserving module extends the core module with personal information about patients, doctors and laboratory employees and builds the full ontology.

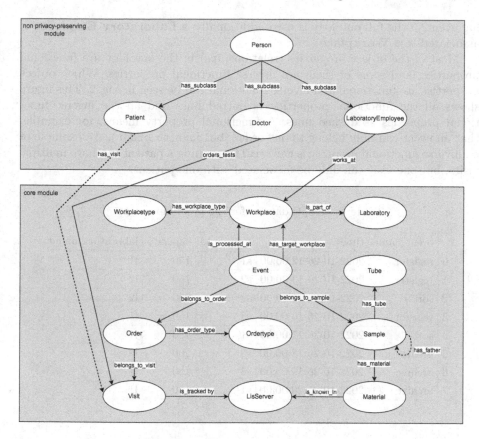

Fig. 2. Concepts and object properties of the ontology, where the dotted lines represent functional properties and the dashed lines represent inverse functional properties.

The ontology contains 15 concepts that will be explained shortly in the following, where each of them contains several data properties, that describe the properties of the concepts and will not be mentioned in the following. The core module consists of eleven concepts, where a **Visit** tracks when a **Patient** visits a **Doctor**, and it is tracked by the **LIS Server**. As long as the non-privacy-preserving module is not included, no personal information of **Patients** nor **Doctors** is included in the **Visit**. One **Visit** can be associated with several **Orders**, each with its own **Ordertype**. The **Events**, which build the foundation to create the XES files, are also associated with an **Order** as well as a **Sample** where a **Sample** can be a sample of a body fluid which is stored in a certain **Tube** and consists of a certain **Material**, for example blood. Additionally, these **Materials** are stored in the **LIS Server**. Each **Event** is processed at a certain **Workplace** with a **Workplacetype** in a **Laboratory**, and an **Event** can also have a target **Workplace**, if the event type, for example, is a sorting event. If the full ontology is used additionally, a **Laboratory Employee** is associated to a **Workplace**.

Most of the object properties (relationships) in the ontology are functional properties, and some of them are inverse functional properties. Which object properties are functional and inverse functional can be seen in Fig. 2. This figure shows all the functional properties as dotted lines and all the inverse functional properties as dashed lines. A functional property means, for example, that an event can only belong to one order (`belongs_to_order`). An example of an inverse functional property is `has_visit`, meaning a patient can have multiple visits, but one visit can only be associated with one patient.

Table 1. Sample dataset for the proof-of-concept.

	event_name	time	sample_id	capacity	laboratory_name
0	register	2022-10-26 12:00:00	s1	150	l1
1	register	2022-10-26 13:00:00	s2	150	l2
2	sort	2022-10-26 15:00:00	s2	200	l2
3	register	2022-10-26 16:00:00	s3	150	l1
4	sort	2022-10-26 17:00:00	s1	150	l1
5	archive	2022-10-26 18:00:00	s2	200	l2
6	archive	2022-10-26 19:00:00	s3	150	l1
7	archive	2022-10-26 20:00:00	s1	150	l1

Example Minimal Dataset. A proof-of-concept has been conducted using a small example dataset. Table 1 shows a simplified database table storing data from the Event, Sample, Workplace, and Laboratory concepts. In the real world dataset, the data from these concepts is distributed over different tables. However, to explain the functionality of the pipeline, this suffices.

3.2   Semantic Header and Database Mapping

Different SQL queries have been implemented to fit the privacy-preserving and the full ontology. The semantic header for the example dataset is presented in Listing 1.1. It captures the mapping of the domain ontology to a relational database, where the alias represents the data property in the according domain ontology.

```
SELECT e.name AS has_event_name,
    e.time AS has_time,
    s.sampleid AS has_sample_id,
    w.capacity AS has_capacity,
    l.name AS has_laboratory_name
FROM event e
LEFT JOIN sample s USING sampleid
LEFT JOIN workplace w USING wpid
LEFT JOIN laboratory l USING labid
```

Listing 1.1. Sample SQL query including the semantic header information.

3.3   SPARQL Query Parsing

In order to dynamically create custom event logs, SPARQL queries need to be parsed, as can be seen in Listing 1.2 and 1.3. Listing 1.2 represents the SPARQL query, which queries the domain ontology.

```
PREFIX lab: <http://stiwa.org/laboratory>
SELECT *
WHERE { ?event lab:has_time ?time .
    FILTER (?time < "2022-10-26_19:00:00"^^xsd:dateTime) .
};
```

Listing 1.2. Sample SPARQL query

Furthermore, Listing 1.3 shows the parsed SPARQL query used to filter the dataset accordingly.

```
{
    "prefix": {
        "lab": "http://www.test.at/sample_ontology"
    },
    "select": [],
    "where": {
        "time": "lab:has_time"
    },
    "filter": [ {
        "time": {
            "operation": "<=",
            "value": "2022-10-26 19:00:00",
            "type": "xsd:dateTime"
        }
    } ]
}
```

Listing 1.3. Parsed SPARQL query.

Additionally, Listing 1.4 shows a more complex SPARQL query operating on the ontology introduced in Sect. 3.1. It contains a filter operation on the date of birth column and only includes the date of birth column in the event log, besides the mandatory fields, like activity, case identifier and timestamp.

```
PREFIX lab:  <http://stiwa.org/laboratory>
SELECT ?dob
WHERE {
    OPTIONAL{ ?patient lab:has_date_of_birth ?dob . }
    FILTER (?dob < "2000-01-01"^^xsd:date)
}
```

Listing 1.4. Sample SPARQL query on the ontology, introduced in Sect. 3.1

3.4 Directly-Follows Graph

Using the provided dataset and queries, the prototype is executed using parts of the ontology from Fig. 2 and an XES file is created that can be imported in any process mining tool. An example of such an XES file is shown in Lisitng 1.5, where the reference to the domain ontology is implemented with help of the XES semantic extension. Each "semantic:modelReference" contains the URI of the according concept or data property in the ontology. The displayed XES sample does not include any extension declarations, but the semantic, concept and time extensions have been used within the implementation of this prototype. For this proof-of-concept DISCO is used to create a DFG from the resulting XES file, which is shown in Fig. 3.

```
<log xes.version="2.0" xes.features="nested-attributes"
xmlns="http://www.xes-standard.org/">
  <trace>
    <string key="concept:name" value="1" />
    <string key="semantic:modelReference"
    value="http://sample.org/lab#has_sample_id" />
    <event>
      <string key="semantic:modelReference"
      value="http://sample.org/lab#Event" />
      <date key="time:timestamp" value="2022-10-15 08:18:04">
        <string key="semantic:modelReference"
        value="http://sample.org/lab#has_timestamp" />
      </date>
      <string key="concept:name" value="example">
        <string key="semantic:modelReference"
        value="http://sample.org/lab#has_event_type" />
      </string>
    </event>
  </trace>
</log>
```

Listing 1.5. Example for a resyulting XES file including the domain ontology references.

4 Discussion

Although focused on the laboratory domain, we want to highlight the following two key features of our approach to event log extraction from databases:

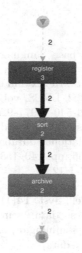

Fig. 3. Resulting DFG, after importing the generated XES file into Disco.

(1) By mapping the domain ontology to the relational database model, we enable *multi-perspective process analysis*. This approach also described by Calvanese et al. [3] works very well for the laboratory domain.

(2) When understanding the meaning of the data, analysts can tailor their datasets, e.g., to privacy needs. For our laboratory domain ontology, we create *privacy by design* when we hand out only the *core module* part to the analysts.

4.1   Future Work

The minimalistic mapping example, i.e., the semantic header in Listing 1.1, only maps data properties. Enhancing the semantic header, especially for object properties, can facilitate the use of ontology-inferred information for XES file creation. Parsing modules could be extended to support a broader range of SPARQL query variants, including different filtering options and the integration of the "GROUP BY" clause. Additionally, optimizing memory usage for extensive datasets could involve generating custom SQL queries based on SPARQL queries within the XES creation module.

Acknowledgements. We thank STIWA for their input in creating a laboratory domain ontology and the provision of extensive real-world datasets. This work was partly funded by BMK, BMAW, and the State of Upper Austria in the frame of the SCCH competence center INTEGRATE (no. 892418) part of the FFG COMET Competence Centers for Excellent Technologies Programme and by the FFG BRIDGE project AK-Graph (no. 883718).

References

1. Information technology - Database languages SQL - Part 1: Framework (SQL/Framework) (2023). https://www.iso.org/standard/76583.html
2. Câmpeanu, C., Salomaa, K., Yu, S.: Regex and extended regex. In: Champarnaud, J.M., Maurel, D. (eds.) CIAA 2002. LNCS, vol. 2608, pp. 77–84. Springer, Berlin (2003). https://doi.org/10.1007/3-540-44977-9_7
3. Calvanese, D., Montali, M., Syamsiyah, A., van der Aalst, W.M.P.: Ontology-driven extraction of event logs from relational databases. In: Reichert, M., Reijers, H. (eds.) BPM 2016. LNBIP, vol. 256, pp. 140–153. Springer, Cham (2016). https://doi.org/10.1007/978-3-319-42887-1_12
4. Chandrasekaran, B., Josephson, J., Benjamins, V.R.: What are ontologies, and why do we need them? IEEE Intell. Syst. **14**(1), 20–26 (1999)
5. Fahland, D.: Data storage vs data semantics for object-centric event data (2022). https://multiprocessmining.org/2022/10/26/data-storage-vs-data-semantics-for-object-centric-event-data/
6. Gamma, E., et al.: Design Patterns: Elements of Reusable Object-Oriented Software. Addison-Wesley Professional Computing Series (1995)
7. Helm, E., Buchgeher, G., Ehrlinger, L.: Online plausibility checks for patient pathways with medical ontologies. In: 5th International Workshop on Process-Oriented Data Science for Healthcare (PODS4H22), Co-Located with ICPM 2022 (2022)
8. Kingsley, O., et al.: Semantic-based process mining technique for annotation and modelling of domain processes. Int. J. Innov. Comput. Inf. Control **16**(3), 899–921 (2020)
9. Knoll, D., Waldmann, J., Reinhart, G.: Developing an internal logistics ontology for process mining. Procedia CIRP **79**, 427–432 (2019)
10. Leonardi, G., Striani, M., Quaglini, S., Cavallini, A., Montani, S.: Towards semantic process mining through knowledge-based trace abstraction. In: Ceravolo, P., van Keulen, M., Stoffel, K. (eds.) SIMPDA 2017. LNBIP, vol. 340, pp. 45–64. Springer, Cham (2019). https://doi.org/10.1007/978-3-030-11638-5_3
11. Li, G., de Murillas, E.G.L., de Carvalho, R.M., van der Aalst, W.M.P.: Extracting object-centric event logs to support process mining on databases. In: Mendling, J., Mouratidis, H. (eds.) CAiSE 2018. LNBIP, vol. 317, pp. 182–199. Springer, Cham (2018). https://doi.org/10.1007/978-3-319-92901-9_16
12. Munoz-Gama, J., et al.: Process mining for healthcare: characteristics and challenges. J. Biomed. Inform. **127**, 103994 (2022)
13. Nykänen, O., et al.: Associating event logs with ontologies for semantic process mining and analysis. In: Proceedings of the 19th International Academic Mindtrek Conference, Tampere, Finland, pp. 138–143. ACM (2015)
14. Polleres, A., Hogan, A., Delbru, R., Umbrich, J.: RDFS and OWL reasoning for linked data. In: Rudolph, S., Gottlob, G., Horrocks, I., van Harmelen, F. (eds.) Reasoning Web 2013. LNCS, vol. 8067, pp. 91–149. Springer, Heidelberg (2013). https://doi.org/10.1007/978-3-642-39784-4_2
15. RDFlib Working Group: RDFlib (2022). https://rdflib.dev
16. Soltani, M., Kahani, M., Behkamal, B.: ONT-OCEL: an ontology-based representation for OCEL. In: CEUR Workshop Proceedings, Hersonissos, Greece, 29 May 2023, vol. 3447, pp. 90–100. CEUR-WS.org (2023)
17. Uschold, M., Gruninger, M.: Ontologies: principles, methods and applications. Knowl. Eng. Rev. **11**(2), 93–136 (1996)

18. Verbeek, H.M.W., Buijs, J.C.A.M., van Dongen, B.F., van der Aalst, W.M.P.: XES, XESame, and ProM 6. In: Soffer, P., Proper, E. (eds.) CAiSE 2010. LNBIP, vol. 72, pp. 60–75. Springer, Heidelberg (2011). https://doi.org/10.1007/978-3-642-17722-4_5
19. W3C SPARQL Working Group: SPARQL 1.1 Query Language (2018). https://www.w3.org/TR/sparql11-query
20. Wynn, M.T., et al.: Rethinking the input for process mining: insights from the XES survey and workshop. In: Munoz-Gama, J., Lu, X. (eds.) ICPM 2021. LNBIP, vol. 433, pp. 3–16. Springer, Cham (2022). https://doi.org/10.1007/978-3-030-98581-3_1

Clinical Event Knowledge Graphs: Enriching Healthcare Event Data with Entities and Clinical Concepts - Research Paper

Milad Naeimaei Aali[1][✉], Felix Mannhardt[2], and Pieter Jelle Toussaint[1]

[1] Norwegian University of Science and Technology, Trondheim, Norway
milad.naeimaei@ntnu.no
[2] Eindhoven University of Technology, Eindhoven, The Netherlands

Abstract. Clinical processes include admission, discharge, medication administration, diagnostic testing, and others. Process mining promises to provide insights for improving such processes. An issue in analyzing clinical processes is that recorded events concerning the treatment of patients are often not only related to the patients themselves, but also the event and activities terminology need to be interpretable globally in different health organizations. Specifically, in the case of multimorbidity, it is expected that clinical events recorded for a patient relate to multiple disorders and are linked to many different clinical concepts from various medical specialties. This hampers the application of process mining as extracting a single-entity event log gives an incomplete view of the patient trajectory, and relating events and activities to clinical terminology understood by medical professionals is complex. We propose to address these issues by building a clinical event knowledge graph that combines multi-entity event data from clinical systems with clearly defined clinical terms from coding systems such as ICD10-cm and a systematically organized collection of medical terms such as SNOMED CT. Our contribution is a framework that facilitates building such a clinical event knowledge graph. We evaluate the proposed framework by showing the feasibility of applying it to the MIMIC-IV dataset. We validated a set of process-related questions on multi-morbid patients with clinical experts. By leveraging the graph, these questions can be answered at the abstraction level of clinical terms. This may facilitate the involvement of medical professionals in the analysis, leading to the enhanced management of healthcare processes.

Keywords: Healthcare · Process Mining · multi-entity event data · clinical concepts

1 Introduction

The healthcare system is one of the essential organizations in each society, and it is necessary for individuals' well-being and quality of life. Therefore, improving the quality of healthcare services is a crucial objective, particularly for multi-morbidity patients. Because, the group of patients with multi-morbidity, which is the co-occurrence of multiple chronic conditions in the same person [1] is a growing [1]. Multiple disorders with overlapping symptoms need to be managed by different medical specialties and various medications. One of the approaches for improving quality of services in healthcare is improving its clinical process because it plays a pivotal role in the healthcare ecosystem.

A clinical process refers to a sequence of events in diagnosing, treating, and managing a patient's medical condition [2], and sometimes, the term "care path-ways" is used instead of clinical processes. Improving clinical processes means delivering more efficient healthcare, improving patient outcomes, and enhancing operational performance within healthcare organizations. So, to fulfill this pur-pose, process mining [2, 3] is one of the practical techniques that can be deployed.

Process mining uses event log data [3] to discover, monitor, and improve pro-cesses. Events are related to a set of steps with well-defined labels (i.e., activities) that occur in a specific order (based on their timestamps) and are related to one or more entities. This research aims to introduce a framework to address two challenges in healthcare process mining to get a better understanding of pro-cess mining tasks in healthcare that may ultimately lead to improved clinical processes: (**CH1**) connecting entities and (**CH2**) linking terminology.

Connecting Entities. It is not always straightforward to connect events to clinical entities. For example, we have patients' diagnosis data in the healthcare domain that stores each patient's disorders. Still, these disorders that can poten-tially be used as a new entity do not relate to events, as shown in Fig. 1. It is impossible to directly connect events to disorders through patients because we connect all activities to all disorders. In contrast, in health organizations, specific activities may occur, for example, for treating a disorder or a specific collection of disorders. Transforming single-entity event data to multi-entity event data [4, 5] can give us more valuable insights into complex care pathways involving multiple disorders, as in multi-morbid patients, than single-entity event data [6].

Linking Terminology. Linking activities and entities to clinical terminology can help us to have standardized and globally accepted clinical processes that are interpretable in different healthcare systems. It also can help us to stan-dardize the segmentation of clinical processes. Also, the hierarchy of concepts can allow us to represent the various abstract levels of processes. Examples of sources for standardized clinical terminology are, e.g., Systematized Nomencla-ture of Medicine Clinical Terms (SNOMED CT) [7], International Classification of Diseases Clinical Modification (ICD CM) [8], and diagnosis-related group (DRG). As shown in Fig. 1, we have two types of terminology linkage: Entities Terminology Linkage (**CH2.1**) and Activities Terminology Linkage (**CH2.2**).

Based on these challenges, our research question is formulated as: *How can we connect relevant healthcare entities to events and link them to clinical ter-minology to provide better insights into multi-morbid patient clinical processes?.* Section 2 provides an overview of relevant literature that has tackled similar research questions to ours. In Sect. 3, we introduce our preliminary formalization.

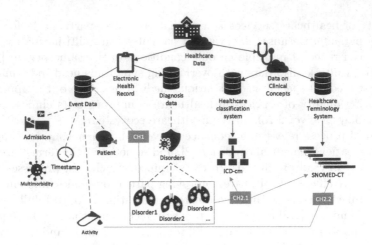

Fig. 1. How can we leverage additional clinical data sources such as terminologies and clinical entities for process mining to enhance the analysis of multi-morbid patient trajectories?

Section 4 delves into our response to the research question, outlining the framework known as the Clinical Knowledge Event Graph. Our evaluation of this framework is detailed in Sect. 5, followed by a thorough discussion of the results in Sect. 6. Finally, we draw our paper to a close in Sect. 7, where we elucidate the forthcoming steps in the utilization of the proposed clinical EKG.

2   Related Work

We review literature related to the challenges of connecting entities to events and linking terminology with event data.

In [9], Rebmann et al. propose a method to transform single-dimensional event data to multi-entity event data automatically. They uncovered multi-entity event data by semantic analysis of textual attributes. Based on our mentioned challenges, This research only wanted to answer the CH1. They could discover multi-entity event data. However, the discovered new entities come from the event's label and not from another data source, including a potential entity with no relationship between it and events in the event log.

Calvanese et al. [10] proposed a methodology named OnProm to extract of event logs from legacy information systems. In that approach, after understanding the details of the process, a conceptual model (UML class diagram) and formal knowledge representation models for the conceptual model (OWL2 QL ontology) are created. Then the facts over the conceptual or formal knowledge representation model were represented using RDF, a collection of subject-predicate-object triples. Then the map between the facts of the legacy information system and the conceptual model is created using SPARQL and SQL query. Finally, entities, events, and attributes are specified using the OnProm tools, and the event log will be extracted. Further, in [11] Xiong et al. leveraged the OnProm framework to create multi-entity event logs from legacy information systems. This research also touches CH1 but has the limitation that the process needs to be known in advance, e.g., the potential entities.

In another related work, [12,13] propose a model in which event log activities are related to ICD9 code to change the level of abstraction by grouping and slicing activities. This research could answer CH2.2. But they must still explain how they connect event log activities to ICD9 terminology.

In summary, the challenge of both satisfying entity connection and terminology linkage has not yet been fully addressed. In the next section, we introduce preliminaries and define required concepts.

3   Preliminaries

We utilize a graph database in the development of the proposed clinical EKG. This database allows us to consolidate information from various sources, including event data, diagnosis data, and terminologies, within a graphical structure. Additionally, it simplifies the process of process mining by leveraging meaningful and semantically driven relationships between nodes and graphs. This, in turn, facilitates the creation of intricate and adaptable queries. The graph database also supports the storage of hierarchical terminology data, such as SNOMED-CT and ICD-10, and streamlines data navigation through path-based traversals. Furthermore, it streamlines the storage of entity attributes, enabling us to manage patient-related information, such as symptoms, onset age, causes, prevalence, and other pertinent semantic details, which in turn provides us with more valuable insights.

Several graph models can be used for building the graph, such as LPG (Labeled Property Graph) and RDF (Resource Description Framework). LPG is a collection of interconnected nodes (vertices) by relationships (directed edges); on the other hand, RDF is a collection of interconnected resources (subject-object) by predicates. We chose the LPG model since it is optimized for querying complicated relationships [4]. We provide the essential ingredients for LPGs following the definitions of an EKG made in [14].

When building the proposed clinical EKG we obtain several such LPGs from different sources and need to combine them into a single LPG with clearly defined node and relationship labels that extend the basic labels {*Event, Entity*} defined for event knowledge graphs [14]. Therefore, we define basic composition operations on LPGs.

Definition 1 (Union of two LPGs [14]**).** *Let $G_1 = (N_1, R_1, \lambda_1, \#_1)$ and $G_2 = (N_2, R_2, \lambda_2, \#_2)$ be two LPGs defined over the same universe of labels and attributes but with disjoint set of nodes ($N_1 \cap N_2 = \emptyset$) and relations ($R_1 \cap R_2 = \emptyset$). The union of G_1 and G_2 is denoted as $G_1 \cup G_2 = (N_1 \cup N_2, R_1 \cup R_2, \lambda_{1 \cup 2}, \#_{1 \cup 2})$ with $\lambda_{1 \cup 2}(n) = \lambda_1(n)$ if $n \in N_1$ and $\lambda_{1 \cup 2}(n) = \lambda_2(n)$ otherwise and $\#_{1 \cup 2}$ defined respectively.*

The union of two LPGs provides us with a single graph when combining data from two sources, but does not connect nodes in N_1 to nodes in N_2 or vice versa. For this we define the concept of a constrained node mapping with which new relations are built between nodes based on a specific mapping function over their attributes.

Definition 2 (Constrained Node Mapping). *Let $G = (N, R, \lambda, \#)$ be a LPG. A constrained node mapping identifies new relationships $r_{csn} \in N \times N$ that are added to the LPG by using a mapping function $csn : N \times N \to \{0, 1\}$ returning if nodes are related to each other (1) or not (0).*

Constraint node mapping functions facilitate building the relationship between nodes with various labels and can be obtained from data, domain knowledge, expert knowledge, dataset data, documents, and sometimes trained machine learning models. We stress that domain knowledge is a critical component of healthcare [15] and encompasses any knowledge and expertise necessary to understand and operate effectively within the healthcare industry. This knowledge includes familiarity with medical terminology, clinical procedures, treatment options, disorder states, the healthcare system, and various healthcare technologies such as electronic health records (EHRs), medical devices, and telemedicine platforms. We kept the constrained node mapping deliberately general since we do not want to constrain the information used, e.g., a constraint mapping may be based directly on a certain attribute $csn_{icd}(n_1, n_2) = 1$ if and only if $\#(n_1, Disorder) = \#(n_2, ICDCode)$ but could also take into account more complexity relations such as the existing relationships. We can now use the defined concept to extend an LPG with new relationships.

Definition 3 (LPG extension). *Let $G = (N, R, \lambda, \#)$ be a LPG. Given csn be a constraint node mapping. Given $x \in \Lambda_R$ be a label for new relationships identified by csn. We use csn to extend G with new relationships and define the LPG extended by csn as $G_{csn} = (N, R \cup R_{csn}, \lambda', \#')$ such that:*

$$R_{csn} = \{(n_1, n_2) \in N \times N \mid csn(n_1, n_2) = 1\}$$

and for any $r \in R_{csn} : \lambda'(r) = x$ and otherwise for $r \in R: \lambda'(r) = \lambda(r)$. Analogously, we may add attributes to the new relationship through extended function $\#'$ which we omit for the sake of space.

Next, we show how our proposed framework builds a LPG that provides the clinical EKG.

4   Clinical Event Knowledge Graph

In this section, we describe the proposed framework for building a clinical event knowledge graph that addresses the challenges we identified for advancing process mining in healthcare. We take the union of all LPGs representing different parts of the clinical data and provide several constrained node mappings that identify new relationships to be added to build the clinical EKG. To simplify the presentation, we assume that all possible labels and attributes are already present in the universes Λ_N, Λ_R, as well as A and U.

We consider four different types of inputs extracted from various sources as the main ingredients of our proposed framework: event data, diagnosis data, ICD-10-CM classes, and SNOMED-CT concepts. Event and diagnosis data are extracted from the electronic health records of the health organization we want to study. For obtaining ICD-10-CM data, we leverage the healthcare classification system published by the World Health Organization[1]. The concepts of the SNOMED-CT terminology system can be obtained from the SNOMED International[2].

4.1 Initial Node Creation

In the first step, we create individual graphs for each of the considered inputs that only contain the considered nodes, their node labels, and attributes without any relationship. For each of the source we list the set of node labels $\Lambda'_N \subset \Lambda_N$ and describe which nodes are created:

- **Event LPG.** The initial event LPG G_{evt} is created from an event table extracted from the hospital information system. We consider the following set of node labels: $\Lambda_{evt} = \{Log, Event, Entity, Activity\}$, analogous to [14] and define two types of entities: *Patients* and *Admissions* through the use of attributes. We then create nodes for each event, each patient, and each admission in the event table as well as a single node for the log and activity nodes for each distinct event label.
- **Diagnosis LPG:** Hospital data contains information on the set of diagnosis codes associated with a patient from which we create G_{dia}. We define the node label $\Lambda_{dia} = \{Disorder\}$ and create diagnosis nodes for each individual diagnosis made for patients in the event table.
- **ICD-10-CM LPG:** We create G_{icd} with the information on ICD codes such that we have node labels $\Lambda_{icd} = \{ICD\}$ and each relevant individual ICD code as node.
- **SNOMED-CT LPG:** We extract a subset of concepts from SNOMED-CT to G_{sno} that are relevant to our data and define node labels $\Lambda_{sno} = \{Concept\}$ and create nodes for each relevant concept.

4.2 Adding Intra-graph Relationships

We need to add relationships to each of the initial LPGs that can be obtained from within the input data. Each relationship is labelled and we provide the set of labels as well as the mapping criteria in Table 1. For example, the event LPG has the same set of relationship labels $\{HAS, CORR, DF, \ldots\}$ as defined

---

[1] https://icd.who.int/browse10/2019/en.
[2] https://browser.ihtsdotools.org/.

in [14]. For each of the defined relationships we specify a constraint node mapping (CNM) and add the relationships to the respective LPG by extension as defined in Definition 3. These CNMs are dependent on the use case and available data.

Table 1. Intra-graph relationships and constrained node mapping.

First Node n_1	Relationship Label	Second Node n_2	CNMs
Log	:HAS	Event	$\#(n_1, LogID) = \#(n_2, EventLog)$
Event	:CORR	Entity (Patient, Adm)	$\#(n_1, Entity1ID) = \#(n_2, EntityID)$ $\#(n_1, Entity2ID) = \#(n_2, EntityID)$
Event	:OBSERVED	Activity	$\#(n_1, EventAct) = \#(n_2, ActivityID)$
Event	:DF	Event	$\#(n_1, EntitiyID) = \#(n_2, EntitiyID)$ $\#(n_1, time) < \#(n_2, time)$ $\#(n_1, time) \not< \#(n_3, time) \not< \#(n_2, time)$
Activity	:DF_C	Activity	$\#(n_1, EvActID) = \#(n_2, EvActID)$ $\#(n_1, time) < \#(n_2, time)$ $\#(n_1, time) \not< \#(n_3, time) \not< \#(n_2, time)$
Patient	:POSES	Admission	$\#(n_1, AdmID) = \#(n_2, PatientID)$
Admission	:OWNS	Disorder	$\#(n_1, DisorderID) = \#(n_2, AdmID)$
Concept	:ANCESTOR_OF	Concept	$\#(n_1, ConceptID) = \#(n_2, ConceptID)$

4.3   Deriving Inter-graph Relationships of the Clinical EKG

In the last step, we combine all individual LPGs into a clinical EKG by taking the union of all individual LPGs $G_{cEKG} = G_{evt} \cup G_{dia} \cup G_{icd} \cup G_{sno}$. Now, we still need to derive the inter-graph relationships to connect nodes of the previously separate graphs. To derive the necessary inter-graph relationships we define, again, a constraint node mapping function and extend G_{cEKG} with the following relationships:

- **Between the ICD nodes and the Concept nodes** we employed *ICDCM DIAGNOSIS MAP 2022* [8] dataset for adding the relationship between ICD and Snomed-CT concepts with label *CONNECTED_TO*.
- **Between the Diagnosis nodes and the ICD nodes** we can use data already available since hospitals often use ICD code in their system. This creates the relationship *LINKED_TO*.
- **Between the Activity nodes and the Concept nodes** we used a manual approach by using domain knowledge and the SNOMED-CT browser to create the relationship *MAPPED_TO*. Note that this step may be partially automated through string matching but likely still requires domain knowledge.

- **Between the Event nodes and the Diagnosis nodes** we could use a supervised machine learning approach to map *Event* nodes in Event data to *Diagnosis* nodes in Diagnosis data. Because it is possible to extract a dataset whose features are event activity values and its classes are disorders from the electronic health record data. This relationship is labelled as *BOND*.

This provides us with the final clinical EKG integrating events with clinical terminology and classification of disorders. Next, we evaluate our proposed framework on a real-life case.

5   Evaluation

We evaluate the feasiblity and effectiveness of our framework by applying it on a real-life case and discussing its ability to answer a set of process questions. In Fig. 2, we illustrated our evaluation approach. We created a set of questions based on the challenges 1 and 2 and verified their usefulness with a clinical expert in the obesity clinical of a Norwegian hospital. Then, we realized our developed framework in a graph database management system and translated the process questions into graph database queries and visualize the results in different formats. In the setup section, we evaluate the effectiveness of our framework by utilizing a carefully selected dataset, which serves as a foundation for assessing its performance and capabilities.

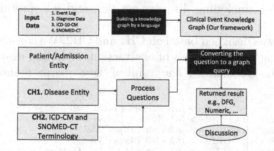

Fig. 2. Our evaluation setup based on process questions and instantiating the clinical EKG for a real-life dataset.

5.1   Setup

For our evaluation we leverage MIMIC-IV to extract the event logs data and diagnosis data from. MIMIC-IV is a freely available database including de-identified clinical records from patients admitted to ICUs. It contains data from over 300,000 ICU admissions from 2008 to 2019 for Beth Israel Deaconess Medical Center in Boston, Massachusetts [16].

5.2 Creating a Clinical EKG for MIMIC-IV

For extraction events, MIMIC-IV dataset was used. We created two entities based on the attributes *PATIENT_ID* and *ADMISSION_ID* stored in the MIMIC-IV dataset. Nodes were created for each distinct event, entity, and admission. Then, an intra-data constrained node mapping between these node types was uncovered. Finally, the relationships based on constrained node mappings were applied between nodes.

For extracting the ICD10 graph, we considered the *D_ICD_DIAGNOSES* table in the MIMIC-IV dataset. For creating the SNOMED-CT graph, we used The SNOMED CT International Edition; we considered the *DESCRIPTION* and the *TEXT_DEFINITION* tables from it to extract nodes, and the *RELATIONSHIP* table to find intra-data constrained node mapped.

Then, we added the relationship based on inter-graph constrained node mapping to obtain a clinical EKG for MIMIC-IV.

5.3 Process Questions and Results

As outlined in Fig. 2, we designed two process questions based on the identified challenges. For the significance and relevance of these questions to care pathways of multi-morbid patients, we interviewed three health experts in a Norwegian health organization; they confirmed that answering these questions aligns with their health organization's interests.

Q1: What is the patient's care pathway with an ID of 1, featuring different levels of abstraction, including disorder entities, and interpretable on a global scale?

This question was designed based on CH1 and CH2. We consider two different queries representing different levels of abstraction, including disorder entity and interpretable on the global scale. The result of these queries is shown in Figure 3.

```
MATCH p=(e1)−[r: DF]−> (e2)
MATCH p1=(e2: Event) −[: CORR]−> (n1: Subject {Type: "Subject"})
MATCH p2=(e1: Event) −[: CORR]−> (n1: Subject {Type: "Subject"})
MATCH p3=(e2: Event) −[: CORR]−> (n2:Visit {Type: "Visit"})
MATCH p4=(e1: Event) −[: CORR]−> (n2:Visit {Type:"Visit"})
MATCH p5=(e2: Event) −[: CORR]−> (n3: Concept {Type: "Concept"})
MATCH p6=(e1: Event) −[: CORR]−> (n3: Concept {Type: "Concept"})
match p7=(e1)−[:OBSERVED]−>(a1)−[:MAPPED_TO]−>(m1)
match p8=(e2)−[:OBSERVED]−>(a2)−[:MAPPED_TO]−>(m2)
RETURN p p1, p2, p3, p4, p5, p6, p7, p8 ;
```

```
MATCH p=(e1)−[r:DF]−>(e2)
MATCH p1=(e2: Event) −[: CORR]−> (n1: Subject {Type: "Subject"})
MATCH p2=(e1: Event) −[: CORR] −> (n1:Subject {Type: "Subject"})
MATCH p3=(e2: Event) −[: CORR]−> (n2:Visit {Type: "Visit"})
MATCH p4=(e1: Event) −[: CORR]−> (n2: Visit {Type: "Visit"})
MATCH p5=(e2: Event) −[: CORR]−> (n3: Concept {Type: "Concept"})
MATCH p6=(e1: Event) −[: CORR]−> (n3: Concept {Type: "Concept"})
match p7=(e1)−[:OBSERVED]−>(a1)−[:MAPPED_TO]−>(m1)−[:ANCESTOR_OF]−>(m3)
match p8=(e2)−[:OBSERVED]−>(a2)−[:MAPPED_TO]−>(m2)−[:ANCESTOR_OF]−>(m4)
RETURN p p1, p2, p3, p4,p5,p6,p7,p8;
```

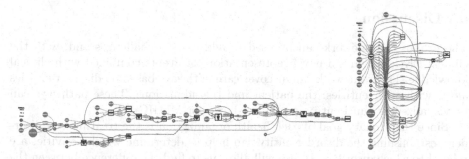

Fig. 3. The result of the second query (The right) obtained from Neo4j, then represented in Graphviz, shows a higher level of abstraction than the first query because it includes fewer activities than the first query (The left).

Q2: What is the care pathway for a specific disorder, such as "Infection of bloodstream SCTID: 431193003," featuring globally accepted activities that have been categorized and segmented in a standardized manner?

This question was also created based on both challenges. First, we implement a query that shows multi-entity care pathways for "Infection of bloodstream SCTID: 431193003," featuring globally accepted activities that have been categorized and segmented standardized as show in Figure 4. Then, we added a line in a query to consider only activities related to the "Transfer summary report."

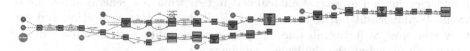

Fig. 4. Query's output categorizes each activity into three distinct groups: Transfer summary report, Laboratory test findings, and Microbiology report, each assigned a unique color. (Color figure online)

```
MATCH p=(e1)−[r:DF]−>(e2)
MATCH p1=(e2: Event) −[:CORR]−> (n1: Subject {Type: "Subject"})
MATCH p2=(e1: Event) −[:CORR]−> (n1: Subject {Type: "Subject"})
MATCH p3=(e2: Event) −[:CORR]−> (n2: Subject {Type: "Visit"})
MATCH p4=(e1: Event) −[:CORR]−> (n2: Subject {Type: "Visit"})
MATCH p5=(e2: Event) −[:CORR]−> (n3: Subject {Type: "Concept"})
MATCH p6=(e1: Event) −[:CORR]−> (n3: Subject {Type: "Concept"})
MATCH p7=(e1)−[: OBSERVED]−>(a1)−[:MAPPED_TO]−> (m1)
MATCH p8=(e2)−[: OBSERVED]−>(a2)−[:MAPPED⁻TO]−> (m2)
MATCH p9=(e1)−[: OBSERVED]−>(a1)−[:TYPE_OF]−> (m3)
MATCH p10=(e2)−[: OBSERVED]−>(a2)−[:TYPE_OF]−> (m4)
where m4.termA= "Transfer summary report"
RETURN p, p1, p2, p3, p4, p5, p6,p7, p8, p9,p10;
```

Next, we focus on the analysis and interpretation of the obtained results.

6   Discussion

The proposed framework can be used to address the challenges and, with the clinical EKG, provides a novel representation for events combined with clinical knowledge. The framework can discover care pathways based on disorder entities along with other entities: the patient and the admissions. These pathways can be visualized as multi-entity graphs as shown for MIMIC-IV.

Since the primary goal of each health organization is the treatment of disorders, establishing the disorder entity can help us determine which activities are related to which disorders. It also will allow us to find the difference between the treatment of one disease to another and how much variation there is in treating certain disorders. The proposed clinical EKG provides access to this information through the lens of clinical terminologies and connecting events to disorders. This is important in the context of multi-morbid patients who experience a different range of symptoms due to multiple disorders. Mapping the disorders referenced in event data to SNOMED-CT concepts help us to find the care pathways of disorders by SNOMED-CT concepts which are universal in all health organizations. This enables interpretation of care pathways by different hospitals in a coherent manner. It also facilitates excluding querying the events at a preferred abstraction level by considering different levels of SNOMED-CT concepts in the query.

Whereas we acknowledge that limitation that we only evaluated our framework on MIMIC-IV, we used standardized representations for clinical knowledge which suggest that our work can be applied in other health organizations. A broader evaluation in several clinical settings showing the general applicability would be important but is inherently difficult due to data protection and privacy concerns. Still, overall our study shows feasibility and usefulness of the framework regarding the challenges we identified.

7   Conclusion

This research proposes to connect relevant healthcare entities such as disorders to events and to link them to clinical terminologies such as ICD-10-CM and SNOMED-CT. Such linkage is facilitated by providing a framework for building a clinical EKG and applied in the context of multi-morbid patients. The clinical EKG can provide better insight into healthcare process mining by facilitating querying of multi-entity event data through the lens of clinical terminology that is standardized across health organizations.

There are still limitations that we need to address in future work. Linking individual events to entities such as disorders is complex and could be automated through machine learning. Similarly, the manual mapping of activities to SNOMED-CT terminology could be automated. Since we argue that the clinical EKG should be accessible for clinical experts who are not experts in graph database querying, a natural language interface to the query language would be a valuable and necessary prerequisite for adoption. Ultimately, ontological reasoning based on LPG and RDF can be researched in future work.

Reproducibility. Our implementation of clinical EKGs is available[3]. We used SQL queries on MIMIC-IV to extract single patient entity event data, diagnoses data, and clinical entity. To extract SNOMED-CT data we used SQL on the SNOMED CT RF2 database. We deployed Cypher queries to store the clinical event data graph in Neo4J and Graphviz in Python to visualize results.

References

1. Marengoni, A., et al.: Aging with multimorbidity: a systematic review of the literature. Ageing Res. Rev. **10**(4), 430–439 (2011)
2. Munoz-Gama, J., et al.: Process mining for healthcare: characteristics and challenges. J. Biomed. Inform. **127**, 103994 (2022)
3. Van Der Aalst, W.: Process Mining: Data Science in Action, vol. 2. Springer, Heidelberg (2016). https://doi.org/10.1007/978-3-662-49851-4
4. Esser, S., Fahland, D.: Multi-dimensional event data in graph databases. J. Data Semant. **10**(1–2), 109–141 (2021)
5. van der Aalst, W.M.P.: Object-centric process mining: dealing with divergence and convergence in event data. In: Ölveczky, P., Salaün, G. (eds.) SEFM 2019. LNCS, vol. 11724, pp. 3–25. Springer, Cham (2019). https://doi.org/10.1007/978-3-030-30446-1_1
6. Naeimaei Aali, M., Mannhardt, F., Toussaint, P.J.: Discovering care pathways for multi-morbid patients using event graphs. In: Munoz-Gama, J., Lu, X. (eds.) ICPM 2021. LNBIP, vol. 433, pp. 352–364. Springer, Cham (2022). https://doi.org/10.1007/978-3-030-98581-3_26
7. SNOMED International and the College of American Pathologists. SNOMED CT (2021). https://www.snomed.org/get-snomed
8. World Health Organization. International Statistical Classification of Diseases and Related Health Problems. https://icd.who.int/
9. Rehmann, A., Rehse, J. R., Van der Aa, H.: Uncovering object-centric data in classical event logs for the automated transformation from XES to OCEL. In: Di Ciccio, C., Dijkman, R., del Río Ortega, A., Rinderle-Ma, S. (eds.) BPM 2022. LNCS, vol. 13420, pp. 379–396. Springer, Cham (2022). https://doi.org/10.1007/978-3-031-16103-2_25
10. Calvanese, D., et al.: Ontology-based data access for extracting event logs from legacy data: the onprom tool and methodology. In: Abramowicz, W. (ed.) BIS 2017. LNBIP, vol. 288, pp. 220–236. Springer, Cham (2017). https://doi.org/10.1007/978-3-319-59336-4_16
11. Xiong, J., et al.: A virtual knowledge graph based approach for object-centric event logs extraction. In: Montali, M., Senderovich, A., Weidlich, M. (eds.) ICPM 2022. LNBIP, vol. 468, pp. 466–478. Springer, Cham (2023). https://doi.org/10.1007/978-3-031-27815-0_34
12. Rabbi, F., Lamo, Y., MacCaull, W.: A model based slicing technique for process mining healthcare information. In: Babur, Ö., Denil, J., Vogel-Heuser, B. (eds.) ICSMM 2020. CCIS, vol. 1262, pp. 73–81. Springer, Cham (2020). https://doi.org/10.1007/978-3-030-58167-1_6
13. Rabbi, F., Fatemi, B., MacCaull, W.: Analysis of patient pathways with contextual process mining. In: HEDA@Petri Nets. CEUR Workshop Proceedings, vol. 3264. CEUR-WS.org (2022)

---

[3] https://github.com/mnaeimaei/ClinicalEventKnowledgeGraphs.

14. Fahland, D.: Process mining over multiple behavioral dimensions with event knowledge graphs. In: van der Aalst, W.M.P., Carmona, J. (eds.) Process Mining Handbook. LNBIP, vol. 448, pp. 274–319. Springer, Cham (2022). https://doi.org/10.
1007/978-3-031-08848-3_9
15. Beerepoot, I., et al.: The biggest business process management problems to solve
before we die. Comput. Ind. **146**, 103837 (2023)
16. Johnson, A.E.W., et al.: MIMIC-IV, a freely accessible electronic health record
dataset. Sci. Data **10**(1), 1 (2023)

Error-Correcting Methodology for Evaluating Compliance to Clinical Guidelines: A Case Study on Rectal Cancer

Mariachiara Savino[1]([✉])(iD), Carlos Fernandez-Llatas[2]([✉])(iD), Roberto Gatta[3](iD),
Giuditta Chiloiro[4](iD), Silvia Di Franco[1](iD), Gema Ibanez-Sanchez[2](iD),
Zoe Valero-Ramon[2](iD), Maria Antonietta Gambacorta[4](iD),
Vincenzo Valentini[4](iD), and Andrea Damiani[5](iD)

[1] Diagnostica per Immagini, Radioterapia Oncologica ed Ematologia,
Università Cattolica del Sacro Cuore, Rome, Italy
mariachiara.savino@unicatt.it
[2] SABIEN-ITACA, Universitat Politècnica de València, Valencia, Spain
cfllatas@itaca.upv.es
[3] Department of Clinical and Experimental Sciences, University of Brescia,
Brescia, Italy
[4] Diagnostica per Immagini, Radioterapia Oncologica ed Ematologia, Fondazione
Policlinico Universitario Agostino Gemelli IRCCS, Rome, Italy
[5] Gemelli Generator Real World Data, Fondazione Policlinico Universitario Agostino
Gemelli IRCCS, Rome, Italy

Abstract. In a clinical setting, physicians often need to tailor general clinical guidelines to match the specific characteristics of individual patients, resulting in deviations from the guidelines. Process mining provides a range of tools to evaluate how well patient pathways align with clinical guidelines. In this work we implement a novel conformance checking method that employs error-correcting techniques to provide a degree of deviation from the clinical guidelines. The described method allows the set of corrective actions to be defined interactively and the cost of each of them to be adjusted on the basis of clinical knowledge. We test the error-correction algorithm on a real-world cohort of locally advanced rectal cancer patients treated at Fondazione Policlinico Universitario A. Gemelli IRCCS to assess the degree of compliance to the European Society of Medical Oncology guidelines, translated into a computer-interpretable version with Pseudo-Workflow formalism. Using this approach, it is possible to extensively analyze the compliance of clinical treatments, from the control-flow to the data perspective, and to discover the most common types of deviations in our cohort.

Keywords: Conformance Checking · Rectal Cancer · Process Mining · Healthcare · Error-Correcting · Guidelines Compliance

---

M. Savino and C. Fernandez-Llatas—Contributed equally to this paper.

J. De Smedt and P. Soffer (Eds.): ICPM 2023 Workshops, LNBIP 503, pp. 309–320, 2024.
https://doi.org/10.1007/978-3-031-56107-8_24

1 Introduction

The wide implementation of evidence-based medicine (EBM) has led to the development of protocols and clinical guidelines (CG) to standardize diagnosis and treatment of a medical condition. CG are protocols usually defined by consensus of medical groups that describe the best practices in care and diagnosis processes. According to EBM principles, the adherence of the treatment to the CG is crucial for ensuring the quality of the care and to the continuous adaption and improvement. So, measuring the deviations on single patients with respect to CG can be a very interesting way to assess the status of the patient or even to adapt and improve the process incorporating more evidence-based knowledge. Process mining, with conformance checking algorithms, allows to evaluate the adherence of real patient processes to CG and to understand major deviations [8]. However, healthcare processes defined in CG strongly depend on decisions made by physicians on the basis of clinical experience and patient's conditions; therefore, when developing and using conformance checking techniques in healthcare, it is essential to consider the unique aspects of this domain and make appropriate modifications [13].

In a clinical context not all types of deviations have the same severity, some deviations have a greater impact on the patient's clinical pathway than others. For example, during cancer treatment, the radiotherapy dose can be slightly increased for selected patients to improve treatment effectiveness. Although this adjustment exceeds the ranges defined in the guidelines, the decision is based on the patient's specific condition and the doctor's clinical knowledge and judgement. In such cases, the deviation from the guidelines may be considered negligible compared to other deviations that may occur. To address this issue, conformance checking methods should include a measure of severity associated with each type of deviation by incorporating the healthcare professionals' knowledge into the analysis [10]. Within the alignments context, some techniques have been developed to assign distinct costs to various types of deviations, such as "Move in model" and "Move in log" [1].

Moreover, traditional algorithms prioritize the control-flow, i.e. the order of events in the traces, ignoring the attributes associated with the events. Recently, a few approaches have been published that combine the data perspective in the alignment-based analysis [3,12], some of which also consider soft constraints by exploiting fuzzy logic [17,18].

In this work we implement and test an error-correcting method [5] that employs the Edit Distance to quantify the extent of the patient's deviation from the CG through the integration of healthcare professionals' knowledge. In this implementation we not only take into account the control-flow change of the process, but also, the differences in the case variables. The algorithm differs from previous works by allowing for the definition of dynamic cost functions that depend on specific attributes of the trace like radiotherapy dose or chemotherapy drugs. Any type of correction and cost function can be defined, enabling a comprehensive evaluation of patient compliance from the control-flow to the data perspective.

We implement the error-correction algorithm in R and validate it on a real-world cohort of locally advanced rectal cancer patients, treated at the Fondazione Policlinico Universitario A. Gemelli IRCCS, to assess the compliance of patient pathways to the European Society of Medical Oncology (ESMO) guidelines for rectal cancer treatment. The application of the error-correcting algorithm provides clinicians with a more detailed overview of compliance and the identification of most common types of deviations.

The remainder of the paper is organized as follows. Section 2 describes the methodology of our work. Section 3 presents and discusses the results. Section 4 concludes the paper.

2   Methodology

In this section we describe the methodology to conduct our study. First, we describe how ESMO guidelines were translated into a computer-interpretable version, then we present the dataset and how the patients' pathways were extracted from the hospital databases. Finally, the implementation of the error-correction algorithm for conformance checking analysis is discussed.

2.1   Computer-Interpretable Version of ESMO Guidelines

For locally advanced rectal cancer patients, the ESMO guidelines [9], published in 2017, provide two different treatment options: (i) Neoadjuvant chemoradiotherapy (nCRT) followed by TME surgery or conservative approach, (ii) short-course radiotherapy (SCRT) followed by TME surgery. In the case of nCRT (also known as long-course radiotherapy), the guidelines prescribe radiotherapy treatment with a delivered dose in the range of 45–54 Gray followed by chemotherapy with 5-Fluorouracil or Capecitabine. On the other hand, SCRT requires a delivered dose of 25 Gray. In the present work, we have excluded adjuvant therapies to simplify the presentation of the results. Additionally, the level of scientific evidence for adjuvant therapies in rectal cancer is generally lower compared to colon cancer [9].

To assess the adherence of our population, the ESMO guidelines were translated into a computer-interpretable version using Pseudo-Workflow (PWF) [11], a formalism used by pMineR software [7]. Previous studies employed PWF and pMineR software to conduct conformance checking analysis in the oncological domain [11, 14–16]. PWF describes CG in terms of two basic components: nodes (or states) and rules (or triggers). For each rule, a condition is tested, and if the condition is met, an effect is produced that changes the state of the patients. This rule structure is repeated to represent all the ESMO guidelines recommendations, resulting in a final XML file that can be interpreted by pMiner software to generate a workflow diagram and to assess compliance.

2.2   Data Extraction

All adult patients with a histological diagnosis of locally advanced rectal cancer treated at Fondazione Policlinico Universitario A. Gemelli IRCCS from January 2000 to December 2021 were included in the study. We also considered patients treated before the publication of the ESMO guidelines in 2017, in order to get insights into the practices of treatment approaches prior to the establishment of the standardized guidelines.

Clinical data were automatically extracted from the radiotherapy department's database using the hospital's data science facility Gemelli Generator Real World Data (G2 RWD) [2] and shaped in the form of an event log. Table 1 shows the list of events and attributes in our final event log. For chemotherapy we created two types of events to separate patients that correctly received 5-Fluorouracil or Capecitabine, as prescribed by CG, from patients that did not. We also created different types of events for surgery according to the type of local surgery.

Table 1. Event log structure: types of events and corresponding attributes.

Event types	Event names	Event attributes
Clinical staging	Staging_C	TNM risk category
Neoadjuvant radiotherapy	Nad_rt	Total delivered dose
Neoadjuvant chemotherapy with 5-FU/Capecitabine	Nad_ct	Oxaliplatin
Neoadjuvant chemotherapy without 5-FU and Capecitabine	Nad_ct_OUT	Oxaliplatin
TME Surgery	Surgery_TME	
Surgery other than TME	Surgery_OUT	
Conservative approach	Conservative_approach	

2.3   Error-Correction Method

The error-correction method we implemented is based on Edit Distance, a metric used to measure the similarity between two sequences by counting the minimum number of operations (such as adding, deleting, or substituting an element) required to transform one sequence into the other. Error-correction methods have already been implemented in previous studies to correct a real trace on the basis of a process model and to determine the distance between two processes [5,6].

In this work, we implemented the algorithm described in [5] to provide a degree of deviation from CG. The error-correction method aims to find the local optimal sequence of corrections that transforms a specific trace according to a process model. The algorithm selects the set of corrections that has the lower penalty cost among all possible sets and the final cost can be used to express the deviation degree from the process model (Fig. 1).

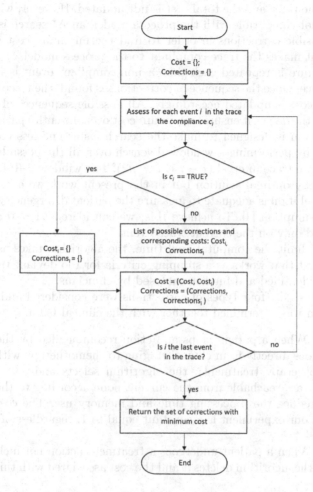

Fig. 1. Flowchart presenting the error-correction algorithm.

As preliminary steps, a collaboration with the clinical team is required in order to define a fixed set of operations that could be used for trace correcting and to associate penalty costs with each type of correction, based on the severity of the deviation. Deviation costs determined with the clinical team represent healthcare providers' knowledge of the process and can provide valuable insights into the underlying reasons for deviations. However, objective validation of these costs, which also takes into account different clinical outcomes, is crucial to ensure that the results obtained do not reflect only the views of a single clinical team. This validation process will be a focus of future analyses.

For each event i in the trace, the conformance checking algorithm implemented in pMineR software evaluates adherence to the guidelines expressed in PWF. When the current event is compatible with the guidelines, no correction is applied to the trace and the total cost is not updated. However, when the current event is not compatible with the process model, an A* search is performed among all possible corrections in order to find the minimum cost sequence of operations that makes the trace compliant to the process model.

The procedure is repeated each time a non-compliant event is identified in the patient trace. Once the sequence of corrections is found, the trace is corrected and the total cost is updated accordingly. All possible sequences of corrections are tested and the one that ensures minimum cost over the entire path is selected.

The algorithm is designed to make the search faster and less computationally intensive, by performing a windowed search over all the possible correction operations in the trace interval $(i - \mu1, i + \mu2)$. The window $(-\text{Inf}, \text{Inf})$ would ensure a globally optimal solution but in the present work we assumed that a local optimal solution is adequate to measure the patient divergence with acceptable time consumption [4]. To achieve this, we considered $\mu1 = 0$ and $\mu2 = 0$ and we focused only on the current trace event.

In order to limit the computational time, the algorithm takes as input also a maximum cost that works as a stopping criteria for too deviant traces. These traces can be identified and further analysed by clinicians.

In our case study, four types of corrections were considered and the cost of each correction was determined together with the clinical team:

1. **Insertion.** When a patient skips an action recommended by the guidelines (e.g. if he goes directly from clinical staging to chemotherapy without undergoing radiotherapy treatment), the algorithm selects and adds only those actions that are reachable from the current node according to the guidelines model, to reduce the processing time and memory use. The cost of adding an event in our experiment is a constant equal to 1, regardless of the type of event.

2. **Deletion.** When a patient undergoes a treatment action not included in the guidelines, the algorithm deletes it and the cost associated with this correction is 0.35.

3. **Radiotherapy dose modification.** Some patients have a radiotherapy event that deviates from ESMO guidelines due to a dose value outside the prescribed range for chemoradiotherapy (45–54 Gy). In this case, the algorithm could apply a corrective action only on the dose attribute so that it would be in the accepted range. In our case study we defined a trapezoidal membership function (m) that determines how much each radiotherapy dose value complies with the guidelines (Fig. 2). When the dose is in the range defined by the guidelines the membership function is equal to 1 whereas it decreases linearly when the deviation increases. The slope when the dose is over 54 Gy is lower than when the dose is under 45 Gy to highlight how an increase in the radiotherapy dose is a less significant deviation than its decrease, with

reference to treatment efficacy. The cost of this type of correction is then computed as 1 − m, as described in [18].

4. **Oxaliplatin deletion.** ESMO guidelines prescribe only 5-FU or Capecitabine for the chemotherapy treatment. Nevertheless, some patients in our cohort participate into internal protocols and receive also an addition of Oxaliplatin. In such cases by changing the value of the Oxaliplatin attribute from 1 to 0 the chemotherapy event becomes compliant to guidelines. We associated a cost of 0.2 to this deviation, as it is actually an intensification of the treatment.

After applying a correction, if the resulting trace no longer complies with the guidelines, its cost is multiplied by 10 in order to penalise it in the choice of the final sequence of operations.

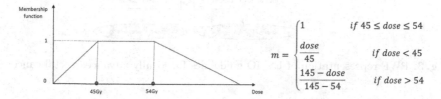

$$m = \begin{cases} 1 & \text{if } 45 \leq dose \leq 54 \\ \dfrac{dose}{45} & \text{if } dose < 45 \\ \dfrac{145 - dose}{145 - 54} & \text{if } dose > 54 \end{cases}$$

Fig. 2. Membership function defining radiotherapy dose compliance.

3   Results

The PWF diagram corresponding to the computer-interpretable version of ESMO guidelines is shown in Fig. 3, boxes represent rules and ovals represent status.

The guidelines define two treatment options for locally advanced rectal cancer patients: SCRT followed by TME surgery or nCRT followed by TME surgery or conservative approach.

The final event log included 4217 events associated to 1082 locally advanced rectal cancer patients treated in Fondazione Policlinico Gemelli IRCCS from January 2000 to December 2021.

We applied the algorithm described in Sect. 2.3 to the final cohort and obtained that 886 (81.88%) patients out of 1082 received a treatment with a degree of deviation greater than zero, whilst 196 (18.11%) patients out of 1082 received a fully compliant treatment with a zero degree of deviation. The median value and the interquartile range of the deviation degree were 0.20 (2.69), showing that although the percentage of non-adherent treatment pathways is high, deviations from ESMO guidelines are quite small (the median value is 5% of the maximum cost calculated in our cohort).

In order to further investigate the compliance in our population, Fig. 4 displays the density plot of deviation degree among non compliant patient pathways. Three main peaks appear in the distribution centered at 0.01, 0.2 and 2.70.

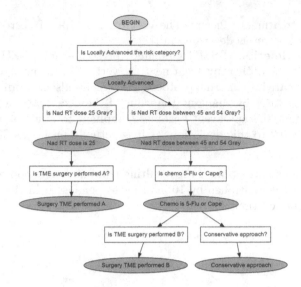

Fig. 3. PWF representation of ESMO guidelines for locally advanced rectal cancer.

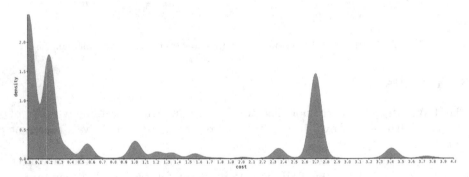

Fig. 4. Density distribution of deviation degree in our population.

For each trace, the error-correction algorithm outputs not only the cost but also the corresponding list of corrective actions. Through this information we were able to investigate the most common types of deviations from guidelines in our cohort:

- **Peak 1:** deviation degree = 0.01. 286 (32.28%) out of 886 not compliant traces had a very small deviation degree, equal to 0.01, that corresponds to a correction action of: "radiotherapy dose modification by 1 Gy". All these patients received cancer treatment fully compliant with the guidelines, except for the radiotherapy dose of 55 Gy, which was 1 Gy higher than the guidelines recommendations.
- **Peak 2:** deviation degree = 0.20. 186 (20.99%) out of 886 not compliant traces had a deviation degree equal to 0.20 that corresponds to a correction action of

"Oxaliplatin deletion". These treatment pathways were fully compliant with the guidelines, except for the addition of Oxaliplatin during chemotherapy.

– **Peak 3:** deviation degree = 2.70. 164 (18.51%) out of 886 not compliant traces had a chemotherapy treatment with drugs not prescribed by guidelines ('Nad_ct_OUT' event). In such cases, the error-correction algorithm transforms the trace according to the guidelines by applying the following sequence of corrections: "Deletion of Nad_ct_OUT event", "Deletion of Surgery_TME event", "Addition of Nad_ct event", "Addition of Surgery_TME event" (Fig. 5a). These corrections result in a deviation degree of 2.70 but it's an overestimate of the real one, 1.35, that can be obtained by considering at each step of the correction algorithm both the current and the previous events, by setting $\mu1 = 1$. When considering also the previous event, the set of correction is: "Deletion of Nad_ct_OUT event", "Addition of Nad_ct event" (Fig. 5b).

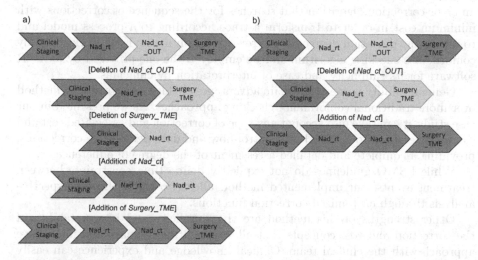

Fig. 5. Example of trace correction using a) $\mu1 = 0$ and $\mu2 = 0$, cost = 2.70; b) $\mu1 = 1$ and $\mu2 = 0$, cost = 1.35.

A previous study of conformance checking conducted on the same cohort [15] showed how a fraction of patients deviates from ESMO guidelines during their treatment pathways due to the existence of internal protocols that lead to treatment choices different from guidelines recommendations. Most of these protocols involve a boost of radiotherapy or chemotherapy, which was also confirmed by the error-correction algorithm that identified "radiotherapy dose modification" and "oxaliplatin deletion" as the most common types of corrections. However, the degree of deviation calculated for patients with these types of corrections is really low when compared to the others. In fact, during the cost definition phase, the physicians agreed on the low severity of these deviations, that are within the research protocols in use at the hospital.

The algorithm we implemented has a significant computational cost. In our case study it took 4 h to analyse the entire cohort of 1082 patients, that can be considered an affordable time for the achieved result. In order to limit the processing time the algorithm focuses only on the current not compliant event, ignoring any corrections on previous or following events. Moreover, we defined a maximum cost of 10 that works as stopping criteria: when it is achieved, the trace correction stops reporting an intermediate solution that can be further analysed by the clinical team. In our case study, the maximum cost was never reached.

4   Conclusions

Our work aimed to evaluate the degree of compliance to the ESMO guidelines for locally advanced rectal cancer treatment in a real-world cohort of patients from Fondazione Policlinico Universitario A. Gemelli IRCCS. We implemented an error-correction algorithm that searches for the sequence of corrections with minimum cost in order to transform a trace according to a process model and to return the deviation degree. The error-correction method can work with any conformance checking algorithm and we employed the one provided by pMineR software for its simplicity and ease of interpretation by clinicians.

Generalisability is one of the main advantages of this error-correcting method over more traditional conformance checking approaches. As we presented in our case study, it can take into account any type of correction and associated cost and can be generalised to include both control-flow and data perspective corrections, providing a complete and detailed assessment of the degree of adherence.

While ESMO guidelines do not explicitly define time constraints between treatment events, our implemented method allows to enable time perspective analysis through customized correction functions.

Other strengths of this method are the simplicity and interpretability of the correction and cost concepts that allow a multidisciplinary and interactive approach with the clinical team. Clinical knowledge and experience can easily be incorporated into the definition of costs for different types of corrections that are specified by physicians on the basis of severity.

One of the main limitations of this algorithm is the computational cost. It can be computationally intensive, particularly when applied to large and complex patient traces. However, in our specific case study, it was not a limitation because the patient traces were not very long. Nevertheless, the elaboration time can increase significantly as the number of events to be corrected in the traces increases and various techniques may be implemented to optimize the error-correction computation, e.g. parallel computing would allow multiple traces to be processed simultaneously.

Further studies are needed to investigate and improve the analysis with regard to:

1. The cost of any deviation from the guidelines and subsequent correction depend strongly on the type of clinical outcome being considered, the weight

of a missing surgery might be different when considering overall survival or disease free survival. As next steps, machine learning techniques can be used for automatic tuning of deviation costs in order to identify the types of deviations that impact most on specific clinical outcomes.

2. Some types of deviations, such as increasing the dose of radiotherapy or adding oxaliplatin to chemotherapy, are considered by the clinical team as positive deviations that represent an intensification of the treatment with an increased probability of favourable prognosis. Therefore, the error-correction algorithm can be modified to also accept positive deviations, i.e. improvements over guidelines recommendations.

References

1. Adriansyah, A.: Aligning observed and modeled behavior. Ph.D. thesis 1 (research TU/e/graduation TU/e), Mathematics and Computer Science (2014). https://doi.org/10.6100/IR770080
2. Damiani, A., et al.: Building an artificial intelligence laboratory based on real world data: the experience of gemelli generator. Front. Comput. Sci. **3**, 768266 (2021). https://doi.org/10.3389/fcomp.2021.768266
3. Felli, P., Gianola, A., Montali, M., Rivkin, A., Winkler, S.: Data-aware conformance checking with SMT. Inf. Syst. **117**, 102230 (2023). https://doi.org/10.1016/j.is.2023.102230
4. Fernandez-Llatas, C.: Interactive process mining in healthcare, pp. 184–200. Springer (2021)
5. Fernandez-Llatas, C., et al.: Interactive process mining in surgery with real time location systems: interactive trace correction. In: Fernandez-Llatas, C. (ed.) Interactive Process Mining in Healthcare, pp. 181–202. Springer, Cham (2021). https://doi.org/10.1007/978-3-030-53993-1_11
6. Fernández-Llatas, C., Benedi, J.M., García-Gómez, J.M., Traver, V.: Process mining for individualized behavior modeling using wireless tracking in nursing homes. Sensors **13**(11), 15434–15451 (2013). https://doi.org/10.3390/s131115434
7. Gatta, R., et al.: pMineR: an innovative R library for performing process mining in medicine. In: ten Teije, A., Popow, C., Holmes, J., Sacchi, L. (eds.) AIME 2017. LNCS, vol. 10259, pp. 351–355. Springer, Cham (2017). https://doi.org/10.1007/978-3-319-59758-4_42
8. Gatta, R., et al.: What role can process mining play in recurrent clinical guidelines issues? A position paper. Int. J. Environ. Res. Public Health **17**(18), 6616 (2020). https://doi.org/10.3390/ijerph17186616
9. Glynne-Jones, R., et al.: Rectal cancer: ESMO clinical practice guidelines for diagnosis, treatment and follow-up. Ann. Oncol. **28**, iv22–iv40 (2017). https://doi.org/10.1093/annonc/mdx224
10. Grüger, J., Geyer, T., Kuhn, M., Braun, S.A., Bergmann, R.: Weighted violations in alignment-based conformance checking. In: Montali, M., Senderovich, A., Weidlich, M. (eds.) ICPM 2022. LNBIP, vol. 468, pp. 289–301. Springer, Cham (2022). https://doi.org/10.1007/978-3-031-27815-0_21
11. Lenkowicz, J., et al.: Assessing the conformity to clinical guidelines in oncology: an example for the multidisciplinary management of locally advanced colorectal cancer treatment. Manag. Decis. **56**(10), 2172–2186 (2018). https://doi.org/10.1108/MD-09-2017-0906

12. Mannhardt, F., De Leoni, M., Reijers, H.A., Van Der Aalst, W.M.: Balanced multi-perspective checking of process conformance. Computing **98**, 407–437 (2016). https://doi.org/10.1007/s00607-015-0441-1
13. Munoz-Gama, J., et al.: Process mining for healthcare: characteristics and challenges. J. Biomed. Inform. **127**, 103994 (2022). https://doi.org/10.1016/j.jbi.2022.103994
14. Placidi, L., et al.: Process mining to optimize palliative patient flow in a high-volume radiotherapy department. Tech. Innov. Patient Support Radiat. Oncol. **17**, 32–39 (2021). https://doi.org/10.1016/j.tipsro.2021.02.005
15. Savino, M., et al.: A process mining approach for clinical guidelines compliance: real-world application in rectal cancer. Front. Oncol. **13**, 1090076 (2023). https://doi.org/10.3389/fonc.2023.1090076
16. Tavazzi, E., Gerard, C.L., Michielin, O., Wicky, A., Gatta, R., Cuendet, M.A.: A process mining approach to statistical analysis: application to a real-world advanced melanoma dataset. In: Leemans, S., Leopold, H. (eds.) ICPM 2020. LNBIP, vol. 406, pp. 291–304. Springer, Cham (2021). https://doi.org/10.1007/978-3-030-72693-5_22
17. Wilbik, A., Vanderfeesten, I., Bergmans, D., Heines, S., Turetken, O., van Mook, W.: Towards a flexible assessment of compliance with clinical protocols using fuzzy aggregation techniques. Algorithms **16**(2), 109 (2023). https://doi.org/10.3390/a16020109
18. Zhang, S., et al.: Fuzzy multi-perspective conformance checking for business processes. Appl. Soft Comput. **130**, 109710 (2022). https://doi.org/10.1016/j.asoc.2022.109710

2nd International Workshop Education Meets Process Mining (EduPM 2023)

2nd International Workshop Education meets Process Mining (EduPM 2023)

Process Mining is a powerful interdisciplinary tool to analyze and enhance processes in many fields, such as healthcare or finance. Education is no exception. Recent approaches to process mining proposed for learning analytics, curricular analytics, or MOOC analytics are just a few examples of how process mining can be used to provide insights into learning processes. However, Education as a discipline contributes to process mining by providing best practices for teaching and methodologies for creating new educational artifacts that improve teaching and assessment of process mining across a spectrum of education levels.

The International Workshop "Education meets Process Mining" aims to provide a high-quality forum for researchers, educators, and practitioners interested in the intersection of education and process mining. The interdisciplinary nature of EduPM is framed in the following two directions. Process Mining for Education (PM4Edu) is concerned with investigating how process mining techniques can be used to address some of the challenges in education. This covers process mining for learning analytics, curricular analysis, student trajectories, MOOCs, blended courses, etc. Process Mining Education (Edu4PM) is concerned with improving the teaching of process mining. This includes, among other things, new learning strategies tailored to process mining, new tools to automatically assess specific process mining topics, systematic studies on how process mining is taught in different educational programs, and new curricula on process mining.

The call for papers solicited two types of contributions: regular papers and Show&Tell submissions. Regular papers make a research contribution to one of the topics listed above. They were evaluated based on their significance, originality, technical quality, and potential to generate relevant discussion. Show&Tell submissions are non-research contributions that give authors the opportunity to present an item or initiative of interest to the EduPM community. They include experiential cases, educational resources, innovative tools, and lightning presentations of tentative or preliminary work, ideas, and collaborative opportunities.

The second edition of EduPM received 15 submissions, of which nine were regular papers and six were Show&Tell contributions. After a through review by the program committee members, four regular submissions were accepted for full-paper presentation. Additionally, after careful consideration by the workshop chairs, two Show&Tell submissions were invited for a short presentation. Below, we briefly describe the papers included in these proceedings.

The paper by Maldonado et al. explores the application of process mining techniques, specifically trace ordering for anomaly detection (TOAD) and hierarchical agglomerative trace clustering (HATC), to detect collusion in online exams. The authors also highlight the challenges and limitations of these methods, including the configuration of parameters and dealing with the lack of negative examples in the data. Preliminary results suggest that HATC might be more effective in identifying collusion clusters.

Still, a teacher-in-the-loop approach is essential to tune the parameters and interpret the results.

The paper by Rafiei et al. describes how event data derived from student exams can be used to analyze the study paths of higher education students and provide guidance for their study planning. Process and data mining techniques are used to investigate the impact that specific sequences of courses taken by students have on academic success. Based on this analysis, the authors use decision trees to generate recommendations to support students in making informed decisions about their course selection and study plans.

The paper by Potena et al. presents a case study using educational process mining techniques to analyze students' careers at an Italian university. The results reveal trends in curriculum compliance, exam patterns, and graduation times. A predictive model is used to identify critical factors that impact the students' graduation time. The insights from this approach can be used to guide educators and universities to improve the success rate of students.

Finally, the paper by Delcoucq explores how gamification, intended as the integration of game mechanisms into the practice of teaching process mining, can promote active learning and enhance the understanding of complex concepts. The paper details gamification strategies that might be useful for process mining and discusses their potential benefits and limitations.

In addition to research contributions, the workshop featured two engaging Show&Tell presentations. The first focused on the newly introduced Celonis Rising Stars Program, an online teaching initiative supporting individualized learning journeys. The second presentation issued a compelling call for cross-university curricular analysis, delving into the requirements and challenges in undertaking such a comprehensive analysis.

Finally, the workshop included a presentation by Gert Janssenswillen of the results of the brainstorming workshop on "best practices for teaching process mining", which was organized the weekend before the workshop as an activity of the Scientific Research Community on Process Mining. The talk presented the main outcome of the brainstorming, namely the design of a 'game plan' for a process mining case that should serve as a modular tool for process mining educators to design their courses. The presentation was followed by an open discussion with all workshop participants on the predicted usefulness of such a resource and the challenges it could help overcome.

We would like to thank all the members of the EduPM 2023 Program Committee for their efforts in reviewing the papers. Our sincere thanks go to all the authors and the workshop participants, who contributed with their work and the lively discussions on the workshop day. A special note of gratitude goes also to the organizing committee of ICPM 2023 for the successful edition of the conference.

November 2023

Jorge Munoz-Gama
Francesca Zerbato
Gert Janssenswillen
Wil van der Aalst

Organization

Workshop Chairs

Jorge Munoz-Gama   Pontificia Universidad Católica de Chile, Chile

Francesca Zerbato   University of St. Gallen, Switzerland

Gert Janssenswillen   Hasselt University, Belgium

Wil van der Aalst   RWTH Aachen University, Germany

Program Committee

Wil van der Aalst   RWTH Aachen University, Germany

Mitchel Brunings   Eindhoven University of Technology, The Netherlands

Andrea Burattin   Technical University of Denmark, Denmark

Daniel Calegari   Universidad de la República, Uruguay

Jerome Geyer-Klingeberg   Celonis SE, Germany

Luciano Hidalgo   Pontificia Universidad Católica de Chile, Chile

Gert Janssenswillen   Hasselt University, Belgium

Manuel Lama Penin   University of Santiago de Compostela, Spain

Sander Leemans   RWTH Aachen University, Germany

Xixi Lu   Utrecht University, The Netherlands

Niels Martin   Hasselt University, Belgium

Jorge Munoz-Gama   Pontificia Universidad Católica de Chile, Chile

Peter Reimann   University of Sydney, Australia

Manuel Resinas   University of Seville, Spain

Marcos Sepúlveda   Pontificia Universidad Católica de Chile, Chile

Pnina Soffer   University of Haifa, Israel

Emilio Sulis   University of Turin, Italy

Ernest Teniente   Universitat Politècnica de Catalunya, Spain

Boudewijn Van Dongen   Eindhoven University of Technology, The Netherlands

Francesca Zerbato   University of St. Gallen, Switzerland

Exploring Gamification in Process Mining Education: Towards a Playful and Engaging Approach

Landelin Delcoucq[✉]

University of Mons (UMONS), Mons, Belgium
landelin.delcoucq@umons.ac.be

Abstract. This article explores how gamification, i.e. the integration of game elements, of the teaching of Process Mining enhances its effectiveness. By combining traditional academic teaching with game elements, gamification stimulates student engagement, facilitates understanding of complex concepts and encourages active learning. This article defines what gamification is (what), what it can bring to the teaching of Process Mining (why), how it can be implemented (how) as well as its limitations and how its development can be envisaged based on strong theoretical concepts and data gathered from the audience concerned.

Keywords: Teaching · Gamification · Process Mining

1 Introduction

In the maze of technical subjects such as Process Mining, teaching can sometimes seem like a complex quest to capture students' attention and stimulate their desire to learn. But what if learning became as captivating as a gaming adventure? It is in this exploration of educational possibilities that gamification comes into its own, transforming concepts into challenges, courses into quests and students into enthusiastic gamers.

Teaching technical subjects related to Process Mining presents specific challenges for teachers including:

- Complexity of technical concepts: Process Mining concepts, such as algorithms, data preprocessing techniques, and visualization methods, can be complex and abstract. Teachers need to find ways to make these concepts accessible and understandable for students new to the field.
- Rapid evolution of the field: The field of Process Mining is constantly evolving, with new techniques, methods and tools emerging regularly. Teachers need to keep up to date of the latest advances and adapt to new trends to ensure the relevance and quality of their teaching.
- Accommodating different levels of competence: Students may have varying levels of competence in Process Mining techniques and tools. Teachers must adapt their teaching to take into account these differences and provide adequate support to each student, offering differentiated learning activities.

J. De Smedt and P. Soffer (Eds.): ICPM 2023 Workshops, LNBIP 503, pp. 325–335, 2024.
https://doi.org/10.1007/978-3-031-56107-8_25

- Availability of appropriate tools and data: Process mining often involves the use of specific tools and software for data analysis. Teachers must ensure that students have access to these tools and provide them with relevant data sets for their practical learning activities.
- Integrating theory and practice: Process mining is based on a solid theoretical foundation, but it is also essential to link these theoretical concepts with practical applications to help students understand how Process Mining techniques are used in real-life contexts. Teachers need to find a balance between theory and practice in their teaching.

Traditional teaching approaches, such as lectures and case studies, may not be sufficiently involving to enable a thorough understanding of Process Mining concepts. It is therefore crucial to explore new pedagogical approaches which offer a fun, interactive and practical learning experience to help students to assimilate Process Mining concepts in an effective and sustainable way.

This innovative teaching approach should involve students by making them active in their learning using interactive methods, stimulating challenges and hands-on activities that encourage students [13]. It needs to provide opportunities for active learning, where students can manipulate, solve problems, make decisions and directly experience Process Mining concepts. This is supported by the fact that they learn best when they are involved in concrete and hands-on activities [27]. Innovative teaching approaches should help students to develop the analytical skills needed to apply Process Mining techniques and should encourage collaboration between students, promoting the exchange of ideas, team problem-solving and effective communication. By adopting innovative pedagogical approaches that address these needs, teachers will facilitate students learning of Process Mining and effectively prepare them to apply these concepts in real-life situations [9].

Gamification, defined as the strategic integration of game mechanisms into non-game environments, aims to increase user engagement, motivation and participation [4]. This interactive and engaging pedagogical tool, can make a significant contribution to this innovative approach. It can be designed to be used in groups, encouraging cooperation, discussion and the sharing of knowledge. This enables students to work together, explore different perspectives and strengthen their collective understanding of Process Mining concepts. Gamified content can offer challenges that encourage students to use their analytical thinking to analyze, identify patterns, detect anomalies and draw relevant conclusions and they can be designed to represent the different stages of Process Mining, enabling students to discover and apply key concepts in a practical, tangible way.

The aim of this article is to answer the what, why and how of gamifying the teaching of Process Mining. In addition to bibliographical references, the hypotheses put forward are based on the responses of 52 bachelor's and master's students in civil engineering in computer science and management at the University of Mons who took part in gamified learning activities as well as a group of 17 students from Poznan University of Technology following a course focusing on cyber-security and Process Mining.

After this introduction, which deals with the what, this paper will be structured as follows: Sect. 2 will give a detailed presentation of the mechanics that can be used to gamify a Process Mining learning activity, with a concrete example. This section refers to the how. Section 3 looks at the theoretical benefits of using gamification to teach Process Mining. This section will answer why. In Sect. 4, we will look at the points to consider when designing a gamified activity, and discuss the main issues involved. The final section concludes the article with a look ahead.

2   Gamification Strategies for Process Mining

The aim of this section is twofold. Firstly, we will take stock of the best-known and most effective gamification methods and techniques. Secondly, these approaches will be applied concretely to the case of Process Mining. These strategies are carefully designed to optimize user engagement, motivation and learning, while facilitating a better understanding of the processes being analyzed [13].

2.1   Competitions and Rankings

The incorporation of a competitive dimension, through rankings and leaderboards, to Process Mining, arousing a desire for performance among students. Indeed, 85% of the students questioned found that competition is a source of motivation. The principles of flow theory [17] offer guidelines to balance challenges and skills, ensuring a rewarding and motivating experience. Furthermore, coopetition, by encouraging cooperation between students while maintaining friendly competition, can foster a positive and collaborative learning environment [2]. For example, each student, divided into teams, carries out process analyses. Each performed analysis is assessed in terms of the accuracy of the results, the time taken to complete them and the complexity of the problems solved. These measurable criteria help to quantify user performance. A league table can then be drawn, enabling everyone to see where they stand. An important and necessary comment on this strategy is that it is vital to ensure that the competition is not overwhelming, as it could generate anxiety or discourage some less competitive users.

2.2   Objectives and Rewards

The introduction of specific objectives and the distribution of rewards are proving to be essential elements in boosting student motivation in process analysis. By breaking down the process into achievable mini-goals, gamification creates a structure that transforms complex tasks into achievable steps. This approach [19] to self-determination theory suggests that satisfying basic psychological needs such as competence and autonomy is essential for nurturing intrinsic motivation [27]. The distribution of rewards, whether virtual (badges, points, etc.) or linked to concrete advantages (access to advanced functions, for example), further amplifies this motivating dynamic. Rewards act as positive reinforcements, strengthening the desired behaviours. For example, an objective might be to complete the analysis of notebook production processes in less than 45 min. This kind of specific objective provides students with a clear short-term direction, avoiding potential confusion and frustration.

2.3   Quests and Missions

The creation of quests and missions transforms process analysis into an interactive adventure, stimulating the exploration of various aspects of the processes. This approach can be enhanced by narrative scenarios that emotionally connect users to tasks and improve perceived relevance. Concepts [18] from experiential learning theory explain how these missions can encourage active reflection and learning, by providing a practical and engaging experience. For example, students could be asked to solve the mystery of delays in the notebook production process by collecting data, modeling the process and carrying out the analysis that identifies the critical points. These missions are based on narrative scenarios, which will be described later in this section, which add an element of intrigue and emotion to the activity, allowing users to project themselves into concrete and motivating situations.

2.4   Playful Micro-interactions

Micro-interactions are small animations, visual reactions and feedback that occur in response to the user's actions, adding a fun and interactive dimension to the whole experience. The integration of playful micro-interactions can add a touch of fun and dynamism to the user experience. These elements can increase engagement and make the overall experience more enjoyable [26]. By combining serious learning with fun elements, users are more likely to stay engaged and extend their participation over time. For example, when the user successfully completes a process analysis, a celebratory animation can be displayed, accompanied by a festive sound to reinforce a feeling of satisfaction.

2.5   Narrative Progression

By incorporating a narrative structure [28], characters and stakes, gamification can create a deeper and more meaningful context for exploring processes. Building a narrative progression involves creating a story around the process analysis. This story will therefore introduce fictional characters who interact with the processes, challenges to overcome and issues to address. The introduction of a narrative has several advantages. Firstly, it gives an emotional dimension to the activity, the emotional connection between the students and the characters/situations. This can make the teaching more immersive and stimulating, while creating a feeling of attachment to it that encourages memorisation. For example, students may be given the role of detectives tasked with solving complex process-related problems with the help of fictional characters representing one algorithm or another, or explorers navigating through uncharted territory equipped with X-OR and X-SPLIT enabling them to model the given situation. The implausibility of narrative contexts is not a hindrance, since only 16% of students pay attention to its realism.

2.6 Personalising the Experience

Integrating the personalising of the experience is a strategy that strengthens student engagement and investment in the learning activity. It does this by enabling students to shape and adapt their virtual environment according to their preferences and skills. Customization can take a number of forms. Students may be able to choose the types of quests or challenges that best match their interests. For example, an optimization-oriented user might focus on challenges related to process improvement, while another student might choose an activity related to process modeling. This approach greatly stimulates student motivation but is double-edged since, as in the example mentioned above, if it is fully applied, it does not guarantee that all students will acquire all the knowledge required. As well as a skills-based aspect, customisation can involve the visual and interactive elements of the interface. Students could be allowed to choose themes, colors and avatars that reflect their personal style. This visual customization creates a sense of ownership and identity, which can strengthen the emotional bond with the application.

3   Contribution of Gamification to Process Mining

The integration of gamification strategies in the context of Process Mining has a major impact on the teaching of the latter. This impact [4] can take the form of a significant increase in user engagement, improved learning and a deeper understanding of the subject matter. By using elements of game design, gamification can transform a potentially complex and even austere activity into a motivating and interactive experience. This section examines the positive effects of gamification and highlights the benefits observed after justifying the appropriateness of this approach to the specific characteristics of teaching of the Process Mining.

As mentioned in the introduction, the three main challenges in teaching Process Mining, which were highlighted by the students interviewed, relate to the applicative nature of the discipline (in particular the use of tools), the rapid evolution of the discipline and the technical complexity of implementing its methods. Gamification offers clear possibilities to make it easier to get to grips with the tools in a personalized way (particularly the badge system). Because they need to be renewed frequently (to maintain a level of interest), gamified activities can keep pace with developments in the discipline. When it comes to complex technical content, the use of narrative or immersive processes can offer a simplified understanding through the prism of a new point of view.

3.1 Improving Active Learning

Gamification encourages active participation of students, which considerably improves learning. Game design elements such as quests, missions and specific objectives stimulate engagement and motivate users to actively solve problems related to Process Mining. The principles of active learning theory [1] are in line with and underline the benefits of gamification for learning. This theory advocates the importance of active engagement, reflection and practical application to facilitate the acquisition of knowledge. As the section above shows, gamification encourages these three elements by encouraging students to actively solve Process Mining challenges, applying their skills and developing new concepts.

3.2 Strengthening User Engagement

One of the major contributions of gamification is to boost user engagement by integrating the elements described in the previous section. The theory of self-determination [3,5] describes, in particular, the way in which gamification reinforces students' intrinsic motivation. This theory highlights the fact that individuals are motivated primarily by three feelings: being able to act on their own (autonomy), being capable (competence) and interacting (social connection). Gamification, by offering specific challenges and objectives, gives users a degree of control over their actions, and therefore autonomy. Virtual rewards, on the other hand, reinforce the feeling of competence when users achieve their goals. Co-operation or co-operative activities offer a variety of interactions (adversaries/partners).

Another theory [22], that of the behavior of organisms, once again highlights the link between gamification and reinforcement of commitment. According to this theory, behaviors followed by positive rewards are more likely to be repeated. By incorporating reward mechanisms into gamification, users are encouraged to participate more fully in the learning activity in order to obtain these positive reinforcements.

3.3 Increasing Understanding of Processes

Gamification, by introducing the elements outlined above, can significantly enhance the understanding of processes. By offering practical scenarios to students and encouraging them to solve concrete problems, gamification adds a layer of meaning to analysis activities, making it easier to understand complex processes.

Experiential learning theory [16] supports the positive effect of gamification on the understanding of the processes studied, and therefore on the analysis that can be made of them. By offering students practical challenges, scenarios outside the conventional academic framework and specific assignments, gamification encourages learning by doing. Users gain a deeper understanding of processes by solving real-life problems rather than simply absorbing theoretical information. Even if the scenarios may seem peculiar or even totally implausible (cf. the example of the explorers navigating through uncharted territory equipped with X-OR and X-SPLIT), a real-life setting reinforces understanding.

The storytelling elements [24] of gamification can improve student engagement and understanding. The interactive approach helps students to grasp complex interactions and sequences of events within a process.

3.4 Promoting Ongoing Commitment

Gamification, by offering progression mechanisms and ongoing rewards, can keep students actively and continuously engaged [20]. Elements such as those described in the previous section encourage users to return regularly to achieve new goals and maintain their position, creating a more sustained learning experience. Students are motivated to stay in touch with the rest of the learning group or to go as far as possible in the reward system [6]. Gamification of learning activities can keep student interest high by constantly proposing new and varied challenges and diversifying the objectives to be achieved, 96% of students were more interested in the proposed learning activity than in other learning activities in the same course. These challenges, updated on a regular basis, avoid monotony and keep students alert to learning issues. In addition, anticipating new challenges stimulates long-term commitment [7].

Another aspect [15] is real-time feedback and public recognition. These two elements are of significant importance in ongoing engagement. Indeed, students are positively impacted by receiving immediate feedback on their actions and by seeing their achievements celebrated by their peers. This reinforces their sense of achievement and encourages them to continue their involvement.

4 Limitations and Points of Attention

The process of gamifying learning linked to Process Mining as described in this article nevertheless has its limitations and requires precautions to be taken on certain specific points. Therefore, this section will be divided into two parts. The first will focus on the elements of gamification on which the teacher must place particular emphasis, otherwise gamification may fail. The second will deal with the limitations of the gamification process and the situations in which it is not advisable to use it.

4.1 Points of Attention

The gamification of learning activities must be carried out in an informed way and must take into account the possible alterations to teaching associated with transforming it into the form of a game. The main concern is that students may be tempted, consciously or unconsciously, to manipulate the data in their possession, the results or the presentation of their analyses in order to gain an advantage [14]. In the test group of students selected, 78% felt that the competitive aspect of the activity was more important than its educational aspect. To avoid this problem, it is crucial that the teacher establishes clear protocols and intermediate verification stages.

Another point of attention concerns responsibility and the healthy nature of competition [23]. The aim of gamification is to create friendly competition between students but, for the same reasons as mentioned in the previous paragraph, this can become excessive and lead to some participants becoming discouraged or even dropping out. Among the panel surveyed, 12% of students felt uncomfortable with the competition at least once during the proposed learning activity. The teacher's role is to strike a balance between maintaining respect between participants and encouraging them to compete [10].

The final point concerns the conception of the activity itself and the difficulty in balancing long-term and immediate learning. Students will be tempted to work on the surface, quickly but sufficiently to obtain the reward (badge, next test, first place, etc.) to the detriment of a more in-depth and systematic approach. It is important that the teacher succeeds in instilling the idea that gamification is a pretext for learning and not an end in itself [25].

4.2   Limitations

The main objective of this article is to highlight the clear benefits of gamification of learning activities linked to Process Mining, however there are some limitations to this process:

- Objective creep [11]: If the gamification process is not properly aligned with the objectives of the learning activity, students will focus on the rewards and fun elements rather than the actual understanding and analysis of the comps. This could compromise the effectiveness of the analysis.
- Sensitivity to Individual Preferences [12]: Each student has individual preferences when it comes to the game elements that motivate them. What works for one student may not work for another. Therefore, some students may not respond positively to gamified elements, reducing their potential engagement. An alternative to this limitation is to diversify the nature of the activities on offer as much as possible.
- Temporary effects [21]: Gamification elements can lead to temporary engagement effects. Once the students have achieved all the rewards or reached the highest levels, their motivation to participate may wane. The sustainability of engagement must be carefully considered to avoid rapid decline. An important note is that this phenomenon is also present in conventional academic teaching, where motivation is linked to passing the exam and not to acquiring the desired skills.
- Visual overload [8]: Adding gamified elements such as badges, points and leaderboards can potentially create visual overload in the student interface. Too much gamified information can confuse the experience and distract users from the main objective. Even more so for students with attention deficit disorders. This aspect needs to be taken into account right from the design stage of the learning activity, in order to offer a visually coherent package.

- Maintenance and evolution [12]: Gamification requires ongoing maintenance to remain effective and attractive. Gamified elements should be updated regularly to avoid stagnation and obsolescence. In addition, it's important to plan the evolution of gamification in line with the changing needs of students and the objectives of the learning activity.
- Cognitive overload [8]: Excessive use of gamification elements can potentially lead to cognitive overload for students. Too much information, rewards and notifications can make the experience confusing and distract students from the main objective of analyzing processes. A balanced, minimalist design is essential to avoid this overload.

5   Conclusion and Perspectives

In this article, we have shown that gamification is an effective and relevant solution for revitalizing the teaching of technical subjects, particularly Process Mining, and stimulating active learning. The innovative pedagogical approach described is a combination of playful elements and classic academic concepts of transmissive teaching. It offers a new dimension to education, transforming classrooms into captivating educational playgrounds. Gamification provides a new way of overcoming the traditional challenges of teaching Process Mining, by appealing to students' natural curiosity and encouraging them to explore, experiment and collaborate. By focusing on active learning and active participation, gamification bridges the gap between theory and practice, creating a more immersive and rewarding educational experience.

However, it is essential to bear in mind that gamification is not the ultimate solution and is far from being a turnkey solution. PRecaution, consideration and long-term design are necessary and vital to avoid potential pitfalls such as discouragement, diversion from initial objectives, dependence on achievement marks or student confusion. In addition, a personalised approach that takes account of students' individual preferences can maximise the effectiveness of gamification.

The stated aim of this article was to answer the three questions about gamification: what, why and how. The first question was addressed by referring to the existing literature and clearly defining the concepts involved. The second question was addressed by highlighting five major aspects of teaching for which gamification provides a new and effective solution. This new and effective solution translates into the implementation of how-to methods, which answers the third question. These methods, which have been theorised and tested in numerous learning contexts, are clearly described and illustrated in the field of Process Mining.

The perspectives for gamification in the teaching of Process Mining are twofold. Firstly, there are currently no independent gamification tools (online games, board games, card games, etc.) developed for the exclusive and specific use of Process Mining teaching. Secondly, one of the aspects of gamification is the personalization of learning paths. In this area, Process Mining allows the learner to act as a disciple in his own right, and thus participate in the gamification process.

Finally, gamification does not and will never replace teaching expertise. It should be seen as an effective way of captivating and motivating learners. The thoughtful integration of gamification into mainstream academic teaching will enable teachers to produce generations of Process Mining experts who are motivated, curious and well prepared for the ever-changing realities of technology.

References

1. Bonwell, C.C., Eison, J.A.: Active learning: creating excitement in the classroom. 1991 ASHE-ERIC higher education reports. ERIC (1991)
2. Csikszentmihalyi, M., Abuhamdeh, S., Nakamura, J.: Flow. In: Csikszentmihalyi, M. (ed.) Flow and the Foundations of Positive Psychology, pp. 227–238. Springer, Dordrecht (2014). https://doi.org/10.1007/978-94-017-9088-8_15
3. Deci, E.L., Ryan, R.M.: Self-determination theory: a macrotheory of human motivation, development, and health. Can. Psychol. **49**(3), 182 (2008)
4. Deterding, S., Dixon, D., Khaled, R., Nacke, L.: From game design elements to gamefulness: defining "gamification". In: Proceedings of the 15th International Academic MindTrek Conference: Envisioning Future Media Environments, pp. 9–15 (2011)
5. Gagne, M., Chemolli, E., Forest, J.: Les méthodologies associées à la théorie de l'autodétermination/methodologies associated with the theory of self-determination. In: La théorie de l'autodétermination: Aspects théoriques et appliqués/The Theory of Self-Determination: Theoretical and Applied Aspects, pp. 33–58. De Boeck Superieur (2016)
6. Hamari, J.: Do badges increase user activity? A field experiment on the effects of gamification. Comput. Hum. Behav. **71**, 469–478 (2017)
7. Huang, B., Hew, K.F., Lo, C.K.: Investigating the effects of gamification-enhanced flipped learning on undergraduate students' behavioral and cognitive engagement. Interact. Learn. Environ. **27**(8), 1106–1126 (2019)
8. Huber, M.Z., Hilty, L.M.: Gamification and sustainable consumption: overcoming the limitations of persuasive technologies. In: Hilty, L.M., Aebischer, B. (eds.) ICT Innovations for Sustainability. AISC, vol. 310, pp. 367–385. Springer, Cham (2015). https://doi.org/10.1007/978-3-319-09228-7_22
9. Ke, F.: A qualitative meta-analysis of computer games as learning tools. In: Handbook of Research on Effective Electronic Gaming in Education, pp. 1–32 (2009)
10. Kim, T.W., Werbach, K.: More than just a game: ethical issues in gamification. Ethics Inf. Technol. **18**(2), 157–173 (2016)
11. Klein, G.: Viewing gamification design limitations and weaknesses through a pandemic lens. Societies **11**(4), 137 (2021)
12. Landsell, J., Hägglund, E.: Towards a gamification framework: limitations and opportunities when gamifying business processes (2016)
13. Malone, T.W., Lepper, M.R.: Making learning fun: a taxonomy of intrinsic motivations for learning. In: Aptitude, Learning, and Instruction, pp. 223–254. Routledge (2021)
14. Marczewski, A.: The ethics of gamification. XRDS: Crossroads ACM Mag. Stud. **24**(1), 56–59 (2017)
15. Mazarakis, A.: Using gamification for technology enhanced learning: the case of feedback mechanisms. Bull. IEEE Tech. Committee Learn. Technol. **4**(17), 6–9 (2015)

16. McCarthy, M., et al.: Experiential learning theory: from theory to practice. J. Bus. Econ. Res. (JBER) **8**(5) (2010)
17. Nakamura, J., Csikszentmihalyi, M.: Flow theory and research. In: Handbook of Positive Psychology, vol. 195, p. 206 (2009)
18. Nikitina, K.: Educational game analysis using intention and process mining. In: CEUR Workshop Proceedings, pp. 117–125 (2020)
19. Ryan, R.M., Deci, E.L.: Intrinsic and extrinsic motivations: classic definitions and new directions. Contemp. Educ. Psychol. **25**(1), 54–67 (2000)
20. Sailer, M., Hense, J.U., Mayr, S.K., Mandl, H.: How gamification motivates: an experimental study of the effects of specific game design elements on psychological need satisfaction. Comput. Hum. Behav. **69**, 371–380 (2017)
21. Sánchez-Mena, A., Martí-Parreño, J.: Gamification in higher education: teachers' drivers and barriers. In: Proceedings of the International Conference the Future of Education, pp. 180–184 (2016)
22. Skinner, B.F.: The Behavior of Organisms: An Experimental Analysis. BF Skinner Foundation (2019)
23. Thorpe, A.S., Roper, S.: The ethics of gamification in a marketing context. J. Bus. Ethics **155**, 597–609 (2019)
24. Tondello, G.F., Mora, A., Marczewski, A., Nacke, L.E.: Empirical validation of the gamification user types hexad scale in English and Spanish. Int. J. Hum Comput Stud. **127**, 95–111 (2019)
25. Versteeg, M., et al.: Ethics & Gamification design: a moral framework for taking responsibility. Master's thesis (2013)
26. Werbach, K., Hunter, D., Dixon, W.: For the Win: How Game Thinking Can Revolutionize Your Business, vol. 1. Wharton Digital Press, Philadelphia (2012)
27. Wouters, P., Van Nimwegen, C., Van Oostendorp, H., Van Der Spek, E.D.: A meta-analysis of the cognitive and motivational effects of serious games. J. Educ. Psychol. **105**(2), 249 (2013)
28. Zichermann, G., Cunningham, C.: Gamification by Design: Implementing Game Mechanics in Web and Mobile Apps. O'Reilly Media Inc., Sebastopol (2011)

Process Mining Techniques for Collusion Detection in Online Exams

Andrea Maldonado[1,2]([⊠]), Ludwig Zellner[1]([⊠]), Sven Strickroth[1],
and Thomas Seidl[1,2]

[1] Ludwig-Maximilians-Universität München, Munich, Germany
{maldonado,zellner,seidl}@dbs.ifi.lmu.de, sven.strickroth@ifi.lmu.de
[2] Munich Center for Machine Learning (MCML), Munich, Germany

Abstract. Honesty and fairness are essential. As many skills, practicing those values starts in the classroom. Whether students are examined online or on-site, only testing their knowledge righteously, educators can assess their skills and room for improvement. As online exams increase, we are provided with more suitable data for analysis. Process mining methods as anomaly detection and trace clustering techniques have been used to identify dishonest behavior in other fields, as e.g. fraud detection. In this paper, we investigate collusion detection in online exams as a process mining task. We explore trace ordering for anomaly detection (TOAD) as well as hierarchical agglomerative trace clustering (HATC). Promising preliminary results exemplify, how process mining techniques empower teachers in their decision making, while via flexible configuration of parameters, leaves the last word to them.

Keywords: Collusion Detection · Hierarchical Agglomerative Clustering · Positive Unlabeled Data · Teacher in the Loop

1 Introduction

The COVID-19 pandemic forced many activities to conform to social distancing. This included teaching and studying in the academic area. Along with it came the examination of course material. Due to the new examination environment, forms of cheating increased, especially regarding collusion between students [31]. Different types of dishonesty in the academic community are defined by Fraser [13]: Sometimes cooperation is tolerated in some contexts as students benefit intellectually from working together. However, colluding in the context of students' individual examinations is certainly not allowed and can be seen as a form of plagiarism. The author does not mention contract cheating which also gained popularity in the last years [30]. Furthermore, "abusing" AI technologies such as ChatGPT is also a current issue. With this work, we want to advance research to support teachers in detecting collusion in the context of online exams. Thus, we limit the scope of this work to this type of dishonesty.

A. Maldonado and L. Zellner—Equal contribution.

J. De Smedt and P. Soffer (Eds.): ICPM 2023 Workshops, LNBIP 503, pp. 336–348, 2024.
https://doi.org/10.1007/978-3-031-56107-8_26

As technology advances, it has become easier for students to cheat by copying and pasting content from the internet or their peers. This undermines the integrity of the academic system and reduces the effectiveness of assessing students' knowledge and skills. Teachers are hardly able to proctor online exams. While attempting to prevent dishonesty, teachers must balance their strategy against limiting possibilities for students to solve an exam effectively, respecting students' right to privacy at home and data analysis in the light of the data protection legislation [3]. Nevertheless, illegal collusion in an exam can be pursued retrospectively because online exams yield the potential of logging a student's answering process. Online exams are carried out using specialized e-assessment systems or customized Learning Management Systems such as Moodle [26]. There are several properties that such systems need to fulfill for an exam (This list is non exhaustive but tailored for this work): Primarily, they need to store the answers for each assignment in a safe way. For contestation protection also intermediate responses with timestamps for each user need to be stored. What is logged highly depends on the used tool and the freedoms a tool offers, such as opening several assignments in tabs in parallel or enforcing a sequential order. There are many different kinds of actions by students, that can be recorded, but only some are essential for such an analysis. This minimalist set of an entry comprises the submission of a task with a student id, a task label, and an associated timestamp. Therefore, this work relies on this minimalist set of data. Certainly, *Process Mining* provides great means to analyze and evaluate this type of data, as it resembles the fundamental data structure utilized in this research area.

We class this work among *positive unlabeled learning*. In this type of binary classification task, negative examples are missing, and access to positive or labeled data [5] is scarce. In the context of collusion detection, this means that a few colluding students have already been detected by a teacher, but proper data, with which we can conclude that a student did not collude, does not exist. In our specific case, this stems from the fact that submissions that are equal to a sample solution and, thus, yield the maximum score does not exhibit clear collusion characteristics. It also brings up the question of what these characteristics may be. In any case, we cannot and do not want to replace teachers with our work but enhance and support them with adequate semi-automated methods and rely on appropriately set parameters that require a knowledgeable user, i.e., a teacher, in the loop.

The contributions of this work are as follows: We frame collusion detection in online exams as a process mining task (1). In this context, we explore techniques and configuration parameters for trace clustering and anomaly detection methods (2). We present preliminary results and discuss the advantages and disadvantages of this framing and challenges for evaluation of the exam collusion detection problem (3).

In Sect. 2, we discuss publications that already address collusion detection and put our work into context. Section 3 defines the aforementioned minimal data requirements and knowledge of applied methods. How a micro-cluster detection method, namely TOAD, and trace clustering can be applied for collusion detection is explained in Sect. 4. Section 5 comprises the applicability and restrictions of our work. We conclude with Sect. 6 and give a prospect regarding potential in future work.

2   Related Work

Since 2007, first methods to analyze logs in the educational area have been systematically mentioned in the context of respective conferences [24]. Bogarín et al. [6] summarized first approaches, introduced *Educational Process Mining (EPM)* and differentiated between discovery and conformance checking techniques. Putting our goal and work into context, this would correspond to conformance checking in a computer-based assessment, whereas conformance follows a different track in comparison to its traditional meaning.

As EDM (Educational Data Mining) and LA (Learning Analytics) have gained increasing attention since 2006 [24] and produce highly usable data for EPM, a fusion of both areas stands to reason. *Process Mining*-based approaches have been used to support learning platforms and improve the quality of university education: Hobeck et al. [16] conducted a case study which demonstrated the potential to translate student trajectories into curriculum recommendations. Fortenbacher et al. [12] created LeMo, a tool on a meta-level which supports teachers in analyzing user behavior, which focused on user-paths in learning platforms. A similar approach was presented by Hidalgo and Munoz-Gama [15], where the authors applied event-abstraction techniques to understand behavioral dynamics of learners in Massive Open Online Courses (MOOCs). Wagner et al. [29] studied planning and monitoring with a combination of rule-based support and process mining techniques. Umer et al. [28] also combined machine learning with process mining techniques. In aformentioned works, the common goal is to improve students learning experience in MOOCs. Additionally, Rohani et al. [23] employed a method developed by Matcha et al. [21] discovering student's learning strategies in a online visual programming course. While there are many approaches to extract supportive information for teachers and students to extend their knowledge and subsequently improve course design, another important area is the detection of student's behavioral patterns, especially in exams. Bala et al. [2] pursued this goal and focus on open-questioned examinations, aiming to discover correlations between the extracted patterns and final grades. A related field where also exam-based behavioral patterns are used is the detection of collusion in online exams.

Exam collusion detection became particularly popular with the COVID-19 pandemic, where often unproctored exams needed to be conducted. In related research there are approaches that do not collect data during exams. Instead, they compare the achieved score of an exam to the previous academic achievements or other previously collected data and find outliers using a regression model (e. g., [9,10,14]). An overview over statistical strategies to detect impersonation and prohibited communication between students is given by Küppers et al. [19]. They differentiate between in-situ and a-posteriori analysis detection. For the former some software for proctoring or locking down the computers during the exam phase has to be installed on the students computer. The latter can be indicated by using *Process Mining* techniques. They confirm our point of view that many methods can only be used for an indication of collusion but not to prove it automatically.

Student behavior for collusion detection, on which we rely in this work, is used in the following two works: Cleophas et al. [8] analyzed a two-fold approach. First, they introduce Jaccard similarity in essay-style answers given in the exam and evaluate them in heat maps. Secondly, similar to our work, they proposed a metric called *Average Absolute Deviation (AAD)* to identify when two students have worked on the same task in a specific time frame for the first time logging the starting and the end time of it. The main problem with AAD is that even if the AAD is relatively high, collusion could still have taken place.

Langerbein et al. [20] proposed to use a hierarchical clustering approach with calculating a similarity based on the achieved points in the same assignment and the number of times two students submitted their solution within the very same one-minute-interval. A one-minute-interval is obtained by dividing the 70 min exam into 70 intervals. This procedure poses the problem that students could have colluded but, by chance, do not fall within the same one-minute-interval. Therefore, these students will not be detected. Oppositely, in our work, we use configurable time windows, which are not discretized. Furthermore, Becker and Meng [4] utilized matrix multiplication to detect similarities between test takers. In contrast to our approach, they do not use time to validate their results, which may lead to uncertainties in multiple cases.

Ingrisone and Ingrisone [18] examine hierarchical agglomerative clustering (HAC) in respect of its applicability to detect collusion in online exams. They use *Gower's similarity coefficient* as a distance metric from [11] and automatically divide their test set into two clusters, namely collusion and non-collusion. As Küppers et al. [19] found out, the challenge is that cheating attempts depend on various factors and can only be indicated. A final decision has to be made by the teacher and should not be assessed automatically.

3   Preliminaries

3.1   Event Logs

In process mining, an event log L is a data set consisting of multiple events. An event is the smallest unit of an event log. It describes the execution of an activity in a process. An *event* has three minimal components: case id c, activity id a and timestamp t, usually expressed as $e = (c, a, t)$. The *case id* c is used to identify which execution this event belongs to. An *activity id* a of an event describes the activity executed at this event. Frequently, a case consists of different activities. The *timestamp* t of an event tells the execution time of this event. A trace is an ordered collection of multiple events which records one execution instance of a process. We denote a trace as $c = \langle e_1, ..., e_n \rangle$, where $\#_{case}(e) := c$, $\#_{act}(e) := a$ and $\#_{time}(e) := t$, as in [17].

3.2   Process Mining Tasks

Trace Ordering for Anomaly Detection (TOAD). The idea behind Trace Ordering for Anomaly Detection [22] is to find micro-clusters in subspaces of temporal activity relations based on density. By computing temporal deviation signatures for each activity relation in a case and applying a density-based clustering method, here OPTICS [1], the authors identify and visualize micro-cluster of traces with higher relative density as anomalies, as shown in Fig. 1.

While the majority of non-deviating traces assembles a large shallow trough, collective anomalies present as deep indentations to the otherwise smooth baseline. The more similar a set of traces is, the denser is the cluster and thus the deeper the trough in the plot. Regarding parameters, TOAD relies mainly on the minimum number of points for a neighborhood $MinPts$. It controls the granularity of the plot, determining the trace ordering. A higher value increases the smoothness.

Hierarchical Agglomerative Trace Clustering (HATC). Hierarchical agglomerative clustering (HAC) [18] gradually generates clusters by merging nearest objects, so that smaller clusters are merged into large ones. In trace clustering approaches [25] observations to be clustered correspond to event log traces. Thus, in this work we focus on Hierarchical Agglomerative Trace Clustering. Usually, HATC results show the hierarchy of the clusters in dendrograms, as shown in Fig. 2. To measure the proximity between two observations, HATC requires the definition of a *distance metric*. Standard distances, like values difference, can asses the dissimilarity using subtraction for continuous variables e.g. timestamps. We aggregate distances over all tasks to compare submissions.

To regard different types of variables, as e.g. categorical and continuous we use composite distance metric. Next, we need to choose a *clustering method* determining how two clusters, i.e., observations will be compared. E.g. single-link compares two clusters using the smallest minimum pairwise distance. Other options include complete-link, average-link and Ward's method. Finally, we choose a *threshold*, by which the "dendrogram is cut" horizontally and a number of clusters emerge from the structure.

4   Exam Collusion as a Process Mining Task

4.1   Mapping Online Exam Data to Event-Logs

The data originates from an exam of an introductory programming course, in which students had to work on fill-in-the-gap assignments, single-response and multiple-response questions. Usually, exams contain multiple task groups, which contain multiple singular tasks. We focus on singular tasks. During that exam the GATE system [27] stores the current response for an task, when students explicitly click on the "submit" button. Then, the students' inputs are stored as the current response together with meta-data such as user ID, task ID, and timestamp. These entries are highly suitable to be represented as events in process mining tasks. We note that responses can be submitted multiple times for a single task by a single user, either to update the response or to save it again. Furthermore, tasks can be submitted in any order. We denote the submission for one exam by one student as $c = \langle e_1, ..., e_n \rangle$.

For the rest of this work: User ID, as *case id*, identifies the user, who submits a certain response. Task ID, as *activity id*, maps a response to its corresponding task. Both elements are associated with a submission timestamp and may also be associated with additional attributes, denoted as $\#_{add}(e)) := r$, e.g. achieved points, current response, task group id.

4.2 Mapping Collusion Detection to Process Mining Tasks

Colluding groups of students present in data as collective anomalous behavior [7], where such certain traces are similar to each other and dissimilar to the rest. In order to grasp similarity between submissions, we focus on both temporal and textual distances between events.

TOAD [22]. Building on the trace notion, presented in Sect. 3.1, we describe a trace in terms of its activities and duration between their corresponding events as follows: $c{:}\#_{act}(e_0) \xrightarrow{\#_{time}(e_1) - \#_{time}(e_0)} \#_{act}(e_1) \cdots \#_{act}(e_{n-1}) \xrightarrow{\#_{time}(e_n) - \#_{time}(e_{n-1})} \#_{act}(e_n)$.

For example, in an exam which contains three tasks a, b, and c, two students would be represented by traces $U_1 : a \xrightarrow{5} b \xrightarrow{7} c \xrightarrow{5} a \xrightarrow{2} b \xrightarrow{2} c$ and $U_2 : b \xrightarrow{10} a \xrightarrow{2} b \xrightarrow{3} c \xrightarrow{2} a \xrightarrow{2} b \xrightarrow{2} c$. Student U_1 submits a response for task a first and takes 5 time units to submit a response for task b afterwards. Using TOAD in the domain of collusion detection in online exams, the parameter $MinPts$ is directly linked to the minimum number of students expected in a collusion group. As this is subject specific, it is essential for the teacher to set this parameter to a suitable value. E.g. $MinPts = 3$ means that the smallest collusion group is expected to have at least three members.

HATC. To use HATC for collusion detection in online exams, we define a *time-based distance* metric as follows. Similarly to the trace notion, presented in Sect. 3.1, we denote the descriptor for a task response submission $c_a : ((\#_{time}(e_i), \#_{add}(e_i)), ...(\#_{time}(e_j), \#_{add}(e_i)))$, where $\#_{case}(e_i) = \#_{case}(e_j) = c$ and $\#_{act}(e_i) = \#_{act}(e_j) = a$. $\#_{add}(e_i))$ denotes a submission associated additional attribute. For example, comparison of task b between two students U_1 and U_2 would be represented by: $U_{1,b} : ((5, \text{"ABC"}), (19, \text{"AX"}))$ and $U_{2,b} : ((0, \text{"ABC"}), (12, \text{"DEF"}), (19, \text{"AX"}))$ Comparing each set of pairs, here six pairs, we compute similarity distances for each submission between students and choose the minimum distance of all pairs to represent the distance between two task submissions, here $(U_{1,b} : (19, \text{"AX"})$ and

$U_{2,b}$: (19, "AX")). Next, the teacher chooses a time window e.g. 1 time unit, which is used as a threshold. If the time minimal difference for an task between students is within that time window, e.g. 60 s, the distance for that task is 0, otherwise 1. We aggregate these results for all tasks for one pair of students, and define this as their time-based distance. By taking additional attributes into account, we enhance the time-based distance to be more strict and specific. In this case, we denote it *strict-distance*. We use the time-based result and multiply it by 0 if the value for a certain additional attribute is the same or by 1 if not. Thus, we give more weight to textual overlap.

Consistent similar task submissions from different students are indicators of collusion. To find such groups of students, whose submissions are consistently most similar to each other, we use single-link as a linkage criterion for the clustering method. Single-link compares two clusters using the smallest minimum pairwise distance. Note that pairwise here refers to pairs of students over all tasks. Finally, the teacher sets a suitable threshold value in relation to the reachability distance in the dendrogram to identify potential collusion groups. Note that on the one hand, if the value is too high, all students will be grouped to the same cluster. On the other hand, if the value is too low, even collusion between students with very similar distance results will not be identified.

Ideally, by observing the dendrogram, the teacher is able to identify a big leap in the reachability distance on the y-axis and use it as a preliminary threshold. It is possible for the teachers to adjust this parameter as it seems suitable for their specific case.

5   Preliminary Results and Discussion

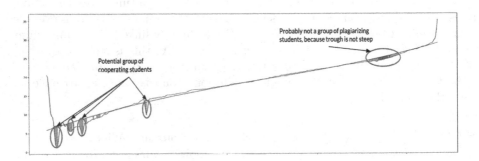

Fig. 1. Preliminary results for TOAD with a reasonable amount of $MinPts = 3$ (find a group of at least 3 students). The x-axis shows student ids and the y-axis represents the reachability distance.

This work examines the applicability of two different process mining approaches, namely TOAD and a variant of HATC, to event log data. The corresponding code base is accessible on GitHub.[1] focuses on detecting groups of colluding

---

[1] https://github.com/lmu-dbs/collusion_det_on_exams.

students. The former approach, *time-based*, is purely based on time information, and the latter, *strict* combines time and text similarity in a distance metric. Our work reveals advantages and limitations in a setting, where minimal information is available. This way it can be applied in a wide range of contexts. Following, we present preliminary experiments and results.

5.1 Preliminary Experiments and Results

A) The dataset in this work only consists of students who have consented to be protocolled. *B)* Furthermore, *groundtruth* comprises students, who have been validated by the teacher as colluding and confessed to collusion after inquiring. To clarify the terminology for the upcoming section, we define the set of true positives (TP) as detected students who exist in the groundtruth, false positives (FP) as detected students who do not exist in the groundtruth, true negatives (TN) as undetected students which do not exist in the groundtruth and false negatives (FN) as undetected students which exist in the groundtruth. The latter three terms must be considered in the context of positive unlabeled data, because of *A)* and *B)*. This highlights the importance of the *teacher in the loop*, further discussed in Sect. 5.2. We execute our experiments on a PC with an Intel i7-8600 CPU and 32 GB RAM.

The application of TOAD, i.e., an anomaly detection method that relies on time data, results in a reachability plot (s. Fig. 1). The interpretation of this plot is essential to decide whether a group of students has been cheating. As this method orders students by their reachability regarding time differences, we are searching for steep but small troughs at the left and right margins of the plot. Wide and flat troughs would represent the main behavior of many students and, hence, do not filter small, cooperating groups. We observe that there are three corresponding troughs on the left-hand side of the plot and a more central one. Unfortunately, this result only shows a minor overlap with the groundtruth consisting of 29 students. We detect 28 students from which only 38 % coincide with the groundtruth (TP). Please note that we deal with positive unlabeled data meaning that there may be cooperations between students that have not been recorded on the groundtruth and that negative examples cannot be labeled. Even so, this method is highly applicable regarding execution time since one run takes approximately 1.5 s.

Applying HATC yields a more promising result. It is important to mention that the number of parameters to be set is higher with this approach (s. Sect. 4.2). Our experimental settings comprise many variants of these parameters, and we show an excerpt of the most insightful outcomes. Values on the vertical axis represent the distance value between submissions on the horizontal axis. Figure 2a shows a variant with strict distance representing equality of a student's input at an assignment combined with a time window of 60 s in which two students have to submit a specific assignment to the GATE system. We visually analyze the resulting dendrogram, as in [20], and set the distance threshold at the position that yields the highest difference to the next distance, i.e., at 13. Compared to Fig. 2b, we use time-based distance only (excluding a student's input) and a time window of three minutes. Since distance continuously decreases in the dendrogram, we set the distance threshold at an equal level, 13. Every student pair that yields a distance lower than the given threshold is considered for potential collusion. Please note, that the threshold is set by the teacher and can be adapted.

With the first setting, we get 11 TP, and the second setting yields 23 TP. It seems that the second setting outperforms the first, but it is obvious that there is a high difference in recall. The second experiment yields a total number of 279 detected students (including TP and FP), which is certainly not justifiable, whereas the first experiment yields 34 detected students. We want to emphasize that in addition to the eleven true positives, we reexamined our results with the lecturer, from whom we obtained the data. We verified that this approach detected twelve additional colluding students, which yields 23 TP in total for 34 detected students. For this approach, one execution takes 4 s. Please note that the preprocessing step, in this case, took approximately 3 h and was conducted over night.

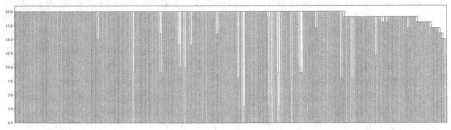

(a) HATC dendrogram using a strict distance, and time window of 60 sec.

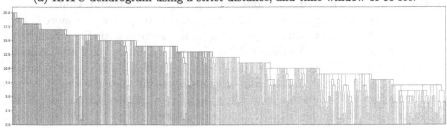

(b) HATC dendrogram using time-based distance, and time window of 180 sec.

Fig. 2. HATC dendrogram using single-link clustering strategy.

5.2   Evaluation Challenges and Opportunities

Ethical Considerations and Boundary Conditions. The evaluation of a detection system indicating collusion poses some significant problems. For instance, there may be concerns regarding student data privacy or even false accusations of collusion. To ensure that data privacy is not violated, students must be asked for consent to use traces, produced during the exam, for developing such systems.

Furthermore, the risk of accusing somebody falsely and the consequences of that should play an essential role in an a-posteriori decision. Therefore, the final decision should and can only be made by the corresponding teacher, who has to analyze the results of a collusion detection method. The method itself should only be seen as a tool making suggestions based on indicators when these indicators strongly depend on the parameter values given by the teacher. Thus, a workflow where the system relies on a *teacher in the loop* is not to be understood as a disadvantage but as an essential improvement for the task at hand.

The approaches we analyze presume some conditions to be fulfilled. First and foremost, at least the colluding students must be contained in the dataset because the method relies on pairwise comparison. This is not easy to achieve since not every student agrees with being observed and recorded. Moreover, the quality of the outcome is limited by the number of tasks in which the candidates cooperated. Less collusion leads to a higher distance, possibly resulting in a higher distance not satisfying the given threshold. Then again, the concept of a *teacher in the loop* proves advantageous because the resulting dendrogram indicates collusion by providing distances. Hence, a teacher may successively inspect students with an increasing distance up to the point where the content or time-based similarity differs widely.

Technical Evaluation. To facilitate aforementioned analysis an approach should consist of an intuitive visualization. Thereby, teachers are able to get a quick and overarching understanding of the current status and can react accordingly. This visualization is based on the findings after applying the approach. These findings, again, depend on the parameter configurations the teacher is making. Hence, the method itself has to be highly transparent and comprehensible.

Another critical aspect is that a method in this context has to operate on positive unlabeled data. The more similar a student's solution is to a sample solution, the more difficult it gets to prove a potential collusion because, at least regarding the content of a submission, it can not be differentiated between well-prepared and colluding students. We derive from this fact that a validating instance is of the essence here. However, timestamps can be used in any case, whereby our approach can still be applied but without the textual input as a resource. Beyond that, it is possible to include many other attributes dependent on the logging system.

Overall, both analyzed approaches possess advantages and drawbacks. TOAD, for example, is faster in its execution when HATC requires three hours of pre-processing in our case, albeit this still is not a critical duration. Additionally, HATC provides the teacher with much more flexibility regarding the configuration. Furthermore, it is a comprehensible method because of its simplicity. HATC proves to be more suitable for our case.

6   Conclusion

In this work, we analyzed two approaches to detect student collusion in online exams in the context of process mining and experimented on a real-world dataset. Tested approaches comprise TOAD and HATC in a collection of parameter varieties, including pure time-based distances, as well as stricter composite distance metrics.

Given the diversity of examination procedures and assignments, as well as considering the severity of a collusion accusation, teachers need to understand and configure parameter values for their specific case. For instance, not all assignments require the same time amount or can vary across different students [20]. Thus, explainable parameters are key, and the lack thereof puts TOAD in the rear. HATC, with very strict parameter settings, prevents teachers from false accusations since it proposes collusion groups with a high cluster confidence. Our work exemplifies the great potential of applying Educational Process Mining.

Despite already promising results, we plan on exploring different datasets and further configurations in experiments thoroughly. Specially, we plan to investigate further a possible differentiation of parameter importance. Additionally, due to the lack of true labels, i.e., positive unlabeled data, open challenges for training and validation remain. Finally, since the concept of a *teacher in the loop* is essential, the investigation of this problem in the context of Active Learning stands to reason.

References

1. Ankerst, M., Breunig, M.M., Kriegel, H.P., Sander, J.: OPTICS: ordering points to identify the clustering structure. ACM SIGMOD Rec. **28**(2), 49–60 (1999)
2. Bala, S., Revoredo, K., Mendling, J.: Process mining for analyzing open questions computer-aided examinations. In: Montali, M., Senderovich, A., Weidlich, M. (eds.) ICPM 2022. LNBIP, vol. 468, pp. 565–576. Springer, Cham (2022). https://doi.org/10.1007/978-3-031-27815-0_41
3. Barrio, F.: Legal and pedagogical issues with online exam proctoring. Eur. J. Law Technol. **13**(1) (2022)
4. Becker, K., Meng, H.: Identifying statistically actionable collusion in remote proctored exams. J. Appl. Test. Technol. **23**, 54–61 (2022)
5. Bekker, J., Davis, J.: Learning from positive and unlabeled data: a survey. Mach. Learn. **109**, 719–760 (2020)
6. Bogarín, A., Cerezo, R., Romero, C.: A survey on educational process mining. Wiley Interdisc. Rev. DMKD **8**(1), e1230 (2018)
7. Chandola, V., Banerjee, A., Kumar, V.: Anomaly detection: a survey. ACM Comput. Surv. (CSUR) **41**(3), 1–58 (2009)
8. Cleophas, C., Hönnige, C., Meisel, F., Meyer, P.: Who's cheating? Mining patterns of collusion from text and events in online exams. INFORMS Trans. Educ. **23**(2), 84–94 (2023). https://doi.org/10.1287/ited.2021.0260
9. D'Souza, K.A., Siegfeldt, D.V.: A conceptual framework for detecting cheating in online and take-home exams. Decis. Sci. J. Innov. Educ. **15**(4), 370–391 (2017). https://doi.org/10.1111/dsji.12140

10. Fask, A., Englander, F., Wang, Z.: On the integrity of online testing for introductory statistics courses: a latent variable approach. PARE **20**(1), n10 (2015)
11. Finch, H.: Comparison of distance measures in cluster analysis with dichotomous data. J. Data Sci. **3**(1), 85–100 (2005)
12. Fortenbacher, A., et al.: LeMo: a learning analytics application focussing on user path analysis and interactive visualization. In: Proceedings of the IDAACS, vol. 2 (2013)
13. Fraser, R.: Collaboration, collusion and plagiarism in computer science coursework. Inform. Educ. Int. J. **13**(2), 179–195 (2014)
14. Harmon, O.R., Lambrinos, J.: Are online exams an invitation to cheat? J. Econ. Educ. **39**(2), 116–125 (2008). https://doi.org/10.3200/jece.39.2.116-125
15. Hidalgo, L., Munoz-Gama, J.: Domain-driven event abstraction framework for learning dynamics in MOOCs sessions. In: Montali, M., Senderovich, A., Weidlich, M. (eds.) ICPM 2022. LNBIP, vol. 468, pp. 552–564. Springer, Cham (2022). https://doi.org/10.1007/978-3-031-27815-0_40
16. Hobeck, R., Pufahl, L., Weber, I.: Process mining on curriculum-based study data: a case study at a German university. In: Montali, M., Senderovich, A., Weidlich, M. (eds.) ICPM 2022. LNBIP, vol. 468, pp. 577–589. Springer, Cham (2022). https://doi.org/10.1007/978-3-031-27815-0_42
17. Huser, V.: Process mining: discovery, conformance and enhancement of business processes (2012)
18. Ingrisone, S.J., Ingrisone, J.N.: Hierarchical agglomerative clustering to detect test collusion on computer-based tests. EM:IP **42**(3), 39–49 (2023)
19. Küppers, B., Opgen-Rhein, J., Eifert, T., Schroeder, U.: Cheating detection: identifying fraud in digital exams. Eur. J. High. Educ. IT (2019)
20. Langerbein, J., et al.: A data mining approach for detecting collusion in unproctored online exams. In: Proceedings of the EDM (2023)
21. Matcha, W., Gašević, D., Uzir, N.A., Jovanović, J., Pardo, A.: Analytics of learning strategies: associations with academic performance and feedback. In: LAK (2019)
22. Richter, F., Lu, Y., Zellner, I., Sontheim, J., Seidl, T.: TOAD: trace ordering for anomaly detection. In: Proceedings of the ICPM. IEEE (2020)
23. Rohani, N., Gal, K., Gallagher, M., Manataki, A.: Discovering students' learning strategies in a visual programming MOOC through process mining techniques. In: Montali, M., Senderovich, A., Weidlich, M. (eds.) ICPM 2022. LNBIP, vol. 468, pp. 539–551. Springer, Cham (2022). https://doi.org/10.1007/978-3-031-27815-0_39
24. Romero, C., Ventura, S.: Educational data mining and learning analytics: an updated survey. WIREs Data Min. Knowl. Discov. **10**(3), e1355 (2020). https://doi.org/10.1002/widm.1355
25. Song, M., Günther, C.W., van der Aalst, W.M.P.: Trace clustering in process mining. In: Ardagna, D., Mecella, M., Yang, J. (eds.) BPM 2008. LNBIP, vol. 17, pp. 109–120. Springer, Heidelberg (2009). https://doi.org/10.1007/978-3-642-00328-8_11
26. Strickroth, S., Kiy, A.: E-Assessment etablieren: Auf dem Weg zu (dezentralen) E-Klausuren. In: Lehre und Lernen entwickeln. No. 6 in Potsdamer Beiträge zur Hochschulforschung, Universitätsverlag Potsdam (2020). https://doi.org/10.25932/publishup-49303
27. Strickroth, S., Olivier, H., Pinkwart, N.: Das GATE-System: Qualitätssteigerung durch Selbsttests für Studenten bei der Onlineabgabe von Übungsaufgaben? In: Proceedings of the DELFI (2011). https://dl.gi.de/handle/20.500.12116/4740
28. Umer, R., Susnjak, T., Mathrani, A., Suriadi, S.: On predicting academic performance with process mining in learning analytics. JRIT **10**(2), 160–176 (2017)

29. Wagner, M., et al.: A combined approach of process mining and rule-based AI for study planning and monitoring in higher education. In: Montali, M., Senderovich, A., Weidlich, M. (eds.) ICPM 2022. LNBIP, vol. 468, pp. 513–525. Springer, Cham (2022). https://doi.org/10.1007/978-3-031-27815-0_37
30. Walker, M., Townley, C.: Contract cheating: a new challenge for academic honesty? J. Acad. Ethics **10**, 27–44 (2012)
31. Watson, G., Sottile, J.: Cheating in the digital age: do students cheat more in on-line courses? In: Proceedings of the SITE. AACE (2008)

Evidence-Based Student Career and Performance Analysis with Process Mining: A Case Study

Domenico Potena[1], Laura Genga[2(✉)], Annalisa Basta[1], Chiara Mercati[1], and Claudia Diamantini[1]

[1] Università Politecnica delle Marche, Ancona, Italy
[2] Eindhoven University of Technology, Eindhoven, The Netherlands
l.genga@tue.nl

Abstract. Educational process mining aims at leveraging data generated during students' learning processes to extract evidence-based insights supporting the continuous improvements of educational programs. In this work, we showcase the application of educational process mining techniques to analyze students' careers at an Italian university, focusing on their progression and outcomes. The study uncovers trends in compliance with curriculum requirements, exam-taking patterns and graduation times. Predictive models are then employed to elucidate the impact of different factors, e.g., the number of exams passed during the first year, on graduation times. These findings provide insights for educational institutions seeking support mechanisms to improve students' success rates.

Keywords: Educational process mining · Curriculum Mining · Student performance analysis

1 Introduction

Today's universities are making continuous efforts to improve their educational programs. This challenge is of particular importance for Italian universities, given that approximately 40% of students do not successfully finish their studies and only 30% manage to graduate within a year following the standard duration of their degree programme.

In recent years, the Italian Ministry of University and Research has introduced tools and metrics for the assessment of study programmes to support universities in identifying possible causes of students' failures. With the context of this study, we focus on the following indicators used to evaluate the *output* of universities in terms of students' careers.

1. **Early**: students who took their degree within the standard duration of the degree programme are considered early graduated (iC02 indicator). For a bachelor degree it is 3 academic years, i.e., 3 years and 6 months.

J. De Smedt and P. Soffer (Eds.): ICPM 2023 Workshops, LNBIP 503, pp. 349–360, 2024.
https://doi.org/10.1007/978-3-031-56107-8_27

2. **One year late:** students who graduated within one year after the period above-mentioned (iC17 indicator).
3. **Late:** students that took more than 1 year beyond the normal duration.

Although the aforementioned indicators offer universities a way to assess their educational system, they provide an aggregated view of the students' behaviours which offers little support in understanding possible causes of students' delays. To uncover possible obstacles for students, one has to understand how they progress during their studies and whether they can complete their courses within the intended timeframe.

In this paper, we showcase the application of *Educational Process Mining* (EPM) techniques to address these challenges in a real-world case study. The goal of EPM is to uncover patterns and trends within educational data to understand how educational processes are carried out and identify improvement opportunities [5]. Our analysis belongs to the so-called "curriculum mining" branch of EPM, whose goal consists in analyzing data related to students' *careers*, i.e. the sequence of registrations of credits-bearing activities, to determine valuable insights on the curricula chosen by students. More precisely, we apply EPM techniques to i) compare students' careers to the *study program*, which represents the order in which exams should be taken according to the curriculum's coordinators, focusing on detecting differences between *early* and *late* students, and ii) determine whether and how students' progression in the first year impacts their graduation time. Unlike previous work in curriculum mining, we consider not only information related to when a student passed a course but all the activities surrounding the exam taking process. Indeed, a student may attempt an exam multiple times before passing the course. We argue that this data can provide us with in-depth insights into the actual effort a student puts in preparing a course and to which extent one or more courses act as bottlenecks hampering students' preparation for other courses. The analysis provided us with valuable insights into common bottlenecks in students' careers.

The rest of this manuscript is organized as follows. Section 2 describes the case study and the research design. Section 3 discusses the obtained results. Section 4 provides an overview of relevant related work, while Sect. 5 draws some conclusions and delineates future work.

2 Study Design

2.1 Case Study: Bachelor Program of an Italian University

Our study focuses on a 3-year Bachelor's Degree program from an Italian university. We analyzed the administration documents to derive the study program for each bachelor year (e.g., Fig. 1 shows the first year). For privacy reasons, we used the X_Y anonymization convention, where X is a progressive letter identifying the name of the course and Y identifies the semester. Courses with a logical sequence have the same letter X, e.g., Physics 1 and Physics 2.

We aim to answer the following questions:

- **Question 1:** Are students following the study program more likely to graduate on time?

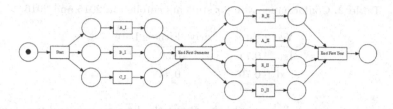

Fig. 1. Study program: first year

Table 1. Indicators students enrolled in 2015 and 2016

Academic Year	Students	Early	One year late	Late
2015–2016	98	37.75%	38.77%	23.46%
2016–2017	93	46.23%	30.10%	23.65%

- **Question 2:** Which courses are the bottlenecks of the curriculum?
- **Question 3:** How does the students' progression in their first year impact the final grade and the graduation time?

The dataset contains 191 students enrolled in the academic years 2015/2016 and 2016/2017, and graduated. We only considered these two years because then the slightly changed between 2017 and 2018. The dataset has been pre-processed together with domain experts to remove outliers and wrong samples. Table 1 shows that only a small percentage of the graduated students managed to complete their studies on time (the 37.75% and the 46.23%, respectively), which suggests that the current setting of the program may involve important bottlenecks, thus making this a suitable case study for our analysis.

For each student, we have the year of enrollment, the overall duration of the graduation process in days and the grade for each exam the student passed. Moreover, for each exam that the student booked for, we also have information about the status and its timestamp. In this paper, we consider the following statuses: *Booked, Passed, Failed, Absent, Withdrawn*. Note that "Absent" means that the student has booked the exam but did not show up; while "Withdrawn" means that the student showed up but decided to withdraw. To gain a better understanding of when activities are carried out w.r.t. the academic year, we have inserted in the log four artificial activities as a time reference to indicate the end of each semester and year: "End first semester", "End first year", "End third semester" and "End second year".

2.2 Methodology

The following subsections delve into the approach adopted for each question.

RQ1: Students' Career Process Analysis. The first question determines whether adhering to the proposed study program increases the likelihood that students will graduate on time.

Table 2. Conformance rate for students enrolled in 2015 and 2016

Year	Fitness Early	Fitness Late
1st	0.74	0.59
2sd	0.70	0.44

The focus of analysis is on processes about the first and second years, as the third year offers more flexibility in class choices. Consequently, an individual's performance is influenced by their personal choices rather than the structure of the study program. For RQ1, the event log contains a trace for each student, where activities are passed exams. First, we employ *conformance checking* techniques [1] to quantify the overall degree of compliance of actual students' careers to the study program for each academic year, underlying the difference between the categories of early and late students. Then, we employ *process discovery* techniques to derive a process model describing the *actual* behaviours of early and late students to gain insights on which process behaviours from the study program are followed or violated by the two categories of students. We used the *Infrequent Inductive Miner* algorithm (IM) [16], a process discovery technique commonly used in literature that can cope with infrequent behaviour and large event logs while ensuring soundness. The IM requires to set a threshold determining how much process behavior should be filtered out. We tested a range of threshold from 0 to 0.9, selecting the best trade-off between fitness and precision.

RQ2: Exam Taking Process. Here, we delve into those exams showing a potential bottleneck behaviour (e.g., low passing rate). The aim is to analyze the actual efforts put into the *preparation* of these exams. To this end, we leverage information about when the student starts and ends the process of studying for an exam, considering how many times an exam has to be retaken before succeding. We created an event log for each analyzed exam, where the student identifier is used as case id, the status correlated to each exam is used as activity, with the corresponding timestamp. Activities represent the path each student follows from first booking the exam to passing it: "Booked", "Passed", "Failed", "Absent", "Withdrawn". Activities, except passed, can occur several times consecutively. We then used the IM to extract the exam preparation process.

RQ3: Prediction. The goal of this analysis consists in assessing the impact of the students' progression during the first year on their final graduation performance. In particular, we analyzed the impact of the number of passed exams and the average grade on students' likelihood to graduate on time by means of a logistic regression model.

3   Results

3.1   Students' Career Processes

Table 2 shows the conformance rate achieved over the whole log (191 students) looking at the fitness, for early and late students, for the first and the second

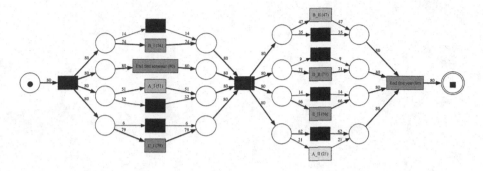

Fig. 2. Model extracted for the first year of the Early students

year. In both cases, early students show a much higher level of compliance than late students, which suggests the higher the conformance to the study program, the higher the probability that the student will graduate on time.

We extracted the process models for both categories of students using the IM implementation in the Pm4Py library[1]. Figure 2 shows the model extracted for the early students, which resembles the study program presented in Fig. 1. Edge labels correspond to the number of students following the corresponding path. At the beginning of the process, all parallel activities can be skipped, except "End first semester". The fact that "End first semester" is in parallel with other courses indicates that some students manage to take them before the end of the first semester, while others don't. Almost all students pass B_I and C_I within the first semester, while slightly fewer students pass A_I. In the second semester, only 26% of students pass A_II, which is the advanced level of A_I.

The model extracted for late students is shown Fig. 3. The pass rate of all exams in the first semester drops dramatically, especially for A_I from 63.75% (for early students) to only 8.89%. This leads to A_II disappearing from the model, which means that none (or very few) students took this exam in the first year. Furthermore, in the second semester, students who pass B_II are far less than those who pass D_II and E_II.

Regarding the models for the second year, shown in Fig. 4 and Fig. 5, the differences are less evident. In both processes, there are still exams that students did not manage to pass in the first year. However, there are many more first-year exams in the process model related to late students than in the early ones. Notably, few of the late students pass A_I by the second year, confirming that it is a course to focus on. M_II would also seem difficult to pass. In fact, it is found only in the process model related to early students, while less than 40% of students passed it. G_I, N_II and O_II drop sharply moving from early to late students model, i.e., from 55.20%/85.23%/69.32% to 8.00%/10.00%/17.78%, respectively. Finally, about half of the students passed F_I e H_I.

---

[1] https://pm4py.fit.fraunhofer.de/.

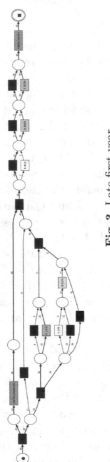

Fig. 3. Late first year

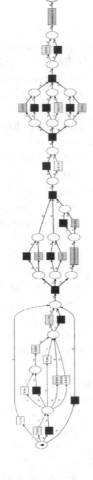

Fig. 4. Early second year

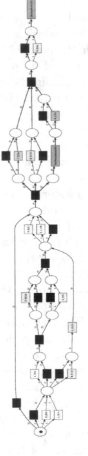

Fig. 5. Late second year

Table 3. Percentage of absent, failed and withdrawn student for each exam

Exam	Absent/Success	Failed/Success	Withdrawn/Success
A_I	68.89%	166.17%	4.2%
B_I	75.99%	133.66%	11.39%
C_I	41.38%	0%	12.81%
A_II	74.5%	80.75%	2.25%
B_II	93.63%	21.57%	17.89%
D_II	9.56%	0%	14.46%
E_II	74.15%	0%	0%
F_I	20.78%	34.96%	9.05%
G_I	6.22%	0%	37.06%
H_I	4.39%	231.22%	0.24%
M_II	47.75%	12.5%	5.75%
N_II	27.32%	147.07%	10.49%
O_II	16.23%	13.25%	11.59%

Summarizing, exam A_I appears to be a bottleneck since fewer students take it, both for early and late students. Consequently, also A_II represents an issue. In the same way, exam M_II can be considered a bottleneck. If we consider only the late students, also B_I, B_II, G_I, N_II and O_II exams appear to be bottlenecks.

3.2 Exam Taking Process

The previous analysis highlighted some exams which are frequently taken by the students later than expected. However, these results do not tell us whether the students decided to postpone the exam preparation at a later stage in their career or whether, instead, they started to prepare on time but encountered challenges in succeding. The goal of this section is to gather more detailed insights on which exams are actual bottlenecks, in the sense that their preparation takes much longer than expected, possibly hampering the preparation of other exams.

Table 3 shows, for each exam, the percentage of *absent*, *failed* and *withdrawn* students, out of the total number of students who passed the exam (i.e., 191 students). Note that cell values may exceed 100% because a student may be absent, withdrawn or fail the exam even several times before passing.

Critical exams, i.e., exams a percentage of students that have failed them over 100%, are highlighted in grey. For the first year, these are A_I and B_I. Other exams showing concerning trends are A_II and B_II, since many students registered for the exam but chose not to attend. In the second year, we can observe a critical situation for exams H_I because the failure rate is greater than 200%, and N_II with a failure rate of 147.07%.

To delve into students' preparation process for these exams, we mined the process models corresponding to the taking process of the detected critical

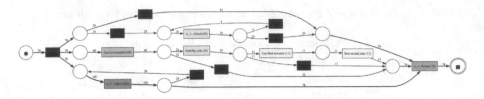

Fig. 6. A_I Early

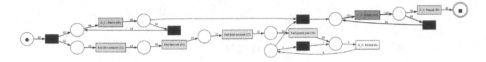

Fig. 7. A_I Late

exams, then compared the obtained models for early and late students. For the sake of space, in the following, we only show the results obtained for the processes of one of the detected critical exams, i.e., A_I.

Figure 6 represents the process of students who graduated on time taking the exam A_I. This process shows three groups of parallel activities. In the first group, we can see a loop of students that are absent, suggesting that they studied for the exam but they did not think they were prepared enough to pass it. However, this loop can also be skipped: in fact, there are students who manage to pass the exam the first time they take it. The second group of activities adds the time perspective to the analysis: half of the students (53.33%) pass the exam by the first year, 28.33% by the end of the third semester, and the rest by the end of the second year. In the last group there is a loop for the students who took the exam but failed. The process ends with the "Passed" activity for all the students.

Figure 7, represent the same process but refers to students who did not graduate on time. Many more unprepared students do not show up or fail the exam, compared to the model in Fig. 6. Moreover, most students pass the exam after the end of second year.

The analysis of the two models shows that early students take the exam earlier. In fact, there are few absentees and many take the exam within the first semester (even if they fail it). We derive that such students start studying as early as the course progresses. As for late students, more than 71% take the exam after the end of the second year. Considering that if a student books for an exam, has started or plans to start studying it, then it follows that late students have longer preparation time.

3.3   Predicting Students' Outcome

This subsection addresses the third RQ, aimed at understanding to which extent students' progression in their first year impacts their graduation performance.

Table 4. Logistic regression results

	Model 1st semester	Model 1st year
F1Score	0.71	0.81
# Exams	2.50	3.74
Average exam grade	3.73	2.97

The above analysis shows that many students, especially *late* ones, do not manage to take first-year exams within the time window as defined in the study program. Hence, we were interested in uncovering potential relations between the number of exams passed during the first year and the final students' outcome. In addition, we considered also the exam grade. A high grade can certainly mean that the student is good, but it can also mean a long time to study at their best. Furthermore, we observed that many students take exams multiple times, possibly to obtain a higher grade, spending more time at preparing for an exam, which in turn may lead to some delay in their graduation.

For this analysis, we built two logistic regression models, for the first semester and the first year, respectively. We used a binary variable representing whether the student graduated on time or not as the dependent variable. As independent variables, we considered the number of exams passed and the average grade achieved. We used the implementation of the logistic regression offered by the *scikit-learn* library[2], using the default dataset split parameter (i.e., 70% of the data used for training, 30% for testing).

Table 4 shows the logistic regression performance for both models, together with the values assigned to the coefficient of each dependent variable. Both models performed reasonably well in terms of F1-score. The F1-score achieved is 0.71 and 0.81 for the model of first semester and of first year, respectively.

Looking at the coefficients, when considering the first semester, the average grade seems to have a stronger impact than the number of exams. However, when considering the entire year, taking more exams seems to be more important than aiming for a high grade. A possible explanation for these results is that in the first semester, there are only three exams, and even if a student fails to do them all, there is still time to recover and to graduate on time. However, missing too many exams in the first year might lead to too many exams to recover in the other two years, which poses some challenges for graduating on time.

4   Related Work

Educational Data Mining (EDM) is an emerging discipline that aims to understand and improve students' learning process [18,20]. Our work is mainly related to EDM approaches that analyze students' academic performance and their failure. A popular trend in this respect consists in modeling students according to

---

[2] https://scikit-learn.org/stable/.

predefined features and applying machine learning to predict student's performance [10–13,15,21]. Many of these studies provide a perspective complementary to the one provided by our analysis, taking into account factors external to the graduation process itself. Even studies centered on the graduation process usually perform a data-oriented analysis, in which students' behaviors are encoded in terms of features without considering the study program's underlying structure. In this respect, our work is similar to the one in [9], which proposes to model and analyze students' careers. They introduce the notion of *ideal career* that corresponds to the career of a graduated student who took each exam just after the end of the corresponding course. Different metrics are used to measure the distance between each student's career and the ideal one (e.g., the Bubblesort distance). Compared to our approach, the work in [9] does not exploit the potentialities of process-based analysis in modeling students' behaviors. In particular, they do not infer any model representing the overall students' behaviors. In contrast, we exploit process formalisms to model the manifesto of study programs that explicitly accounts for parallelisms, thus allowing us to obtain a more accurate evaluation of the difference between single careers and the ideal path.

The application of process mining techniques to educational data, referred to as *Educational Process Mining* (EPM) [5], is a subject that has been recently gaining increasing interest. EPM has been applied to deal with different educational problems, such as on-line learning environments [6,17,23], computer-supported collaborative learning tools [4,19], professional training [3,7]. However, only a few works investigated the applications of EPM to curriculum mining. [22] propose a set of patterns modeling typical constraints of academic curricula and use these patterns to analyze the graduation process. However unlike the present work, they do not infer the process model representing students' careers and do not focus on delay analysis. Our approach is similar to [14], in analyzing the exam-taking process and program study compliance. However, [14] do not consider differences between early and late students.

In [2], authors apply process mining techniques to analyze event log data generated within educational information systems, with the purpose of understanding students' behavior during online learning. The work differs from ours in two main ways: (i) it is based on the concept of digital twin for the representation of students' activities and (ii) its focus is on the single course while ours is on the entire career. To the best of our knowledge, [8] is the only work that considers the entire student's career. In particular, it applies process discovery techniques to curriculum event logs with the purpose of characterizing behaviors of students that performed best/worst in terms of years required to complete the graduation process and final grade. In this work, we shift the focus to classes of students defined accordingly to the indicators defined by the Italian Minister of Education. Moreover, we investigate students' compliance with the study program and the students' delays in taking their exams.

5   Conclusion and Future Works

This study has delved into the landscape of students' career processes. Process mining techniques allowed us to map out students' journeys. We were able to identify typical students' process behaviours, which, in turn, allowed us to gather interesting insights into which paths from the ideal study program are usually followed and which ones are violated for the two categories of students under analysis. Our exploration of early and late students' behaviours concerning the curriculum revealed distinctive patterns and bottlenecks, notably revolving around specific exams such as A_I and A_II. These exams impact students' graduation times, making them key areas for attention and intervention. We also delved into the exam preparation process for the identified critical exams, uncovering insightful patterns in how the two analyzed categories of students usually prepare for these exams. Finally, we exploited logistic regression to quantify the impact of the number of exams taken in the first year and the average grade on the overall students' graduation performance. Moreover for the regression model we plan to consider additionally explanatory variables, such as the subject group of the exam. In conclusion, this research opens doors and encourages future analysis to improve the quality of education by predicting the students' academic performance and supporting those in the risk group. In future work, we plan to extend the students' samples with additional enrollment years and different courses, to determine to which extent we can determine similar or different patterns. Furthermore, we intend to investigate how to convert the insights derived from this kind of analysis in actionable recommendations that can support the students in determining the best path to follow at different moments of their career, keeping into account their current progression.

References

1. Adriansyah, A., van Dongen, B.F., van der Aalst, W.M.P.: Conformance checking using cost-based fitness analysis. In: 2011 IEEE 15th International Enterprise Distributed Object Computing Conference, pp. 55–64. IEEE (2011)
2. Azeta, A., Agono, F., Adesola, F., Nwaocha, V., Tjiraso, S.: A process mining framework for analysing students' behaviours using digital twin. Available at SSRN 4331450 (2022)
3. Bergenthum, R., Desel, J., Harrer, A., Mauser, S.: Learnflow mining. In: DeLFI 2008: Die 6. e-Learning Fachtagung Informatik, pp. 269–280. Gesellschaft für Informatik eV (2008)
4. Bergenthum, R., Desel, J., Harrer, A., Mauser, S.: Modeling and mining of learnflows. In: Jensen, K., Donatelli, S., Kleijn, J. (eds.) Transactions on Petri Nets and Other Models of Concurrency V. LNCS, vol. 6900, pp. 22–50. Springer, Heidelberg (2012). https://doi.org/10.1007/978-3-642-29072-5_2
5. Bogarín, A., Cerezo, R., Romero, C.: A survey on educational process mining. Wiley Interdisc. Rev. Data Min. Knowl. Discov. 8(1), e1230 (2018)
6. Bogarín, A., Romero, C., Cerezo, R., Sánchez-Santillán, M.: Clustering for improving educational process mining. In: Proceedings of International Conference on Learning Analytics and Knowledge, pp. 11–15. ACM (2014)

7. Cairns, A.H., Gueni, B., Assu, J., Joubert, C., Khelifa, N.: Analyzing and improving educational process models using process mining techniques. In: Proceedings of International Conference on Advances in Information Mining Management, pp. 17–22 (2015)
8. Cameranesi, M., Diamantini, C., Genga, L., Potena, D.: Students' careers analysis: a process mining approach. In: Proceedings of International Conference on Web Intelligence, Mining and Semantics, p. 26. ACM (2017)
9. Campagni, R., Merlini, D., Sprugnoli, R., Verri, M.C.: Data mining models for student careers. Expert Syst. Appl. **42**(13), 5508–5521 (2015)
10. Dekker, G.W., Pechenizkiy, M., Vleeshouwers, J.M.: Predicting students drop out: a case study. In: International Working Group on Educational Data Mining (2009)
11. Gowda, S.M., Baker, R.S.J.D., Pardos, Z., Heffernan, N.T.: The sum is greater than the parts: ensembling student knowledge models in ASSISTments. In: Proceedings of KDD Workshop on Knowledge Discovery in Educational Data (2011)
12. Guruler, H., Istanbullu, A., Karahasan, M.: A new student performance analysing system using knowledge discovery in higher educational databases. Comput. Educ. **55**(1), 247–254 (2010)
13. Herzog, S.: Measuring determinants of student return vs. dropout/stopout vs. transfer: A first-to-second year analysis of new freshmen. Res. High. Educ. **46**(8), 883–928 (2005)
14. Hobeck, R., Pufahl, L., Weber, I.: Process mining on curriculum-based study data: a case study at a German university. In: Montali, M., Senderovich, A., Weidlich, M. (eds.) ICPM 2022. LNBIP, vol. 468, pp. 577–589. Springer, Cham (2022). https://doi.org/10.1007/978-3-031-27815-0_42
15. Lassibille, G., Navarro Gómez, L.: Why do higher education students drop out? Evidence from Spain. Educ. Econ. **16**(1), 89–105 (2008)
16. Leemans, S.J.J., Fahland, D., van der Aalst, W.M.P.: Discovering block-structured process models from event logs containing infrequent behaviour. In: Lohmann, N., Song, M., Wohed, P. (eds.) BPM 2013. LNBIP, vol. 171, pp. 66–78. Springer, Cham (2014). https://doi.org/10.1007/978-3-319-06257-0_6
17. Mukala, P., Buijs, J.C.A.M., Leemans, M., van der Aalst, W.M.P.: Learning analytics on coursera event data: a process mining approach. In: Proceedings of International Symposium on Data-Driven Process Discovery and Analysis, pp. 18–32 (2015)
18. Peña-Ayala, A.: Educational data mining: a survey and a data mining-based analysis of recent works. Expert Syst. Appl. **41**(4), 1432–1462 (2014)
19. Reimann, P., Frerejean, J., Thompson, K.: Using process mining to identify models of group decision making in chat data. In: Proceedings of International Conference on Computer Supported Collaborative Learning, pp. 98–107. International Society of the Learning Sciences (2009)
20. Romero, C., Ventura, S.: Educational data mining: a survey from 1995 to 2005. Expert Syst. Appl. **33**(1), 135–146 (2007)
21. Romero, C., Ventura, S., Espejo, P.G., Hervás, C.: Data mining algorithms to classify students. In: Proceedings of International Conference on Educational Data Mining, pp. 8–17 (2008). www.educationaldatamining.org
22. Trcka, N., Pechenizkiy, M.: From local patterns to global models: towards domain driven educational process mining. In: Proceedings of International Conference on Intelligent Systems Design and Applications, pp. 1114–1119. IEEE (2009)
23. Vidal, J.C., Vázquez-Barreiros, B., Lama, M., Mucientes, M.: Recompiling learning processes from event logs. Knowl.-Based Syst. **100**, 160–174 (2016)

Extracting Rules from Event Data
for Study Planning

Majid Rafiei[1]([⊠])[iD], Duygu Bayrak[1][iD], Mahsa Pourbafrani[1][iD],
Gyunam Park[1][iD], Hayyan Helal[2][iD], Gerhard Lakemeyer[2][iD],
and Wil M.P. van der Aalst[1][iD]

[1] Chair of Process and Data Science, RWTH Aachen University, Aachen, Germany
majid.rafiei@pads.rwth-aachen.de
[2] Knowledge-Based Systems Group, RWTH Aachen University, Aachen, Germany

Abstract. In this study, we examine how event data from *campus management systems* can be used to analyze the study paths of higher education students. The main goal is to offer valuable guidance for their study planning. We employ process and data mining techniques to explore the impact of sequences of taken courses on academic success. Through the use of decision tree models, we generate data-driven recommendations in the form of rules for study planning and compare them to the recommended study plan. The evaluation focuses on RWTH Aachen University computer science bachelor program students and demonstrates that the proposed course sequence features effectively explain academic performance measures. Furthermore, the findings suggest avenues for developing more adaptable study plans.

Keywords: Event Data · Decision Trees · Campus Management Systems · Machine Learning

1 Introduction

In higher education, study programs have specific examination regulations covering various aspects, such as degree requirements, grading criteria, thesis guidelines, and module grade cancellation procedures. These regulations provide guidelines for students to follow throughout their studies. For example, the examination regulation for the RWTH Bachelor computer science program of 2018 mandates that students must have accumulated a minimum of 120 credit points (CP) before registering for the thesis. With such requirements in mind, students can choose different paths and courses based on their interests. The examination regulations often include a recommended study plan to guide students in completing their compulsory courses in the most suitable order.

Following the recommended study plan can be beneficial for timely graduation, assuming all required courses are successfully completed. However, students have different capacities to handle the workload suggested by the study plan each semester, leading some to deviate from it and lose its guidance. Therefore, assistance and guidance are necessary to help students effectively plan their studies.

J. De Smedt and P. Soffer (Eds.): ICPM 2023 Workshops, LNBIP 503, pp. 361–374, 2024.
https://doi.org/10.1007/978-3-031-56107-8_28

One way to provide this assistance is by analyzing historical study path data, which can reveal characteristics of successful paths resulting in good overall GPAs. By extracting insights from such data, we can generate rules or recommendations to support students in making informed decisions about their course selection and study plans.

This paper focuses on utilizing event data from Campus Management Systems (CMS) to understand how students progress in their study programs. Various feature extraction methods capture the course sequence. Decision tree models trained with these features and Key Performance Indicators (KPIs) like GPA provide data-driven study planning recommendations to students. We evaluate the proposed features and models using data from computer science bachelor program students at RWTH Aachen University. The results show that the features effectively explain academic performance measures, like overall GPA and course grades. Comparing different features and models reveals their similar predictive effectiveness. We extract study planning rules from the models and discuss characteristics of study paths leading to positive or negative academic outcomes. Adhering to the recommended course sequence correlates with academic success, but deviations can also lead to positive outcomes, providing opportunities for more flexible study plans.

The remainder of this paper is structured as follows. In Sect. 2, we provide preliminaries. Section 3 outlines the related work. We introduce the used dataset in Sect. 4. Our main contributions are highlighted in Sect. 5. In Sect. 6, we present the evaluation, and Sect. 7 concludes the paper.

2   Preliminaries

Event Data (Log). Process mining utilizes event data which is a collection of events, where each event has the following essential attributes: *case-id, activity*, and *timestamp* [1]. The case-id identifies the instance, the activity represents the action, and the timestamp records the activity's time. Additional attributes like resources, costs, and people may provide contextual information. See Table 1 for a sample event log. Events represent specific activities in the process, and multiple events form a case. Using timestamps, we create traces, representing each case's activity sequence. For example, the trace $\sigma = \langle op, pp, pa, sh \rangle$ corresponds to the activities for order (case) with id 1 in Table 1. Event logs can be represented as multisets of traces, such as $L = [\langle op, pp, pa, sh \rangle^2]$ for Table 1.

Directly Follows Graph (DFG). DFGs are forms of process models, represented as directed graphs, where nodes are activities and edges signify the *directly-follows* relationship between activities. Fake start and end activities connect all first and last activities. DFG discovery involves counting how often one activity follows another. Figure 1 displays the DFG discovered from the event log $L = [\langle a, b, d \rangle^{10}, \langle a, b, c, d \rangle^{20}, \langle a, c, d \rangle^5]$.

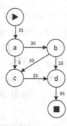

Fig. 1. The DFG discovered from event log $L =$ [$\langle a, b, d \rangle^{10}, \langle a, b, c, d \rangle^{20},$ $\langle a, c, d \rangle^{5}$].

Table 1. A fragment of an event log.

Order ID	Customer ID	Activity	Timestamp
1	1	Order placement (op)	01-04-2023 16:02:00
1	1	Picking products (pp)	01-04-2023 19:46:00
2	2	Order placement (op)	01-04-2023 20:13:00
1	1	Packing (pa)	02-04.2023 08:07:00
2	2	Picking products (pp)	02-04.2023 08:35:00
2	2	Packing (pa)	02-04.2023 09:21:00
1	1	Shipping (sh)	02-04.2023 10:05:00
2	2	Shipping (sh)	02-04.2023 10:05:00

Decision Tree. A Decision Tree is a tree-based structure used for classification tasks. It has internal nodes representing decision points and leaf nodes representing decision outcomes. In classification, the model predicts a class label for input data by considering descriptive attributes [8]. Various techniques exist for selecting the best attribute for a split in a decision tree, e.g., *Information Gain* [9] or *Gini Index* [4].

3 Related Work

A comprehensive survey of process mining techniques in the educational context can be found in [3]. In the first categories of studies, students are grouped based on academic performance indicators, like course grades, and specific process models (e.g., DFG) are discovered for each group. The relation between students' usage of the online educational system and their grades is explored in [7] and [6], with consistent findings that actively engaged students to achieve better grades. These studies focus on applying process mining to analyze student groups individually.

Besides analyzing different student groups, study paths derived from CMSs and curriculum mining techniques are employed. The main focus in the second category of studies is on the recommendation and improvement of the study path. In [2], the effectiveness of a curriculum is evaluated by comparing predefined study paths with actual study paths taken by students, focusing on first-time course enrollments and excluding retakes. Results indicate the need for potential curriculum modifications, as some courses were not taken in the predefined semester. In [11], the authors discuss using process mining, particularly process discovery, on curriculum data to uncover study paths followed by students. They propose the development of a course recommender system by comparing processes followed by successful and less successful students. Also, in [5], the authors utilize process mining techniques to discover process models and gain insights regarding typical patterns followed by students.

In [12], the authors explored three different sequence-based course recommendation systems, including one based on process mining. Despite [11], in this approach, a process model was not discovered, but a causal footprint approach [1] for conformance checking was utilized to compute the similarity between a student and successful students based on their study paths. The recommendations were based on the taken courses by successful students with similar paths. Data mining techniques predict academic performance using diverse factors. They are also used to analyze demographics, digital footprints, and academic indicators, e.g., grades [10,13].

Our research utilizes process and data mining techniques to explore connections between courses using event data from a CMS. Unlike previous studies, we focus on students' study paths across multiple courses, including the impact of retaking courses. Our aim is to support students starting their studies by suggesting appropriate courses. Additionally, we analyze study path characteristics related to academic performance, distinguishing our approach from comparing actual study paths to recommended plans.

student-id	course-id	credit	time-start	time-end	semester	grade	final -status	gender	nationality	study-time
331322	course-107	8	05.02.19	08.02.19	1	3.3	PASSED	gender-2	country 1	3.0027
331324	course-107	8	05.02.19	08.02.19	1	3	PASSED	gender-2	country 1	3.0027
331354	course-107	8	05.02.19	08.02.19	1	1.7	PASSED	gender-2	country 2	3.0027
...	...	...	...	...	...	...	...	...	...	...

Fig. 2. Fragment of a larger event log. Each row corresponds to an event.

4   Dataset Description

Descriptive analysis is performed to gain insights into different aspects of the data. We analyze event data extracted from RWTH Aachen University's CMS, comprising exam attempts and grade entries of computer science bachelor's students. The data covers the period from the winter semester 2018/19 to the summer semester 2021, focusing on students following the examination regulations of 2018. Filtering ensures the inclusion of only exams aligned with mandatory courses for the Computer Science Bachelor's program. The cleaned event data consists of 10751 events, 1411 students, and 18 courses.

Figure 2 shows a fragment of the event data, where each row represents an event indicating an exam taken by a student. This includes both passed and failed exam attempts. Each event has the presented attributes in Table 2. We consider the student-id attribute as the case identifier. The exam attempts for specific courses, identifiable by the course-id attribute, are considered as activities. Timestamp options include the exam date or a coarser-grained timestamp, such as the semester.

By assuming the exam date, i.e., the time-start attribute, as the timestamp attribute, we get the dotted chart shown in Fig. 3. In this chart, each dot refers to an event (exam attempt). The dots are aligned horizontally according to the timestamp and vertically according to the case, i.e., dots in a single horizontal line represent a single student and define a trace.

From left to right, we can spot six groups, each representing an exam period. The first exam period will take place between January and April 2019. The second period is from July to October 2019, and so on. In addition, we can see three student cohorts. The first began its studies in the winter semester of 2018/19 and has study IDs ranging from 328954 to 342392. The second cohort began a year later, in winter semester 2019/20, and covered IDs 343430-365485. The third and final cohort, which covers IDs 369089-386368, began in the winter semester 2020/21.

Table 2. Event attributes of the event data.

Attributes	Explanation
Student-id	the anonymized unique ID of the student that took the exam
Course-id	the anonymized name of the course
Credit	the number of ECTS-points assigned to the course
Time-start	the date when the exam was written
Time-end	the date of exam result published to CMS
Semester	semester counter value when the student took the exam
Grade	the grade of the exam attempt (can be missing)
Final-status	the status of the exam result (PASSED or FAILED)
Gender	the anonymized gender of the student taking the exam
Nationality	the anonymized nationality of the student taking the exam (country-1 or other)
Study-time	student's study duration (years) at the time of data extraction from the CMS

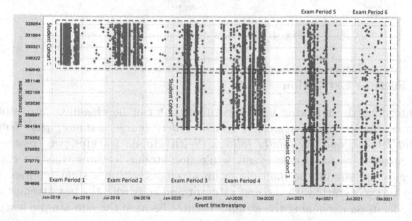

Fig. 3. Dotted chart showing exam attempt events of computer science bachelor students. The dotted chart was created using ProM Lite 1.3.

5 Approach

Figure 4 provides an overview of our approach to discovering study planning rules from event data. We utilize decision trees for their interpretability and feature interaction capturing. Each path from the root to a leaf node in the trained decision tree can be translated into a rule. The discovered rules depend on the chosen descriptive features and label attributes. For example, using course semesters as descriptive features and overall GPA as the label attribute, a rule can suggest an excellent GPA if specific courses are taken in certain semesters. Our focus is mainly on order-related descriptive features, considering that recommended study plans often rely on course order.

5.1   Running Example

We illustrate different feature types using the student example from Table 3. In this case, the student's course sequence includes taking courses 1 and 2 in semester 1, course 3 in semester 2, retaking

Table 3. Study path of an example student.

Semester	1	2	3	4	5
Courses	course-1	course-3	course-1	-	course-4
	course-2				course-5

course 1 in semester 3 (after previously failing it in semester 1), not taking any courses in semester 4, and finally taking courses 4 and 5 in semester 5.

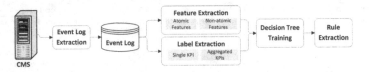

Fig. 4. Overview of the approach.

5.2   Feature Extraction

We introduce the following set of features that can be classified into atomic and non-atomic: *course semester, course order, course distance, path length, directly follows,* and *eventually follows.* With atomic features, we treat each exam attempt as an atomic event, while non-atomic features consider course life cycles and summarize multiple exam attempts within a single course. The course life cycle starts with the first attempt and ends with the last attempt. We mainly focus on explaining the atomic features because the non-atomic features are incremental extensions of the atomic features.

Atomic Course Semester (a-cs-): A course semester feature describes the semester in which a particular course was taken. It includes the course ID and an index value indicating the corresponding semester. This binary feature is set to true if the specified course was taken in the specified semester. In our example, the extracted course semester features are as follows: *a-cs-course-1-1 = true, a-cs-course-2-1 = true, a-cs-course-3-2 = true, a-cs-course-1-3 = true, a-cs-course-4-5 = true,* and *a-cs-course-5-5 = true.* All other features with different index values for those mentioned courses have the value false.

Atomic Course Order (a-co-): This feature captures the order of taken courses. It consists of the course ID and an index value specifying the order value of that course. The order value starts with one for the first course taken and increases for subsequent courses in the order they were taken. For our student example, the atomic course order features extracted are as follows: *a-co-course-1-1 = true, a-co-course-2-1 = true, a-co-course-3-2 = true, a-co-course-1-3 = true, a-co-course-4-4 = true,* and *a-co-course-5-4 = true.* Features with different index values for these courses have the value false. Note that course-4 and course-5 have the order value 4, even though they were taken in semester 5. The course order feature only captures course order and ignores any breaks between semesters.

Atomic Course Distance (a-cd-): This feature captures the number of semesters between each course and the first course taken. The feature includes the course ID and an index value indicating the semester distance. The first course taken has a distance of 0, courses taken in the subsequent semester have a distance of 1, and so on. In our example, *a-cd-course-1-0 = true, a-cd-course-2-0 = true, a-cd-course-3-1 = true, a-cd-course-1-2 = true, a-cd-course-4-4 = true,* and *a-cd-course-5-4 = true.* Every feature with other index values for those courses has the value false.

Atomic Path Length (a-pl-): The Path length feature focuses on measuring the number of edges that need to be traversed to go from one node to another in the DFG. Nodes representing courses taken in the same semester are arranged in parallel and share the same predecessor and successor nodes. The path length between these parallel nodes is set to zero, indicating that they are taken in the same semester. Therefore, the Path length feature captures the number of semesters that elapse between taking one course and taking another course, while disregarding any semester breaks when calculating the semester distance. If no path exists between two courses, the path length feature gets -1.

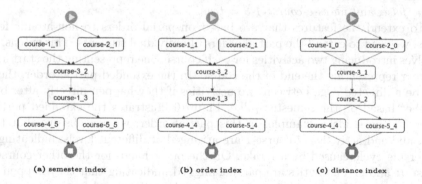

(a) semester index   (b) order index   (c) distance index

Fig. 5. Partial orders of our student example obtained using different indices in the node names.

Note that to avoid loops in DFGs due to retaking courses after a failure, we include the previously introduced indices, i.e., semester, order, and distance, in activity names. Moreover, to be able to model concurrency, we convert DFGs to partial orders. Figure 5 depicts partial orders for our student example using different indices. Consequently, we define three different types of this feature: atomic path length with semester-index (a-pl-s), atomic path length with order-index (a-pl-o), and atomic path length with distance-index (a-pl-d).

Atomic Directly Follows (a-df-): This feature indicates whether one course is directly followed by another course or not. The directly follows features are binary, representing the edges in the partial order. If there is a directed edge between two courses in the partial order, the corresponding directly follows feature will have a value of true. Note that similar to the path length feature, since we consider three different types of partial orders, we also consider three different types of this feature including a-df-s (for semester-index), a-df-o (for order-index), and a-df-d (for distance-index). In our running example, for instance, a-df-s-$course$-1-1 $\rightarrow$ $course$-3-2 = $true$. The courses not directly following each other get the value $false$.

Atomic Eventually Follows (a-ef-): This feature captures whether a course was eventually taken after another course. This feature tries to capture long-distance relations between courses. Again similar to the path length and directly follows features, we consider three different types of this feature including a-ef-s (for semester-index), a-ef-o (for order-index), and a-ef-d (for distance-index). The values of this feature are also binary. For instance, in our running example, considering semester as the index, a-ef-s-$course$-1-1 $\rightarrow$ $course$-3-2 = $true$. The courses not eventually following each other get the value $false$.

We extend the atomic features to incorporate the non-atomic definitions by introducing two features for each course, representing the start and end. The index values in these features indicate the semester, order, or distance values of the start and end, respectively. For our student example, the extracted non-atomic course semester features are: na-cs-s-$course$-1-1 = $true$, na-cs-e-$course$-1-1 = $false$, and na-cs-e-$course$-1-3 = $true$.

To extend the features that are based on parial orders to non-atomic features, we need to extend the partial orders of individual students. This extension involves introducing two activities for each course: one representing the start and another representing the end of the course. In the extended partial order, there will be a directed edge between two activities if they happen directly after one another based on the semester value. Figure 6 illustrates the extended partial order for the student example. In this partial order, we can observe that the start and end activities of course-1 are arranged at different levels, indicating a longer life cycle caused by a retake. On the other hand, for the other courses, the start and end activities are parallel aligned, indicating that they happen at the same time. Note that for non-atomic partial-order-based features, since we already have the start and end indicators, we do not face the loop issues due to retaken courses. Thus, we do not need indices for the courses.

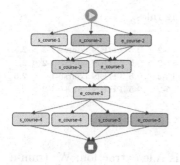

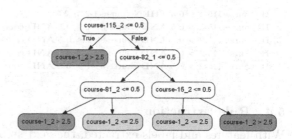

Fig. 6. Partial order of student example including the concept of course life cycles.

Fig. 7. Decision tree trained using atomic course semester features and 2-level course-1-2 grade label.

5.3 Label Extraction

To extract labels that capture academic performance, we need to establish metrics for measurement. One can consider two different groups: aggregate KPIs and single KPIs. The former assesses performance at a broader study level, while the latter focus on individual courses. In each group, we can define different KPIs. For instance, in the aggregated group, we can define three different KPIs: time-to-degree, overall GPA, and dropout. Also, in the single group, we can consider the course grade and pass/fail status as two different KPIs.

Some of the above-mentioned metrics are not applicable to our data due to our data limitations. For instance, the available data do not contain information about a student's graduation. The data only consists of exam attempts and grade entries of mandatory courses, excluding electives, courses in the applied subject area, and the thesis. Therefore, it is not possible to determine whether a specific student has already graduated or calculate their time-to-degree using the available data.

At the same time, since we follow the same approach for extracting rules from different label features, we only focus on the overall GPA and course-grade metrics. The grades and consequently overall GPAs in German universities are based on a 1-5 scale, where the lower grades are considered better, and 4.0 is considered as the passing threshold. We can group the overall GPA into different levels. For instance, a four-level classification is as follows: excellent ($GPA \leq 1.5$), good ($1.5 < GPA \leq 2.5$), satisfactory ($2.5 < GPA \leq 3.5$), and sufficient ($3.5 < GPA \leq 4.0$), and a two-level classification is as follows: good ($GPA \leq 2.5$) and satisfactory ($2.5 < GPA \leq 4.0$).

Table 4. The five study planning rules.

1. **IF** course-115-2 $\leq$ 0.5 **THEN** course-1-2 > 2.5
2. **IF** course-115-2 > 0.5 **AND** course-82-1 $\leq$ 0.5 **AND** course-81-2 $\leq$ 0.5 **THEN** course-1-2 > 2.5
3. **IF** course-115-2 > 0.5 **AND** course-82-1 $\leq$ 0.5 **AND** course-81-2 > 0.5 **THEN** course-1-2 $\leq$ 2.5
4. **IF** course-115-2 > 0.5 **AND** course-82-1 > 0.5 **AND** course-15-2 $\leq$ 0.5 **THEN** course-1-2 $\leq$ 2.5
5. **IF** course-115-2 > 0.5 **AND** course-82-1 > 0.5 **AND** course-15-2 > 0.5 **THEN** course-1-2 > 2.5

5.4 Rule Extraction

With features and labels extracted, the next step is rule extraction. We train a decision tree using the descriptive features and labels, then convert each root-to-leaf path into a rule. For instance, using the atomic course semester feature and a 2-level course grade label for course 1 taken in the second semester, we can obtain the tree shown in Fig. 7. To prevent overfitting in decision trees, we determine the maximum depth through experimentation and accuracy assessment. Note that in the decision nodes, if a course is taken in the specified semester, then *course semester <= 0.5* is evaluated as False. This decision tree can be translated into five study planning rules, which correspond to the paths from the root to any leaf node, Table 4. Note that not all rules may be equally relevant, as some may cover only a few instances or have low accuracy. Thus, we use a relevancy measure combining both the accuracy of the rules and the number of instances covered by the rule.

The extracted rules can be interpreted as follows: (1) If a student takes course-1 in the second semester without concurrently enrolling in course-115, it is anticipated that their grade in course-1 will be greater (worse) than 2.5, (2) If a student takes course-1 in semester 2 and enrolls in course-115 in the same semester and does not enroll in course-81 concurrently and course-82 in the preceding semester, it is foreseen that their grade in course-1 will exceed 2.5, signifying a below-average performance, (3) In contrast to rule 2, if the student concurrently enrolls in course-81 while having taken course-1 and course-115, their grade in course-1 is expected to be 2.5 or less, suggesting a better performance, (4) If a student concurrently enrolls in course-1 and course-115, has previously taken course-82, and doesn't take course-15 concurrently, they are projected to receive a grade in course-1 of 2.5 or less, and (5) If the student also takes course-15 concurrently with the rest except course-82, and course-82 is taken in semester 1, it is expected that their grade in course-1 will be greater than 2.5. Next, we evaluate the performance of each decision tree model trained on different feature and label combinations.

6   Evaluation

We developed a tool to train decision tree models on various features and discover rules from these models to predict good/bad grades in different courses. The source code is available on Github (https://github.com/m4jidRafiei/AIStudyBuddy-RuleExtractor). Note that here we only show the results for course grade metrics.

Table 5. Mean accuracy, precision, and recall values (%) of predicting the grade of different courses.

	Course-45	Course-115	Course-71	Course-131
Accuracy	67 ± 5	68 ± 1	60 ± 3	69 ± 2
Precision (Grade $\leq$ 2.5)	67 ± 6	62 ± 1	57 ± 3	67 ± 2
Precision (Grade $>$ 2.5)	76 ± 8	76 ± 2	64 ± 2	73 ± 4
Recall (Grade $\leq$ 2.5)	86 ± 8	78 ± 1	60 ± 4	75 ± 6
Recall (Grade $>$ 2.5)	45 ± 17	60 ± 2	61 ± 5	64 ± 5

6.1   Course Grade Prediction

In this subsection, we predict course grades based on a two-level class (grade $\leq$ 2.5 and grade $>$ 2.5) using the dataset from Sect. 4. Features are extracted following the approach in Subsect. 5.2. We focus on four key courses (IDs 45, 115, 71, and 131) frequently taken in different study stages. To train and evaluate decision tree models using the different datasets, we use a 4-fold cross-validation. In each iteration, we specify one fold as the test set and train a decision tree model on the remaining 3 folds. We evaluate the trained model on the test set, retain the evaluation score, and discard the model. Finally, we compute the average performance of the model using the evaluation scores of each iteration.

We use consistent hyperparameters for all decision tree models, including the Gini Index for splitting. The stopping criteria are a maximum tree depth of 5, a minimum of 1 sample per leaf node, and a minimum of 2 samples to split an internal node. We evaluate performance using accuracy, recall, and precision. Table 5 summarizes the performance metrics. Generally, average accuracy values are observed to be above 65%, except for models predicting grades for course-71, which began with an accuracy of 55%. Notably, the features were less successful in accounting for the grades in course-71 compared to the other three courses, as revealed by the mean precision and recall values.

For all four courses, the models struggled to accurately identify students with a course grade higher than 2.5, as reflected by mean recall values of 60% or lower. Nonetheless, with a mean precision of at least 64% across all four courses, the models tended to be correct when they did predict a grade above 2.5. Regarding the prediction of grades lower or equal to 2.5, models forecasting grades for course-45 and course-131 showed good performance, with average precision and recall values exceeding 67%. For course-115, the models performed well in detecting students with a grade lower or equal to 2.5, indicated by a mean recall of 78%, but with a reduced precision of 62%.

6.2   Extracting Rules

We analyze study planning rules for distinguishing good and bad course-131 grades. Specifically, we focus on rules extracted from the model trained on atomic course semester features to predict the fourth-semester course grade for course-131. See Fig. 8 for a visual representation of the trained model. The three most relevant study planning rules based on a combined measure of sample count and accuracy are presented in Table 6.

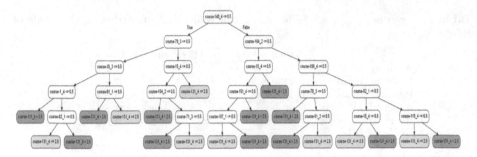

Fig. 8. Decision Tree to predict the grade for course-131 taken in 4th semester. For readability, we removed "cs-" in the feature prefix.

Table 6. The three most relevant study planning rules.

1. **IF** course-140-4 > 0.5 **AND** course-104-2 > 0.5 **AND** course-106-4 > 0.5 **AND** course-82-1 > 0.5 **AND** course-115-4 ≤ 0.5 **THEN** class: course-131-4 ≤ 2.5
2. **IF** course-140-4 ≤ 0.5 **AND** course-78-3 ≤ 0.5 **AND** course-15-3 ≤ 0.5 **AND** course-1-4 ≤ 0.5 **THEN** class: course-131-4 > 2.5
3. **IF** course-140-4 > 0.5 **AND** course-104-2 ≤ 0.5 **AND** course-15-4 > 0.5 **THEN** class: course-131-4 > 2.5

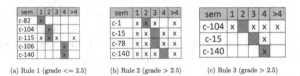

(a) Rule 1 (grade <= 2.5)   (b) Rule 2 (grade > 2.5)   (c) Rule 3 (grade > 2.5)

Fig. 9. Comparison of three most relevant atomic course semester rules (for predicting the grade of course-131) with suggested semesters by the university. The suggested semester is highlighted in orange. Rule conditions are indicated by a "x".

Rule 1 indicates that to achieve a grade below 2.5 in course-131 during the fourth semester, the student should take courses 106 and 140 concurrently. They should also enroll in courses 82 and 104 during the first and second semesters. However, they should avoid taking course-115 concurrently with course-131 and enroll in it in any semester other than the fourth.

Figure 9(a) shows the recommended study plan compared to rule 1 conditions. The alignment between the rule's conditions and the advised study plan is evident, except for course-115. The model indicates that students can be flexible with course-115 scheduling without affecting course-131 performance. This suggests a positive outcome if course-115 is not taken alongside course-131.

Rules 2 and 3 prescribe study paths anticipated to have poor grades (above 2.5) in course-131. Rule 2 predicts a bad grade if courses 1 and 140 are not undertaken in parallel with course-131 in the fourth semester, and if courses 15 and 78 are not taken directly prior in the third semester. Figure 9(b) depicts these conditions and demonstrates their alignment with the deviation from the study plan for courses 15, 78, and 140. However, the condition concerning course-

1 does not conflict with the proposed study plan, as its enrollment is suggested for the second semester.

On the other hand, Rule 3 forecasts a bad grade if courses 15 and 140 are undertaken concurrently with course-131, and if course-104 is not enrolled in the advised second semester. As depicted in Fig. 9(c), course-140 is suggested for concurrent enrollment with course-131 in the study plan, but course-15 is advised to be taken prior to course-131.

7 Conclusion

Our study used process and data mining techniques to investigate the impact of course sequences on academic success by generating data-driven study planning recommendations for computer science bachelor program students at RWTH Aachen University. These findings point to the possibility of developing more adaptable study plans. One limitation is that we focused on students who studied for the standard three-year period at RWTH Aachen University, which may not fully capture the long-term impact of study planning rules on academic performance. We lack information about holiday semesters, which can affect the accuracy of exam result assignments. Additionally, our analysis focused solely on mandatory courses in the computer science bachelor program, excluding elective courses, required courses from outside computer science, and the thesis which could affect the GPA. Our future steps include investigating the impact of the time between grade publication and the next exam on student performance, investigating elective course combinations that lead to better academic performance, and considering alternative classification models to uncover additional study planning rules.

Acknowledgement. The authors gratefully acknowledge the financial support by the Federal Ministry of Education and Research (BMBF) for the joint project AIStudyBuddy (grant no. 16DHBKI016).

SPONSORED BY THE
Federal Ministry
of Education
and Research

References

1. van der Aalst, W.M.P.: Process Mining - Data Science in Action, 2nd edn. Springer, Heidelberg (2016)
2. Bendatu, Y., Yahya, B.N.: Sequence matching analysis for curriculum development. Jurnal Teknik Industri **17** (2015)
3. Bogarín, A., Cerezo, R., Romero, C.: A survey on educational process mining. Wiley Interdisc. Rev. Data Min. Knowl. Discovery **8**, e1230 (2017)
4. Breiman, L.: Classification and Regression Trees. Routledge, Milton Park (2017)
5. Cameranesi, M., Diamantini, C., Genga, L., Potena, D.: Students' careers analysis: a process mining approach. In: Proceedings of the 7th International Conference on Web Intelligence, Mining and Semantics. ACM (2017)
6. Cenka, B.A.N., Santoso, H.B., Junus, K.: Analysing student behaviour in a learning management system using a process mining approach. Knowl. Manage. E-Learn. **14**(1), 62–80 (2022)

7. Etinger, D.: Discovering and mapping LMS course usage patterns to learning outcomes. In: Ahram, T., Karwowski, W., Vergnano, A., Leali, F., Taiar, R. (eds.) IHSI 2020. AISC, vol. 1131, pp. 486–491. Springer, Cham (2020). https://doi.org/10.1007/978-3-030-39512-4_76

8. Maimon, O.Z., Rokach, L.: Data Mining with Decision Trees: Theory and Applications, vol. 81. World Scientific, Singapore (2014)

9. Quinlan, J.R.: Induction of decision trees. Mach. Learn. **1**, 81–106 (1986)

10. Romero, C., Ventura, S.: Educational data mining: a review of the state of the art. IEEE Trans. Syst. Man Cybern. Part C: Appl. Rev. **40**, 601–618 (2010)

11. Wang, R., Zaiane, O.R.: Discovering process in curriculum data to provide recommendation. In: Educational Data Mining (2015)

12. Wang, R., Zaïane, O.R.: Sequence-based approaches to course recommender systems. In: Hartmann, S., Ma, H., Hameurlain, A., Pernul, G., Wagner, R.R. (eds.) DEXA 2018. LNCS, vol. 11029, pp. 35–50. Springer, Cham (2018). https://doi.org/10.1007/978-3-319-98809-2_3

13. Yagci, M.: Educational data mining: prediction of students' academic performance using machine learning algorithms. Smart Learn. Environ. **9**, 11 (2022)

8th International Workshop on Process Querying, Manipulation, and Intelligence (PQMI 2023)

8th International Workshop on Process Querying, Manipulation, and Intelligence (PQMI 2023)

The aim of the Eighth International Workshop on Process Querying, Manipulation, and Intelligence (PQMI 2023) was to provide a high-quality forum for researchers and practitioners to exchange research findings and ideas on methods and practices in the corresponding areas. *Process Querying* combines concepts from Big Data and Process Modeling & Analysis with Process Intelligence and Business Process Analytics to study techniques for retrieving and manipulating models of processes, both observed in the real world as per the recordings of IT systems, and envisioned as per their design in the form of a conceptual representation. The ultimate aim is to systematically organize and extract process-related information for subsequent use. *Process Manipulation* studies inferences from real-world observations for augmenting, enhancing, and redesigning models of processes with the ultimate goal of improving real-world business processes. *Process Intelligence* looks into the application of representation models and approaches in Artificial Intelligence (AI), such as knowledge representation and reasoning, search, automated planning, natural language processing, explainable AI, autonomous agents, and multi-agent systems, among others, for solving problems in process mining, that is automated process discovery, conformance checking, and process enhancement, and vice versa using process mining techniques to tackle problems in AI.

Techniques, methods, and tools for process querying, manipulation, and intelligence have several applications. Examples of practical problems tackled by the themes of the workshop include business process compliance management, business process weakness detection, process variance management, process performance analysis, predictive process monitoring, process model translation, syntactical correctness checking, process model comparison, infrequent behavior detection, process instance migration, process reuse, and process standardization.

PQMI 2023 attracted ten high-quality submissions. Each paper was reviewed by at least three members of the Program Committee. The review process led to five accepted papers.

The keynote "Mining the Process of Process Mining: Navigating Cognition of Process Miners in Action" by Irit Hadar was canceled since the speaker was not able to attend the workshop and present the keynote, due to the situation in Israel. Tian Li, Gyunam Park, and Wil van der Aalst contributed a paper that addresses the declarative process modeling problem in object-centric settings, and a graphical constraint-checking technique for process executions extracted from object-centric event data. The paper by Gyunam Park, Sevde Aydin, Cüneyt Uğur, and Wil van der Aalst presents a case study using the after-sales service process of Borusan Cat within Borusan Group, and highlights the applicability of applying object-centric process mining techniques in practice, by focusing on the ability to conduct multidirectional analyses for a more profound understanding of the analyzed context. The paper by Ava Swevels, Dirk Fahland, and Marco Montali presents a semantic header that defines how extracted legacy data maps to OCED concepts and the domain-specific reference ontology using PGschema. The paper by Viki Peeva and Wil van der Aalst focuses on local process models, small models designed to explain sub-behaviors within the process, and proposes a three-step pipeline for grouping similar local process models using various model similarity measures. The usefulness of the technique is demonstrated through a real-life case study. Finally, the paper by Mohammadreza Fani Sani, Michal Sroka, and Andrea Burattin explores the integration of Large Language Models (LLMs) in process mining and robotic process automation (RPA), and presents an approach to generating event logs from fine-grained tasks recorded based on user actions using LLMs. We hope the reader will enjoy reading the PQMI papers in these proceedings to learn more about the latest advances in research in process querying, manipulation, and intelligence.

October 2023   The PQMI Workshop Organizers

Organization

Workshop Organizers

Artem Polyvyanyy	University of Melbourne, Australia
Claudio Di Ciccio	Sapienza University of Rome, Italy
Antonella Guzzo	University of Calabria, Italy
Arthur ter Hofstede	Queensland University of Technology, Australia
Renuka Sindhgatta	IBM Research, India

Program Committee

Agnes Koschmider	Kiel University, Germany
Ahmed Awad	University of Tartu, Estonia
Anna Kalenkova	University of Adelaide, Australia
Chiara Di Francescomarino	Fondazione Bruno Kessler-IRST, Italy
Fabrizio M. Maggi	Free University of Bozen-Bolzano, Italy
Hagen Völzer	University of St. Gallen, Switzerland
Han van der Aa	University of Mannheim, Germany
Kanika Goel	Queensland University of Technology, Australia
Luigi Pontieri	National Research Council, Italy
María Teresa Gómez-López	University of Seville, Spain
Minseok Song Pohang	University of Science and Technology, South Korea
Eugenio Vocaturo	National Research Council, Italy
Pablo David Villarreal	Universidad Tecnológica Nacional, Argentina
Rong Liu Stevens	Institute of Technology, USA
Seppe Vanden Broucke	Katholieke Universiteit Leuven, Belgium

LLMs and Process Mining: Challenges in RPA

Task Grouping, Labelling and Connector Recommendation

Mohammadreza Fani Sani[1(✉)], Michal Sroka[1], and Andrea Burattin[2]

[1] Microsoft Development Center Copenhagen, Copenhagen, Denmark
{mfanisani,misroka}@microsoft.com
[2] Technical University of Denmark, Kgs. Lyngby, Denmark
andbur@dtu.dk

Abstract. Process mining is often used to identify opportunities for process automation leading to improved efficiency and cost savings. Robotic process automation (RPA) is a fast-growing area that provides tremendous productivity growth to a growing number of companies across many industries. RPA tools allow users to record their work and then propose areas for automation, and produce scripts to automate work. Recording how a process is conducted, coupled with process mining techniques, offers the most detailed view of what process is followed, how well it is followed, and whether there are areas for automation or improvement in process or policies. However, the main challenge to deriving these insights is the need for grouping fine-grained recorded tasks into events, giving them names, and proposing how to automate those high-level tasks. In this paper, we propose a framework for using large language models (LLMs) to assist users in these steps, by leveraging their natural language understanding and generation capabilities. We first address the problem of event log generation, which is an input of automation techniques, by using LLMs to group and label tasks based on their semantic similarity and context. We then tackle the problem of connector recommendation by using LLMs to recommend best plugins to automate tasks. We evaluate our approach on a real publicly available dataset, and show that it can improve the quality and efficiency of event log generation and connector recommendation, compared to the baseline methods.

Keywords: Process Mining · Large Language Models · Robotic Process Automation

1 Introduction

Process mining is a data science field that aims to discover, monitor, and improve business processes based on event data produced by information systems supporting process executions. Process mining consists of several tasks, such as *process discovery*, *conformance checking*, and *process enhancement*. Process discovery generates a process model from event logs, conformance checking compares

J. De Smedt and P. Soffer (Eds.): ICPM 2023 Workshops, LNBIP 503, pp. 379–391, 2024.
https://doi.org/10.1007/978-3-031-56107-8_29

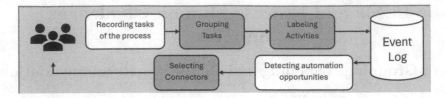

Fig. 1. Schematic view of process automation. We first need to gather an event log from the users' process recordings. Thereafter, detecting automation opportunities for automation and select the corresponding connectors for recommendations. In blue, the activities tackled by this paper. (Color figure online)

the logs and model, and process enhancement provides insights for improvement [1].

One of the applications of process mining is process automation, which aims at increasing the performance and efficiency of processes by automating manual and repetitive tasks. Process automation can increase business processes' efficiency, quality, and reliability by using software robots or *connectors* that can execute tasks automatically or semi-automatically. For example, in an invoice processing scenario, a connector can extract the relevant information from a scanned document and store it in a database, or send an email notification to the customer. To do that it is usually required to provide event logs that capture the execution of the process instances and to select the corresponding connectors that enable the integration of different services and applications in the automation workflow.

Preparing event logs and selecting connectors are not trivial tasks, and often involve manual effort and domain knowledge from users. For example, users need to group their recorded tasks into activities, which are the basic units of analysis in process mining, and label them with meaningful names that reflect their semantics and goals. These steps are crucial for producing high-quality data (necessary to obtain reliable results) yet can be challenging as, for example, grouping tasks and labeling the activities can be inconsistent and error-prone, especially for complex and heterogeneous processes that involve multiple users, systems, and data sources. Moreover, users must select the most suitable connectors for automating the activities, among the hundreds of available options, depending on the functionality, compatibility, and security of the services and applications involved. These steps can be time-consuming and may limit the potential benefits of process automation.

Figure 1 provides a schematic view of process automation. To automate a process, we usually need to collect an event log which is usually done by several users collaboratively. We record all the tasks that different users do. Afterward, the users should group the tasks into activities, and label the activities by different words. After that we obtain an event log. If we find some places for automation we can recommend the connectors for each activity.

To overcome these challenges, in this paper, we propose a novel approach incorporating large language models (LLMs) to assist users in task grouping, labeling, and connector recommendation. LLMs are neural network models trained on massive amounts of text data. They can perform various natural language understanding and generation tasks, such as answering questions, summarizing texts, or generating sentences [2]. We leverage the LLMs' capabilities to analyze the event data, generate meaningful labels, and recommend relevant connectors, based on natural language prompts and queries. We use GPT 3.5 Turbo [3] and GPT-4 [4] as an example of LLMs, but our approach can be generalized to other LLMs as well.

Our approach consists of three main steps:

1. Task grouping: We use LLMs to cluster the tasks into activities, based on their similarity in terms of data, system, and user. We describe the tasks' attributes, their time, and their order in a natural language prompt and ask the LLM to assign a cluster label to each task. We then aggregate the tasks with the same cluster label into an activity.
2. Labeling: We use LLMs to generate meaningful labels for the activities, based on their cluster labels and task attributes. We use LLM to generate a short and descriptive label for the activity.
3. Connector recommendation: We use LLMs to recommend the most suitable connectors for automating the activities, based on their labels, task attributes, and available connectors.

We evaluate our approach on a real publicly available dataset, which contains event logs from 50 different business processes [5]. We compare our approach with the baseline method, based on traditional clustering, string matching, and ranking algorithms leveraging process discovery and conformance checking [6]. We measure the quality and efficiency of our approach in terms of accuracy, completeness, consistency, and time. We show that our approach can improve the quality and efficiency of task grouping, labeling, and connector recommendation, compared to the baseline method.

The contributions of this paper are as follows:

- We propose a novel approach to use LLMs for task grouping, labeling, and connector recommendation in process mining, which can assist users in preparing event logs and selecting connectors for process automation.
- We evaluate our approach on a real, publicly available dataset, and show that it can improve the quality and efficiency of the process automation steps, compared to the baseline methods.

The rest of the paper is organized as follows. Section 2 reviews the related work on process mining, process automation, and LLMs. Section 3 describes the preliminaries and the notation used in the paper. Section 4 presents the proposed approach for task grouping, labeling, and connector recommendation. Section 5 reports the evaluation results, then, Sect. 6 discusses the limitations and the future work of our approach and finally, Sect. 7 concludes the paper.

2   Related Work

Several research has been done in the areas of recommender systems and process automation in process mining. A comprehensive survey of these systems is available in [7].

In [8], the authors present a process mining technique to enable effective RPA activities toward process improvement. Moreover, [9] discusses the capabilities of processes-based techniques with RPA and proposes an automatable indicator system as well as RPA activities to maximize the automation investment.

In [10], a survey on task mining has been reported and several applications and challenges in front of this research are represented. The authors in [11], present an unsupervised approach for task recognition from user interaction streams. Moreover, [12] has proposed a tool to record the interactions with user interfaces and to generate an event log that can be used to bridge the gap between process mining and RPA by detecting the tasks that can be automated. Furthermore, in [6], we propose to use process models and their conformance for recommending connectors. This approach requires some training event logs and discovers models for each connector. Thereafter, for each process instance, we recommend the connectors that their models are fitted more to it.

Several recent works analyzed the interaction of LLMs and process mining. For example, in [13] authors focused on conversation agents; [14] focus on specific prompt strategies similarly to what is reported in [15] (where the focus is also on abstraction). Other work focused on explainability of prediction results in process mining [16]. Authors of [17] identify six research directions where LLMs can be useful tools in BPM.

3   Preliminaries

In this section, we formalize the main concepts necessary to define a task, a recording, a grouping of tasks, labeling, and connector recommendation.

To capture how a process is executed by different users, they record the required tasks regarding that process. For each task, different information is captured such as the tools that are used, the input data, the action that is done, etc. In the following, we formally define a task.

Definition 1 (Task). *A task $s=(a_1, a_2, \ldots, a_n, \tau)$ is a tuple of attribute values, with domains $a_i \in \mathrm{dom}(a_i)$ and $\tau \in \mathbb{T}$ where $\mathbb{T}$ is the time domain with discrete time units. Let $\mathcal{TK}$ be the universe of tasks and $s \in \mathcal{TK}$ be a task. The projector operator π can be used to access specific components of the tuple: $\pi_i(s)=a_i$ returns the attribute value of attribute A_i and $\pi_\tau(s)$ returns the execution time of s.*

Given a set $\mathcal{S}$ of elements, we apply the Kleene operator to it $\mathcal{S}^*$ to indicate all possible sequences comprising all elements of $\mathcal{S}$. An element $S=\langle s_1, \ldots, s_m \rangle \in \mathcal{S}^*$ is therefore a sequence of elements each of which belongs to $\mathcal{A}$. As shortcuts, we use the length operator $|S|=m$; indexes: $S_i=s_i$; and $S^{first}=s_1$, $S^{last}=s_m$. The concatenation of two sequences s_1 and s_2 is defined as $s_1 \cdot s_2$.

A record is a sequence of tasks that are sorted based on their execution times.

Definition 2 (Record). *Let $\mathcal{TK}$ be the universe of tasks, $\mathcal{I}$ be the universe of recording ids, and $\mathbb{T}$ be the time domain with discrete time units. A record $r = (id, S)$ is a tuple where $id \in \mathcal{I}$ is the recording identifier for this sequence and $S \in \mathcal{TK}^*$ is a finite sequence of tasks which are ordered by execution time: $\forall_{i,j \in \{1, \ldots, |S|\}} i < j \implies \pi_\tau(s_i) \leq \pi_\tau(s_j)$.*

In task grouping, the goal is to convert low-level behavior to higher-level. To achieve this, we segment and group the tasks of each record. In the following, we formally define task grouping.

Definition 3 (Task grouping). *Let $\mathcal{R}$ be the universe of records achievable from the universe of tasks $\mathcal{TK}$ and the universe of recording ids $\mathcal{I}$; then let $(id, S) \in \mathcal{R}$ be a record. We can define $TG : \mathcal{R} \to \mathcal{P}(\mathcal{TK}^*)$[1] as a task grouping function. This function receives a record and returns a set of sequences of tasks such that, given a record $r = (id, S)$ and the resulting grouping $g = TG(r)$ we have that $g_1 \cdot g_2 \cdot \ldots \cdot g_{|G|} = S$ and*

$$\forall_{i,j\in\{1,\cdots,|g|\}} \left(\pi_\tau(g_i^{first}) < \pi_\tau(g_j^{first}) \implies \pi_\tau(g_i^{last}) < \pi_\tau(g_j^{first})\right) \wedge$$
$$\left(\pi_\tau(g_i^{first}) > \pi_\tau(g_j^{last}) \implies \pi_\tau(g_i^{first}) < \pi_\tau(g_j^{last})\right)$$

In other words, the task grouping splits a sequence of tasks into several subsequences of its tasks. However, the concatenation of all subsequences should recreate the original sequence and, for any two subsequences S_i and S_j, all the tasks S_i should be executed before all the tasks of S_j, or all of them should be executed after the tasks in S_j.

After grouping the tasks, we must also provide a descriptive name for each group. We call this part *labeling* and define it in the following.

Definition 4 (Labeling). *Let $\mathcal{I}$ be the universe of recording ids, $\mathcal{TK}$ be the universe of tasks, and $\mathcal{A}$ be the universe of activity names (to an abstraction level that is meaningful to the end-user). We define $L : \mathcal{TK}^* \to \mathcal{A}$ as a labeling function that assigns an activity name to a sequence of tasks.*

Using the labeling function, we can generate an event log from the recordings. The procedure of converting task attributes to event log attributes with high-level activities is out of the scope of the paper. However, in the following, we formally define an event log, following the typical definitions found in the literature.

Definition 5 (Event log). *Let $\mathcal{C}$ be the universe of case identifiers, $\mathcal{A}$ the universe of activity names, and $\mathcal{X} = \mathcal{N} \times \mathcal{V}$ the set of extra attributes (each comprising a name in $\mathcal{N}$ and a value in $\mathcal{V}$). The event universe $\mathcal{E} = \mathcal{C} \times \mathcal{A} \times \mathcal{P}(X)$ is the set of all possible events. From the event universe, it is possible to extract traces as sequences of events that share the same case identifier. An event log is then a multi-set of traces.*

It is possible to see a direct mapping from the concepts in record, tasks (grouping), and labeling into the definition of event log. Specifically, the recording ids (of records) are the case identifiers (of event logs) which are producing traces (of event logs), and tasks in records are grouped and labelled, and these labels are activity names (in event logs).

---

[1] With $\mathcal{P}(A)$ we indicate the powerset of A: the set of all possible subsets of A.

After generating an event log and finding the automation opportunities, we may need to select some connectors for the automation. As there could be many available connectors, having a connector recommender that suggests the ideal recommender is valuable. In the following, we formally define a connector recommender.

Definition 6 (Connector recommender). *Let $\mathcal{A}$ denote the universe of activity names and let Γ be the universe of connectors. We define $CR : \mathcal{A}^* \to \mathcal{P}(\Gamma)$ as a* connector recommender *that receives a sequence of activities and returns a set of connectors that could replace the sequence of activities. Finally, we can use CR_k to denote a recommender that returns exactly k connectors.*

4 Using LLM for Task Grouping, Labeling, and Connector Recommendation

In this section, we aim to explain how, by using LLMs, we are able to group the tasks, label appropriate activities to each group, and recommend some connectors for each trace. We aimed to design a workflow that requires business knowledge. Consequently, the designed workflow can be used for different business recordings.

The schematic view of the proposed workflow is shown in Fig. 2. We separate the proposed method into *Preparation* and *Application* phases. In the preparation phase, the goal is to generate a template for the future prompts. The key to high quality results from LLM is a process of improving this template called prompt engineering [18]. In the prompt, we should describe the assignment (i.e., the role of LLM), what are inputs, and how we expect to have outputs. Depending on the assignment, we can have zero to few examples to let LLM understand the task more.

One aspect that should be considered in the preparation phase is that different LLMs may need different prompt engineering styles. In this paper, we consider GPT-4-32K-0314 and GPT-3.5-Turbo-16K models.

In the application phase, we use the designed template and fill it with the values of inputs for the new cases. The filled template is given to LLM and it returns the expected output.

The proposed workflow, can be used for different assignments and in this paper, we used it for task grouping, labeling, and connector recommendation.

5 Evaluation

We applied these methods on a public dataset reflecting real life scenarios, containing 50 processes labelled by humans [5]. For each process, we have at least 3 cases manually labelled. The labels include how tasks should be grouped and named. The dataset includes ids of step, process, and recording and label event names. It also contains some columns like *StepName* which is the name of the step that can be from one of 19 different options, e.g., *Press button in window*.

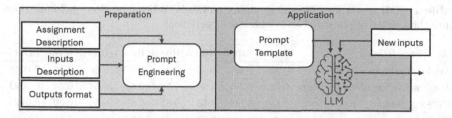

Fig. 2. The schematic view of process workflow to use LLMs for RPA.

StepDescription, which is a more detailed description of the step, e.g., *Button 'New Tab' in Window 'Process-Microsoft Edge'*, or ApplicationProcessName, which is the process name, taken from the opened application, e.g., *msedge*. For details, we refer the reader to [19]. Moreover, a filtered version of this dataset is preprocessed and labeled for evaluating the connector recommendation[2]. The prompt templates that we used for the experiments can be found in https://github.com/mfanisani/LLM4RPA.

We utilized LLMs for task grouping, labeling, and connector recommendation assignments. Thus, we provided a prompt template for each assignment, and we used two configurations of OpenAI as the LLMs, i.e., GPT-3.5-Turbo (*GPT3.5* in short) [3] and *GPT-4* [4]. In the following, for each assignment, we first explain the experimental metrics. Then, for each task, we provide the evaluation results. Because the LLM output is non-deterministic, we repeat the experiments for each assignment 6 times.

5.1 Task Grouping Experiments and Results

To evaluate the quality of the proposed task grouping, we compared the groups suggested by the LLM method with human labels from the dataset. A metric widely used for measuring how the quality of clusters compares with expected clustering is Normalized Mutual Information (NMI) [20]. It is based on the mutual information measure, which quantifies how much information is shared by two random variables. NMI normalizes the mutual information by some function of the entropy of the two clustering, so that the score ranges from 0 to 1. NMI is often used to evaluate the performance of clustering algorithms when the true labels are known.

We can compute the NMI using the following formula

$$\text{NMI}(U, V) = \frac{2 \times I(U, V)}{H(U) + H(V)} \tag{1}$$

where U and U are two clustering outputs for the same data set, $I(U, V)$ is the mutual information between U and V, and $H(U)$ and $H(V)$ are the entropy of

---

[2] The dataset and its filtered version are available via https://github.com/microsoft/50BusinessAssignmentsLog and https://github.com/nikraftarf/Recommender-System-Based-on-processMining/tree/main/Data, respectively.

Table 1. NMI scores for different grouping methods. Where the Error column represents the margin of error at 1.984 confidence coefficient.

Grouping Method	Run 1	Run 2	Run 3	Run 4	Run 5	Run 6	Mean	Error*
ApplicationProcessName	0.36	0.36	0.36	0.36	0.37	0.36	0.36	0.0016
ApplicationParentWindowName	0.55	0.54	0.54	0.54	0.54	0.54	0.54	0.0023
GPT3.5 Turbo	0.58	0.59	0.56	0.61	0.59	0.59	0.59	0.0123
GPT4	0.75	0.76	0.75	0.76	0.74	0.74	0.75	0.0060

U and V, respectively. A higher NMI indicates a better agreement between the clustering 's outputs, while a lower NMI indicates a worse agreement.

As a baseline we consider grouping tasks when the user changes their focus. The change of focus can manifest itself in changing of the window in focus, or changing the window name. The former is represented in the dataset as changes of ApplicationProcessName column, and the latter as ApplicationParentWindowName.

Task grouping is the first task in the pipeline as indicated on the diagram in Fig. 1. The quality of task grouping strongly depends on the considered input data as described in Definition 3. For grouping and labelling, we use the following columns: *StepId, StepName, StepDescription, ApplicationProcessName,* and *ApplicationParentWindowName.* then, for each step, we concatenate the mentioned values into a concatenated string as the representative of the step.

Thereafter, we formulate a prompt template including instructions, knowledge about task grouping, and a few examples to understand the response and the expected outputs. As a result, for each row of input data representing a task, we obtain a predicted label. If multiple consecutive tasks are assigned the same label, we consider them as a group, i.e., a high-level event.

Table 1 shows the results of comparing human-assigned and LLM-generated groups. We run the experiments 6 times and report the average values and Error*. The results indicate that ApplicationProcessName as a baseline performs the poorest with an average score of 0.36, and ApplicationParentWindowName gives a much better estimate with an average NMI score of 0.54. The results from GPT 3.5 Turbo, are better than both baselines and offer a stable increase in quality across all experiments. We achieved the best results by using *GPT*4 that outperforms all others by a large amount, obtaining an average NMI score of 0.75. It indicates that using LLMs improves the quality of *task grouping* assignment.

5.2   Group Labelling Experiments and Results

To evaluate the quality of the label generated for each event, i.e., a group of tasks, we are using three metrics to measure different types of similarities. To check for *syntactical similarity*, we used BLEU score [21] and normalized Levenstein distance [22]. Moreover, to assess *semantic similarity*, we used the *cosine similarity* between the embedding generated using text-embedding-ada-002 model for both the generated and expected labels.

Table 2. Examples of labels given by human experts and generated by *GPT4*.

Id	Label	Cosine Similarity	BlEU	Normalized Levenstein
1	*Human*: Open the attendance sheet *GPT4*: Open Attendance Sheet	0.96	0.71	0.16
2	*Human*: Go to approval app *GPT4*: Search for Approval App	0.95	0.5	0.44
3	*Human*: Open email app. *GPT4*: Access Gmail	0.86	0	0.71
4	*Human*: Create a report *GPT4*: Create Power BI report	0.86	0.5	0.53
5	*Human*: Create a tasks through roadmap app. *GPT4*: Add task to project	0.82	0	0.68
6	*Human*: Find the email notification regarding daily attendance and verify it *GPT4*: Get email notification	0.84	0.12	0.71

Table 3. The Similarity of labels that are assigned by humans and the ones predicted by GPT.

Label Similarity Metric		Run 1	Run 2	Run 3	Run 4	Run 5	Run 6	Avg	Stdev	Error
BLEU	*GPT3.5*	0.39	0.39	0.39	0.39	0.39	0.39	0.39	0.0	0.0
	GPT4	0.41	0.41	0.41	0.43	0.43	0.41	0.42	0.0103	0.0168
Cosine Similarity	*GPT3.5*	0.81	0.81	0.81	0.81	0.81	0.81	0.81	0.0012	0.0010
	GPT4	0.83	0.83	0.83	0.83	0.83	0.83	0.83	0.0005	0.0004
Normalised Levenstein	*GPT3.5*	0.87	0.89	0.88	0.85	0.87	0.85	0.87	0.0141	0.0114
	GPT4	0.86	0.88	0.87	0.86	0.87	0.86	0.87	0.0062	0.0050

The comparison of the human assigned labels and LLM-generated labels using different measures is presented in Table 3. The high cosine similarity scores indicate that, using LLM models, we provide activity labels that are semantically similar to the ones that were assigned by humans. It should be noted that by using the proposed approach, we can save a considerable amount of post-processing time as different users may assign different labels to a group. Note that using LLM lets us have labeling in a central way. It is also worth to mention that the syntactical similarity is relatively low. By investigating the labels, we found that it is mainly because of humans and GPT models may use different words to name the same activity. Selected examples of human and LLM-generated labels are presented in Table 2. For example, in the sixth example, the human and LLM-based labels are semantically very close; however, their syntactical similarity is quite low due to the chosen wordings. Moreover, the results indicate that GTP3.5 and GPT4 generated comparable quality of labels for the events.

5.3   Connector Recommendation Experiments and Results

In the last assignment, to recommend connectors, we use cr_k with different k-values from 1 to 5 (cf. Definition 6). To evaluate the accuracy of the connector recommendation, we have used the following formula:

Table 4. Comparing the retrive rate of using process discovery [6] and LLM methods when different number of connectors are recommended.

Connector	Records#	Retrive Rate										
		K=1			K=2			K=3			k=5		
		PD	GPT3.5	GPT4	PD	GPT3.5	GPT4	PD	GPT3.5	GPT4	PD	GPT3.5	GPT4
Approvals	7	57	100	86	71	100	100	71	100	100	100	100	100
googlecalendar	6	50	50	17	50	67	67	67	67	67	100	83	83
Microsoftforms	5	60	60	100	60	60	100	80	60	100	100	60	100
Office365users	4	75	100	100	75	100	100	100	100	100	100	100	100
onenote	4	25	50	100	25	50	100	50	50	100	50	50	100
Outlook	5	60	0	80	60	60	80	80	60	100	80	60	100
Planner	5	60	60	100	80	60	100	80	60	100	100	60	100
rss	4	0	25	50	0	25	50	0	25	50	25	25	50
Sendmail	5	20	60	60	80	100	60	80	100	100	100	100	100
Sharepoint	4	40	75	100	40	100	100	60	100	100	60	100	100

$$RetrieveRate = \frac{|\{\text{Labeled Connector}\} \cap \{\text{Recommended Connectors}\}|}{|\{\text{Recommended Connectors}\}|} \quad (2)$$

The higher value means a more accurate recommendation.

To generate the prompt template for the connector recommendation assignment, we only used *StepName, StepDescription, ApplicationProcessName, ApplicationParentWindowName* columns of all steps that belong to a record as the inputs. We gave all the mentioned data as a concatenated string for each record. The results of using LLM for connector recommendation are presented in Table 4. Here, we compared the result of the proposed approach with the method that is presented in [6](i.e., *PD*). In most cases, we have a higher *Retrieve Rate* using LLM models. Specifically, for $k<3$, LLM could be considered as the best method. However, by increasing k, we do not have that much improvement.

Note that to use the method that is proposed in [6], we need some training recordings, and adjusting process models using different parameters of process discovery algorithms that can be time consuming. However, using LLMs, we do not need to have any labeled data, and the only requirement is having the list of available connectors for the recommendation. Moreover, using the method that is presented in [6], we only benefit from control-flow information, however, using LLM, we benefit from more data attributes.

6   Discussion

The results of experiments indicate that we can use LLMs for automating many process mining and automation activities. The task grouping and labeling that are covered in this paper can be challenging and error-prone. Different users, may group tasks with different granulates and use different labels. Note that even small difference in the labels (e.g., "send email" and "sending email") leads to having more than one activity in the event log.

Although the results indicate that we have high accuracy in the given tasks, it is suggested not to remove the users from the process. We recommend to use

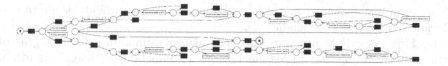

Fig. 3. The process model (in the Petri net description) discovered on projected event log of *Office365users* connector.

LLMs as a method to recommend grouping, labels, and connectors, and the user selects to confirm them. The initial exploration of the baseline Process Discovery (PD) method has yielded results not exceptionally off compared to those of the LLM, particularly evident with higher K values (cf. Table 4) by incorporating additional top connectors. Delving into the realm of explainability, it's essential to consider the differences in how the two approaches convey their results. The Process Models generated through the PD Method offer a level of explainability and the capability of comparing the models underlying different connectors, which contrasts with the self-explanation of the GPT model. Though it is possible to ask GPT models for an explanation of the results, their actual effectiveness remains to be assessed. For example, Fig. 3 presents the process model that will be used for the *Office365users* connector. For the process instances that belong to this connector, we usually have similar results using both approaches.

Additionally, the Process Discovery method is capable of computing the conformance of execution with respect to the reference model, thus providing a measure of the "confidence" of the trace to the reference. While the PD method has already demonstrated good performance from this point of view, LLMs are fundamentally incapable of expressing any confidence level for the results they provide, thus challenging their trustworthiness with their human operators.

An interesting point of comparison arises in terms of data ingestion capabilities. The GPT model possesses the capacity to assimilate a broader spectrum of information, as opposed to the process discovery, which can ingest only event logs (i.e., data referring to the control-flow). This aspect opens the discussion on the varying degrees to which each approach can accommodate and incorporate the available data. From this point of view, LLMs outperform process mining-based systems and certainly can serve as inspiration to improve process discovery algorithms.

7   Conclusion and Future Work

In this paper, we proposed to use LLMs for assisting users in process mining and automation tasks, such as task grouping, event labeling, and connector recommendation. We showed that LLMs can leverage their natural language understanding and generation capabilities to produce high-quality and semantically coherent outputs, based on the recorded data of user activities. We evaluated our approach on a real publicly available dataset, and compared it with the baseline method. We found that by using LLMs we are able to improve the quality and efficiency of task grouping and event labeling, as well as provide accurate and relevant connector recommendations.

Looking towards future prospects, the idea of combining the strengths of both process mining and LLMs emerges as a compelling avenue. This fusion could potentially yield results that surpass the capabilities of each method in isolation. A noteworthy distinction lies in the nature of the dataset: the wealth of textual information available can be harnessed by the LLM but not as readily by process mining. This discrepancy underscores the unique advantages and considerations of each approach.

References

1. van der Aalst, W.M.P.: Process Mining - Data Science in Action, 2nd edn. Springer, Heidelberg (2016). https://doi.org/10.1007/978-3-662-49851-4
2. Kasneci, E., et al.: ChatGPT for good? On opportunities and challenges of large language models for education. Learn. Individ. Differ. **103**, 102274 (2023)
3. OpenAI: Gpt-3.5 turbo: a large language and code model with function calling data. https://platform.openai.com/docs/models/gpt-3-5 (2023)
4. OpenAI: GPT-4 technical report. CoRR **abs/2303.08774** (2023)
5. Sroka, M., Fani Sani, M.: Recording of 50 business assignments (2023)
6. Fani Sani, M., Nikraftar, F., Sroka, M., Burattin, A.: Behavioral recommender system for process automation steps. In: Proceedings of the DATA, Scitepress (2023)
7. Eili, M.Y., Rezaeenour, J., Fani Sani, M.: A systematic literature review on process-aware recommender systems. CoRR **abs/2103.16654** (2021)
8. Geyer-Klingeberg, J., Nakladal, J., Baldauf, F., Veit, F.: Process mining and robotic process automation: a perfect match. In: Proceedings of the Co-located Events with BPM, vol. 2196 of CEUR Workshop Proceedings, pp. 124–131 (2018)
9. Wanner, J., Hofmann, A., Fischer, M., Imgrund, F., Janiesch, C., Geyer-Klingeberg, J.: Process selection in RPA projects - towards a quantifiable method of decision making. In: Proceedings of the ICIS, Association for Information Systems (2019)
10. Mayr, A., Herm, L., Wanner, J., Janiesch, C.: Applications and challenges of task mining: a literature review. In: Proceedings of the ECIS (2022)
11. Rebmann, A., van der Aa, H.: Unsupervised task recognition from user interaction streams. In: Indulska, M., Reinhartz-Berger, I., Cetina, C., Pastor, O. (eds.) Advanced Information Systems Engineering. CAiSE 2023. LNCS, vol. 13901, pp. 141–157. Springer, Cham (2023). https://doi.org/10.1007/978-3-031-34560-9_9
12. Choi, D., R'bigui, H., Cho, C.: Enabling the gab between RPA and process mining: user interface interactions recorder. IEEE Access **10**, 39604–39612 (2022)
13. Jessen, U., Sroka, M., Fahland, D.: Chit-chat or deep talk: prompt engineering for process mining. CoRR **abs/2307.09909** (2023)
14. Berti, A., Qafari, M.S.: Leveraging large language models (LLMS) for process mining (technical report). CoRR **abs/2307.12701** (2023)
15. Berti, A., Schuster, D., van der Aalst, W.M.P.: Abstractions, scenarios, and prompt definitions for process mining with LLMS: a case study. CoRR **abs/2307.02194** (2023)

16. Stevens, A., Smedt, J.D.: Explainable artificial intelligence in process mining: assessing the explainability-performance trade-off in outcome-oriented predictive process monitoring. CoRR **abs/2203.16073** (2022) Withdrawn

17. Vidgof, M., Bachhofner, S., Mendling, J.: Large language models for business process management: opportunities and challenges. CoRR **abs/2304.04309** (2023)

18. White, J., et al.: A prompt pattern catalog to enhance prompt engineering with ChatGPT. arXiv preprint arXiv:2302.11382 (2023)

19. Sroka, M., Fani Sani, M.: 50 business assignments log (2022)

20. Cover, T.M., Thomas, J.A.: Elements of Information Theory. Wiley, Hoboken (2006)

21. Papineni, K., Roukos, S., Ward, T., Zhu, W.J.: Bleu: a method for automatic evaluation of machine translation. In: Proceedings of the ACL. (2002) 311–318

22. Yujian, L., Bo, L.: A normalized Levenshtein distance metric. IEEE Trans. Pattern Anal. Mach. Intell. **29**(6), 1091–1095 (2007)

Checking Constraints for Object-Centric Process Executions

Tian Li[(✉)], Gyunam Park, and Wil M. P. van der Aalst

Process and Data Science Group (PADS), RWTH Aachen University, Aachen,
Germany
{tian.li,gnpark,wvdaalst}@pads.rwth-aachen.de

Abstract. Conformance-checking techniques reveal the deviations
between event data and the desired process specification, which can be
expressed as a process model or a set of rules. State-of-the-art approaches
assume a single case identifier, i.e., each case in the business process is
associated with only one object. In contrast, processes in real life usually
involve multiple object types. For instance, an order management process
involves object types such as orders, items, and packages. These objects
interact with one another, e.g., packing multiple items from the inventory
to create a package. Existing techniques may provide misleading insights
when applied to such object-centric event data. We address the issue
by extracting process executions (cases) from the object-centric event
log and representing constraints using *Object-Centric Constraint Models*
(OCCMs). In this way, we handle cardinality, temporal, and performance
constraints. Compared to procedural languages like Petri nets, the declarative nature of OCCMs provides more flexibility in modeling constraints,
and constraint checking delivers more comprehensive *diagnostics that go
beyond isolated cases*. The proposed method has been implemented as a
ProM plug-in that supports the extraction of process executions, user-
defined OCCMs, and constraint-checking. The feasibility of the proposed
approach has been evaluated with other state-of-the-art approaches.

Keywords: Process Mining · Conformance Checking · Constraint
Checking · Object-Centric

1 Introduction

Process mining techniques aim to analyze event data recorded in the information systems and gain insights into business processes. Identifying unexpected
or undesired deviations in processes is critical to mitigating risks or bottlenecks,
thus monitoring the operational issues is essential for companies and organizations to maintain operational efficiency.

State-of-the-art constraint-checking/conformance-checking techniques are
based on a *single case notion* in the event data, i.e., an event is associated with
one object of a unique type (case notion). However, in real-life processes stored
in ERP systems, one event can be associated with different objects of multiple
types. For example, a simplified recruitment process is illustrated in Fig. 1. The

© The Author(s), under exclusive license to Springer Nature Switzerland AG 2024
J. De Smedt and P. Soffer (Eds.): ICPM 2023 Workshops, LNBIP 503, pp. 392–405, 2024.
https://doi.org/10.1007/978-3-031-56107-8_30

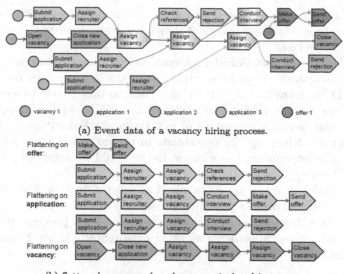

(a) Event data of a vacancy hiring process.

Flattening on offer:

Flattening on application:

Flattening on vacancy:

(b) flattened sequences based on a particular object type.

Fig. 1. Real-life event data for the recruitment process and flattened event data with one object type.

organization opens a new vacancy based on specific needs. Candidates who are interested in the position send applications before the submission deadline. After several rounds of reference checking or interviews, one candidate is hired for the vacancy.

In this process, events can be associated with multiple objects of different types, and each event may have multiple preceding and succeeding events. Therefore, the whole process is not a collection of homogeneously typed event sequence assumed in traditional process mining settings. To bridge this gap between object-centric settings and traditional conformance-checking techniques, the flattening approach [1] is currently used. It first chooses an object type as a case notion, then produces sequences of events related to the lifecycle of objects of this type. As illustrated in Fig. 1b, each case notion provides a sequential event sequence, describing the lifecycle of each object of the selected type. However, there are drawbacks to flattening event data in object-centric settings. To illustrate the problem, we showcase three example constraints as follows:

- constraint 1: *Open vacancy* should be later followed by *Close vacancy*.
- constraint 2: *Close new application* should be preceded by at least one *Submit application*.
- constraint 3: *Submit application* should happen within two months after *Open vacancy*.

When flattening with object type vacancy, constraint 1 is satisfied as *Open vacancy* is followed by *Close vacancy* afterward. However, constraint 2 is violated since *Close new application* is not preceded by any *Submit application*, and constraint 3 is also violated due to the absence of *Submit application* after *Open vacancy*. The underlying reason is that flattening removes activities not related to the object type, thus constraints that involve multiple object types can not be accurately checked.

To tackle the aforementioned problems, we propose a constraint-checking technique that operates in object-centric settings, which provides two key contributions: **1)** We introduce an extraction technique that is able to identify process executions from an *Object-Centric Event Log (OCEL)* [5] using one leading object type and multiple secondary object types. **2)** We outline three different constraint models to specify constraints in the extracted process execution. The approach is implemented as a plugin in the ProM package "ObjectCentricConstraintChecking".

The remainder of the paper is organized as follows. In Sect. 2 we discuss the related work, then we present preliminaries and the notion of process executions in Sect. 3. In Sect. 4, we formalize the constraint models for process execution. In Sect. 5, we evaluate our approach with other existing techniques. Finally, Sect. 6 concludes the paper.

2   Related Work

The importance of constraint monitoring and follow-up process redesign has long been recognized by the industry. In [11], a technique was proposed to derive monitoring queries from a process model and monitor control-flow deviations. A run-time framework based on Linear Temporal Logic (LTL) was introduced [9]. On the whole, the majority of work for constraints in the process still revolves around traditional event data using a single case notion such that the event data present a sequential structure.

Due to the drawbacks of flattening with a single case identifier when dealing with object-centric event data, there have been a few studies highlighting handling event data with multiple dimensions [2]. A method to model business processes based on artifacts was discussed in [6]. A method to model and reason over object-centric behavioral constraints was proposed in [4]. Jalali et al. [8] tracked rules defined for process instances by considering multiple perspectives. In [7], the authors convert the multi-dimensional event log to graph-based data models and retrieve behavioral insights, such as direct-follow-relations.

3   Preliminaries

Given a set X, the power set $\mathcal{P}(X)$ denotes the set of all possible subsets. A sequence $\sigma = \langle x_1, \ldots, x_n \rangle$ assigns an order to elements of X, and $len(\sigma) = n$ is the length of σ. X^* denotes the set of all sequences over X.

A graph is a tuple $G = (V, E)$ where V is a set of nodes and $E \subseteq V \times V$ is a set of edges. In an undirected graph, $\forall_{v,v' \in V} : (v, v') \in E \leftrightarrow (v', v) \in E$. For two distinct nodes $v, v' \in V$, $path(v, v') = \{\langle (v, v_1), (v_1, v_2), \ldots, (v_{k-1}, v_k), (v_k, v') \rangle \in E^*\}$ denotes the set of all possible paths between them. $conn(v, v') = true$ if and only if nodes v and v' are connected, i.e., $path(v, v') \neq \emptyset$. For two connected

Table 1. Example object-centric event log L_1.

Event	Object type			Event type	Timestamp
	Order	Item	Package		
e1	o1	i1, i2		Place order	2019-01-12 09:36:06
e2	o1	i1		Item out of stock	2019-01-12 10:01:02
e3	o1	i2		Pick item	2019-01-12 10:06:58
e4	o1	i1		Reorder item	2019-01-12 11:59:42
e5	o2	i3		Place order	2019-01-12 13:13:19
e6	o1	i1, i2		Pay order	2019-01-12 15:31:07
e7	o2	i3		Pick item	2019-01-12 16:36:52
e8	o1	i2	p2	Create package	2019-01-14 09:12:35
e9	o1, o2	i1, i3	p1	Create package	2019-01-14 11:01:29
e10	o1		p2	Package delivered	2019-01-15 12:36:01
e11	o1, o2		p1	Package delivered	2019-01-15 15:44:53
e12	o2			Payment reminder	2019-01-22 09:15:41
e13	o2			Pay order	2019-01-23 17:21:56

nodes v and v', the distance in between is the length of the shortest path $dist(v, v') = len(\sigma)$ such that $\sigma \in path(v, v') \land \forall_{\sigma' \in path(v,v')} \; len(\sigma') \geq len(\sigma)$.

Definition 1 (Object-Centric Event Log (OCEL)). *Let $\mathbb{U}_e$ be the universe of events, $\mathbb{U}_{etype}$ be the universe of event types (i.e., activities), $\mathbb{U}_{time}$ be the universe of timestamps, $\mathbb{U}_o$ be the universe of objects, and $\mathbb{U}_{ot}$ be the universe of object types. An object-centric event log is a tuple $L = (E, O, \pi_{etype}, \pi_{otype}, \pi_{omap}, \pi_{time}, <)$, where:*

- *$E \subseteq \mathbb{U}_e$ is a set of events,*
- *$O \subseteq \mathbb{U}_o$ is a set of objects,*
- *$\pi_{etype} \colon E \to \mathbb{U}_{etype}$ is the function associating an event to an event type,*
- *$\pi_{otype} \colon E \to \mathbb{U}_{ot}$ is the function associating an object to an object type,*
- *$\pi_{omap} \colon E \to \mathcal{P}(O)$ is the function associating an event to a set of related objects,*
- *$\pi_{time} \colon E \to \mathbb{U}_{time}$ is the function associating an event to a timestamp,*
- *$<$ is a total order on the events.*

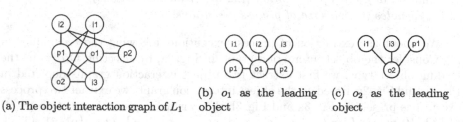

(a) The object interaction graph of L_1

(b) o_1 as the leading object

(c) o_2 as the leading object

Fig. 2. Object interaction graph and two subgraphs extracted with leading object type.

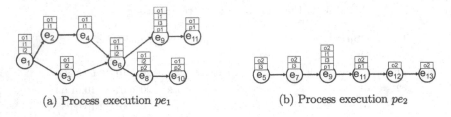

(a) Process execution pe_1 (b) Process execution pe_2

Fig. 3. Process executions extracted from corresponding object interaction graphs.

An example OCEL L_1 is present in Table 1, where we only keep the event id, object type, event type, and timestamp. There are multiple objects, including $i1, i2, i3, o1, o2, p1, p2 \in \mathbb{U}_o$.

Definition 2 (Object Interaction Graph). *Let $L = (E, O, \pi_{etype}, \pi_{otype}, \pi_{omap}, \pi_{time}, \leq)$ be an OCEL, its object interaction graph $OG_L = \{O, I\}$ where O is a set of objects and $I = \cup_{e \in E}\{(o_1, o_2) \mid o_1, o_2 \in \pi_{omap}(e) \wedge o_1 \neq o_2\}$.*

The object interaction graph of an OCEL consists of nodes of all the objects, and every pair of objects co-occurring in the set of related objects of an event is connected with an undirected edge. The object interaction graph of L_1 has been illustrated in Fig. 2a. The degree of dependency between objects can be measured by the distance in the object interaction graph. For example, items $i1$ and $i3$ are associated with order $o2$, while item $i2$ is not. This association is reflected in the graph as the distance between $i1/i3$ and $o2$ is 1, whereas the distance between $i2$ and $o2$ is 2.

Then we introduce the case concept, i.e., process executions in object-centric event data. Then we explain an extraction technique to extract process executions from OCEL.

Definition 3 (Process Execution). *Let $L = (E, O, \pi_{etype}, \pi_{otype}, \pi_{omap}, \pi_{time}, <)$ be an object-centric event log, and $OG_L = (O, I)$ be the object interaction graph of L. A process execution $pe = (E', O', R')$ is a tuple where:*

- *$E' \subseteq E$ is a set of events,*
- *$O' \subseteq O$ forms a connected subgraph in OG_L.*
- *$R' \subseteq \{(e, e') \in E' \times E' \mid \exists_{o' \in O'}\exists_{\langle e_1,...,e_n \rangle = trace(o')}\exists_{1 \leq i < n}e = e_i \wedge e' = e_{i+1}\}$ is the set of process flow relation (i.e. direct-follow-relations),*
  $\mathbb{U}_{pe}$ denotes the universe of process executions.

We adopt the extraction of process executions following the techniques in [3]. Consider the object interaction graph in Fig. 2a, by selecting Orders as the leading object type, we first extract two object interaction graphs depicted in Fig. 2b and Fig. 2c. Based on the object interaction graph, we extract two process executions present in Fig. 3a and Fig. 3b. For instance, process execution $pe_1 = (E, O, R)$ where $E = (\{e_1, e_2, e_3, e_4\ e_6, e_8\ e_9, e_{10}, e_{11}\}, O = \{o1, i1, i2, i3, p1, p2\}, R = \{(e_1, e_2), (e_1, e_3), (e_2, e_4), (e_3, e_6), (e_4, e_6), (e_6, e_8), (e_6, e_9), (e_8,$

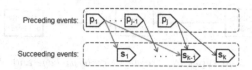

Fig. 4. Sorted events of preceding/succeeding event types in process execution *pe*.

e_{10}), $(e_9, e_{11})\}$. In order to formalize the semantics of constraint models in the next section, we introduce several notations for process executions.

Definition 4 (Notations for Process Executions). *Let $pe = (E, R, O)$ be a process execution, $et \in \mathbb{U}_{etype}$ be an event type, $e \in E$ be an event in pe. We introduce the following notations:*

- $pre_e(E) = \{e' \in E \mid conn(e', e) = true\}$ *is the set of events in pe preceding e, from which e is reachable,*
- $suc_e(E) = \{e' \in E \mid conn(e, e') = true\}$ *is the set of reachable events succeeding e,*
- $all_{et}(E) = \{e' \in E \mid \pi_{etype}(e') = et\}$ *is the set of events corresponding to event type et,*
- $first_{et}(E) = e$ *such that $\pi_{etype}(e) = et \wedge \not\exists_{e' \in E} \ \pi_{etype}(e') = et \wedge e' < e$ is the first event of type et in p. $first_{et}(E) = \perp$ denotes the absence of events of type et,*
- $last_{et}(E) = e$ *such that $\pi_{etype}(e) = et \wedge \not\exists_{e' \in E} \ \pi_{etype}(e') = et \wedge e' > e$ is the last event of type et in p. $last_{et}(E) = \perp$ denotes the absence of events of type et.*

As for pe_1 depicted in Fig. 3a, $pre_{e_3}(E) = \{e_1\}$ is the set of events preceding e_3, $suc_{e_3}(E) = \{e_6, e_8, e_9, e_{10}, e_{11}\}$ is the set of events succeeding e_3. $all_{Pick\ item}(E) = \{e_3\}$ is the set of events that execute *Pick item*. $first_{Create\ package}(E) = e_8$ is the first event in pe_1 that executes *Create package*. $last_{Package\ delivered}(E) = e_{11}$ is the last event in pe_1 that executes *Package delivered*.

4 Object-Centric Constraint Model

In this section, we explain how to model the constraints for process executions using graphical notation. We first introduce the process flow cardinality and temporal constraint models to describe the constraints from a behavioral perspective. Each constraint has a preceding event type, a succeeding event type, and constraint information that enforces the restrictions between them. Afterward, we focus on the performance constraints w.r.t. an event type in the process executions. Each constraint has one event type and constraint information that specifies the performance requirements.

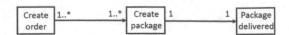

Fig. 5. A CCM for event types *Place order*, *Create package* and *Package delivered*.

4.1   Process Flow Constraint Model

In the process execution extracted from object-centric event data, the same event type may occur repeatedly. For example, one *Place order* event is later followed by several *Create package* events, as the items from one order may be packed and sent in different packages. Likewise, one *Create package* may be preceded by multiple *Place order* events, as a package may contain items from different orders.

The above examples are abstracted and present in Fig. 4. Given a process execution $pe = (E, O, R)$, we abstract two event types, i.e., the preceding event type *Pre* and succeeding event type *Suc*, such that $Pre = \{p \in E \mid \pi_{type}(p) = pre\}$ is the set of events of type *pre*, and $Suc = \{s \in E \mid \pi_{type}(s) = suc\}$ is the set of events of type *suc*. We sort the events in *Pre* and *Suc* based on their timestamps. A preceding event $p \in Pre$ is connected to a succeeding event $s \in Suc$ if $conn(p, s)$ is true. As depicted, a preceding event p_1 is connected to succeeding events s_1 and s_{k-1} (edges in blue), which indicates that events s_1 and s_{k-1} are the connected succeeding events for p_1. We introduce cardinality types to indicate the allowed number of connected succeeding events after each preceding event or the required number of connected preceding events before each succeeding event.

Definition 5 (Process Flow Cardinality Constraint Model (CCM)). *Let $A \subseteq \mathbb{U}_{etype}$ be the set of event types, and $C \subseteq \mathbb{U}_{ct}$ be the set of cardinality types. A process flow cardinality constraint model $CCM = (V, C_{cd}, L_{pre\_cd}, L_{suc\_cd})$ is a graph where:*

- *$V \subseteq A$ is a set of nodes,*
- *$C_{cd} \subseteq V \times V$ is the set of cardinality edges that connect a preceding event type to a succeeding event type,*
- *$L_{pre\_cd} \in C_{cd} \rightarrow \mathcal{P}(\mathbb{N})$ maps edges to the cardinality of the preceding event types,*
- *$L_{suc\_cd} \in C_{cd} \rightarrow \mathcal{P}(\mathbb{N})$ maps edges to the cardinality of the succeeding event type.*

Figure 5 depicts a process flow cardinality constraint model $CCM = (A, C_{cd}, L_{pre\_cd}, L_{suc\_cd})$ with $A = \{Place\ order,\ Create\ package,\ Package\ delivered\}$, $C_{card} = \{c_1 = (Place\ order,\ Create\ package),\ c_2 = (Create\ package,\ Package\ delivered)\}$. $L_{pre\_cd}(c_1) = \mathbb{N}^+$ (denoted as 1..*) indicates that each event executing *Create package* is preceded by at least one event executing *Place order*. $L_{suc\_cd}(c_1) = \mathbb{N}^+$ indicates that each event executing *Place order* is succeeded by at least one event executing *Create package*. $L_{pre\_cd}(c_2) = \{1\}$ (denoted as 1..1) indicates that each event executing *Package delivered* is preceded by exactly one event executing *Create package*. $L_{suc\_cd}(c_2) = \{1\}$ indicates that each event executing *Create package* is succeeded by exactly one event executing *Package delivered*.

Definition 6 (Conformance of CCM). *Let* $CCM = (V, C_{cd}, L_{pre\_cd}, L_{suc\_cd})$ *be a process flow cardinality constraint model, and* $pe = (E, O, R)$ *be a process execution. pe satisfies* $c_{cd} = (et_1, et_2) \in C_{cd}$, *if and only if:*

- $\forall_{e \in all_{et_1}(E)} \mid suc_e(all_{et_2}(E)) \mid \in L_{suc\_cd}(c_{cd}),$
- $\forall_{e' \in all_{et_2}(E)} \mid pre_{e'}(all_{et_1}(E)) \mid \in L_{pre\_cd}(c_{cd}).$

For each constraint in CCM, the preceding event type et_1 defines the events set $all_{et_1}(E)$, while the succeeding event type et_1 defines the events set $all_{et_2}(E)$. For each preceding event $e \in all_{et_1}(E)$, it is checked whether the number of succeeding events of type et_2 is within the allowed number. Likewise, for each succeeding event $e' \in all_{et_2}(E)$, it is checked whether the cardinality constraint is satisfied.

For example, consider the process execution pe_1 in Fig. 3a, event e_1 that executes *Place order* is succeeded by events e_8 and e_9 that executes *Create package*. Both e_8 and e_9 that execute *Create package* are preceded by e_1 that executes *Place order*. Likewise, the cardinalities between event type *Create package* and *Package delivered* are also satisfied. Therefore, process execution pe_1 satisfies the CCM in Fig. 5.

Subsequently, we introduce a model that reflects the temporal constraints between a pair of events in the process execution. For instance, items from one order may be sent with multiple packages, and the timely delivery of all goods guarantees customer satisfaction. Therefore, we define the process flow temporal constraint model to enforce that the time between two specific events must conform to predefined time frames, e.g., it is required that the last *Package delivered* should take place within a week after the *Place order*.

Definition 7 (Process Flow Temporal Constraint Model (TCM)). *Let* $A \subseteq \mathbb{U}_{etype}$ *be the set of event types,* $U \in \{seconds, minutes, hours, days, weeks, months\}$ *be the time unit, and* $P \in \{first, last\}$ *be the set of temporal patterns. A process flow temporal constraint model* $TCM = (V, C_{tp}, L_{pt}, L_{tp})$ *is a graph where:*

- $V \subseteq A$ *is a set of nodes,*
- $C_{tp} \subseteq A \times A$ *is the set of temporal edges,*
- $L_{pt} \in C_{tp} \to P \times P$ *maps temporal edges to temporal pattern,*
- $L_{tp} \in C_{tp} \to \mathbb{R} \times \mathbb{R} \times U$ *maps temporal edges to time frames.*

Figure 6 depicts a process flow temporal constraint model $TCM = (V, C_{tp}, L_{pt}, L_{tp})$ with $A = \{Place\ order, Package\ delivered\}$, $C_{tp} = \{c_1 = (Place\ order, Package\ delivered)\}$. $L_{pt}(c_1) = (first, last)$ indicates that we select the first event in the process execution that executes *Place order* and the last event in the process execution that executes *Package delivered*. $L_{tp}(c_1) = (0, 3, days)$

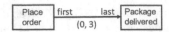

Fig. 6. A TCM for event types *Place order* and *Package delivered*.

indicates that the time frames between the first *Place order* and the last *Package delivered* should be within three days.

Definition 8 (Conformance of TCM). *Let* $TCM = (V, C_{tp}, L_{pt}, L_{tp})$ *be a process flow temporal constraint model, and* $pe = (E, O, R)$ *be a process execution. For* $c_{tp} = (v_1, v_2) \in C_{tp}$, *pe satisfies if and only if:*

- $L_{pt}(c_{tp}) = (first, first)$: $\pi_{time}(first_{v_1}(E)) - \pi_{time}(first_{v_2}(E)) \in L_{tp}(c_{tp})$,
- $L_{pt}(c_{tp}) = (first, last)$: $\pi_{time}(first_{v_1}(E)) - \pi_{time}(last_{v_2}(E)) \in L_{tp}(c_{tp})$,
- $L_{pt}(c_{tp}) = (last, first)$: $\pi_{time}(last_{v_1}(E)) - \pi_{time}(first_{v_2}(E)) \in L_{tp}(c_{tp})$,
- $L_{pt}(c_{tp}) = (last, last)$: $\pi_{time}(last_{v_1}(E)) - \pi_{time}(last_{v_2}(E)) \in L_{tp}(c_{tp})$.

For each constraint in the model, the preceding event type v_1 with the preceding pattern determines which preceding event to take and the succeeding event type v_2 with the succeeding pattern determines the corresponding succeeding event. It is checked whether the time gap between the two events satisfies the temporal constraint.

For instance, consider the process execution pe_1 in Fig. 3a. Event e_1 that executes *Place order* is succeeded by events e_{10} and e_{11} that execute *Package delivered*. In this scenario, e_1 is chosen as the preceding event, and e_{11} is chosen as the last succeeding *Package delivered*. The time frame is calculated based on their timestamps. Since the time in between is less than three days, pe_1 satisfies TCM.

Definition 9 (Performance Constraint Model (PCM)). *Let* $A \subseteq \mathbb{U}_{etype}$ *be the set of event types,* $\mathbb{U}_{tp}$ *be the universe of time performance types,* $OT \subseteq \mathbb{U}_{ot}$ *be the set of object types,* $T \subseteq \mathbb{U}_{tp}$ *be the time performance types,* $U \in \{seconds, minutes, hours, days, weeks, months\}$ *be the time unit,* F *be the frequency performance type, and* $C \subseteq \mathbb{U}_{ct}$ *be the set of cardinalities. A performance constraint model* $PCM = (V, E_{ot}, E_t, E_{fq}, L_{ot}, L_t, L_{fq})$ *is a graph where:*

- $V \subseteq A \times OT \times T \times F$ *is a set of nodes,*
- $E_{ot} \subseteq V \times OT$ *is the set of cardinality edges,*
- $E_t \subseteq V \times T$ *is the set of time edges,*
- $E_{fq} \subseteq V \times F$ *is the set of frequency edges,*
- $L_{ot} \in E_{ot} \rightarrow \mathcal{P}(\mathbb{N})$ *maps cardinality edges to object cardinality, i.e., the allowed number of associated objects for this object type,*
- $L_t \in E_t \rightarrow \mathbb{R} \times \mathbb{R} \times U$ *maps time edges to time frames,*
- $L_{fq} \in E_{fq} \rightarrow \mathcal{P}(\mathbb{N})$ *maps frequency edges to frequency value.*

Figure 7 defines a $PCM = (V, E_{ot}, E_t, E_{fq}, L_{ot}, L_t, L_{fq})$ where $V = \{$ *Create package, Waiting time, Item, Order, Frequency*$\}$, $E_{ot} = \{e_1 = ($ *Create package,*

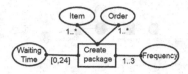

Fig. 7. A PCM for event type *Create package*.

Order), $e_2 = (Create\ package,\ Item)\}$, $E_t = \{e_3 = (Create\ package,\ Waiting$ *time*)$\}$, $E_{fq} = \{e_4 = (Create\ package,\ Frequency)\}$, $L_{ot}(e_1) = \mathbb{N}^+$ and $L_{ot}(e_2) = \mathbb{N}^+$ indicates that the number of items and orders should be greater than 1, $L_t(e_3) = (0,\ 24,\ hours)$ indicates the waiting time, $L_{fq}(e_5) = 1..3$ implies that the occurrence of *Create Package* in the process execution should lie between one to three times. Consider the process execution pe_1 in Fig. 3a. Events e_8 and e_9 correspond to event type *Create package*, thus the frequency of this event type satisfies the constraint. Event e_9 is associated with two item objects and one order object, while event e_8 is associated with one item and one order object, thus the constraint on object frequency is satisfied. Moreover, since the waiting time for e_8 and e_9 falls within 24 h, pe_1 satisfies the PCM.

Next, we define the Object-Centric Constraint Model (OCCM) models, which relate multiple behaviors in process executions through a combination of process flow modeling and performance modeling.

Definition 10 (Object-Centric Constraint Model (OCCM)). *An object-centric constraint model OCCM = (TCM, CCM, PCM) is a hybrid graph where:*

- *$CCM = (V,\ C_{cd},\ L_{pre\_cd},\ L_{suc\_cd})$ is a process flow cardinality constraint model,*
- *$TCM = (V',\ C_{tp},\ L_{pt},\ L_{tp})$ is a process flow temporal constraint model,*
- *$PCM = (V'',\ E_{ot},\ E_t,\ E_{fq},\ L_{ot},\ L_t,\ L_{fq})$ is a performance constraint model.*

An object-centric constraint model OCCM combines constraints on the process flow, but also constraints of certain event types that should be satisfied in the process execution. A process execution conforms to the object-centric constraint model $OCCM = (CCM,\ TCM,\ PCM)$ if and only if it satisfies each constraint in CCM, TCM and PCM.

We implement the checking of constraints as a ProM plugin, which enables the user to 1) extract process executions based on a leading object type 2) configure the constraint model based on Definition 5, Definition 7 and Definition 9 3) evaluate the violations of the constraint model in each process execution according to Definition 6 and Definition 8.

5   Implementations and Evaluations

In this section, we first introduce the implementations of the approach and then evaluate its feasibility by comparing it with other existing techniques.

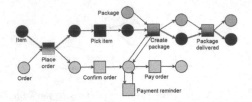

Fig. 8. An order management process: It begins with the event type "Place order", which involves the placement of an order with multiple items. Once the order has been confirmed, the items in the order are picked from inventory and packed into a package. Finally, the "Package delivered" and "Pay order" events mark the completion of the process.

5.1 Implementations

The approach presented before has been implemented as a ProM plug-in, which supports the following functions: **1)** The extraction of process executions from object-centric event logs. **2)** User-defined graphical OCCM. **3)** Constraint checking and violation diagnosis for the extracted process executions.

5.2 Evaluations

Based on the implementation, we evaluate the ability of our approach by comparing it with other state-of-the-art models that model the same constraints. Figure 8 is an *Object-Centric Petri Nets (OCPNs)* [2] that illustrates the simplified process model of an order management process. We illustrate the following five constraints for the extracted process executions in Fig. 9:

- Constraint 1: *Pick item* should be preceded by precisely one *Place order*. Place order could be succeeded by arbitrary number of *Pick item*.
- Constraint 2: the final *Pay order* after the first *Payment reminder* should occur within two weeks.
- Constraint 3: the allowed number of item objects associated with *Create package* should be less than five.
- Constraint 4: the allowed frequency of *Payment reminder* is less than or equal to two times.
- Constraint 5: the waiting time for *Reorder item* should be less than one day.

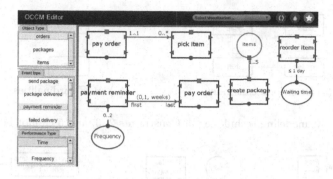

Fig. 9. OCCM in the ProM plug-in.

Next, we evaluate the ability of the OCCM by comparing it with other models that describe the aforementioned constraints in the process.

Figure 10 is the graphical notations of Declare templates. The response constraint in Fig. 10a approaches constraint 1 by specifying that if *Pick item* occurs, *Place order* occurs beforehand. However, it could not imply the allowed number of *Pick item* after *Place order*, or the allowed number of *Place order* before *Pick item*. As for the atMostTwo constraint in Fig. 10b, it approaches constraint 4 by requiring that *Payment reminder* occurs no more than two times in each case. Declare template is incapable of describing constraints 2, 3, and 5. The isolated case notion does not consider the interaction of different object types, and the performance-related constraints are not specified.

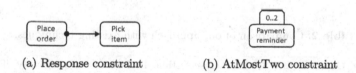

(a) Response constraint   (b) AtMostTwo constraint

Fig. 10. Declare templates. Constraints 2, 3, and 5 cannot be modeled.

There are other declarative-based techniques that address the drawbacks of using single-case notions. Figure 11 employs OCBC models to describe the constraints in the event log. This technique relates events in the log through a data perspective. One major drawback is that the temporal constraint, such as constraint 2, is missing due to the absence of process executions. Also, time and frequency performance constraints are missing in OCBC.

Another recent technique uses object-centric constraint graphs (OCCGs) to evaluate constraints based on the metrics of the entire object-centric event log, i.e., the technique does not pinpoint violations for single process execution. As depicted in Fig. 12a, the model describes that a simple causal relation between two event types regarding an item object should hold for all events of type *Place order*. Due to the absence of a process execution notion, it assigns an object type

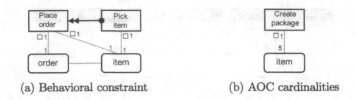

(a) Behavioral constraint   (b) AOC cardinalities

Fig. 11. OCBC modeling technique [4]. Constraints 2, 3, and 5 cannot be modeled.

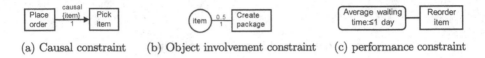

(a) Causal constraint   (b) Object involvement constraint   (c) performance constraint

Fig. 12. OCCGs modeling technique [10]. Constraints 1, 2, and 4 cannot be modeled.

label for the ordering relation. However, when multiple object types interact, the technique is not suitable for modeling specific cardinality or temporal constraints between two events. Thus constraints 1 and 2 are not represented, and frequency constraint 4 is not possible.

In summary, the declarative approach ignores object-centric settings and fails to reflect performance, cardinality, and temporal constraints. In contrast, OCBC and OCCG modeling techniques partly address the issue while not considering constraints for each single process execution, whereas our modeling technique can explicitly represent one-to-many and many-to-many relations on a more granular level. The comparison is summarized in Table 2.

Table 2. Comparison of our approach with existing techniques.

Techniques	Object-centric Settings	Case Notion	Performance	Cardinality	Temporal
Declare [4]	–	✓	–	–	–
OCBC [4]	✓	–	–	✓	–
OCCG [10]	✓	–	✓	–	–
Our work	✓	✓	✓	✓	✓

6   Conclusion

In this paper, we proposed a novel graphical constraint-checking technique for process executions extracted from object-centric event data. The declarative nature of our approach enables a more flexible constraint modeling than procedural languages such as Petri nets. We implemented the language as an editor in ProM, which supports designing models to describe constraints for process executions. One future research direction is to scale the atomic events to non-atomic as the event data in real life can have a non-zero execution duration. Additionally, we plan to extend the approach for more complex constraints, such that deviations on the attribute levels can be detected.

References

1. van der Aalst, W.M.P.: Object-centric process mining: dealing with divergence and convergence in event data. In: Olveczky, P., Salaun, G. (eds.) Software Engineering and Formal Methods. Lecture Notes in Computer Science(), vol. 11724, pp. 3–25. Springer, Cham (2019). https://doi.org/10.1007/978-3-030-30446-1_1
2. van der Aalst, W.M.P., Berti, A.: Discovering object-centric petri nets. Fundam. Informaticae **175**(1–4), 1–40 (2020)
3. Adams, J.N., Schuster, D., Schmitz, S., Schuh, G., van der Aalst, W.M.P.: Defining cases and variants for object-centric event data. In: ICPM, pp. 128–135. IEEE (2022)
4. Artale, A., Kovtunova, A., Montali, M., van der Aalst, W.M.P.: Modeling and reasoning over declarative data-aware processes with object-centric behavioral constraints. In: Hildebrandt, T., van Dongen, B., Roglinger, M., Mendling, J. (eds.) Business Process Management. Lecture Notes in Computer Science(), vol. 11675, pp. 139–156. Springer, Cham (2019). https://doi.org/10.1007/978-3-030-26619-6_11
5. Berti, A., van der Aalst, W.M.P.: OC-PM: analyzing object-centric event logs and process models. Int. J. Softw. Tools Technol. Transf. **25**(1), 1–17 (2023)
6. Bhattacharya, K., Gerede, C.E., Hull, R., Liu, R., Su, J.: Towards formal analysis of artifact-centric business process models. In: Alonso, G., Dadam, P., Rosemann, M. (eds.) Business Process Management. Lecture Notes in Computer Science, vol. 4714, pp. 288–304. Springer, Berlin (2007). https://doi.org/10.1007/978-3-540-75183-0_21
7. Esser, S., Fahland, D.: Multi-dimensional event data in graph databases. J. Data Semant. **10**(1–2), 109–141 (2021)
8. Jalali, A., Johannesson, P.: Multi-perspective business process monitoring. In: Nurcan, S., et al. (eds.) Enterprise, Business-Process and Information Systems Modeling. Lecture Notes in Business Information Processing, vol. 147, pp. 199–213. Springer, Berlin (2013). https://doi.org/10.1007/978-3-642-38484-4_15
9. Maggi, F.M., Montali, M., Westergaard, M., van der Aalst, W.M.P.: Monitoring business constraints with linear temporal logic: an approach based on colored automata. In: Rinderle-Ma, S., Toumani, F., Wolf, K. (eds.) Business Process Management. Lecture Notes in Computer Science, vol. 6896, pp. 132–147. Springer, Berlin (2011). https://doi.org/10.1007/978-3-642-23059-2_13
10. Park, G., van der Aalst, W.M.P.: Monitoring constraints in business processes using object-centric constraint graphs. In: Montali, M., Senderovich, A., Weidlich, M. (eds.) Process Mining Workshops. Lecture Notes in Business Information Processing, vol. 468, pp. 479–492. Springer, Cham (2022). https://doi.org/10.1007/978-3-031-27815-0_35
11. Weidlich, M., Ziekow, H., Mendling, J., Günther, O., Weske, M., Desai, N.: Event-based monitoring of process execution violations. In: Rinderle-Ma, S., Toumani, F., Wolf, K. (eds.) Business Process Management. Lecture Notes in Computer Science, vol. 6896, pp. 182–198. Springer, Berlin (2011). https://doi.org/10.1007/978-3-642-23059-2_16

Analyzing an After-Sales Service Process Using Object-Centric Process Mining: A Case Study

Gyunam Park[1(✉)], Sevde Aydin[2], Cüneyt Uğur[3], and Wil M. P. van der Aalst[1]

[1] Process and Data Science Group (PADS), RWTH Aachen University, Aachen, Germany
{gnpark,wvdaalst}@pads.rwth-aachen.de
[2] Gebze Technical University, Darica, Turkey
s.aydin2019@gtu.edu.tr
[3] AI and Process Automation Department, Borusan Cat - R&D, Digital and Technology, Istanbul, Turkey
cugur@borusan.com

Abstract. Process mining, a technique turning event data into business process insights, has traditionally operated on the assumption that each event corresponds to a singular case or object. However, many real-world processes are intertwined with multiple objects, making them object-centric. This paper focuses on the emerging domain of object-centric process mining, highlighting its potential yet underexplored benefits in actual operational scenarios. Through an in-depth case study of *Borusan Cat*'s after-sales service process, this study emphasizes the capability of object-centric process mining to capture entangled business process details. Utilizing an event log of approximately 65,000 events, our analysis underscores the importance of embracing this paradigm for richer business insights and enhanced operational improvements.

Keywords: Object-Centric Process Mining · Case Study · After-Sales Service Process

1 Introduction

Process mining leverages event data from operational processes to gain insights [1]. This includes techniques such as process discovery, which automatically derives process models from event data; conformance checking, which compares the recorded event log with the process model; process enhancement, which augments the process model with frequency and performance details; and predictive process monitoring, which foresees the remaining time and potential risk of an ongoing case. Companies like Siemens, Uber, BMW, and Bosch have effectively employed process mining, achieving substantial savings amounting to millions of Euros [12].

In process mining, there is a prevalent assumption that each event corresponds directly to a singular, specific case. Consider a healthcare scenario: an event, like registration, refers directly to a single patient. Yet, this assumption often does not hold in real-world contexts. Instead, many business processes, in reality, are shaped by the interactions of several intertwined objects, making them *object-centric* [3]. For example, an omnipresent Purchase-To-Pay (P2P) process encompasses multiple object types,

J. De Smedt and P. Soffer (Eds.): ICPM 2023 Workshops, LNBIP 503, pp. 406–418, 2024.
https://doi.org/10.1007/978-3-031-56107-8_31

including purchase orders, goods receipts, and invoices. An event within such processes can relate to multiple objects of distinct types. For instance, event *verify goods receipts* in a P2P process might correspond to multiple goods receipts and the associated purchase order. Similarly, an event *three-way matching* relates to an invoice, its relevant goods receipts, and the corresponding purchase order to confirm the invoice's amount.

Object-centric process mining deviates from the conventional assumption that each event is tied to only one case or object. Rather, it allows an event to connect with multiple objects. This approach grants analysts the adaptability to select their preferred object and event perspectives for various analyses. It also captures the complexity of object interactions, enabling a deeper analysis of intertwined business processes, and leverages multi-dimensional data models for a more precise representation of business processes [2].

In recent years, various tools and techniques tailored for object-centric process mining have emerged [7,8,11]. However, while this paradigm holds great potential, the corresponding tools and techniques have not been widely applied. Therefore, there is a need for documented real-life applications of these concepts.

This paper presents a case study using the after-sales service process of *Borusan Cat* within *Borusan Group*. As one of *Caterpillar Inc.*'s 160 dealers - a global frontrunner in construction and mining equipment manufacture - *Borusan Cat* operates in six countries with a workforce exceeding 3,000. They cater to three primary sectors: construction, mining, and energy & transportation within these nations. Our study utilizes an event log containing around 65,000 events, aiming to present the findings, underscoring the potential of object-centric process mining in a service process context.

The structure of this paper is as follows: Sect. 2 details the background of the case study. Next, Sect. 3 outlines the planning of the case study, introducing the process and defining the goals for analysis. Afterward, Sect. 4 describes the extraction of the object-centric event log. Then, Sect. 5 introduces our data preprocessing strategies. In Sect. 6, we delve into the mining and analysis phase. Next, Sect. 7 discusses both implemented and prospective improvement strategies. Finally, Sect. 8 concludes the paper.

2 Background

This section presents the context of the company and the process where the proposed case study is performed. Moreover, we introduce a process mining methodology used to conduct our case study.

2.1 Company

The Borusan Group[1] stands as one of Türkiye's most distinguished conglomerates, boasting a workforce of more than 12,000 in 12 countries spanning three continents. As a dealer of *Caterpillar Inc.* and numerous leading brands, *Borusan Cat* serves the construction, resource, energy, and transportation industries. With a team of more than 3,000 employees in six countries, the company provides machinery, generators, and spare parts sales, complemented by after-sales support. Beyond offering Cat construction equipment and generator rental services, *Borusan Cat* delivers holistic solutions to enterprises in the construction, mining, energy, marine, and oil sectors.

---

[1] https://www.borusan.com/en/home.

Driven by its goals of amplifying operational excellence and enhancing customer satisfaction, *Borusan Cat*'s process excellence team has analyzed the after-sales service process, focusing on Key Performance Indicators (KPIs) such as chargeable working hours, deviations between actual and planned hours, technician turnaround durations, technician productivity, their time optimization, and operational effectiveness at client locations based on daily technician activities. These established KPIs serve as a compass to oversee the after-sales service process.

2.2   Process Description

Figure 1 shows a data model of the after-sales service process. A customer issues a work order that may encompass multiple order items, e.g., each item for an issue. A schedule is created for each order item and can be allocated to several technicians, while a technician is involved in multiple schedules. In other words, the relationship between schedules and technicians is many-to-many.

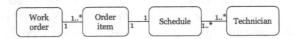

Fig. 1. A data model of the after-sales service process

Figure 2 shows the reference process model for the process where a single techni-cian handles a single schedule. Note that the reference model does not describe the pro-cess where multiple technicians handle multiple schedules. First, a schedule is assigned to a technician based on customer information (name, location, and job description) and work order details (order number and item number) from the SAP system. Upon the start time of the assigned schedule, the system initiates the SCHEDULER START activity. When the end time of a technician's schedule approaches, the system activates the SCHEDULER END activity. Technicians must complete all customer-related activ-ities within this scheduled timeframe. Work completed within this period is deemed *normal work*, while any extra work outside this timeframe is termed *overwork*.

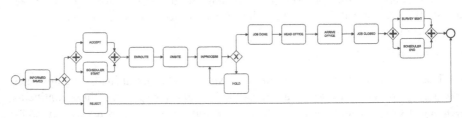

Fig. 2. Reference process model in BPMN notations

Technicians can either accept or decline the assigned schedule for various reasons (e.g., adverse weather and equipment unavailability). An ACCEPT activity is recorded for acceptance, and REJECT for declination. After accepting, the technician sets out for the customer's location, marking the ENROUTE status on their mobile app. After arriving at the customer's location, the technician updates the status to ONSITE. The technician begins to work on the order, indicating this with the INPROCESS status. If a technician pauses their work, they select the HOLD status. Upon finishing the job, the technician selects JOB DONE. The technician updates the HEAD OFFICE status as they head back. Upon return, the technician marks ARRIVE OFFICE. If all tasks for a customer are finished on the same day, the technician updates the status to JOB CLOSED. After service provision, technicians send an evaluation survey to customers, denoted by the SURVEY SENT activity.

2.3 Methodology

To apply process mining successfully, the process mining discipline provides several project methodologies aiming at supporting the application of process mining in organizational contexts. For instance, the L^* life-cycle model [1] and the Process Mining Project Methodology (PM^2) [6] provide clear guidance to practitioners on how they implement process mining projects which aim to improve process performance and compliance to rules and regulations.

To apply object-centric process mining in an organizational setting, we extend PM^2 to guide the organization that seeks to apply object-centric process mining. The renewed methodology consists of five stages.

1. **Planning**: this stage is to set up the project and determine the object-centric analysis' goals that need to be answered at the end of the project in a way that improves the process performance.
2. **Extraction**: this stage is to extract the event data from the information system and obtain the object-centric event log.
3. **Data Preprocessing**: this stage is to prepare the event data so that the following mining and analysis techniques can produce optimal results.
4. **Mining and Analysis**: this stage is to apply object-centric process mining techniques to the preprocessed event data and get insights into the interaction among various object types which answer the object-centric analysis' goals.
5. **Improvement**: this stage transforms actionable insights into actual management actions that support the process to improve performance and compliance.

In the following sections, we apply each step to the after-sales service process of *Borusan Cat*.

3 Planning

First, the design of our case study was influenced by the insights given by our partners at the company. We initiated a set of focused panel discussions to familiarize ourselves with the complexity of the scheduling process and how object-centric process mining could best be applied to it.

From our early interactions with company stakeholders, we discovered that they already employed a traditional process mining infrastructure. This system was primarily centered on analyzing a single schedule by a single technician. However, our discussions spotlighted the challenges and inadequacies of using traditional process mining approaches for analyzing the multi-faceted nature of the after-sales service process, i.e., the many-to-many relationships between schedules and technicians (cf. Fig. 1). Moreover, the existing approaches did not provide insights into severe deviations and potential bottlenecks arising from the multi-faceted relationships between schedules and technicians.

To handle the gap, we have organized our objectives into three main pillars:

- Transparency: To establish clear insight into the process, especially focusing on the multi-faceted interactions between schedules and technicians.
- Compliance monitoring: To detect and understand deviations from established business rules, focusing on the rules defined over the interaction of schedules and technicians.
- Efficiency analysis: To analyze potential bottlenecks in the process, focusing on the bottlenecks that occur at the interaction of schedules and technicians.

4   Extraction

We extracted an Object-Centric Event Log (OCEL) from a database tied to the application *WeKing*. The application serves as an integral tool for *Borusan Cat*'s employees. Managers at *Borusan Cat* use *WeKing* web application (cf. Fig. 3(b)) to allocate schedules, whereas technicians use *WeKing* mobile application (cf. Fig. 3(b)) for real-time status updates. All these interactions are logged in an Oracle database. From the database, we extract event data of schedules and technicians, adhering to the OCEL standard format[2].

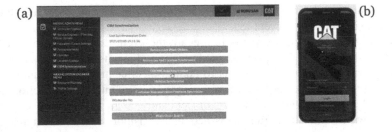

(a)   (b)

Fig. 3. *WeKing* application that supports the after-sales service process: (a) web application and (b) mobile application

Our extraction concentrated on the events occurring in Türkiye from 2023, specifically those related to external after-sales services where technicians visit customer sites. The details of an event, such as customer names and work order descriptions, were extracted.

The resulting dataset comprises 65,774 events associated with 6,483 schedules and 173 technicians. Table 1 shows a fraction of the OCEL in tabular form. The first entry, for instance, showcases an event labeled *e1*, noting the activity *ACCEPT* on *2023-01-02 08:54*. This event refers to technician *4006975* and schedule *3948148*.

---

[2] http://www.ocel-standard.org/.

Table 1. Example object-centric event log of the after-sales service process represented as a table.

Id	Activity	Timestamp	Technician	Schedule
e1	ACCEPT	2023-01-02 08:54	[4006975]	[3948148]
e2	ENROUTE	2023-01-02 08:54	[4006975]	
e3	ONSITE	2023-01-02 12:51	[4006975]	
e4	INPROCESS	2023-01-02 12:51	[4006975]	[3948148]
–	–	–	–	–

5 Data Preprocessing

This section details the preprocessing steps employed on the extracted object-centric event log. First, our dataset contains instances of unfinished process executions. For instance, there are schedules that are still ongoing within the system. To ensure the reliability and accuracy of our analyses, these incomplete executions are omitted from the event log.

Second, certain activities related to schedules and technicians adhere to a specific sequence. For example, the activity ENROUTE should logically precede ONSITE. This is because a technician would only arrive at a customer's site after initiating their journey. Similarly, the SCHEDULER START activity must come before SCHEDULER END. There were instances where these sequences were disrupted due to data recording anomalies. The schedules and technicians involved in these irregularities were filtered out to maintain the integrity of our insights.

Third, our primary attention is on typical scenarios where a single technician is designated to a schedule. We thus exclude schedules that involve multiple technicians from our analysis. Such occurrences are rare and often result from unintended actions by the technicians. The resulting event log contains 57,601 events of 5,566 schedules and 169 technicians.

6 Mining and Analysis

In this section, we conduct various analyses using the preprocessed object-centric event log. First, we compute basic statistics to gain an initial understanding of the process and conduct single-viewpoint analyses focusing on schedules and technicians, respectively. Next, we perform multi-viewpoint analysis using various object-centric process mining techniques to closely analyze the multi-faceted interaction between schedules and technicians. Finally, based on the insights from the multi-viewpoint analysis, we conduct an in-depth analysis to analyze the implications and root causes of the insights to elicit improvements.

6.1 Basic Statistics and Single Viewpoint Analysis

Initially, an explorative analysis was performed with the aim of obtaining a foundational understanding of the process. Figure 4 shows the distribution of schedules and technicians across various regions. Tuzla EP stands out with the largest number of schedules, i.e., 1,336, followed by Istanbul Avrupa, which has 877 schedules. When considering the ratio of schedules per technician, Istanbul Avrupa leads with an average of 39.86 schedules assigned per technician.

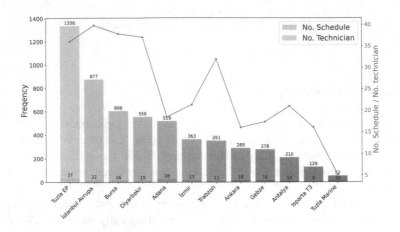

Fig. 4. Distribution of schedules and technicians across regions

Next, we concentrated exclusively on the scheduling process. In this process, *scheduled hours* for every schedule can be computed as the time difference between the SCHEDULER START and SCHEDULER END activities. Concurrently, *actual hours* are inferred from the difference in time between ACCEPT and JOB CLOSED activities. A schedule is considered as *overwork* if the actual hours surpass the scheduled hours. Out of 5,566 total schedules, 4,282 were identified as overwork. For illustrative purposes, schedule 4101760, initially set for 9 h, took a total of 11 h, as demonstrated in Fig. 5(a).

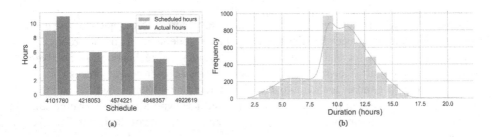

Fig. 5. (a) Overwork schedules and (b) Daily labor hours of a technician

Next, we transition to the technician's viewpoint. First, we have observed that each technician has 340 activities on average. It was deemed ineffective to use technicians as the case notion, given the extensive number of schedules each technician might possess.

To address this, we adopted a new case notion that embodies a technician's daily activities. In this context, each 'case' characterizes a day's worth of a technician's events.

Figure 5(b) unveils the daily labor hours of a technician. Predominantly, their work stretches between 8 to 12 h. However, in about 25% of the instances, the work hours extend beyond 12. Investigating deeper into this anomaly, we discover several underlying causes. Among them, the technician's engagement in a HOLD activity emerged as a significant contributor. Technicians engaged in such activities consistently showed a 3% longer working duration compared to their counterparts without the HOLD activity.

6.2   Multi-viewpoints Analysis Using Object-Centric Process Mining

In our preceding analysis, we examined individual viewpoints (perspectives) of the process related to schedules and daily technician tasks. In the following analysis, we employ object-centric process discovery [4], object-centric constraint monitoring [9], and object-centric performance analysis [10] to analyze the interplay between schedules and technicians. For that, we use OCPA, a Python library supporting object-centric process mining [5].

First, we discover an object-centric Petri net from the extracted object-centric event log. As shown in Fig. 6, the discovered process model shows the interaction between the scheduling process (colored in purple) and the technician process (colored in pink). Note that such interactions were not possible to observe in the reference model described in Fig. 2.

Each schedule has a designated start and end time, represented as SCHEDULER START and SCHEDULER END, respectively. Once accepted by a technician, the schedule is processed by the technician. Upon completion of the schedule, a survey reaches the customer.

The technician's journey begins with accepting a schedule, followed by traveling to the designated site, and ultimately executing the task. Given that a single technician might handle several schedules, this cycle could iterate beginning with the acceptance of a fresh schedule, as illustrated in Fig. 6(a). The cycle concludes when no additional schedules are in the pipeline.

Schedules and technicians intersect at multiple junctures. Their interplay initiates when a technician accepts a schedule and terminates upon its completion. In between, the technician works on the schedule and might occasionally pause it if needed.

The discovered process model unveils several deviations from the reference process model. For instance, Fig. 6(b) suggests that the customer survey is occasionally omitted. Additionally, as pinpointed in Fig. 6(c), a schedule might be halted even before the technician reaches the site. Moreover, Fig. 6(d) indicates scenarios where the survey is dispatched prior to task completion.

Based on the insights derived from the process model, we have designed the following compliance rules and monitored their violations using the approach presented in [9]:

- Compliance rule 1: A survey should be sent per schedule.
- Compliance rule 2: A schedule should not be halted until the technician arrives onsite.

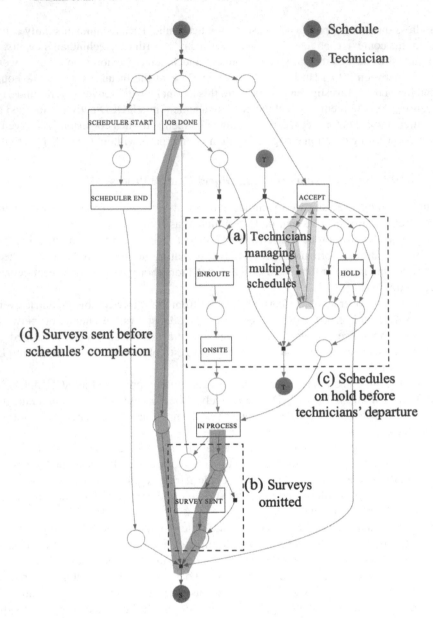

Fig. 6. Discovered process model as an object-centric Petri net [4]

– Compliance rule 3: Surveys should be dispatched after the technician completes the scheduled task.

In 2023, compliance rule 1 was violated 2,222 times, while rules 2 and 3 were violated 144 and 124 times, respectively.

Figure 7 shows object-centric performance metrics. Figure 7(a) measures the duration from activity ENROUTE to activity ONSITE, indicating the technician's travel time to the assigned schedules. With an average time of 2.02 h — notably long given the typical 4-hour planning of a schedule — this metric indicates a severe bottleneck in the process. A minimum time of zero signifies overlooked travel logging or immediate reporting upon arrival, while the upper limit of 12.67 h hints at accidents during transit. Figure 7(b) shows the lagging time of technicians for accepting schedules. The average lagging time is 1.92 h, which indicates the average latency of 1.92 h caused by technicians after the schedule is already started.

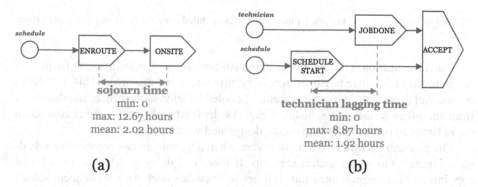

(a)   **(b)**

Fig. 7. Object-centric performance metrics: (a) transit time for a schedule and (b) a latency by technicians for accepting schedules

6.3 In-Depth Analysis

In this section, we delve deeper into the implications of the high transit time of technicians highlighted in the object-centric performance analysis (cf. Fig. 7). As shown in Fig. 8(a), the transit time can account for over 50% of a technician's scheduled time. For example, technician 4760451's schedule was planned for 5 h, yet 4 h (or 80% of the time) were dedicated solely to traveling. Given that the original schedules allocate only a brief period for movement, such timings inevitably result in delays in schedules.

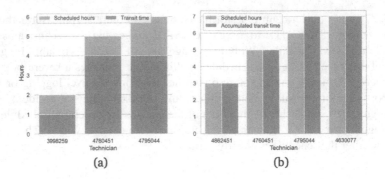

Fig. 8. (a) Scheduled time vs. Transit time and (b) Scheduled time vs. Accumulated transit time

Our investigation with additional data also uncovered that technicians frequently return to the main office to gather necessary equipment and resources. This introduces extra travel time: both from their current scheduled location to the office, and then back from the office to the next scheduled site. As depicted in Fig. 8(b), the accumulated travel time can occasionally surpass the designated work schedule.

The problem becomes even more severe when a technician has consecutive schedules. Figure 9 showcases such a scenario. If there is a delay in a technician's initial appointment due to prolonged travel, it not only pushes back their subsequent schedules, but the following schedules also inherit the amplified delay.

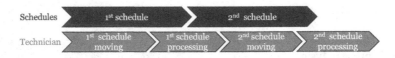

Fig. 9. Impact of accumulated delays on subsequent schedules: The technician started processing the second schedule almost at the end of its scheduled end.

7   Improvements

Our study led to several tangible improvements being incorporated into the organization. We delved into issues surrounding overwork schedules (cf. Subsect. 6.1), uncovering root causes for technician tardiness. As a remedy, the company initiates reminders for technicians via a mobile application, enhancing real-time process oversight. Moreover, to prevent the consequences of high transit time (cf. Subsect. 6.3), the company now factors in technician-customer proximity and assigns work based on anticipated processing time.

We also assess potential improvements, yet to be operationalized. First, evaluating the disparity between overwork schedules and schedule processing times highlighted discrepancies between planned and actual technician schedules. As a result, future schedules will incorporate historical scheduling data for more accurate planning.

Presently, once the dispatcher establishes daily schedules, they remain static, even amid day-to-day shifts. Especially when technicians have multiple daily schedules (cf. Subsect. 6.2), the introduction of a recommendation system could allow dynamic schedule updates based on real-time events.

Our research pinpointed excessive use of the "hold" status by technicians taking unscheduled breaks (cf. Subsect. 6.2). While this has not directly triggered any current improvement actions, it has provided valuable insights into refining the scheduling process.

8 Conclusion

In this case study, we explored the after-sales service process at *Borusan Cat* using object-centric process mining. The analysis has underscored the significance of intertwined processes, most notably, the interaction between schedules and technician activities. Through examining distribution metrics, overwork schedules, and the anomalies found in daily technician activities, we have unfolded some pivotal challenges in the company - particularly the high transit times which, at times, consumed more than half of the technician's scheduled working hours. This led to a domino effect, where one delay translated into cascading delays across subsequent schedules, highlighting the urgent need for process optimization.

With the profound understanding derived from this case study, *Borusan Cat* is now armed with the knowledge to streamline their after-sales service process. First, the introduction of mobile reminders for technicians and geographically strategic task assignments reflect the organization's commitment to addressing the identified transit time issues. Our insights further advocate for the use of historical data in future scheduling and the potential of recommendation algorithms for real-time adaptability.

This work has several limitations. While our case study emphasizes two object types, i.e., schedules and technicians, the after-sales process encompasses additional objects such as work orders and order items. A deeper analysis of the interactions among these objects could yield more comprehensive insights. Additionally, we have not fully harnessed the breadth of emerging techniques in object-centric process mining, such as object-centric conformance checking and variant analysis. Exploring these advanced methods presents a promising avenue for future research.

Acknowledgment. The authors would like to thank the Alexander von Humboldt (AvH) Stiftung for funding this research.

References

1. van der Aalst, W.M.P.: Process Mining: Data Science in Action, 2nd edn. Springer, Cham (2016)
2. van der Aalst, W.M.P.: Object-centric process mining: the next frontier in business performance. White paper, Celonis (2023)
3. van der Aalst, W.M.P.: Object-centric process mining: unraveling the fabric of real processes. Mathematics **11**(12), 2691 (2023)

4. van der Aalst, W.M.P., Berti, A.: Discovering object-centric petri nets. Fundam. Informaticae **175**(1–4), 1–40 (2020)

5. Adams, J.N., Park, G., van der Aalst, W.M.P.: ocpa: a Python library for object-centric process analysis. Softw. Impacts **14**, 100438 (2022)

6. van Eck, M.L., Lu, X., Leemans, S.J.J., van der Aalst, W.M.P.: PM^2: a process mining project methodology. In: Zdravkovic, J., Kirikova, M., Johannesson, P. (eds.) CAiSE 2015. Lecture Notes in Computer Science, vol. 9097, pp. 297–313. Springer, Cham (2015). https://doi.org/10.1007/978-3-319-19069-3_19

7. Fahland, D.: Process mining over multiple behavioral dimensions with event knowledge graphs. In: van der Aalst, W.M.P., Carmona, J. (eds.) Process Mining Handbook. Lecture Notes in Business Information Processing, vol. 448, pp. 274–319. Springer, Cham (2022). https://doi.org/10.1007/978-3-031-08848-3_9

8. Ghilardi, S., Gianola, A., Montali, M., Rivkin, A.: Petri net-based object-centric processes with read-only data. Inf. Syst. **107**, 102011 (2022)

9. Park, G., van der Aalst, W.M.P.: Monitoring constraints in business processes using object-centric constraint graphs. In: Montali, M., Senderovich, A., Weidlich, M. (eds.) ICPM 2022. Lecture Notes in Business Information Processing, vol. 468, pp. 479–492. Springer, Cham (2022). https://doi.org/10.1007/978-3-031-27815-0_35

10. Park, G., Adams, J.N., van der Aalst, W.M.P.: OPerA: object-centric performance analysis. In: Ralyté, J., Chakravarthy, S., Mohania, M.K., Jeusfeld, M.A., Karlapalem, K. (eds.) ER 2022. Lecture Notes in Computer Science, vol. 13607, pp. 281–292. Springer, Berlin (2022). https://doi.org/10.1007/978-3-031-17995-2_20

11. Rebmann, A., Rehse, J., van der Aa, H.: Uncovering object-centric data in classical event logs for the automated transformation from XES to OCEL. In: Ciccio, C.D., Dijkman, R.M., del-Río-Ortega, A., Rinderle-Ma, S. (eds.) BPM 2022. Lecture Notes in Computer Science, vol. 13420, pp. 379–396. Springer, Berlin (2022). https://doi.org/10.1007/978-3-031-16103-2_25

12. Reinkemeyer, L. (ed.): Process Mining in Action: Principles, Use Cases and Outlook. Springer International Publishing, Cham (2020)

Grouping Local Process Models

Viki Peeva[✉] and Wil M. P. van der Aalst

Chair of Process and Data Science (PADS), RWTH Aachen University,
Aachen, Germany
{peeva,wvdaalst}@pads.rwth-aachen.de

Abstract. In recent years, process mining emerged as a proven technology to analyze and improve operational processes. An expanding range of organizations using process mining in their daily operation brings a broader spectrum of processes to be analyzed. Some of these processes are highly unstructured, making it difficult for traditional process discovery approaches to discover a start-to-end model describing the entire process. Therefore, the subdiscipline of Local Process Model (LPM) discovery tries to build a set of LPMs, i.e., smaller models that explain subbehaviors of the process. However, like other pattern mining approaches, LPM discovery algorithms also face the problems of model explosion and model repetition, i.e., the algorithms may create hundreds if not thousands of models, and subsets of them are close in structure or behavior. This work proposes a three-step pipeline for grouping similar LPMs using various process model similarity measures. We demonstrate the usefulness of grouping through a real-life case study, and analyze the impact of different measures, the gravity of repetition in the discovered LPMs, and how it improves after grouping on multiple real event logs.

Keywords: Local process models · Model grouping · Model clustering · Model similarity · Process model comparison

1 Introduction

Process mining is a scientific discipline for discovering, monitoring, and improving processes via readily-available data from different data management systems. The three main pillars of process mining are process discovery, conformance checking, and process enhancement [1]. As the interest in process mining grows, new applications pose new challenges. One such challenge is discovering a single start-to-end model for highly unstructured processes ([19, Figure 7]). To resolve this problem, one usually focuses on frequent behavior because of the 80/20 rule of data variability. However, in some domains, especially ones covering human behavior, the rule does not hold and better solutions are needed. A relatively new field is Local Process Model (LPM) discovery [19], where the idea is to build smaller process models explaining fragments of the behavior instead of one overall model. Yet, current LPM discovery approaches return hundreds or thousands of models for one event log (*model explosion*), with highly similar models

J. De Smedt and P. Soffer (Eds.): ICPM 2023 Workshops, LNBIP 503, pp. 419–430, 2024.
https://doi.org/10.1007/978-3-031-56107-8_32

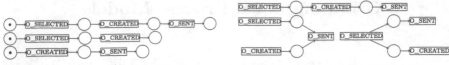

(a) Three highest ranked LPMs discovered by [19].

(b) Three highest ranked LPMs discovered by [16].

Fig. 1. LPMs discovered using [19] and [16] on the filtered and transformed *BPIC2012* event log for resource 10939 as explained in [19].

repeating between them (*model repetition*) as shown in Fig. 1. Although this is desirable in some use cases [7,14], it does not help with a better understanding of highly variable processes.

To alleviate this problem, in this work, we propose a pipeline that groups similar LPMs, and for each group, one representative LPM is chosen. By doing so, highly similar models that describe small differences in behavior are grouped together, allowing analysts to focus on the bigger picture by examining a smaller diverse set of LPMs and only dive deeper into the differences when necessary. More specifically, we start with an LPM discovery approach that returns a set of LPMs. These LPMs are then clustered such that model similarity, using different process model similarity measures, is measured, and for each cluster, a representative LPM is chosen. We evaluate the proposed approach on multiple event logs by comparing model diversity between the originally returned set of LPMs and the representative set obtained after grouping. Additionally, we demonstrate the benefit of clustering LPMs by inspecting a smaller set of models on the *BPIC2012-res10939* event log.

The rest of the paper is structured as follows. In Sect. 2, we introduce the needed preliminaries to follow the rest of the paper. Section 3 introduces what LPMs are and in Sect. 4 we present different process model similarity measures. We explain the framework in Sect. 5 and we present the obtained results in Sect. 6. We conclude the paper with final remarks in Sect. 7.

2   Preliminaries

2.1   General

We define sets ($X = \{a, b\}$), multisets ($M = [a^2, b^3]$), sequences ($\sigma = \langle a, b, c \rangle$), and tuples ($t = (a, b, c)$) as usual. Given a set X, $\mathcal{P}(X)$ is the power set of X, X^* represents the set of all sequences over X, and $\mathbb{M}(X)$ is the set of all multisets over X. We use $\sigma(i)$ to denote the i-th element of the sequence σ and $M(a) = 2$ to denote that item a appears twice in the multiset M.

We use $f(X) = \{f(x) | x \in X\}$ (and $f(\sigma) = \langle f(\sigma(1)), f(\sigma(2)), ..., f(\sigma(n)) \rangle$) to apply the function f to every element in the set X (the sequence σ) and $f_{\upharpoonright X}$ (respectively $\sigma_{\upharpoonright X}$) to denote the projection of the function f (respectively the sequence σ) on the set X.

2.2   Process Mining

Normally, the collected data used for process analysis is transformed in the form of *event logs*. Hence, in Definition 1, we formally define *traces* and *event logs*. Note that although traces are usually defined as sequences of events, in this work, we are only interested in the activity executed by each event.

Definition 1 (Trace, Event Log). *Given the universe of activities* $\mathcal{A}$, *we define* $\rho \in \mathcal{A}^*$ *as a trace, and* $L \in \mathbb{M}(\mathcal{A}^*)$ *as an* event log.

In Definition 2, we define *labeled Petri nets*. Note that a transition $t \in T$ with $l(t) = \tau$ is called silent and that there may be duplicate transitions $t_1, t_2 \in T$ such that $l(t_1) = l(t_2)$.

Definition 2 (Labeled Petri net). *A* labeled Petri net $N = (P, T, F, l)$ *is a tuple, where* P *is a set of places and* T *is a set of transitions such that* $P \cap T = \emptyset$. $F \subseteq (P \times T) \cup (T \times P)$ *is the flow relation, and* $l : T \to \mathcal{A} \cup \{\tau\}$ *the labeling function.*

Now, given a node $x \in P \cup T$, we define the *preset* of x as $\bullet x = \{y \in P \cup T | (y, x) \in F\}$ and the *postset* of x as $x \bullet = \{y \in P \cup T | (x, y) \in F\}$.

To attach behavior to labeled Petri nets we use a *marking* and the *firing rule*. A marking M denotes the state of a Petri net as a multiset of places ($M \in \mathbb{M}(P)$) and the firing rule allows for changes between states (i.e., markings). Given a marking M, a transition t is *enabled* in the marking M if and only if $\bullet t \subseteq M$. If a transition t is enabled in the marking M, it can fire and change the state of the net to a new marking $M' = (M \setminus \bullet t) \cup t \bullet$. We write $M \xrightarrow{t} M'$. A sequence of transitions $\sigma = \langle t_1, \ldots, t_n \rangle \in T^*$ is enabled in M and by firing it marking M' is reached if and only if there exist $M_0, M_1, \ldots, M_n$ such that $M_0 = M$, $M_n = M'$, and $M_{i-1} \xrightarrow{t_i} M_i$ for $1 \le i \le n$. We write $M \xrightarrow{\sigma} M'$.

Now, we formally define an *accepting Petri net* in Definition 3 and the set of all its firing sequences in Definition 4.

Definition 3 (Accepting Labeled Petri Net). *An* accepting labeled Petri net *is a triple* (N, M_i, M_f) *such that* $N = (P, T, F, l)$ *is a labeled Petri net,* $M_i \in \mathbb{M}(P)$ *is the initial marking, and* $M_f \in \mathbb{M}(P)$ *is the final marking.*

Definition 4 (Complete Firing Sequences). *Let* $AN = (N, M_i, M_f)$ *be an accepting Petri net,* $\mathcal{F}(AN) = \{\sigma \in T^* | M_i \xrightarrow{\sigma} M_f\}$ *is the set of complete firing sequences for* AN.

3   Local Process Models

In contrast to process discovery, whose task is to discover one model that explains the traces of an event log from start to end, LPM discovery tries to mine a set of models each matching some particular sub-behavior represented by subsequences in the event log.

LPMs were first introduced in [19] as a replacement for process discovery of highly unstructured processes. However, afterward, the use cases where LPMs are used expanded (e.g., [6,7,10,12–14,17]) and multiple approaches and extensions for LPM discovery followed [3,5,16].

All existing approaches [3,16,19], with the exception of [5], suffer from the *model explosion* problem. The approach in [5] first finds common subsequences and then discovers models on them. This, however, makes it predisposed to similar problems as the traditional process discovery approaches and restricts the set of LPMs use-case scenarios the approach can be applied to. Still, as everyone else, they are prone to the *model repetition* problem. The approach in [19] incrementally extends process trees by adding new nodes, in [3] two existing LPMs (represented with process trees) differing only in one node are joined together to create a larger LPM. In the new model, the differing nodes are added as children to one of the process tree operators. Finally, in [16], LPMs are created by joining place nets together. This makes it clear that all approaches would build highly similar, i.e., repetitive models. Additionally, if one focuses on frequent behavior, the highly similar models would all explain highly similar behavior making highly-ranked models contain clusters of repetitive models. The implementations of [19] and [16] offer a rudimentary grouping of the models. However, it becomes evident this is not sufficient when one considers human analysts manually inspecting and analyzing hundred of LPMs. Therefore, with this work, we try to alleviate this shortcoming of LPM discovery approaches.

In this work, we focus on LPMs discovered with [16]. Therefore, although LPMs can, in general, be represented by any modeling language (Petri nets, process trees, BPMNs, etc.), in this work we restrict to a subclass of accepting labeled Petri nets. We show a few example LPMs in Fig. 1b and we give a formal definition in Definition 5. We use $T_{in} = \{t \in T | \bullet t = \emptyset\}$ to denote the transitions that have an empty preset and we call them *unrestricted transitions*. We define the set of complete valid firing sequences of such LPMs in Definition 6 by restricting that each place in the net can receive at most one token from unrestricted transitions.

Definition 5 (Local Process Models). *A Local Process Model (LPM) is an accepting labeled Petri net $lpm = (N_{lpm}, M_i, M_f)$ such that $N_{lpm} = (P, T, F, l)$ is a labeled Petri net that satisfies the following restrictions:*

1. *$\forall_{x,x' \in P \cup T} \exists_{\langle x_1, \ldots, x_n \rangle}(x = x_1 \wedge x' = x_n \wedge \forall_{1 \leq i < n}((x_i, x_{i+1}) \in F) \vee (x_{i+1}, x_i) \in F))$, i.e., there is only one connected component, and*
2. *$\forall_{p \in P}(\bullet p \neq \emptyset \wedge p\bullet \neq \emptyset)$, i.e., each place has at least one incoming and one outgoing arc,*

and $M_i \in \mathbb{M}(P)$ and $M_f \in \mathbb{M}(P)$ are the initial and final marking. We use $\mathbb{U}_{LPM}$ to denote the universe of such LPMs.

Definition 6 (Local Process Model Behavior). *Given an LPM $lpm = (N_{lpm}, M_i, M_f)$ such that $N_{lpm} = (P, T, F, l)$, we define $\mathcal{F}_{LPM}(lpm) = \{\sigma \in \mathcal{F}(lpm) | \forall_{1 \leq i < j \leq |\sigma|}(\sigma(i) \in T_{in} \wedge \sigma(j) \in T_{in} \implies \sigma(i) \bullet \cap \sigma(j)\bullet = \emptyset)\}$ to be all valid complete firing sequences of lpm.*

The *language* of an LPM *lpm* is obtained by projecting all valid complete firing sequences on the transition labels and removing τ-skips, i.e., $\mathcal{L}(lpm) = \{l(\sigma)_{\restriction A}|\sigma \in \mathcal{F}_{LPM}(lpm)\}$. We use $\mathcal{L}^n(lpm) = \{l(\sigma)_{\restriction A}|\sigma \in \mathcal{F}_{LPM}(lpm) \wedge |\sigma| \leq n\}$ to denote the language restricting to complete firing sequences of length at most n. We can use the language to measure conformance with respect to an event log L and rank the LPMs. The ranking can take into consideration different quality measures, such as fitness, precision, and simplicity. We write $rank_L \in \mathbb{U}_{LPM} \nrightarrow \mathbb{N}$ to denote a ranking function, and $\mathbb{U}_{rank}$ to denote the universe of all such ranking functions.

We later use these definitions to extract features from the LPMs and formalize the different similarity measures.

4 Process Model Similarity Measures

To get an overview of existing similarity measures, we considered multiple survey papers [4,8,9,18,20]. Although there can be small differences in how they categorize different similarity measures, all of them agree, the basic split is into measures that compare the structure of the process model and those that compare the behavior. Subsequently, one can consider the level of abstraction used, e.g., complete language versus weak order relations. Therefore, we choose five representative similarity measures. Before introducing the specific measures, we first define what a similarity measure is in Definition 7.

Definition 7 (Similarity Measure). *A* similarity measure $sim_{name} \in \mathbb{U}_{LPM} \times \mathbb{U}_{LPM} \rightarrow [0, 1]$ *is a function that calculates the similarity between two LPMs. We use 'name' to distinguish a specific measure, and $\mathbb{U}_{sim}$ to denote the universe of all similarity measures.*

To introduce the similarity measures, we assume we are given two LPMs $lpm_A = (N_{lpm}^A, [], [])$ s.t. $N_{lpm}^A = (P_A, T_A, F_A, l_A)$ and $lpm_B = (N_{lpm}^B, [], [])$ s.t. $N_{lpm}^B = (P_B, T_B, F_B, l_B)$. In the following, we illustrate the measures we use in this work with the help of lpm_A and lpm_B.

Transition label comparison is the most simple measure we investigate. The measure calculates the transition label overlap between the models.

$$sim_{transition}(lpm_A, lpm_B) = \frac{2 * |l_A(T_A) \cap l_B(T_B)|}{|l_A(T_A)| + |l_B(T_B)|}$$

Node comparison is somewhat more complex, in that it includes place overlap as well. We use this measure to represent structural measures using abstraction. The measure calculates the similarity between two models by combining transition label comparison and place matching between the nets. We assign to each pair of places a matching gain $g(p_1, p_2) = \frac{1}{2} * \frac{2*|l_A(\bullet p_1) \cap l_B(\bullet p_2)|}{|l_A(\bullet p_1)| + |l_B(\bullet p_2)|} + \frac{1}{2} * \frac{2*|l_A(p_1 \bullet) \cap l_B(p_2 \bullet)|}{|l_A(p_1 \bullet)| + |l_B(p_2 \bullet)|}$ and we use the Hungarian algorithm [11] to solve the assignment problem. We use G_{places} to represent the gain of the optimal assignment.

Then, we define the measure as

$$sim_{node}(lpm_A, lpm_B) = \frac{2 * |l_A(T_A) \cap l_B(T_B)| + 2 * G_{places}}{|l_A(T_A)| + |l_B(T_B)| + |P_A| + |P_B|}$$

Eventually-follow graph similarity is a behavioral abstraction measure that measures the overlap of the eventually-follows relation in the languages of the two models. We calculate it as

$$sim_{efg}^n(lpm_A, lpm_B) = \frac{2 * |EF_A^n \cap EF_B^n|}{|EF_A^n| + |EF_B^n|}$$

such that $EF_A^n = \{(a,b)|\exists_{\rho \in \mathcal{L}^n(lpm_A)}(\exists_{1 \leq i < j \leq |\rho|}(a = \rho_i \wedge b = \rho_j))\}$ and EF_B^n is defined correspondingly.

Full trace matching comparison represents the more sophisticated behavioral measures. We define it as

$$sim_{full}^n(lpm_A, lpm_B) = \frac{2 * G_{traces}}{|\mathcal{L}^n(lpm_A)| + |\mathcal{L}^n(lpm_B)|}$$

where G_{traces} represents the gain of the optimal trace assignment. To calculate the gain between two traces we invert the normalized Levenshtein distance.

Finally *graph edit model comparison* represents sophisticated structural measures. It calculates model similarity by using the graph edit distance (ged) as defined in [2], where the node substitution cost is 1 if the nodes differ in type, i.e., one is a place and the other transitions, or if the compared nodes are differently labeled transitions. The node substitution cost between two places is calculated as $1 - g(p_1, p_2)$, where $g(p_1, p_2)$ is the gain defined as before. The edge substitution cost takes the average of the node substitution cost between the source and sink nodes of the two edges. To convert the ged to a similarity measure, we use the formula below.

$$sim_{ged}(lpm_A, lpm_B) = 1 - ged(lpm_A, lpm_B)$$

In the remainder, we also use the term distance measure, which we always consider to be the inverse of the similarity, i.e., $dist_{name}(lpm_A, lpm_B) = 1 - sim_{name}(lpm_A, lpm_B)$ for any $name \in \{transition, node, efg, full, ged\}$

5   Method to Group LPMs

In this work, we propose a three-step pipeline that starts with an event log and a multitude of process model comparison measures and ends with groups of similar LPMs, as shown in Fig. 2. The first step is discovering LPMs (Step 1), which can also be omitted, starting the pipeline with a set of LPMs instead. Then, the models are clustered such that the similarity between them is determined by the previously defined process model similarity measures (Step 2). Finally, for each cluster, we choose a representative model (Step 3).

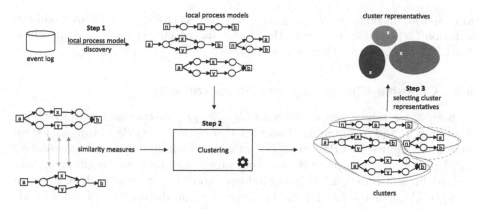

Fig. 2. Illustration of the proposed three-step pipeline.

5.1 Local Process Model Discovery (Step 1)

In the first step, we focus on discovering a set of LPMs LPM_L given an event log L. Although multiple approaches are available, in this work, we use the approach presented in [16]. The produced models are ranked from highest to lowest using a rank function $rank_L$ as previously defined.

5.2 Clustering (Step 2)

In the clustering step, we accept a set of LPMs and a similarity measure and return a set of clusters. We define the *universe of LPM cluster sets* in Definition 8, and a *clustering algorithm* in Definition 9.

Definition 8 (Universe of Local Process Model Cluster Sets). *We define* $\mathbb{U}_{\sqcap} = \{X_{LPM} \subseteq \mathcal{P}(LPM_L) | LPM_L \subseteq \mathbb{U}_{LPM} \wedge \emptyset \notin X_{LPM} \wedge \bigcup X_{LPM} = LPM_L\}$ *to be the universe of LPM cluster sets.*

Definition 9 (Clustering Algorithm). *We define* $clust \in \mathcal{P}(\mathbb{U}_{LPM}) \times \mathbb{U}_{sim} \not\rightarrow \mathbb{U}_{\sqcap}$ *to be a* clustering algorithm. *To denote a clustering algorithm given some set of parameters P, we write $clust_P$.*

The goal of the clustering algorithm is to return the LPMs in homogeneous groups, such that the similarity is high within the individual groups and low between them. One clustering algorithm can produce different cluster sets for the same model set based on the parameters P. In our work, we focus on hierarchical clustering and consider distance threshold and linkage as possible parameters. In particular, we use linkage to determine how the distance between two clusters containing multiple models is calculated and the distance threshold to determine the maximum merging distance. For the traditional hierarchical clustering algorithm, we use the returned clusters in $\sqcap_{LPM_L} = clust_P(LPM_L, sim_{name})$ for an LPM set LPM_L discovered on an event log L and a similarity measure sim_{name}

are pairwise disjoint, i.e., $\forall_{LPM_i, LPM_j \in \sqcap_{LPM_L}} LPM_i \cap LPM_j = \emptyset$. We overload the notation $\sqcap_{LPM_L}(lpm)$ to denote the cluster in the cluster set $\sqcap_{LPM_L}$ in which the LPM lpm belongs. That is, it holds $lpm \in \sqcap_{LPM_L}(lpm) \in \sqcap_{LPM_L}$.

5.3   Choosing Cluster Representatives (Step 3)

In Step 3, we take a set of LPMs $LPM_L \subseteq \mathbb{U}_{LPM}$ discovered on an event log L in Step 1, and a computed cluster set $\sqcap_{LPM_L} = clust(LPM_L, sim_{name})$ from Step 2. We return an LPM set $\sqcap_{LPM_L}^{repr}$ in which we keep only one representative LPM per cluster. In this work, we choose representative models either by taking the highest-ranked LPM in each cluster considering some ranking function $rank_L \in \mathbb{U}_{rank}$ or the LPM with the minimal mean distance to all other LPMs in the cluster. In Definition 10, we formally define *representative projection* as a function that maps a set of LPMs to one model.

Definition 10 (Representative projection). *A representative projection $repr \in \mathcal{P}(\mathbb{U}_{LPM}) \nrightarrow \mathbb{U}_{LPM}$ is a function that takes an LPM set LPM_L and returns one representative LPM. We use $repr_{rank}$ and $repr_{dist}$ to denote the representation projections based on the highest ranking and minimal mean distance respectively.*

Now, for the set of LPMs $LPM_L \subseteq \mathbb{U}_{LPM}$, we create the set $\sqcap_{LPM_L}^{repr_x} = \{repr_x(LPM_i) | LPM_i = \sqcap_{LPM_L}(lpm) \wedge lpm \in LPM_L\}$ and we call it the *cluster representatives*, where $x \in \{rank, dist\}$. This way, we significantly reduce the number of LPMs from the original set LPM_L, but still keep the essence of the entire set.

6   Evaluation Results

The evaluation is performed on six LPM sets, discovered on real event logs. In Table 1, we give a summary of the LPM sets and the corresponding event logs used in the experiments. For clustering, we use the agglomerative clustering algorithm of the `scikit-learn` package [15]. For all experiments, we use the complete linkage and iterate the distance thresholds between 0.1 and 1.0. For each combination of an LPM set, similarity measure, and clustering algorithm parameter, we rerun the clustering 100 times, resulting in 30000 experiments. Whenever single values are shown, the most compact clustering according to the silhouette score was taken unless otherwise specified. All used cluster representatives we calculated using $repr_{dist}$.

Due to space limitations, in the remainder, we only show the results of some of the experiments. All analogous graphs (on other LPM sets, measures, representative choosing strategies, or parameters), together with all resources needed to replicate the experiments, can be found on https://github.com/VikiPeeva/CombiningLPMDandPMSM.

Table 1. Local process model sets used in the evaluation

Event Log	LPM set	Number of models
BPI Challenge 2012	$LPM_{BPIC2012}$	1096
BPI Challenge 2012 - resource 10939	$LPM_{BPIC2012\text{-}res10939}$	4496
BPI Challenge 2017	$LPM_{BPIC2017}$	600
Sepsis	LPM_{Sepsis}	601
Road Traffic Fine Management	LPM_{RTFM}	1694
Hospital Billing	LPM_{HB}	2051

6.1 Case Study

We focus on the *BPIC2012-res10939* event log in this part of the evaluation. In [19], Tax et al. showed how we can use LPMs to see different frequently appearing behavioral patterns that could not be seen on the start-to-end model because of too unstructured behavior. However, as shown in Fig. 1, the highest-ranked models for both [19] and [16] focus on different behavioral variants of *O_SELECTED*, *O_CREATED*, and *O_SENT*. Such repetition appears for lower-ranked models as well. In Fig. 3, we show the three highest-ranked representative LPMs after grouping the original set of LPMs. It is clear that the behavioral span of these three models is significantly larger than the behavior described by the three highest-ranked original models discovered by both Peeva et al. and Tax et al. (see Fig. 1). If we map back the ranks of the three representative models to the original set, one would have to consider 1, 17, and 20 higher ranked, but at the same time, more repetitive models before reaching them.

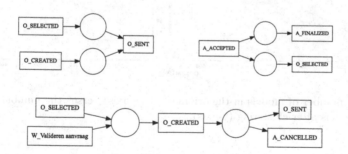

Fig. 3. The three highest-ranked representative LPMs for *BPIC2012-res10939*.

6.2 Local Process Model Diversity Analysis

In Sect. 5, we introduced how to reduce a set of LPMs *LPM* to a subset of representative models $\sqcap_{LPM}^{repr}$ given a cluster set $\sqcap_{LPM}$. In this part, we show how significant is the decrease from the original to the representative set for the most compact clusterings, and whether the set of n highest-ranked LPMs in the representative set is more diverse than the set of n highest-ranked LPMs in the original set.

We start by considering the 5, 10, 20, 50, 100, and 500 highest-ranked LPMs obtained on each of the event logs, that is, the sets $LPM_L^{(5)}$, $LPM_L^{(10)}$, $LPM_L^{(20)}$, $LPM_L^{(50)}$, $LPM_L^{(100)}$, and $LPM_L^{(500)}$, where L represents the event logs in Table 1. In Fig. 4, we illustrate the decrease in the number of LPMs discovered on the *BPIC2012-res10939* and *Sepsis* event logs for the different similarity measures. The number n, denoting the n highest-ranked models in the original set $LPM_L^{(n)}$, is shown on the x-axis and the number of representative models in $\sqcap_{LPM_L^{(n)}}^{repr_{dist}}$, is on the y-axis. It is clear that according to all similarity measures, the most compact clusterings of the LPMs for the *Sepsis* event log tend to have more clusters. Meaning, the original set already contains more diverse LPMs, and correspondingly the decrease in the number of models is lower. On the contrary, when considering the *BPIC2012-res10939* event log, it is noticeable that there is a mismatch between what different similarity measures consider compact grouping. The *node* measure prefers a few clusters, while the *full* measure favors much more clusters. Nevertheless, in both cases, the most conservative reduction still reduces the number of models by at least half. Additionally, it is worth mentioning that although these computations are done for the most compact clusterings in our experiments, in general, the number of clusters is something that can be controlled.

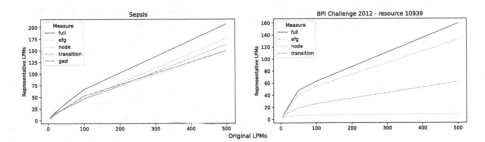

Fig. 4. The number of models in the original set (x-axis) versus the number of representative models after clustering (y-axis).

In the second part, we compare the mean distance between all pairs of the n highest-ranked models in the original sets $LPM_L^{(n)}$, versus the mean distance between all pairs of the n highest-ranked models in the representative sets $(\sqcap_{LPM_L}^{repr_{dist}})^{(n)}$ for $n = \{5, 10, 50, 100\}$. Figure 5 shows the differences between $LPM_L^{(10)}$ and $(\sqcap_{LPM_L}^{repr_{dist}})^{(10)}$ for each of the event logs and the *efg* measure. It is clear that in all cases the mean distance of the representative set is higher than the mean distance on the original set, meaning the set is more diverse. The highest increase can be noticed for the *BPIC2017* event log and the smallest for the *BPIC2012-res10939* event log. The distance increase happens for almost all n, measure and event log combinations, while for a few no significant change could be noticed.

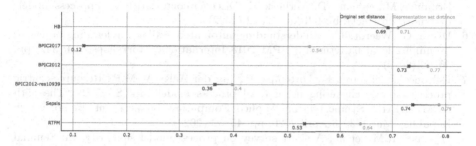

Fig. 5. The mean distance between all pairs of LPMs in the original set $LPM_L^{(10)}$ versus the cluster representative set $(\sqcap_{LPM_L}^{repr_{dist}})^{(10)}$ and the *efg* measure.

7   Conclusion

In this paper, we used process model similarity measures to group similar LPMs together. We proposed a three-step approach consisting of LPM discovery, clustering, and choosing LPM cluster representatives. In the evaluation, we showed how grouping similar LPMs together improves process understandability on a real-life case study and we showcased LPM repetition decrease and diversity improvement on six real event logs.

There are numerous possibilites for future work. Currently, we experimented only on one LPM discovery approach, hence, we can expand this work by considering LPMs discovered with different algorithms. To further advance the method, one can also organize the LPMs in each cluster set in hierarchies for more structured navigation between the models. Additionally, the framework could be extended with new similarity measures and different clustering algorithms. Finally, a natural extension would be to test whether LPMs can be used to compare process model similarity measures in an unsupervised manner.

SPONSORED BY THE

Federal Ministry
of Education
and Research

Acknowledgment. We thank the Alexander von Humboldt (AvH) Stiftung for supporting our research. The authors gratefully acknowledge the financial support by the Federal Ministry of Education and Research (BMBF) for the joint project AIStudyBuddy (grant no. 16DHBKI016).

References

1. van der Aalst, W.M.P.: Process Mining - Data Science in Action, Second Edition
2. Abu-Aisheh, Z., Raveaux, R., Ramel, J., Martineau, P.: An exact graph edit distance algorithm for solving pattern recognition problems. In: ICPRAM 2015, vol. 1, pp. 271–278 (2015)

3. Acheli, M., Grigori, D., Weidlich, M.: Efficient discovery of compact maximal behavioral patterns from event logs. In: CAiSE 2019 (2019)

4. Becker, M., Laue, R.: A comparative survey of business process similarity measures. Comput. Ind. **63**(2), 148–167

5. Brunings, M., Fahland, D., Verbeek, E.: Discover context-rich local process models (extended abstract). In: ICPM-D 2022 (2022)

6. Deeva, G., Weerdt, J.D.: Understanding automated feedback in learning processes by mining local patterns. In: BPM 2018 International Workshops, vol. 342, pp. 56–68 (2018)

7. Delcoucq, L., Lecron, F., Fortemps, P., van der Aalst, W.M.P.: Resource-centric process mining: clustering using local process models. In: SAC '20: The 35th ACM/SIGAPP Symposium on Applied Computing, online event, [Brno, Czech Republic], March 30–3 April 2020, pp. 45–52 (2020)

8. Dijkman, R.M., et al.: A short survey on process model similarity. In: Seminal Contributions to Information Systems Engineering, 25 Years of CAiSE, pp. 421–427

9. Dumas, M., García-Bañuelos, L., Dijkman, R.M.: Similarity search of business process models. IEEE Data Eng. Bull. **32**(3), 23–28

10. Kirchner, K., Markovic, P.: Unveiling hidden patterns in flexible medical treatment processes - A process mining case study. In: ICDSST 2018, vol. 313, pp. 169–180 (2018)

11. Kuhn, H.W.: The hungarian method for the assignment problem. In: 50 Years of Integer Programming 1958–2008 - From the Early Years to the State-of-the-Art, pp. 29–47

12. Leemans, S.J.J., Tax, N., ter Hofstede, A.H.M.: Indulpet miner: combining discovery algorithms. In: OTM 2018, vol. 11229, pp. 97–115 (2018)

13. Mannhardt, F., de Leoni, M., Reijers, H.A., van der Aalst, W.M.P., Toussaint, P.J.: Guided process discovery - a pattern-based approach. Inf. Syst. **76**, 1–18

14. Mannhardt, F., Tax, N.: Unsupervised event abstraction using pattern abstraction and local process models. In: RADAR+EMISA 2017, vol. 1859, pp. 55–63 (2017)

15. Pedregosa, F., et al.: Scikit-learn: machine learning in Python. J. Mach. Learn. Res. **12**, 2825–2830

16. Peeva, V., Mannel, L.L., van der Aalst, W.M.P.: From place nets to local process models. In: PETRI NETS (2022)

17. Pijnenborg, P., Verhoeven, R., Firat, M., Laarhoven, H.V., Genga, L.: Towards evidence-based analysis of palliative treatments for stomach and esophageal cancer patients: a process mining approach. In: ICPM 2021, pp. 136–143 (2021)

18. Schoknecht, A., Thaler, T., Fettke, P., Oberweis, A., Laue, R.: Similarity of business process models - a state-of-the-art analysis. ACM Comput. Surv. **50**(4), 52:1–52:33

19. Tax, N., Sidorova, N., Haakma, R., van der Aalst, W.M.P.: Mining local process models. J. Innov. Digit. Ecosyst. **3**(2), 183–196

20. Thaler, T., Schoknecht, A., Fettke, P., Oberweis, A., Laue, R.: A comparative analysis of business process model similarity measures. In: BPM 2016 International Workshops, vol. 281, pp. 310–322 (2016)

Implementing Object-Centric Event Data Models in Event Knowledge Graphs

Ava Swevels[1]([⊠])(iD), Dirk Fahland[1](iD), and Marco Montali[2](iD)

[1] Eindhoven University of Technology, Eindhoven, The Netherlands
{a.j.e.swevels,d.fahland}@tue.nl
[2] Free University of Bozen-Bolzano, Bolzano, Italy
montali@inf.unibz.it

Abstract. Recent advances in object-centric process mining necessitated the standardization of object-centric event data (OCED). An IEEE taskforce has developed a "meta-model" for OCED, but there is no existing reference implementation or automated techniques to transform legacy data into OCED. This task requires domain-specific knowledge about the semantics of the legacy data in order to make explicit how events act on various inter-related data objects and their attributes. We propose a semantic header that defines how extracted legacy data maps to OCED concepts and the domain-specific reference ontology using PG-schema. We automatically translate the header into database queries to construct an event knowledge graph that is compliant with OCED and the domain ontology using a declarative extract-load-transform approach. The approach has been implemented and demonstrated on 7 real-life datasets, making it one of the first attempts to make OCED operational.

Keywords: OCED · Semantic Header · Event Knowledge Graph · PG-Schema · ELT Framework

1 Introduction

The process mining field has recently witnessed a surge in the analysis of real-life processes that (co-)evolve multiple, interrelated objects. Several works have highlighted the intrinsic limitations of conventional case-centric process mining techniques [1,6,11,12] when analyzing and representing such processes. This has fueled the new wave of so-called *object-centric process mining* (OCPM) [2], with some seminal techniques targeting the discovery of process models dealing with multiple objects and their interaction [3,7,16], and some process mining vendors (notably MyInvenio/IBM and Celonis) proposing solutions in this space.

Further research and adoption of OCPM relies on a commonly accepted data model for such processes that can *simultaneously* describe the *structural dimension* (objects, relationships, and their attributes) and the *temporal dimension* (how events create and change structure over time). Although the previously proposed OCEL (object-centric event log) format [13] is a lightweight representation of object-centric event data, it lacks concepts to express the nature and

J. De Smedt and P. Soffer (Eds.): ICPM 2023 Workshops, LNBIP 503, pp. 431–443, 2024.
https://doi.org/10.1007/978-3-031-56107-8_33

changes of relationships. To fill this gap, the IEEE task force on process mining has started an initiative to standardize object-centric event data (OCED). The task force proposed a meta-model[1], and called for reference implementations and techniques to extract OCED event logs from legacy sources; where legacy data is considered non-conforming to the OCED format.

Section 2 recalls the OCED proposal and addresses two-subproblems related to the implementation of OCED along the process mining pipeline: *(i)* how to *represent and store* OCED in a way that enables process mining usage, and *(ii)* how to *transform* data from legacy systems into OCED formatted data. Both subproblems are intertwined with the more general problem of linking legacy data with a corresponding semantic description so that the transformed data conforms to the knowledge of the domain [19,20]. Specifically, the OCED proposal is defined on the level of a "metamodel" and has to be instantiated by refining generic event, object, and relation concepts to obtain the actual data model for a given data set.

We address these challenges by refining the model of *event knowledge graphs* (EKGs) [12], which naturally model events, objects, and their relations for process mining, to the OCED proposal. This allows us to represent and store OCED (and any domain-specific refinement of OCED) as a Property Graph (PG) [8] in a standard graph DB system. Our implementation consists of three steps where the first two steps define the *"semantic header"* of the data, which specifies data representation and transformation in line with data semantics, and the third step performs the transformation on the actual instance-level data:

(1) We formalize the OCED proposal as a PG-schema [5], a recent proposal for modeling graph-based data schemas, providing a common interface for process querying. The schema defines a *base ontology* for representing and transforming OCED, which includes a *semantic layer* (defining the OCED concepts) and a *record layer* (defining concepts for generic data records from a legacy system and how they are related to the semantic layer).
(2) We demonstrate how to use PG-schema's inheritance mechanism to specialize this base ontology into a domain-specific *reference ontology* which also includes a *semantic layer* (defining the domain's semantic objects, events, and relations), and a *record layer* (defining in which legacy records the domain-level concepts are stored). Furthermore, we extend these structural definitions with rules to transform data in the record layer into nodes and relationships of the semantic layer, similar to *ontology-based data access* [19].
(3) We provide a declarative *extract-load-transform* (ELT) framework, called *OCED-PG*. We load the legacy data records into the graph DB as a record layer. We then transform the data records into OCED by automatically translating the transformation rules of step (2) into queries over the record layer.

This paper presents two major contributions: the semantic header and OCED-PG-an ELT framework in a Python library (PromG). All in all, this paper provides one of the first attempts to make OCED operational, and we

---

[1] cf. the *OCED Symposium* ICPM 2022, https://icpmconference.org/2022/program/xes-symposium/.

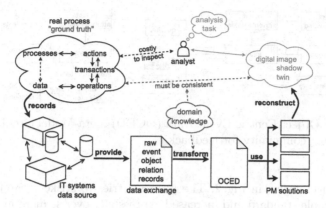

Fig. 1. Data exchange shall support consistent construction of a digital image that is consistent with reality.

do so relying on graph database languages and technologies, avoiding ad-hoc implementations allowing analysts to easily manipulate event data for process mining tasks.

The rest of this paper is structured as follows: Sect. 2 reviews the OCED proposal and discusses the challenges of its implementation. Section 3 presents a concrete realization of a semantic header for OCED using PG-schema. Section 4 gives an overview of OCED-PG. Finally, Sect. 5 evaluates the feasibility of our approach and outlines the conclusions and limitations of this work.

2   Goals and Challenges in Implementing OCED Formats

The technical goal of realizing a standardized OCED format is to provide a unified interface for *data exchange* between source systems and process mining solutions. This goal serves an *analysis goal* as visualized in Fig. 1: an analyst solving a *process analysis task* requires a fundamental understanding of how the actual process operated on the underlying complex data (c.f. Sect. 1). As it is too costly to inspect the reality of the process, the process and data dynamics are recorded in *IT systems*, acting as a *data source* for *(re)constructing a digital image* of the real process. This image *must be consistent* with the process' "ground truth" to let the analyst draw valid conclusions.

Consistency for object-centric processes requires: **(C1)** only showing events, objects, and relationships that were observed in reality (i.e., avoiding convergence and divergence [12]), and **(C2)** representing them in terms of the domain's semantic concepts [9, 19–21].

We now summarize how the OCED proposal aids consistency, and then we identify concrete challenges for implementing any (standardized) data format for OCED for process mining.

2.1   OCED Meta-model

In order to ensure (C1), a working group in the process mining community has been developing a more versatile event log standard [18] resulting in the proposal

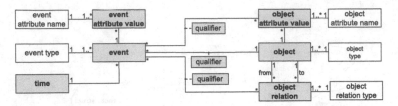

Fig. 2. Draft Object-Centric Event Data (OCED) Meta-Model circulated in the Process Mining community for feedback.

(see footnote 1) shown in Fig. 2. The proposal tries to strike a careful balance between a simple standard and increased expressivity over sequential event logs. It does so by treating events, objects, relations, and their attributes as first-class citizens and by using attributes, relations, and qualified relations between events and objects to capture the structural dimension of the process in a graph-like form [4,14]. The proposal provides a base ontology for events, objects and relations but does not define its semantics as these are domain-specific, and the temporal dimension is only implicitly expressed through timestamps, enabling but not fulfilling (C2).

2.2   Challenge: Storage vs Semantics

Data stored in source systems generally do not even meet criteria (C1) as their data model is optimized for usage rather than analysis: objects are spread across multiple tables, there are no events but only time-stamped records, relations are expressed in various ways, and activities rarely indicate which objects, relations, and attributes were involved [10,16]. Therefore, we argue that generating OCED should address (C1) and (C2) separately (see Fig. 1). First, extract the data from the source systems to generate a "raw record" ground truth of individual observed events, objects, and relations based on knowledge of the source system storage format. Then, use semantic information to transform the raw data into OCED for PM analysis. We focus on (C2) subsequently.

In line with prior literature [9,19–21], we stand for a pragmatic, goal-driven approach, arguing that such a semantics-aware transformation depends on the analysis task: the task determines the level of granularity, detail, and required representation of the data. This already holds for constructing classical event logs, where the analyst may combine multiple attributes to define a suitable case identifier or may refine activities. The range of options for OCED transformation is vast, so an OCED implementation must give the analyst the flexibility to determine how the (extracted) raw data maps to the domain knowledge. This gives the analyst the design space to build their analysis in line with the ground truth. Building on ideas from ontology-based data access [19] and virtual knowledge graphs [20], we propose to create a separate *semantic header* which describes how the raw data maps to (**C2a**) OCED's base ontology, and (**C2b**) to the domain data model of the process, requiring a refinement of OCED to represent specific domain concepts. For automation, the semantic header must be rich enough to enable the **(C2c)** automated transformation from the raw data to a "domain-specific" OCED representation. Notably, pairing raw records with a semantic header file holding the domain knowledge realizes also a *light-weight exchange format for OCED* placing the work intensive transformation to OCED to data import.

In the following, we tackle (C2a) to (C2c) through an entirely graph-based approach. We extend the model of event knowledge graphs [12] to satisfy (C2a) and (C2b). Using a graph-based representation allows us to specify simple declarative transformation rules that we can automatically translate into graph queries for automated translation to satisfy (C2c). Although not as general as full-fledged pipelines for mapping legacy relational data to case-centric [9,10] and object-centric [21] event logs, this results in a pragmatic approach that is fully grounded on graph-based representations, query languages, and underlying graph DB technologies.

3   A Semantic Header for Object-Centric Event Data

In this section, we define the concrete realization of a semantic header for object-centric event data, resorting to the PG-schema approach for property graphs [5]. The semantic header consists of a *(i) base ontology* including a *semantic layer* encoding OCED and a *record layer* encoding raw data records and linking them to the semantic layer, and *(ii)* a *reference ontology* extending the *base ontology* layers with domain-specific records, entities, events, and relations.

3.1   A Gentle Introduction to PG-Schema

A property graph database uses, as main storage mechanism, a property graph (PG), which is a directed multi-graph where nodes represent objects and edges represent relationships. The two main features of PGs is that nodes and relationships come with labels and properties. Labels are used to type elements. While nodes may be typed with multiple labels, each relationship has exactly one. Furthermore, nodes and relationships carry properties, represented as attribute-value pairs. PGs are typically schema-less, and only recent developments, especially PG-schema [5], have highlighted the need to define schemas for PGs.

PG-Schema defines property graph schemas via PG-Types and PG-Keys. PG-Types deal with typing rules for nodes/edges, defining allowed types through admissible combinations of labels and properties in nodes and edges, and also constraining the types of edges that can be connected between nodes of certain types. PG-Keys provide a range of integrity constraints over types, including keys and participation constraints. Our work is currently limited to only include PG-Types, consisting of node types, edge types and graph types. We describe these constructs showing how they can be used to define a schema for EKGs, following the structure presented in [12]; this will also prove useful later, as it will provide the basis for the PG-schema encoding of OCED. A PG-schema for EKGs is given through the declaration of the graph type EKGType, illustrated in Fig. 3. It consists of 3 node types characterized by labels Event, Entity and

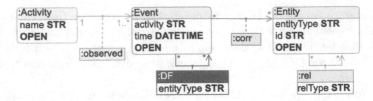

Fig. 3. PG-Schema for graph type EKGType

Activity, for events, activities, and entities respectively, and 4 relationships with labels corr ("event correlated to entity"), df ("event directly followed by event"), rel ("entity related to entity") and observed ("activity observed event").

Node types are defined by their label and properties together with their data type. No other properties or labels can be attached to a node type, unless the keyword OPEN is declared among the properties or labels respectively. Furthermore, a property can be declared as OPTIONAL. Edge types are defined by their source and target node, label and properties. The properties of an edge type and the OPEN keyword are used similarly as with node types.

3.2 Base Ontology

Semantic Layer: Encoding OCED as a PG-Schema. We have formalized and specified the OCED proposal using PG-schema in the *semantic layer* of the

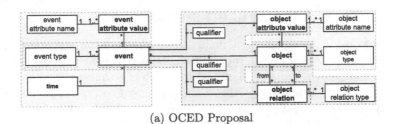

(a) OCED Proposal

(b) Visual representation of PG-Schema of baseOntologyType

Fig. 4. Side-to-side comparison of OCED as meta-model and as PG-Schema

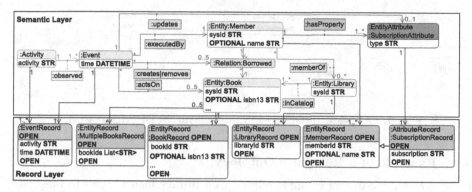

Fig. 5. PG-Schema for libraryType capturing the domain knowledge of a library loan process

base ontology (addressing (C2a)). The resulting graph type baseOntologyType is presented next to the OCED proposal in Fig. 4b (Semantic Layer) using the same color scheme for similar concepts. baseOntologyType stems from EKGType in Fig. 3, and substantially modifies it in the following five aspects. (1) Property entityType is removed from the Entity nodes. Now, we allow for multiple labels, as indicated by the keyword OPEN. Hence, instead of indicating the entity type as a property, it is specified by a dedicated label. In the same way, since there can be several types of events, the Event node now also allows for multiple labels. (2) The attributes of an entity that evolve over time are modeled as separate EntityAttribute nodes. (3) The relationship :rel can be modeled as a relationship, or reified as a :Relation node. In the latter case, edges :from and :to indicate the related entities and the direction of the relationship. The way in which entities are related depends on the domain context and should be specified by a label. Therefore, we permit additional labels through OPEN. (4) Since events act not only on entities, but also on attributes and relationships, a relationship is created from Event nodes to Entity nodes, EntityAttribute nodes and Relation nodes. Again, how events act on entities, attributes, and relationships depend on domain context. This qualifier can be set as a label or as a property (cf. OPEN). (5) The DF relation has been removed as this is not part of OCED.

Record Layer. The *base ontology* also consists of a *record layer*, as shown in Fig. 4b (Record Layer). This layer is used to lift raw data records into the graph DB, and link them to the elements of the semantic layer - once the actual instances of the semantic layer are defined, it can hence be removed, or kept for provenance reasons. The record layer has 3 nodes with labels EventRecord, EntityRecord and AttributeRecord, and a relationship with label extractedFrom, indicating where a semantic layer node actually comes from. The nodes are OPEN, implying they can have additional attributes and labels.

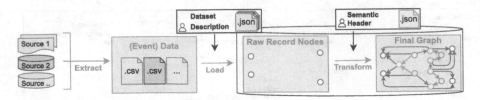

Fig. 6. Overview of OCED-PG, a declarative ELT framework

3.3 Example of a Reference Ontology

From now on, we use an example related to a library loan process to illustrate how OCED-PG works. In this section, we use it to show how the base ontology can be refined into a reference ontology using PG-schema's inheritance mechanism as shown in Fig. 5 (addressing (C2b)).

Specifically, we extend baseOntologyType (Fig. 4b) into libraryType to reflect the semantics of the process. A Library holds Books in its catalog. Events with observed Activities like *borrow, extend, return* and *update membership*, are executed by a Member and act on Books or on the MembershipAttribute (which a Member has as property). The borrowed relation between Books and Members are created or removed by an Event. The record layer reflects the source of the semantic layer nodes. Hence, we consistently refine it as well; i.e. Events and Activities are extracted from EventRecords, Members from MemberRecords, and so on.

4   Framework: OCED-PG

We now explain how actual (event) data can be stored in a graph DB using the semantic header, following Sect. 3. To this end, we define OCED-PG which is a Extract, Load, and Transform (ELT) framework outlined in Fig. 6. The first step is to *extract* the (event) data from different sources into CSV files (see Sect. 4.1). Then we *load* each record of the CSV files as a Record node in the graph database. We ensure that the properties in these nodes are properly names and typed using a data set description file (see Sect. 4.2). Lastly, we *transform* the Record nodes into a new layer in the graph DB that captures the semantic meaning of the records with automatically generated queries (see Sect. 4.3).

4.1 Extracting Data from Legacy Sources

The first step is to extract the original, legacy data, without attached semantics into CSV files. Such data can be taken from multiple sources, for example, SAP systems, production data, or APIs. Data sets may include event and/or entity records. Timestamped event records document changes to the process and associated data. Entity records describe entities with their properties.

For our technical example, we generated, through simulation, three data sets containing *(i)* timestamped records of members executing activities, *(ii)* book records, and *(iii)* member records respectively. An overview is given in Table 1.

Table 1. Overview of the simulated datasets for the library loan example

Events (18616 records)			Library books (5000 records)			Members (1000 records)		
attribute	column	dtype	attribute	column	dtype	attribute	column	dtype
timestamp	time	TIME	libraryId	library	STR	memberId	id	STR
activity	activity	STR	bookId	id	STR	name	name	STR
memberId	member	STR	isbn13	isbn13	STR	subscription	type	STR
bookIds	book ids	List[STR]	...	...	...			
membership	type	STR						

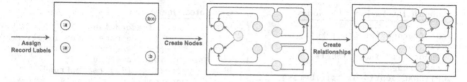

Fig. 7. Overview of the different transformation rules in the Transform step

4.2 Load Data

After extraction, we *load* the data set records into corresponding nodes of a graph DB. This is automated using *dataset description files* containing a description of each record attribute. Each attribute is described by its attribute name, the corresponding column name, the datatype (see Table 1) and, optionally, a string format to parse timestamp attributes. Each data set is *loaded* as follows: *(i)* using a description file, the corresponding data set is loaded into memory; *(ii)* for each attribute, the corresponding column is renamed to comply with the syntactical rules of the graph DB; *(iii)* each record from the data set is loaded as a Record node into the graph DB; *(iv)* timestamp attributes are converted to date (time).

4.3 Transform

The last step of OCED-PG is to *transform* the raw Record nodes into an EKG using the semantic header (addressing (C2c)). The semantic header is concretely stored as a JSON document that contains the definition of the reference ontology (using the (OCED) constructs from the base ontology as supertypes). We extend these structural definitions with three types of transformation rules: *(i)* rules to assign labels to raw Record nodes; *(ii)* rules to create, from record layer nodes, so-called *semantic nodes*, i.e., instances of the types defined in the semantic and domain layers, *(iii)* rules to create relationships between semantic nodes. Rules of these three distinct types are applied in cascade, following the order shown in Fig. 7 (record nodes are in gray). We detail next how these rules are formed.

Assign Record Labels Rules. Since Record nodes may contain different types of data, they are distinguished through specific labels. The semantic header includes, for each type of record, a label, the required and optional attributes, and optionally a condition using the pattern shown in Listing 1.1(a). The transformation rule is automatically translated into a query that identifies all Record nodes with the correct attributes and then assigns the appropriate label.

(a) Semantic Header Input for Record Nodes

```
(record:$record_labels
    WHERE $condition
    {$required_attributes,
    OPTIONAL $optional_attributes})
```

Generated Query

```
1  MATCH (record:Record)
2  WHERE $condition
3  AND $required_attributes_not_null
4  SET record:$record_labels
```

(b) Semantic Header Input for Nodes

```
Record: (record:$record_labels)
Semantic Node:
    ($node_name:$node_labels
    $required_attributes,
    OPTIONAL $optional_attributes})
```

Generated Query

```
1  MATCH (record:$record_labels)
2  CREATE/MERGE ($node_name:$node_labels
3              {$set_required_attributes})
4  SET $set_optional_attributes
5  MERGE (record) <- [:extractedFrom]
6      - ($node_name)
```

Listing 1.1. Transformation rule patterns and the generated queries to assign labels to record nodes (a) and to create semantic nodes (b).

Semantic Node Creation Rules. Semantic nodes are created based on their presence in at least one record layer node. The semantic header includes, for each semantic node, its labels, the required attributes, the optional attributes, and from which record node it is extracted, following the pattern in Listing. 1.1(b). The transformation rule is translated into a query that identifies the correct record nodes and then creates or merges a node with the correct labels and attributes. Merging a node means that it is created if it does not exist, otherwise it is retrieved. (E.g., Entity nodes with the same identifier are merged.) Laslty, a extractedFrom relation from the record to the semantic node is merged.

Semantic Relationship Creation Rules. Relationships can be created in two different ways. First, two different semantic nodes are related if they have been extracted from the same Record node. Figure 8 visually shows that the actsOn relationship can be created between Event and Book nodes that are extracted from the same :EventRecord:BookRecord node. Second, nodes can be related based on a subgraph of the semantic layer. For example, domain knowledge is used to determine the coreference constraints indicating that a Member can only borrow a Book from the catalog of a Library if they are a member of that Library (Fig. 8).

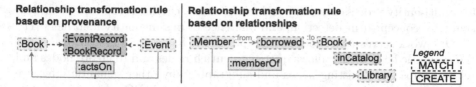

Fig. 8. Example of actsOn and memberOf transformation rules.

Table 2. Type information of EKGs and execution time for 8 datasets

Data set	Source Size (GB)	#node types					#edge types	Memory (GB)	Time (mins)
		:Event	:Activity	:Entity	:Attribute	:Relation			
Library	0.002	1	1	3	1	1	7	1	0.5
BPIC'14	0.08	2	1	7	0	0	11	1	7.7
BPIC'15	0.11	1	1	3	0	0	7	1	4.4
BPIC'16	1.06	4	1	13	0	0	17	5	162.4
BPIC'17	0.29	1	1	5	0	0	4	1	19.7
BPIC'19	0.52	1	1	7	0	0	8	5	31.2
SAP	0.01	1	1	4	0	2	5	1	2.0
Manufacturing	0.03	1	1	4	0	0	1	1	3.7

5   Conclusion and Demonstration

This paper explored the development of a reference implementation for OCED. We proposed a three-layer approach to create a semantic-aware representation and storage system for OCED. We developed OCED-PG, a declarative ELT framework, that maps the raw data to a corresponding EKG, using the semantic header as a basis. The method is robust and extendable due to the flexibility of PG schema and property graphs allowing for alterations or expansions to OCED.

OCED-PG is implemented in a Python library called PromG. It is designed to automatically generate Cypher queries against a Neo4j instance to transform raw data into the semantic domain. We have identified patterns in the transformation rules, providing a simple interface (i.e. the semantic header) for analysts to manipulate event data. We tested OCED-PG on eight different data sets[2] by constructing an EKG for each dataset based on a semantic header, demonstrating the feasibility of our approach. Table 2 gives an overview of the data sets, the domain knowledge applied, the memory allocated, and the execution time.

Our implementation of OCED is not intended to be a data transport format but is designed for analysis. We have established key concepts for specifying semantic headers of process event data, allowing analysts to customize the semantic model for the specific process and analysis without compromising the data storage format. EKGs have already been demonstrated to be beneficial for further enrichment and analysis of the data. Previous research has applied EKGs

---

[2] See https://zenodo.org/record/8296559.

for multi-entity process discovery and conformance checking [12], task identification [15], concept drift detection, and inference of missing entity identifiers [17].

Our work serves as a proof-of-concept, but it has certain limitations. First, the semantic header only allows queries to enrich nodes and to create nodes and relationships from existing nodes and subgraphs; any other semantic inference will require extensions to the semantic header. Second, PG-schema is used as a conceptual idea, but neither the semantic header nor the database actually enforce a schema yet. Third, the implementation is not optimized for efficiency or performance; for instance, since we perform a query for each entry in the semantic header, we have to loop over all the record nodes for each entry in the worst case. Lastly, our method does not take into account streaming data or a standardized import/export for data in an OCED data transport format.

Acknowledgement. The research underlying this paper was partially supported by AutoTwin EU GA n. 101092021.

References

1. van der Aalst, W.M.P.: Object-centric process mining: dealing with divergence and convergence in event data. In: Ölveczky, P.C., Salaün, G. (eds.) SEFM 2019. LNCS, vol. 11724, pp. 3–25. Springer, Cham (2019). https://doi.org/10.1007/978-3-030-30446-1_1
2. van der Aalst, W.M.P.: Twin transitions powered by event data - using object-centric process mining to make processes digital and sustainable. In: ATAED 2023. CEUR Workshop Proceedings, vol. 3424. CEUR-WS.org (2023)
3. van der Aalst, W.M.P., Berti, A.: Discovering object-centric petri nets. Fundam. Inform. **175**(1–4), 1–40 (2020)
4. Angles, R., Gutierrez, C.: Survey of graph database models. ACM Comput. Surv. **40**(1), 1:1–1:39 (2008)
5. Angles, R., et al.: PG-schema: schemas for property graphs. ACM Manage. Data (PACMMOD, 2023) **1**(2), 198:1–198:25 (2023)
6. Artale, A., Kovtunova, A., Montali, M., van der Aalst, W.M.P.: Modeling and reasoning over declarative data-aware processes with object-centric behavioral constraints. In: Hildebrandt, T., van Dongen, B.F., Röglinger, M., Mendling, J. (eds.) BPM 2019. LNCS, vol. 11675, pp. 139–156. Springer, Cham (2019). https://doi.org/10.1007/978-3-030-26619-6_11
7. Barenholz, D., Montali, M., Polyvyanyy, A., Reijers, H.A., Rivkin, A., van der Werf, J.M.E.M.: There and back again - on the reconstructability and rediscoverability of typed Jackson nets. In: Gomes, L., Lorenz, R. (eds.) PETRI NETS 2023. LNCS, vol. 13929, pp. 37–58. Springer, Cham (2023). https://doi.org/10.1007/978-3-031-33620-1_3
8. Bonifati, A., Fletcher, G.H.L., Voigt, H., Yakovets, N.: Querying Graphs. Synthesis Lectures on Data Management. Morgan & Claypool Publishers (2018)
9. Calvanese, D., Jans, M., Kalayci, T.E., Montali, M.: Extracting event data from document-driven enterprise systems. In: Indulska, M., Reinhartz-Berger, I., Cetina, C., Pastor, O. (eds.) CAiSE 2023. LNCS, vol. 13901, pp. 193–209. Springer, Cham (2023). https://doi.org/10.1007/978-3-031-34560-9_12

10. Calvanese, D., Kalayci, T.E., Montali, M., Santoso, A.: OBDA for log extraction in process mining. In: Ianni, G., Lembo, D., Bertossi, L., Faber, W., Glimm, B., Gottlob, G., Staab, S. (eds.) Reasoning Web 2017. LNCS, vol. 10370, pp. 292–345. Springer, Cham (2017). https://doi.org/10.1007/978-3-319-61033-7_9
11. Dumas, M., Fournier, F., Limonad, L., et al.: AI-augmented business process management systems: a research manifesto. ACM Trans. Manag. Inf. Syst. **14**(1), 11:1–11:19 (2023)
12. Fahland, D.: Process mining over multiple behavioral dimensions with event knowledge graphs. In: van der Aalst, W.M.P., Carmona, J. (eds.) Process Mining Handbook. LNBIP, vol. 448, pp. 274–319. Springer, Cham (2022). https://doi.org/10.1007/978-3-031-08848-3_9
13. Ghahfarokhi, A.F., Park, G., Berti, A., van der Aalst, W.M.P.: OCEL: a standard for object-centric event logs. In: Bellatreche, L., Dumas, M., Karras, P., Matulevičius, R., Awad, A., Weidlich, M., Ivanović, M., Hartig, O. (eds.) ADBIS 2021. CCIS, vol. 1450, pp. 169–175. Springer, Cham (2021). https://doi.org/10.1007/978-3-030-85082-1_16
14. Hogan, A., et al.: Knowledge graphs. ACM Comput. Surv. **54**(4), 71:1–71:37 (2022)
15. Klijn, E.L., Mannhardt, F., Fahland, D.: Classifying and detecting task executions and routines in processes using event graphs. In: Polyvyanyy, A., Wynn, M.T., Van Looy, A., Reichert, M. (eds.) BPM 2021. LNBIP, vol. 427, pp. 212–229. Springer, Cham (2021). https://doi.org/10.1007/978-3-030-85440-9_13
16. Lu, X., Nagelkerke, M., van de Wiel, D., Fahland, D.: Discovering interacting artifacts from ERP systems. IEEE Trans. Serv. Comput. **8**(6), 861–873 (2015)
17. Swevels, A., Dijkman, R., Fahland, D.: Inferring missing entity identifiers from context using event knowledge graphs. In: Di Francescomarino, C., Burattin, A., Janiesch, C., Sadiq, S. (eds.) BPM 2023. LNCS, vol. 14159, pp. 180–197. Springer, Cham (2023). https://doi.org/10.1007/978-3-031-41620-0_11
18. Wynn, M.T., et al.: Rethinking the input for process mining: insights from the XES survey and workshop. In: Munoz-Gama, J., Lu, X. (eds.) ICPM 2021. LNBIP, vol. 433, pp. 3–16. Springer, Cham (2022). https://doi.org/10.1007/978-3-030-98581-3_1
19. Xiao, G., Calvanese, D., Kontchakov, R., Lembo, D., Poggi, A., Rosati, R., Zakharyaschev, M.: Ontology-based data access: a survey. In: Artificial Intelligence (IJCAI 2018), pp. 5511–5519. ijcai.org (2018)
20. Xiao, G., Ding, L., Cogrel, B., Calvanese, D.: Virtual knowledge graphs: an overview of systems and use cases. Data Intell. **1**(3), 201–223 (2019)
21. Xiong, J., Xiao, G., Kalayci, T.E., Montali, M., Gu, Z., Calvanese, D.: A virtual knowledge graph based approach for object-centric event logs extraction. In: Montali, M., Senderovich, A., Weidlich, M. (eds.) ICPM 2022. LNBIP, vol. 468, pp. 466–478. Springer, Cham (2022). https://doi.org/10.1007/978-3-031-27815-0_34

2nd International Workshop on Collaboration Mining for Distributed Systems (COMINDS 2023)

2nd International Workshop on Collaboration Mining for Distributed Systems (COMINDS 2023)

Nowadays, business processes tend to be more and more distributed, increasing the need to share information. These collaborative processes are carried out by people, robots, software components, organizations, or business units that want to create new forms of business. Therefore, the monitoring of these collaboration processes through Process Mining opens up the need for tailor-made approaches able to detect issues that typically occur in distributed systems. In this setting, confidentiality, privacy, data heterogeneity, and case correlation are only a few of the issues related to data preprocessing. Likewise, there is a lack of discovery algorithms, conformance techniques, and enhancement approaches. In this direction, the Second Workshop on Collaboration Mining for Distributed Systems (COMINDS 2023) aimed to facilitate the sharing of research findings, ideas, and experiences of new process mining techniques and practices for analyzing collaborative processes. Moreover, it aimed to create a dialogue centered on the development of scientific foundations enabling the application of process mining in such distributed scenarios.

The workshop attracted ten submissions, showing the interest of the research community in the topic. Each submitted paper had a strict peer-review process that involved three reviewers from the program committee. The workshop opened with the keynote entitled "Unraveling the Fabric of Intertwined Processes: How Object-Centric Process Mining is Changing the Way We Improve Operational Processes" from Wil van der Aalst, and continued with the presentation of the five accepted papers, which were also selected for inclusion in these post-proceedings. The articles are briefly summarized below.

The paper by Meroni and Garda presents a technique that exploits the E-GSM declarative modeling language to seamlessly monitor multi-party business processes. The method maps the results of the monitoring, and in particular execution flow violations, from E-GSM back to BPMN diagrams.

The paper by Rott et al. presents a three-step extension to the PM project methodology (PM2) to integrate data across organizational boundaries. The methodology supports data integration for cross-organizational Process Mining, assisting researchers and practitioners in unlocking value potential from analysis.

The paper by Benzin and Rinderle-Ma presents an overview of the potential standard model classes of Petri Nets for collaboration processes to derive design guidelines for collaboration discovery. The results are an extensive review and analysis of such model classes.

The paper by Graves et al. introduces the concept of item quantities to describe the movement of not individually identifiable items across distributed processes. In this regard, the authors present a quantity-related event log and an extension of object-centric Petri nets for quantities uncovering in the logistics domain.

The paper by Peña et al. presents an approach for discovering inter-organizational collaborative business processes. The approach takes as input an XES event log enriched with participant and message information to discover a BPMN 2.0 collaboration process model and corresponding choreography.

We would like to thank all the authors of submitted papers for publication in this proceedings book, and all the Program Committee for their excellent work in reviewing submitted contributions and providing the authors with insightful comments. We also want to thank the ICPM and workshop chairs and the organization for their support in carrying out this workshop.

November 2023

Lorenzo Rossi
Andrea Delgado
Mahsa Pourbafrani

Organization

Workshop Chairs

Lorenzo Rossi   University of Camerino, Italy
Andrea Delgado   Universidad de la República, Uruguay
Mahsa Pourbafrani   RWTH Aachen University, Germany

Program Committee

Andrea Burattin   Technical University of Denmark, Denmark
Chiara Di Francescomarino   Fondazione Bruno Kessler, Italy
Cristina Cabanillas   Universidad de Sevilla, Spain
Daniel Calegari   Universidad de la República, Uruguay
Flavio Corradini   University of Camerino, Italy
Adela del Río Ortega   Universidad de Sevilla, Spain
Marco Franceschetti   University of St. Gallen, Switzerland
Orlenys López Pintado   University of Tartu, Estonia
Fabrizio Maria Maggi   Free University of Bozen-Bolzano, Italy
Giovanni Meroni   Technical University of Denmark, Denmark
Majid Rafiei   RWTH Aachen University, Germany
Barbara Re   University of Camerino, Italy
Hajo Reijers   Utrecht University, The Netherlands
Francesco Tiezzi   University of Florence, Italy
Pascal Poizat   Paris Nanterre University, France

Additional Reviewer

Sara Pettinari

Petri Net Classes for Collaboration Mining: Assessment and Design Guidelines

Janik-Vasily Benzin[✉][iD] and Stefanie Rinderle-Ma[iD]

TUM School of Computation, Information and Technology,
Technical University of Munich, Garching, Germany
{janik.benzin,stefanie.rinderle-ma}@tum.de

Abstract. Collaboration mining develops discovery, conformance checking, and enhancement techniques for collaboration processes. The collaboration process model is key to represent the discovery result. As for process mining in general, Petri Net classes are candidates for collaboration process models due to their analytical power. However, a standard model class to represent collaboration processes is lacking due to the heterogeneity of collaboration and, thus, of collaboration mining techniques. Collaboration heterogeneity requires to cover, for example, intra-organizational collaborations as well as choreographies that span a process across multiple organizations. A standard collaboration model class would advance collaboration mining by focusing discovery through a common target model, supporting comparison, and enabling flexible mining pipelines. To find a standard model class, we aim at capturing collaboration heterogeneity in a meta model, assess Petri net classes as candidates for collaboration process models through the meta model, and derive design guidelines for the collaboration discovery.

Keywords: Collaboration Mining · Collaboration Process Models · Petri Net Classes · Design Guidelines

1 Introduction

Process mining research develops process discovery, conformance checking and enhancement techniques for *process orchestrations* that define what work is done in what order for similar *cases* [2,4,25]. In contrast, collaboration mining research develops the same for *collaboration processes* that define what work is done in what order for *collaborating cases*, i.e., collaboration processes correspond to multiple process orchestrations that collaborate via departments [32], services [22,45], agents [37,47,48], and organizations [14,28,53,55].

For mining process orchestrations the de-facto standard model class is *workflow nets* [3] to represent what work has to be done in what order as, for example, the workflow net concept underlies many models targeted by process discovery techniques [9]. Although declarative process models were also proposed, they

J. De Smedt and P. Soffer (Eds.): ICPM 2023 Workshops, LNBIP 503, pp. 449–461, 2024.
https://doi.org/10.1007/978-3-031-56107-8_34

are by far in the minority [9] and no discovery technique for collaboration processes targeting a declarative model is known to us. Hence, we focus on procedural models in the following. Nevertheless, a de-facto standard model class for collaboration processes is missing, as the model classes targeted by discovery techniques are diverse, e.g., *communication nets* [45] vs. composed *RM_WF_nets* [32]. The heterogeneity of model classes is a consequence of the heterogeneity of collaborations, e.g., *message exchanges* [14] and *handover-of-work* [48], from various perspectives, e.g., *operational* [45] vs. *organizational* [48], and on various granularity levels, e.g., intra-organizational [32] vs. inter-organizational [14].

The goal of this work is to identify potential standard model classes for collaboration processes as *"the choice of target model is very important for the discovery process itself"* [1]. For this, we analyse the collaboration mining literature and related research areas with respect to the collaboration studied and integrate it in a *collaboration process meta model* in Sect. 2. Next, we derive assessment criteria from the collaboration process meta model to assess standard Petri net classes with respect to required properties of a standard model class for collaboration processes and findings from the assessment in Sect. 3. We focus on Petri net classes due to their expressiveness, graphical and integrating[1] nature, formal semantics, analysis techniques, and tool support [3,38,40]. Similar to process mining, collaboration mining starts with discovering a collaboration process model [4] such that the targeted model class determines applicable conformance checking and enhancement techniques. Thus, we translate the assessment findings into design guidelines for process discovery in Sect. 4 and conclude as well as outline future work in Sect. 5.

2   A Collaboration Process Meta Model

The assessment of Petri net classes as standard candidates for collaboration process models in Sect. 3 necessitates an analysis of the heterogeneous collaboration studied in collaboration mining (cf. Sect. 1), as the collaboration determines what must be modelled in a collaboration process model. Due to the heterogeneity in what is considered as a collaboration process (CP), we take an integrating approach to understand what has to be modelled in a collaboration process (CP) model by presenting a collaboration process (CP) meta model.

The meta model integrates specifications of what has to be modelled from research areas that study CP models through a *top-down* approach that starts from scratch and models the CP as it should be executed. In that sense, collaboration mining represents the opposite *bottom-up* approach by assuming the CP has already been running for some time such that event logs can be extracted from information systems supporting the CP. Hence, the CP meta model brings process models from both top-down and bottom-up approaches together and is presented in Sect. 2.1 and instantiated for a real-world CP in Sect. 2.2.

---

[1] Many alternative modelling languages can be transformed into Petri nets [40].

2.1   Elements of the Collaboration Process Meta Model

To guide the integration of existing CP models, the functional, behavioral, informational, operational and organizational process perspectives [25] are depicted in Fig. 1. Aside from the analysis question defining the perspective on a process, the resulting main concept, the concept's abstraction relation instances/concept granularities, and elements of the perspective are presented. Existing work taking the top-down or bottom-up approach identifies a perspective's element as the answer to what is collaborating, i.e., the involved *collaboration concepts* (perspective's elements denoted in blue in Fig. 1).

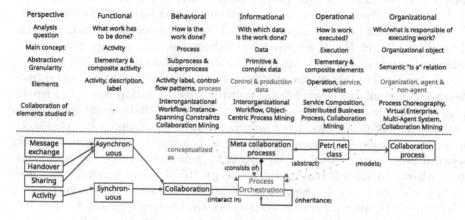

Perspective	Functional	Behavioral	Informational	Operational	Organizational
Analysis question	What work has to be done?	How is the work done?	With which data is the work done?	How is work executed?	Who/what is responsible of executing work?
Main concept	Activity	Process	Data	Execution	Organizational object
Abstraction/ Granularity	Elementary & composite activity	Subprocess & superprocess	Primitive & complex data	Elementary & composite elements	Semantic "is a" relation
Elements	Activity, description, label	Activity label, control-flow patterns, process	Control & production data	Operation, service, worklist	Organization, agent & non-agent
Collaboration of elements studied in		Interorganizational Workflow, Instance-Spanning Constraints Collaboration Mining	Interorganizational Workflow, Object-Centric Process Mining	Service Composition, Distributed Business Process, Collaboration Mining	Process Choreography, Virtual Enterprise, Multi-Agent System, Collaboration Mining

Fig. 1. Process perspectives [25] and research areas that study collaboration between perspective's elements and their relation to the collaboration process meta model.

Existing research areas taking the top-down approach are *interorganizational workflows* [2,8], *process choreographies* [15,16,19,20,36], *virtual enterprises* [13,23,24], *distributed business processes* [12,44], *service compositions* [4,6,42], *multi-agent systems* [46,47], and (process) *instance-spanning constraints* [18,52]. In contrast, the bottom-up approach is taken by *object-centric process mining* [5,10] and *collaboration mining* [14,22,28,32,37,45,48,53,55]. Considering both approaches, collaboration can be the result of multiple organizations (denoted in blue as an element of the organizational perspective in Fig. 1) or an organization's departments (non-agents in Fig. 1) collaborating towards achieving a common business goal. Also, collaboration can be the result of multiple services (element of the operational perspective) or agents (organizational perspective) collaborating to execute a CP. Similarly, collaboration can be the result of multiple objects (informational perspective) collaborating to be processed in a CP. Lastly, collaboration can be the result of multiple process instances (behavioral perspective) collaborating to meet the requirements stated in compliance constraints.

Hence, the main element of the CP meta model defining the various collaboration concepts can be an organization, (non-)agent, services, objects, and process instances. To cover the diverse nature of concepts, we conceptualize all these perspective's elements with their respective process orchestration, e.g., the process orchestration of a particular medical department [32] or of a particular web service [45] (cf. "conceptualized as" relation in dotted blue in Fig. 1). Our process orchestration conceptualization in the CP meta model is in line with top-down and bottom-up approaches, as work for both approaches typically models its collaboration concept by some process orchestration, e.g., the underlying workflow net for each medical department [32] or for each web service [45]. Hence, the *meta collaboration process* that abstracts the Petri net classes modelling the CP in Fig. 1 consists of process orchestrations that interact in various collaborations, i.e., the process orchestrations of a CP collaborate.

Despite the diverse range of represented concepts in terms of process perspective and granularity level, the relationships between process orchestrations in the CP meta model (cf. Fig. 1) are either a collaboration, e.g., two agent's exchange messages, or *inheritance* [11], e.g., a service and its subservice are abstracted into a single service. The inheritance relation between process orchestrations captures the various granularity levels of existing works' collaboration concepts (department vs. organization) in the CP meta model. The collaboration relationship can be generally defined as either asynchronous or synchronous [2] (cf. Fig. 1). *Message exchanges*, e.g., http-messages in web services [45], *handover-of-work* between process orchestrations, e.g., agent A executes activity "a" and hands the work over to agent B that executes activity "b" [48], and *sharing*, e.g., a doctor in a clinic can only do one task at a time [32], are studied for asynchronous collaboration between process orchestrations. On the contrary, synchronous collaboration is studied as an *activity* that is either executed by multiple process orchestrations together, e.g., an internist and a surgeon consult to determine necessary medication for a patient [32], or multiple process orchestrations are referenced in an activity, e.g., the order and package for packing the items of an order [5].

The applicability of the four collaboration types in the CP meta model to a real-world manufacturing CP are shown in the next section.

2.2 Collaboration Process Meta Model Instance in Manufacturing

To show the applicability of the CP meta model, we instantiate it (depicted in Fig. 2) for a real-world manufacturing CP [34]. Note, that the following real-world CP represents only a part of the complexity and heterogeneity of collaboration possible in the real-world, in particular in healthcare, e-Government or similar domains. The CP is a batch production of chess pieces orchestrated by the Cloud Process Execution Engine (CPEE) [35]. The CPEE executes the batch production process orchestration (denoted in blue in Fig. 2) that refers to the top-level orchestration process executed by the CPEE. The batch production produces all chess pieces that are purchased in an order (informational process orchestration related by synchronous collaboration <sync> in Fig. 2). The batch production process orchestration instantiates a production process orchestration for each produced chess piece by message exchange (<msg> relation between batch production and production) that is then executed in parallel by the CPEE. As soon as the production process orchestration is finished, it sends a confirmation message back to the batch production process orchestration. Cardinality constraints for the various collaboration relations are also depicted. For example, a single batch production produces all orders in the CP synchronously.

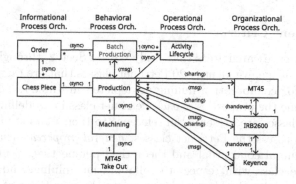

Fig. 2. Selected process orchestrations of a collaboration process meta model instance of the chess piece batch production recorded in [34] as multiple event logs.

Subprocesses instantiated by a behavioral process orchestration, i.e., process orchestrations instantiated with a blocking semantic [35], are a synchronous collaboration, e.g., production and machining in Fig. 2. The CPEE has a fine-grained activity lifecycle model, that is referred to by the activity lifecycle operational process orchestration in Fig. 2. Hence, the respective behavioral and the operational process orchestrations synchronously collaborate by executing the respective activity lifecycle transitions. A MT45 lathe machine, an IRB2600 industrial robot and a Keyence precision measurement machine are responsible for executing the CP. As there is only a single MT45, IRB2600 and Keyence machine, these limited resources are shared by the production process orchestration. The machines are orchestrated by message exchanges, i.e., their process orchestrations collaborate in a <msg> collaboration with the production.

Following the meta model in Fig. 1, the CP meta model instance in Fig. 2 abstracts a concrete Petri net CP model that can be mined for the batch production event logs. Depending on the analysis question motivating the mining of a CP model for the batch production, a subset of process orchestrations can be selected to scope the mined CP model. As it is not clear, what Petri net class should be targeted for the CP model by process discovery (cf. Sect. 1), the next section assesses candidate Petri net classes.

3   Assessment of Petri Net Classes in Modelling Collaboration Processes

As elaborated in Sect. 2.1, capturing CP in their entirety is a challenging task, in particular, w.r.t. the CP model class and the CP discovery technique which are tightly intertwined [1]. Hence, in this section, we assess existing Petri Net classes for their capability of modelling and discovering CPs.

3.1   Assessment Criteria

Given the existing research areas that study CPs in Sect. 2, through snowballing and expert knowledge, we identify 20 Petri net classes that are target candidates as CP models for collaboration mining as depicted in Table 1. The assessment aims to determine the properties of each Petri net class in modelling CP models. The Petri net classes are presented in reference to their main study and year of publication. To assess the Petri net classes, *general properties* characterize the class from a general conceptual and theoretical perspective, *mining properties* characterize the class with respect to collaboration mining, and *collaboration properties* characterize the class with respect to the four types of collaboration occurring in the CP meta model (cf. Fig. 1).

Table 1. Overview of the 20 Petri net model classes with CP modelling assessment.

Class	Main Study	Year	General Properties				Mining Properties				Collaboration Properties			
			Appr.	Turing Compl.	Data	Seman-tics	CP Repr.	PD	Redis-cover.	Sound-ness	Mes-sages	Hand-over	Shar-ing	Acti-vity
Petri Net	[39]	1962	T	−[38]	I	I/T	I	I	−	NA	I	I	I	I
Colored Petri Net	[26]	1981	T	−[26]	E	I	I	I	−	NA	E	E	E	E
Object System	[49]	1996	T	+[27]	E	I	E	I	−	NA	E	E	E	E
Interorgan. Workflow	[2]	1998	T	−[38]	I	I	E	I	−	D	E	I	I	E
Interaction Petri Net	[15]	2007	T	−[38]	I	I	E	[22] [14]	−	?	E[a]	I	I	−
Compositional Service Tree	[6]	2009	T	−[38]	I	I	E	?	−	D	E	I	I	−
υ-PN	[43]	2011	T	−[43]	E	I	I	?	−	U	I	I	I	I
Integrated RM_WF_net	[55]	2013	B	−[38]	I	I	E	[55]	−	D	E	I	E	E
Composed RM_WF_net	[54]	2015	T	−[38]	I	I	E	[31] [32]	−	?	E	I	E	E
Healthcare Petri Net	[33]	2018	T	−[38]	I	I	E	?	−	?	I	E	E	−
Synchronuous Proclet System	[17]	2019	T	−? [17]	E	T	E	?	−	NA	I	I	I	E
t-PNID	[40]	2019	T	−[38]	E	I	E	I	−	U	I	I	I	E
Communication Net	[45]	2019	B	−?	I	I	E	[45]	−	?	E	I	I	−
Top-Level Process Model	[53]	2020	B	−?	I	I	E	[53]	−	D	E	I	I	I
System Net	[41]	2020	B	−?	E	T	E	?	−	NA	E	E	I	I
Object-centric Petri Net	[5]	2020	B	−?	E	I	E	[5]	−	?	I	I	I	E
Industry Net	[29]	2022	T	−?	I	I	E	[28]	−	?	E	I	I	−
Multi-Agent System Net	[48]	2023	B	−[38]	I	I	E	[48]	−	D	I	E	I	I
Generalized Workflow Net	[37]	2023	B	−?	I	I	E	[37]	−	D	E	I	I	E
Typed Jackson Net	[10]	2023	D	[10]	E	I	E	[10]	+	S	I	I	I	E

[a] Interaction Petri nets are the only model class that conceptualizes a message exchange as an atomic, synchronous firing of a transition in a Petri net [15].

General properties of Petri net classes are the *approach* [36], *Turing completeness* [38], ability to represent *data* (cf. control vs. production data in Sect. 2) and the proposed type of *semantics* [50]. To build a CP model, two approaches exist: *(T)op-down* starts from scratch and models the CP manually by starting with the definition of process orchestrations and collaborations and further refining the workflow nets, while *(B)ottom-up* starts with an event log recorded from information systems supporting the CP execution and mines a CP model. Next, Petri net classes can either be Turing complete $(+)$ or not $(-)$. If the Turing completeness is only conjected, the conjecture is denoted with a ?, e.g., $-^?$.

As the ability to represent a concept in a Petri net class can either be $-$, i.e., the class definition prohibits the representation, *(I)mplicit*, i.e., the concept can theoretically be represented in the class, but has no dedicated element in the definition, or *(E)xplicit*, i.e., the concept has a dedicated element in the definition, the properties data, *CP representation* and all four collaboration properties are based on this distinction. Petri net semantics can either be *(I)nterleaving*, i.e., semantics is defined as traces of fired transitions such that transition labels always interleave/are totally ordered, and *(T)rue concurrency*, i.e., semantics is defined as a *causal net* [50] such that transition firings can be partially ordered or "truly concurrent".

Mining properties are the CP representation, *discovery technique (PD)*, *rediscoverability* [7], and *soundness* [2]. As CPs are a composition of process orchestrations, e.g. [2,32], CP representation refers to the representation of workflow net compositions. To mine a CP model that is an instance of the Petri net class, a discovery technique targeting that Petri net class has to either exist, is unknown to exist *(?)*, or is *(I)nherited* from a Petri net subclass. An important and desired property of a Petri net for collaboration mining is its soundness (and generalized definitions such as *identifier soundness* [10]) that can either be *(N)ot (A)pplicable* as the class is too general, unknown *(?)* as a restated definition is missing, *(U)ndecidable* or *(D)ecidable* as a decision problem, and *(S)ound by construction*.

3.2   Findings

From the assessment result in Table 1, we deduce nine findings covering the three property classes general, mining and collaboration.

General: The first finding is that research on candidate Petri net classes started with the top-down approach and has gradually put more focus on the bottom-up approach. The second finding is that for 19 Petri net classes, the approach assessment is straightforward, while the typed Jackson net proposal [10] fuses the top-down with the bottom-up approach by taking both approaches in turn and bringing them together through a framework for rediscoverability. However, their motivation puts more focus on the bottom-up approach. The third finding is the observation that Typed Jackson nets and object-centric Petri nets [5] are the only bottom-up approaches with an explicit data representation, a consequence of recent efforts to mine CP models for the informational process perspective (cf. Fig. 1) in which process orchestrations are objects and collaboration is synchronous. Considering the general properties, a fourth finding is that there is no existing discovery technique that defines a true concurrency semantics for its Petri net class. The fourth finding contrasts a recent effort on true concurrency through *systems mining* by [21] and related efforts on partial order-based process mining [30].

Mining: A fifth finding is that early Petri net classes inherit discovery techniques from later proposals for Petri net subclasses, e.g. the *Colliery technique* [14] is a discovery technique for the Interaction Petri net class, which is a subclass of the interorganizational workflow proposed nine years earlier. The sixth finding is that discovery techniques were only proposed three times for an existing Petri net class proposed in a top-down approach, i.e., the two approaches are brought together through distinct publications in [14,22] for the interaction Petri net, in [31,32] for the composed RM_WF_net, and in [28] for the industry net. We conject that both the interaction Petri net and industry net are equivalent both in terms of the assessment and theoretically, which emphasizes the need for a central Petri net class for collaboration mining to alleviate potential redundancies in research. The seventh finding is that rediscoverability and sound by construction are rare and coincide in typed Jackson nets, although both are important properties. The lack of these properties leaves us in the dark whether instances of the Petri net class can be rediscovered and whether the discovered model of that model class is actually behaviorally sound.

Collaboration: The eighth finding is that colored Petri nets and object systems are the only classes that explicitly represent all four collaboration types, but lack a native discovery technique targeting that class. Although the discovery technique [5] for object-centric Petri nets results in an inherited discovery technique for colored Petri nets, the former class lacks explicit representation of three of the four collaboration types. In contrast, the classes integrated RM_WF_net and composed RM_WF_net targeted by the discovery techniques in [55] and [32] explicitly represent three of the four collaboration types. The multi-agent system net targeted by the agent miner [48] is the only class particularly designed for explicitly representing the missing handover collaboration type, pointing to a potential fused class with explicit representation of all four classes and a discovery technique that comes with it. Overall, the eighth finding highlights that the early classes colored Petri net and object systems are too general and powerful to be targeted by a discovery technique (yet), but proposed subclasses for which a discovery technique exists do not yet come with the explicit modelling of all four collaboration types.

The ninth and final finding is that there is yet no class for collaboration mining that the workflow net constitutes for process orchestration mining. The next section translates the nine findings into design guidelines for collaboration miners.

4   Design Guidelines for Process Discovery

The assessment of existing Petri net classes as standard candidates for CPs Sect. 3 resulted in nine findings that are the foundation of the design guidelines for future process discovery in collaboration mining. The search for the standard Petri net class for collaboration mining continues and underlies the first three guidelines:

G1 Take the balance between (explicit) modelling and decision power of your targeted Petri net class actively into account. Existing discovery techniques target either the one end, e.g. [10] with good decision power on soundness and rediscoverability, but lack of three collaboration types, or the other end of the bargain, [32] with good modelling power, but lack of known decision power on soundness and rediscoverability. A future discovery technique targeting a (potentially new) class that has modelling power to represent all four collaboration types and good decision power not only brings together the top-down and bottom-up approach, but also is applicable to the challenges studied in a diverse range of research areas and their respective application domains (cf. Fig. 1).

G2 Match your discovery technique's design rationale with the properties of existing classes to access the existing theoretical and practical knowledge and improve rather algorithmically instead of by definition of a new class. If a new class is still necessary, take the first guideline into account.

G3 State your targeted class explicitly and formally, as it allows straightforward assessment similar to Sect. 3.1 and is part of the first maturity stage [51] of your discovery technique. Have all four maturity stages in mind.

G4 Think three times about not taking a divide-and-conquer approach to discovery, as the CP is a composition. If you have another approach, motivate it well.

G5 Balance your design guided by the previous four guidelines with your discovery technique's complexity to achieve sufficient efficiency for practical purposes.

By taking these guidelines into account, collaboration mining techniques can be flexibly combined, easily compared and assessed, and come with a well-researched theoretical foundation.

Limitations: Despite the extensive set of covered techniques and research areas, the heterogeneity of collaboration results may result in having missed existing work on collaboration. Also, the set of assessed Petri net classes is likely not completely comprehensive. Hence, a Petri net class might exists already that is the best candidate for a standard CP model. Additionally, the criteria can be further refined to improve the characterization of the standard CP model.

5   Conclusion and Future Work

The integration of heterogeneous collaboration in our CP meta model enables the assessment of existing Petri net classes with respect to properties of a standard model class for CP and can guide new collaboration mining techniques beginning with process discovery. As a clear standard Petri net class for CP is still missing, future techniques should take this lack of standardization into account to advance collaboration mining in a coherent way. Additionally, a fusion of the top-down and bottom-up approach opens up yet to be utilized ways of combining results from both sides. An empirical evaluation of the CP meta model in covering collaboration heterogeneity through case studies in various distributed settings such as e-Government or healthcare and/or through various, applicable real-world datasets can further validate our results and guide the collaboration mining research in dealing with the complexity of collaborations and its heterogeneity.

Acknowledgements. This work has been partly funded by the Austrian Research Promotion Agency (FFG) via the "Austrian Competence Center for Digital Production" (CDP) under the contract number 854187.

References

1. van der Aalst, W.M.P.: On the representational bias in process mining. In: 2011 IEEE WETICE, pp. 2–7, June 2011
2. van der Aalst, W.M.P.: Modeling and analyzing interorganizational workflows. In: Proceedings 1998 ACSD, pp. 262–272 (1998)
3. van der Aalst, W.M.P.: Interorganizational workflows: an approach based on message sequence charts and petri nets. Syst. Anal. Model. Simul. **34**, 335–367 (1999)
4. van der Aalst, W.M.P.: Service mining: using process mining to discover, check, and improve service behavior. IEEE Trans. Serv. Comput. **6**(4), 525–535 (2013)
5. van der Aalst, W.M.P., Berti, A.: Discovering object-centric petri nets. Fundam. Inform. **175**(1–4), 1–40 (2020)
6. van der Aalst, W.M.P., van Hee, K.M., Massuthe, P., Sidorova, N., van der Werf, J.M.: Compositional service trees. In: Franceschinis, G., Wolf, K. (eds.) PETRI NETS 2009. LNCS, vol. 5606, pp. 283–302. Springer, Heidelberg (2009). https://doi.org/10.1007/978-3-642-02424-5_17
7. van der Aalst, W.M.P., Weijters, T., Maruster, L.: Workflow mining: discovering process models from event logs. IEEE Trans. Knowl. Data Eng. **16**(9), 1128–1142 (2004)
8. van der Aalst, W.M.P., Weske, M.: The P2P approach to interorganizational workflows. In: Dittrich, K.R., Geppert, A., Norrie, M.C. (eds.) CAiSE 2001. LNCS, vol. 2068, pp. 140–156. Springer, Heidelberg (2001). https://doi.org/10.1007/3-540-45341-5_10
9. Augusto, A., Conforti, R., Dumas, M., Rosa et al., M.L.: Automated discovery of process models from event logs: review and benchmark. IEEE Trans. Knowl. Data Eng. **31**(4), 686–705 (2019)
10. Barenholz, D., Montali, M., Polyvyanyy, A., Reijers, H.A., et al., H.A.: There and back again. In: Gomes, L., Lorenz, R. (eds.) Application and Theory of Petri Nets and Concurrency. PETRI NETS 2023. LNCS, vol. 13929, pp. 37–58. Springer, Cham (2023). https://doi.org/10.1007/978-3-031-33620-1_3
11. Basten, T., van Der Aalst, W.: Inheritance of behavior. J. Log. Algebraic Program. **47**(2), 47–145 (2001)
12. Borkowski, M., Fdhila, W., Nardelli, M., Rinderle-Ma, S., Schulte, S.: Event-based failure prediction in distributed business processes. Inf. Syst. **81**, 220–235 (2019)
13. Chu, X.N., Tso, S.K., Zhang, W.J., Li, Q.: Partnership synthesis for virtual enterprises. Int. J. Adv. Manuf. Technol. **19**(5), 384–391 (2002)
14. Corradini, F., Re, B., Rossi, L., Tiezzi, F.: A technique for collaboration discovery. In: Augusto, A., Gill, A., Bork, D., Nurcan, S., Reinhartz-Berger, I., Schmidt, R. (eds.) Enterprise, Business-Process and Information Systems Modeling. BPMDS EMMSAD 2022 2022. LNBIP, vol. 450, pp. 63–78. Springer, Cham (2022). https://doi.org/10.1007/978-3-031-07475-2_5

15. Decker, G., Weske, M.: Local enforceability in interaction petri nets. In: Alonso, G., Dadam, P., Rosemann, M. (eds.) BPM 2007. LNCS, vol. 4714, pp. 305–319. Springer, Heidelberg (2007). https://doi.org/10.1007/978-3-540-75183-0_22
16. Decker, G., Weske, M.: Interaction-centric modeling of process choreographies. Inf. Syst. **36**(2), 292–312 (2011)
17. Fahland, D.: Describing behavior of processes with many-to-many interactions. In: Donatelli, S., Haar, S. (eds.) PETRI NETS 2019. LNCS, vol. 11522, pp. 3–24. Springer, Cham (2019). https://doi.org/10.1007/978-3-030-21571-2_1
18. Fdhila, W., Gall, M., Rinderle-Ma, S., Mangler, J., Indiono, C.: Classification and formalization of instance-spanning constraints in process-driven applications. In: La Rosa, M., Loos, P., Pastor, O. (eds.) BPM 2016. LNCS, vol. 9850, pp. 348–364. Springer, Cham (2016). https://doi.org/10.1007/978-3-319-45348-4_20
19. Fdhila, W., Indiono, C., Rinderle-Ma, S., Reichert, M.: Dealing with change in process choreographies: design and implementation of propagation algorithms. Inf. Syst. **49**, 1–24 (2015)
20. Fdhila, W., Rinderle-Ma, S., Knuplesch, D., Reichert, M.: Change and compliance in collaborative processes. In: 2015 IEEE SCC, pp. 162–169, June 2015
21. Fettke, P., Reisig, W.: Systems Mining with Heraklit: The Next Step, June 2022. arXiv:2202.01289 [cs]
22. Gaaloul, W., Baïna, K., Godart, C.: Log-based mining techniques applied to web service composition reengineering. Serv. Oriented Comput. Appl. **2**(2), 93–110 (2008)
23. Garcia, E., Giret, A., Botti, V.: Designing normative open virtual enterprises. Enterp. Inf. Syst. **10**(3), 303–324 (2016)
24. Grefen, P., Mehandjiev, N., Kouvas, G., Weichhart et al., G.: Dynamic business network process management in instant virtual enterprises. Comput. Ind. **60**(2), 86–103 (2009)
25. Jablonski, S., Bussler, C.: Workflow management: modeling concepts, architecture and implementation. ITP New Media (1996)
26. Jensen, K.: Coloured petri nets and the invariant-method. Theor. Comput. Sci. **14**(3), 317–336 (1981)
27. Köhler, M., Rölke, H.: Properties of object petri nets. In: Cortadella, J., Reisig, W. (eds.) ICATPN 2004. LNCS, vol. 3099, pp. 278–297. Springer, Heidelberg (2004). https://doi.org/10.1007/978-3-540-27793-4_16
28. Kwantes, P., Kleijn, J.: Distributed synthesis of asynchronously communicating distributed process models. In: Koutny, M., Kordon, F., Moldt, D. (eds.) Transactions on Petri Nets and Other Models of Concurrency XVI. LNCS, vol. 13220, pp. 49–72. Springer, Berlin, Heidelberg (2022). https://doi.org/10.1007/978-3-662-65303-6_3
29. Kwantes, P.M., Kleijn, J.: On the synthesis of industry level process models from enterprise level process models. In: ATAED@ Petri Nets/ACSD, pp. 6–22 (2018)
30. Leemans, S.J.J., van Zelst, S.J., Lu, X.: Partial-order-based process mining: a survey and outlook. Knowl. Inf. Syst. (2022)
31. Liu, C., Li, H., Zeng, Q., Lu et al., T.: cross-organization emergency response process mining: an approach based on petri nets. Math. Probl. Eng. **2020**, e8836007 (2020)
32. Liu, C., Li, H., Zhang, S., Cheng et al., L.: Cross-department collaborative healthcare process model discovery from event logs. IEEE Trans. Autom. Sci. Eng. **20**(3), 2115–2125 (2023)
33. Mahulea, C., Mahulea, L., García Soriano, J.M., Colom, J.M.: Modular Petri net modeling of healthcare systems. Flex. Serv. Manuf. J. **30**(1), 329–357 (2018)

34. Mangler, J., Ehrendorfer, M.: XES Chess Pieces Production, May 2023. https://zenodo.org/record/7477845
35. Mangler, J., Rinderle-Ma, S.: Cloud Process Execution Engine: Architecture and Interfaces, September 2022. arXiv:2208.12214 [cs]
36. Meyer, A., Pufahl, L., Batoulis, K., Fahland, D., Weske, M.: Automating data exchange in process choreographies. Inf. Syst. **53**, 296–329 (2015)
37. Nesterov, R., Bernardinello, L., Lomazova, I., Pomello, L.: Discovering architecture-aware and sound process models of multi-agent systems: a compositional approach. Softw. Syst. Model. **22**(1), 351–375 (2023)
38. Peterson, J.L.: Petri Nets. ACM Comput. Surv. **9**(3), 223–252 (1977)
39. Petri, C.A.: Kommunikation mit automaten (1962)
40. Polyvyanyy, A., van der Werf, J.M.E.M., Overbeek, S., Brouwers, R.: Information systems modeling: language, verification, and tool support. In: Giorgini, P., Weber, B. (eds.) CAiSE 2019. LNCS, vol. 11483, pp. 194–212. Springer, Cham (2019). https://doi.org/10.1007/978-3-030-21290-2_13
41. Reisig, W.: Composition of component models - a key to construct big systems. In: Margaria, T., Steffen, B. (eds.) ISoLA 2020. LNCS, vol. 12477, pp. 171–188. Springer, Cham (2020). https://doi.org/10.1007/978-3-030-61470-6_11
42. Rinderle-Ma, S., Reichert, M., Jurisch, M.: Equivalence of web services in process-aware service compositions. In: 2009 IEEE ICWS, pp. 501–508, July 2009
43. Rosa-Velardo, F., de Frutos-Escrig, D.: Decidability and complexity of Petri nets with unordered data. Theor. Comput. Sci. **412**(34), 4439–4451 (2011)
44. Schulte, S., Hoenisch, P., Hochreiner, C., Dustdar et al., S.: Towards process support for cloud manufacturing. In: 2014 IEEE 18th EDOC, pp. 142–149, September 2014
45. Stroiński, A., Dwornikowski, D., Brzeziński, J.: A distributed discovery of communicating resource systems models. IEEE Trans. Serv. Comput. **12**(2), 172–185 (2019)
46. Tan, W., Xu, W., Yang, F., Xu, L., et al.: A framework for service enterprise workflow simulation with multi-agents cooperation. Enterp. Inf. Syst. **7**(4), 523–542 (2013)
47. Tour, A., Polyvyanyy, A., Kalenkova, A.: Agent system mining: vision, benefits, and challenges. IEEE Access **9**, 99480–99494 (2021)
48. Tour, A., Polyvyanyy, A., Kalenkova, A., Senderovich, A.: Agent Miner: An Algorithm for Discovering Agent Systems from Event Data, July 2023. arXiv:2212.01454
49. Valk, R.: On Processes of Object Petri Nets (1996)
50. van Glabbeek, R., Vaandrager, F.: Petri net models for algebraic theories of concurrency. In: de Bakker, J.W., Nijman, A.J., Treleaven, P.C. (eds.) PARLE 1987. LNCS, vol. 259, pp. 224–242. Springer, Heidelberg (1987). https://doi.org/10.1007/3-540-17945-3_13
51. van der Werf, J.M.E.M., Polyvyanyy, A., van Wensveen, B.R., Brinkhuis et al., M.: All that glitters is not gold: Four maturity stages of process discovery algorithms. Inf. Syst. **114**, 102155 (2023)
52. Winter, K., Rinderle-Ma, S.: Defining instance spanning constraint patterns for business processes based on proclets. In: Dobbie, G., Frank, U., Kappel, G., Liddle, S.W., Mayr, H.C. (eds.) ER 2020. LNCS, vol. 12400, pp. 149–163. Springer, Cham (2020). https://doi.org/10.1007/978-3-030-62522-1_11
53. Zeng, Q., Duan, H., Liu, C.: Top-down process mining from multi-source running logs based on refinement of petri nets. IEEE Access **8**, 61355–61369 (2020)

54. Zeng, Q., Lu, F., Liu, C., Duan, H., et al.: Modeling and verification for cross-department collaborative business processes using extended petri nets. IEEE Trans. Syst. Man Cybern.: Syst. **45**(2), 349–362 (2015)
55. Zeng, Q., Sun, S., Duan, H., Liu, C., et al.: Cross-organizational collaborative work-flow mining from a multi-source log. Decis. Support Syst. **54**, 1280–1301 (2013)

From Identities to Quantities: Introducing Items and Decoupling Points to Object-Centric Process Mining

Nina Graves$^{(\boxtimes)}$, István Koren , Majid Rafiei ,
and Wil M. P. van der Aalst

Chair of Process and Data Science (PADS), RWTH Aachen University,
Aachen, Germany
{graves,koren,majid.rafiei,wvdaalst}@pads.rwth-aachen.de
https://www.pads.rwth-aachen.de/

Abstract. Logistics processes ensure that the right product is at the right location at the right time in the right quantity. Their efficiency is crucial to industrial operations, as they generate costs while not adding value to the product. Process mining techniques improve processes using real-life data. However, the application of process mining to logistics processes poses several challenges, as (1) recorded material movements refer to quantities of items, not individual objects and (2) the required data are often scattered over several systems requiring additional pre-processing efforts. This work presents the concept of item quantities to describe the movement of not individually identifiable items across distributed processes. Subsequently, we introduce a framework to integrate the explicit consideration of item quantities into process mining, consisting of a quantity-related event log and an extension of object-centric Petri nets as a basis for quantity-dependent process analysis. The analysis of an artificial event log demonstrates the additional insights the consideration of quantities uncovers and highlights the potential for the application of process mining in the logistics domain.

Keywords: Process Mining · Logistics · Material Flow Analysis

1 Introduction

In current times, a swift transformation towards sustainable practices is essential, requiring in-depth analysis and transformation of processes concerning the sourcing, processing, and transporting of material [12]. Process mining is a relatively young discipline, leveraging readily available event data to analyse, monitor, improve and support business processes [2]. Apart from being a growing field for research in academia [9], its industrial adoption is swiftly expanding across various industries [8]. Despite the benefits of process mining for intralogistics [7] as well as inter-organisational processes [13], its application to the logistics domain is relatively low [9].

© The Author(s), under exclusive license to Springer Nature Switzerland AG 2024
J. De Smedt and P. Soffer (Eds.): ICPM 2023 Workshops, LNBIP 503, pp. 462–474, 2024.
https://doi.org/10.1007/978-3-031-56107-8_35

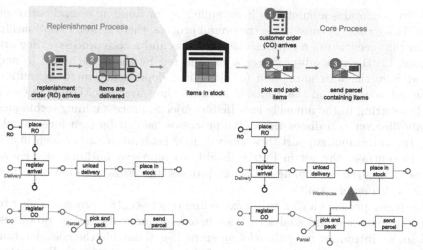

(a) Disconnected OCPN without item IDs.   (b) OCPN extended by a decoupling point indicating a collection of items.

Fig. 1. Example of a quantity-dependent process composed of two decoupled sub-processes.

The main reason for this discrepancy lies in the data availability [15]. The event log used for object-centric process mining, contains information on the execution of an activity linked to at least one individually identifiable object [3]. Process discovery algorithms combine the events referring to the same object to detect dependencies among different activities – this means every object requires one unique identifier for the end-to-end process. There are two requirements data on logistics processes do not necessarily fulfil: First, logistics processes describe material movements, such as the addition or removal of a number of items without necessarily referring to uniquely identifiable objects [5,9]. For example, one book and two cups are added to the warehouse, instead of book-123, cup-456 and cup-789. Secondly, they can be scattered across several systems, even crossing organisational boundaries, leading to the required data being distributed without matching identifiers [4], i.e., the identifiers different organisations use for the same object are different.

Consider, for example, a warehouse management process, as depicted in Fig. 1. The warehouse's core process is fulfilling customer orders (shown on the right of the figure), referring to its three item types: photo albums a, books b, and cups c. Whenever a customer order arrives, the requested number of items is picked from the warehouse and packed into a parcel before it is sent to the customer. When the number of items in the warehouse is low, a replenishment sub-process is executed. This sub-process begins with placing a replenishment order, leading to the delivery of items that are unpacked and placed in the warehouse. All uniquely identifiable objects (replenishment orders, deliveries, customer orders and parcels) are associated with their corresponding events.

One delivery contains a number of items sufficient for fulfilling several customer orders. We see that (1) considering the overall process, there is no 1:1 relationship between the execution of a replenishment process and a core process – they are *decoupled*, (2) the two sub-processes are connected by the items added to and removed from the warehouse, and (3) there is a dependency in the execution of both sub-processes on the available items in the warehouse. Using an event log only referring to the uniquely identifiable objects, process mining techniques can only discover two disconnected sub-processes, as can be seen for example in Fig. 1a, and cannot support their analysis in consideration of non-identifiable items. In contrast, the net in Fig. 1b, is able to represent both a collection of items as well as the decoupling of the two processes by using an additional type of node: a *decoupling point*.

This paper presents a framework extending object-centric process mining to enable the detection and analysis of decoupled, quantity-dependent processes. To do so, we introduce *quantity-relating event logs* to enable the consideration of item quantities as well as an extension of object-centric Petri nets. We further demonstrate the additional insights that can be gained by taking available item quantities at the execution time of events into account using an artificial event log. After presenting related work (Sect. 2), Sect. 3 introduces the preliminaries including items, item collections and quantity operations. Quantity-relating event logs (QELs) and quantity nets are presented in Sect. 4. In Sect. 5, we analyse an artificial QEL to present the benefits and shortcomings of the framework. Section 6 concludes this work.

2   Related Work

The problems of missing or mismatching identifiers and the discovery and analysis of quantity-dependent processes have been addressed in literature. Federated process mining deals with the joint consideration of disconnected processes, described and formalised in [1]. Approaches to match identifiers of distributed processes using EDI messages [6] and leveraging Radio Frequency Identification (RFID) data [10] were discussed in the literature. In [11], the authors introduce an approach in which individually identifiable objects are grouped to map their identifiers to joint identifiers collected from RFID data. All of these methods rely on the existence of the individual and shared identifiers for the relevant entities of the process and allow for a fully end-to-end analysis of each of the relevant entities. In contrast, the authors of [20] present an abstraction-based, privacy-preserving approach to discovering inter-organisational processes. Although the presented procedure allows process analysis without requiring shared end-to-end identifiers, it requires a 1:1 mapping between process executions of the different systems.

A typical example of a quantity-based interdependency of process executions is batch processing. When processing in a batch, an activity or sub-process is executed a predetermined number of times without interruption before the objects are passed on to the next step [19]. Several works aim to discover different types of batched activities, such as [18] or batched sub-processes [17]. All of these approaches assume event data containing an entry for each batched element. The authors of [21] assume a mixture of events referring to batched objects as well as individual ones, the batched ones including the information on the number of batched objects.

Some works explicitly address the logistics-related challenges of process mining. In [5], an approach for the preparation and visualisation of material movement data is presented, allowing for the identification of inefficiencies in the paths the material takes. A methodology combining association rules with process mining to uncover dependencies between processes and performance indicators for supply chains is introduced in [16]. In [14], the authors present an approach to enrich event data with additional information to detect waste in a value stream. We see that existing literature focuses on preparing event data to use out-of-the-box process mining techniques instead of integrating the additionally available data to enhance process mining's capabilities.

3 Preliminaries

This section introduces some general mathematical operations as well as concepts related to object-centric process mining. Function projections, denoted $f \restriction_W$, define the application of a function $f : X \not\to Y$ to a different domain W, with: $dom(f \restriction_W) = dom(f) \cap W$ and $f \restriction_W (x) = f(x)$ for $x \in dom(f \restriction_W)$. A sequence of length n over a set A is denoted $\sigma = \langle a_1, a_2, ..., a_n \rangle \in A^*$, with $\sigma = \langle \rangle$ as the empty sequence and $\sigma_1 \cdot \sigma_2$ the concatenation of sequences. The j-th element of a sequence $\sigma = \langle a_1, ..., a_j, ..., a_n \rangle \in A^*$ is denoted $\sigma[j] = a_j$ and the *prefix* of $\sigma[j]$ is referred to as $\sigma_{:j} = \langle a_1, ..., a_{j-1} \rangle$.

To define an Object-Centric Event Log (OCEL), the basis for object-centric process mining, we introduce the universe of activities $\mathcal{U}_{act}$, the universe of events $\mathcal{U}_{ev}$, the universe of objects $\mathcal{U}_o$, the universe of object types $\mathcal{U}_{ot}$, and the universe of timestamps $\mathcal{U}_{time}$.

Definition 1 (Object-centric Event Log). *An object-centric event log is a tuple $OCEL = (E, O, act, otypes, time, E2O)$, where $E \subseteq \mathcal{U}_{ev}$ is a set of events, $O \subseteq \mathcal{U}_o$ is a set of objects, $act : E \to \mathcal{U}_{act}$ is a function assigning activities to events, $otype : O \to \mathcal{U}_{ot}$ maps each object identifier to an object type, time : $E \to \mathcal{U}_{time}$ assigns a timestamp to each event, and $E2O \subseteq (E \times O)$ describes the relation between events and objects.*

We denote $A(OCEL)$ for the set of activities, and $OT(OCEL)$ as the set of object types. As introduced in [3], Object-Centric Petri Nets (OCPNs) are defined in correspondence to an OCEL by specifying the set of object types $OT(OCEL)$ and the tokens being associated with objects of the log. In addition to a labelled Petri net $N = (P, T, F, l)$, defined in the usual way, OCPNs include a mapping assigning an object type to every place, and a set of variable arcs.

Definition 2 (Object-Centric Petri net). *An object-centric Petri net is a tuple $ON = (N, pt, F_{var})$ where $N = (P, T, F, l)$ is a labelled Petri net, pt : $P \to OT$ maps places onto object types, and $F_{var} \subseteq F$ is a subset of variable arcs.*

Normal arcs describe the removal or addition of a single token, whereas variable arcs indicate a variable number of tokens to be removed or added. The firing of a transition occurs in regard to a *binding* (t, b), which includes the transition to be fired as well as a binding function. The binding defines the sets of tokens to be consumed, $cons(t, b)$, and produced, $prod(t, b)$.

The example presented in the introduction considers two operationally decoupled sub-processes tied by their impact on a known collection of items - a warehouse. We consider *items* to be elements of the process relevant to the control flow that occur in varying quantities. Although each item refers to a particular item type, they differ from objects as they are not described by an identifier but by the quantity they occur in. The universe of item types is denoted $\mathcal{U}_{it}$, and $I \subseteq \mathcal{U}_{it}$ refers to a set of item types. In the logistics domain, we have to distinguish between the demand for items of different types (negative quantity) and the actual presence of such items (positive quantity). Thus, we introduce *item quantities*, which assign a signed integer to each item type.

Definition 3 (Item Quantity). *Let $I \subseteq \mathcal{U}_{it}$ be a finite set of item types. An item quantity $q : I \rightarrow \mathbb{Z}$ is a function that maps each item type $i \in I$ to a signed integer. The set of all possible item quantities over I is denoted $\mathcal{I}(I) = \{q : I \rightarrow \mathbb{Z}\}$. Item quantities can be changed by addition and subtraction, given $q_1, q_2 \in \mathcal{I}(I)$ be two item quantities over $I \subseteq \mathcal{U}_{it}$:*
$q_1 \oplus q_2 = q_3$ *where* $\forall i \in I : q_3(i) = q_1(i) + q_2(i)$, *and*
$q_1 \ominus q_2 = q_3$ *where* $\forall i \in I : q_3(i) = q_1(i) - q_2(i)$.

We use a notation for item quantities similar to multisets but emphasising the difference using different brackets. Some examples for item quantities over $I = \{x, y, z\}$ with $I \subseteq \mathcal{U}_{it}$: $q_1 = [\![\,]\!]$, $q_2 = [\![x, x, x, y]\!]$, $q_3 = [\![x, y^{-1}, y^{-1}, z, z]\!]$, $q_4 = [\![x^3, y]\!]$, and $q_5 = [\![x, y^{-2}, z^2]\!]$. q_1 is an empty item quantity, q_2 and q_4 are two notations for the same item quantity, just as q_3 and q_5. $q_2(y) = 1$ refers to the quantity associated with item type y for q_2, just as $q_3(y) = -2$ for item quantity q_3, and $q_1(y) = 0$ for q_1. The set of all item types q assigns a non-zero quantity to is denoted, $set(q) = \{i \mid q(i) \neq 0\}$, e.g. $set(q_2) = \{x, y\}$ and $set(q_1) = \emptyset$. Examples for operations on item quantities: $q_2 \oplus q_3 = [\![x^4, y^{-1}, z^2]\!]$, $q_4 \ominus q_5 = [\![x^2, y^3, z^{-2}]\!]$, and $q_5 \ominus q_3 = q_1$.

The positive item quantity of q is denoted $q^+ = b\lceil_{\{i \in set(q) \mid q(i) > 0\}}$ and $q^- = q\lceil_{\{i \in set(q) \mid q(i) < 0\}}$ as the negative item quantity of q, e.g. $q_3^+ = [\![x, z^2]\!]$ and $q_5^- = [\![y^{-2}]\!]$. An item quantity $q \in \mathcal{I}(I)$ is considered *fully positive*, iff $q = q^+$ and *fully negative* iff $q = q^-$.

A location or entity dedicated to collecting items, such as a warehouse or a buffer, is referred to as a collection point. Every collection point refers to an item quantity, its *item level*, describing the availability or lack of items of specific item types. We consider a finite set of collection points $CP \subseteq \mathcal{U}_{cp}$ from the universe of collection points.

Definition 4 (Item Levels). *Given a set of item types $I \subseteq \mathcal{U}_{it}$ and a set of collection points $CP \subseteq \mathcal{U}_{cp}$, the mapping $m_q : CP \rightarrow \mathcal{I}(I)$ describes the item levels of the collection points in CP.*

In line with Definition 3, the item level of a particular item type $i \in I$ of collection point $cp \in CP$ is denoted $m_{q,I}(cp)(i)$. Consider, a warehouse $cp \in CP$ containing items of three different types: $I = \{cups, books, albums\}$. Currently, there is a stock of 21 cups and the item level of books lies at $m_{q,I}(cp)(books) = 17$, but a demand for 25 albums. Hence, the item level for the warehouse is $m_{q,I}(cp) = [\![cups^{21}, books^{17}, albums^{-25}]\!]$.

A collection point's item level is changed in a *quantity operation* by adding another item quantity $q \in \mathcal{I}(I)$ to the current item level, denoted $m_{q,I}(cp) \xrightarrow{q} m'_{q,I}(cp)$, where $m'_{q,I}(cp) = m_{q,I}(cp) \oplus q$. After the execution of a quantity operation, the item level of all item types with a negative item quantity $i \in set(q^-)$ is reduced and increased for all available item types $i \in set(q^+)$. The execution of a sequence of quantity operations on the initial item level $m_{q,I}^{init}(cp) \xrightarrow{q_1} m_{q,I}'(cp) \xrightarrow{q_2} ... \xrightarrow{q_n} m''_{q,I}(cp)$, is denoted $m_{q,I}^{init}(cp) \xrightarrow{\sigma} m_{q,I}''(cp)$, with $\sigma = \langle q_1, q_2, ..., q_n \rangle$ describing the sequence of item quantities. Using item quantities, we can now represent collections of items as well as material movements.

4   Quantity-Dependent Process Mining

The underlying concepts of item quantities, collection points, item levels and quantity operations are nothing new: Inventory management is one of the largest areas in logistics. However, current process mining techniques cannot describe item quantities and business processes jointly [9]. This section proposes a framework extending object-centric process mining to (1) connect the execution of events with changes to item levels, (2) detect the item levels of known collection points at the time individual processes are executed, and (3) model decoupled quantity-dependent processes. The framework is based on the assumption that the execution of quantity operations is connected to events described exhaustively in the event log.

4.1   Quantity-Relating Event Logs

Our goal is to define an event log that enables the identification of dependencies between the execution of activities, sub-processes, and item levels without needing identifiers for all items. This requires an event log that connects events to quantity operations and, thereby, describes the item levels' development. We achieve this by adding collection points and item types to the log and mapping quantity operations to events.

Definition 5 (Quantity Event Log). *A quantity-relating event log is a tuple* $QEL = (OCEL, I, CP, eqty)$, *where* $OCEL = (E, O, act, otypes, time, E2O)$ *is an object-centric event log,* $I \subseteq \mathcal{U}_{it}$ *is a set of item types,* $CP \subseteq \mathcal{U}_{CP}$ *is the set of known collection points, and* $eqty : E \to (CP \nrightarrow \mathcal{I}(I))$ *assigns quantity updates to events and collection points.*

As this event log extends usual OCELs, applying other process mining techniques is not limited by using QELs. Table 1 shows a QEL for the example process of

Table 1. Example of a QEL displayed in a single table

events (E, act, time)			eqty		objects (O, otypes, E2O)			
event	activity	timestamp	quantity	cp	RO	CO	delivery	parcel
ev-zz	register co	22.12.2020 12:22	$[\![a^{-3}]\!]$	cp1		co-883		
ev-vl	pick and pack	22.12.2020 12:24	$[\![a^{-3}, b^{-10}]\!]$	cp2		co-882		p-942
ev-tg	send parcel	22.12.2020 12:31						p-941
ev-rg	register co	22.12.2020 13:56	$[\![b^{-3}, c^{-1}]\!]$	cp1		co-884		
ev-pa	send parcel	22.12.2020 13:57						p-942
ev-yq	pick and pack	22.12.2020 14:01	$[\![a^{-3}]\!]$	cp2		co-883		p-943
ev-kj	send parcel	22.12.2020 14:11						p-943
ev-bn	register delivery	22.12.2020 15:19			ro-11		d-11	
ev-iq	pick and pack	22.12.2020 15:23	$[\![b^{-3}, c^{-1}]\!]$	cp2		co-884		p-944
ev-gq	send parcel	22.12.2020 15:39						p-944
ev-id	unpack delivery	22.12.2020 16:12					d-11	
ev-ya	register co	23.12.2020 09:40	$[\![b^{-5}]\!]$	cp1		co-891		
ev-mr	pick and pack	23.12.2020 10:22	$[\![b^{-5}]\!]$	cp2		co-891		p-951
ev-sj	send parcel	23.12.2020 10:38						p-951
ev-oo	place in stock	28.12.2020 10:43	$[\![b^{990}]\!]$	cp2			d-11	
ev-qk	register co	28.12.2020 10:50	$[\![b^{-5}, c^{-3}]\!]$	cp1		co-925		

Fig. 1, in which all information is aggregated into a single table: We see the event details, information on the related quantity operations and the involved objects of the different object types. Please note, that this is only possible as every event only refers to one object of each type and one collection point. We see that the events "register co", "pick and pack" and "place in stock" are associated with quantity operations regarding two different collection points.

As we see in the example log, we cannot determine the item level of the individual collection point based on this information. We, therefore, introduce a preliminary simplification in which we assume the existence of an *init*-event mapping each collection point to its initial item level, dated prior to every other event with a quantity operation. It is clear, that associating the quantity operations with events allows for considering sequences of quantity operations. Using a projection that keeps the sequence's length and summing over each entry's prefix, the quantity level of every collection point can be determined during any event in the log. The left of Fig. 2, shows a sequence σ of 10 entries, each referring to a collection point and an item quantity, derived by ordering the quantity operations according to the timestamp of the corresponding event. By considering the initial item levels $m_{q,I}^{init}(cp_1) = [\![a^{21}, b^{25}, c^{10}]\!]$, and $m_{q,I}^{init}(cp_2) = [\![a^{31}, b^{27}, c^6]\!]$ it is possible to determine the development of each collection point's item level at any time within the sequence, as can be seen on the right.

4.2 Quantity Nets

One of the main benefits of process mining is its ability to identify process models capable of relaying the causalities uncovered by analysing event data – as seen in

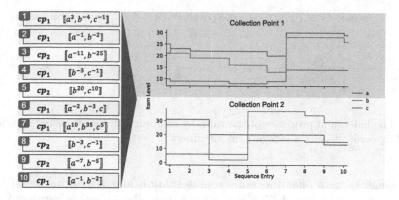

Fig. 2. Sequence of quantity operations (left) and item levels of both collection points with initial levels of $m_{q,I}^{init}(cp_1) = [\![a^{21}, b^{25}, c^{10}]\!]$ and $m_{q,I}^{init}(cp_2) = [\![a^{31}, b^{27}, c^6]\!]$.

the introduction OCPNs are not capable of doing so for non-identifiable items. In this work, we consider a collection of items as a point in which several sub-processes are decoupled, indicating an item quantity-related dependency of their process executions by adding *decoupling points* to OCPNs.

Definition 6 (Labelled Quantity Net). *A labelled quantity net is a tripartite graph* $QN = (P, T, DP, F, F_{var}, pt, l)$, *with* P *a set of places,* T *a set of transitions,* $DP \subseteq \mathcal{U}_{cp}$ *a set of decoupling points,* $F \subseteq ((P \times T) \cup (T \times P) \cup (T \times DP) \cup (DP \times T))$ *a set of arcs,* $F_{var} \subseteq (F \cap ((P \times T) \cup (T \times P)))$ *a subset of variable arcs between places and transitions,* $pt : P \to \mathcal{U}_{ot}$ *a mapping of places to object types,* $l : T \nrightarrow \mathcal{U}_{act}$ *a function assigning activity names to transitions.*

The semantics of OCPNs are described by bindings, which we keep unchanged but refer to the binding function as *place binding*. The binding of the quantity net is composed of the place binding and a valid quantity-binding b^q, thus $b = (t, b^p, b^q)$. A quantity binding is a function $b^q : DP \nrightarrow \mathcal{I}(I)$ describing a quantity item for decoupling points, the semantics of which are considered equivalent to those of quantity operations for collection points. A binding is valid, if it only assigns a function value to places and decoupling points connected to the transition it refers to. Depending on the type of arc, the change in the item level $m_{q,I}(dp) \xrightarrow{q} m'_{q,I}(dp)$ by an item quantity $q \in \mathcal{I}(I)$ is either an addition $m'_{q,I}(dp) = m_{q,I}(dp) \oplus Q$ (incoming arc) or a subtraction $m'_{q,I}(dp) = m_{q,I}(dp) \ominus q$ (outgoing arc). Please note, that these semantics can lead to an increase in the item level if a negative item quantity is subtracted from a negative item level. Figure 3 shows an example, in which, for simplicity, only the transition, decoupling points and quantity binding function (graph notation) are detailed. The execution of b_1 fires transition t_1 and adds $[\![a^2, c]\!]$ to dp_1's current item level, $m_{q,I}(dp_1) \xrightarrow{b_1^q} m'_{q,I}(dp_1) = [\![a^6, b^6, c^3]\!]$, leaving dp_2's item level unchanged. Executing b_2 removes items from dp_1, $m_{q,I}(dp_1)'' = m_{q,I}(dp_1)' \ominus [\![a, b^2]\!]$, and adds $[\![b, c]\!]$ to dp_2, so that $m''_{q,I}(dp_2) = m_{q,I}(dp_2) \oplus b_2^q(dp_2)$.

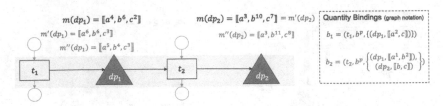

Fig. 3. The individual processes of the running example can be connected through a decoupling point, despite a lack of item identifiers.

As quantity nets offer the same representation and semantics as OCPNs, they do not limit the modelling capabilities, yet offer a further representation of behaviour. The decoupling points represent the connection of otherwise disconnected processes as well as an inter-dependency of a collection of items and the process. We briefly describe a very basic form of discovery by imposing two strong requirements. The first is that only fully positive and fully negative item quantities are included in the QEL. The second is that all events belonging to the same activity must "agree" in their impact on a collection point – there are no quantity operations by events in which one refers to a fully positive, and the other refers to a fully negative item quantity for the same collection point. Given a QEL fulfilling these requirements, the OCPN discovered by the event log can be extended by first adding each collection point as a decoupling point. Subsequently, arcs between the activities referring to at least one quantity operation and the corresponding collection point are added – the arc's direction depends on the sign of the quantity operation.

5   Example Application

The main goal of inventory management is maintaining a continuous capability to meet variable and uncertain demand while minimising cost. Current approaches for inventory management consider specific parameters related to item quantities and lead times. Still, they cannot additionally consider the end-to-end process leading to increases and decreases of stock levels [5]. This section applies the previously introduced framework to increase its comprehension and demonstrate how it enhances process mining's capabilities. To do so, we present an analysis of a simulated QEL[1] describing a typical example for a decoupled process: inventory management. The log describes a process similar to the process used as the running example – the only difference is that customer orders can loop around the activity "pick and pack". Figure 5 shows the corresponding quantity net created by extending the discovered OCPN. The selected log fulfils the criteria for discovering quantity nets, as it has one activity referring to fully positive quantity operations ("place in stock") and another ("pick and pack") with only negative item quantities.

---

[1] Link to the data: https://git.rwth-aachen.de/ninagraves/intro_qrpm.

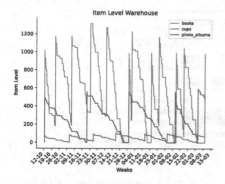

Fig. 4. Warehouse's Item level over time.

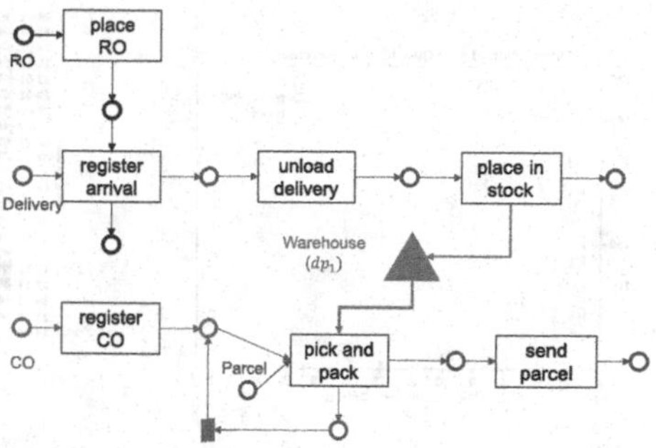

Fig. 5. Quantity net of example process.

The log shows a decoupled process, as significantly more customer orders are processed than replenishment orders placed: One delivery of albums covers about 519 customer orders in a turnover time of 33 days, every delivery of books lasts for about eight business days, and delivered cups last for 17 days. Figure 6 shows the distribution of the number of ordered items per type (only considering orders with a demand for this item type) per customer order – assuming the accumulated item quantities removed regarding the same customer order represent the ordered quantity. The average customer order arrives 15.6 times per business day and refers to an item quantity of 1.35 photo albums, 6.9 books and 0.29 cups. In comparison, 21 deliveries arrived in the same period. Eleven deliveries contain 980 or 990 books, six include 81 or 82 cups, and four deliveries add 556 to 560 photo albums to the warehouse. An overview of the delivered (and assumed to be ordered) items can be found in Fig. 7.

Further process insights can be gained from the QEL by considering the item level of the warehouse at the time specific events were executed. A closer look at the replenishment orders shows that the time between the placement of replenishment orders varies throughout the process, making a time-based dependency unlikely. Taking the item level at the time of each order's placement into account (added as a shade to Fig. 7), we see that the sum of the current item level and the requested quantity appear to be somehow connected, indicating a quantity-related dependency of the event's execution on the item level. This indirect dependency on the item level is not depicted in the quantity net, and further investigation is out of this work's scope.

The process model in Fig. 5 suggests several executions of the activity "pick and pack" regarding the same customer order. For 106 customer orders, the activity was executed several times – removing items from the warehouse and sending a parcel to a customer every time. Closer consideration of the timestamps shows that this behaviour is not distributed evenly over the period but aggregates selectively. By applying standard process mining techniques to detect the waiting times, we further see that the average waiting time of objects before the activity

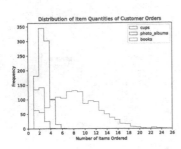

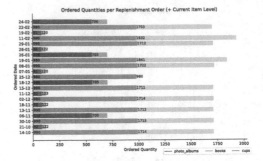

Fig. 6. Demand customer orders.   **Fig. 7.** Ordered items per replenishment order.

"pick and pack" is performed is up to 54% higher than in other periods. The warehouse's item levels reveal that this behaviour coincides with stock-outs of books or albums. Within these periods, only a few customer orders are processed, none leading to a removal of items of the out-of-stock item type. Shortly after, the density of events removing items of this type is higher than usual; this can also be seen in the steep decreases after the arrival of deliveries in Fig. 4.

The example of a quantity-related analysis provided in this section revealed dependencies that could not have been uncovered with standard object-centric process mining techniques. Despite the semantics of the quantity net not being able to depict all of them, they are capable of (1) displaying the two processes as decoupled and (2) depicting the dependency of the execution of the activity "pick and pack" on the collection point's item level.

6   Conclusion

In the high uncertainty and variability within current fast-paced environments, managing logistics processes requires increased transparency over the impacting end-to-end processes [13]. This presentation of early-stage research provides a foundation for the application of process mining for logistics processes by allowing the joint analysis of item quantities and end-to-end processes. The exemplary analysis indicates that the framework can capture direct dependencies between activities and known collection points and its support in revealing further dependencies. The extraction of the required quantity event log, the detection of additional quantity-related dependencies, and supporting software are future research topics. Additionally, the consideration of collection points supports the analysis of process networks, thereby serving as an abstraction for federated process mining. We conclude the presented framework as a promising first step in enabling process mining techniques to consider quantities instead of identities.

Acknowledgement. Funded by the Deutsche Forschungsgemeinschaft (DFG, German Research Foundation) under Germany's Excellence Strategy - EXC-2023 Internet of Production - 390621612. We also thank the Alexander von Humboldt (AvH) Stiftung for supporting our research.

References

1. van der Aalst, W.M.: Federated process mining: exploiting event data across organizational boundaries. In: Proceedings - 2021 International Conference on Smart Data Services, SMDS 2021, pp. 61–71. IEEE (2021)
2. van der Aalst, W.M.: Process mining: a 360 degree overview. In: van der Aalst, W.M.P., Carmona, J. (eds.) Process Mining Handbook. Lecture Notes in Business Information Processing, vol. 448, pp. 3–34. Springer, Cham (2022). https://doi.org/10.1007/978-3-031-08848-3_1
3. van der Aalst, W.M., Berti, A.: Discovering object-centric Petri nets. Fund. Inform. **175**(1–4), 1–40 (2020)
4. Becker, T., Intoyoad, W.: Context aware process mining in logistics. Procedia CIRP **63**, 557–562 (2017)
5. van Cruchten, R.M.E.R., Weigand, H.H.: Process mining in logistics: the need for rule-based data abstraction. In: RCIS Proceedings, pp. 1–9. IEEE (2018)
6. Engel, R., van der Aalst, W.M.P., Zapletal, M., Pichler, C., Werthner, H.: Mining inter-organizational business process models from EDI messages: a case study from the automotive sector. In: Ralyté, J., Franch, X., Brinkkemper, S., Wrycza, S. (eds.) CAiSE 2012. LNCS, vol. 7328, pp. 222–237. Springer, Heidelberg (2012). https://doi.org/10.1007/978-3-642-31095-9_15
7. Friederich, J., Lugaresi, G., Lazarova-Molnar, S., Matta, A.: Process mining for dynamic modeling of smart manufacturing systems: data requirements. Procedia CIRP **107**, 546–551 (2022)
8. Galic, G., Wolf, M.: Global process mining survey 2021 - delivering value with process analytics - adoption and success factors of process mining. Technical report, Deloitte (2021)
9. Garcia, C.D.S., et al.: Process mining techniques and applications - a systematic mapping study. Expert Syst. Appl. **133**, 260–295 (2019)
10. Gerke, K., Claus, A., Mendling, J.: Process mining of RFID-based supply chains. In: 2009 CEC, pp. 285–292. IEEE (2009)
11. Gerke, K., Mendling, J., Tarmyshov, K.: Case construction for mining supply chain processes. In: Abramowicz, W. (ed.) BIS 2009. LNBIP, vol. 21, pp. 181–192. Springer, Heidelberg (2009). https://doi.org/10.1007/978-3-642-01190-0_16
12. Ghisellini, P., Cialani, C., Ulgiati, S.: A review on circular economy. J. Clean. Prod. **114**, 11–32 (2016)
13. Jacobi, C., Meier, M., Herborn, L., Furmans, K.: Maturity model for applying process mining in supply chains. Logist. J. (12) (2020)
14. Knoll, D., Reinhart, G., Prüglmeier, M.: Enabling value stream mapping for internal logistics using multidimensional process mining. Expert Syst. Appl. **124**, 130–142 (2019)
15. Knoll, D., Waldmann, J., Reinhart, G.: Developing an internal logistics ontology for process mining. Procedia CIRP **79**, 427–432 (2019)
16. Lau, H., Ho, G., Zhao, Y., Chung, N.: Development of a process mining system for supporting knowledge discovery in a supply chain network. Int. J. Prod. Econ. **122**(1), 176–187 (2009)
17. Martin, N., Pufahl, L., Mannhardt, F.: Detection of batch activities from event logs. Inf. Syst. **95**, 101642 (2021)
18. Pika, A., Ouyang, C., Ter Hofstede, A.H.M.: Configurable batch-processing discovery from event logs. ACM Trans. Manage. Inf. Syst. **13**(3), 1–25 (2022)

19. Pufahl, L.: Modeling and executing batch activities in business processes. Ph.D. thesis, Universität Potsdam (2018)
20. Rafiei, M., van der Aalst, W.M.: An abstraction-based approach for privacy-aware federated process mining. IEEE Access **11**, 33697–33714 (2023)
21. Wen, Y., Chen, Z., Liu, J., Chen, J.: Mining batch processing workflow models from event logs. Concurr. Comput. **25**(13), 1928–1942 (2013)

Mapping Artifact-Driven Monitoring Results Back to BPMN Process Diagrams

Giovanni Meroni[(✉)] [iD] and Szabolcs Garda

Technical University of Denmark, Kgs. Lyngby, Denmark
giom@dtu.dk

Abstract. Artifact-driven process monitoring is a technique that exploits the E-GSM modeling language to seamlessly monitor multi-party business processes. Despite allowing greater flexibility in monitoring, E-GSM makes the modeling and understanding of monitoring results harder than imperative process modeling languages. To overcome this limitation, methods to automatically transform imperative process models into (E-)GSM models have been introduced. However, to the best of our knowledge, no approach to show monitoring results obtained with artifact-driven monitoring over the original imperative process model has been proposed. In this paper, we propose a method to map the results, and in particular execution flow violations, back to BPMN diagrams.

Keywords: Process monitoring · E-GSM · BPMN

1 Introduction

Business process monitoring is the phase of the BPM lifecycle devoted to oversee to which extent process executions conform to the planned behavior [5]. This is particularly relevant whenever a multi-party process takes place. In this context, none of the involved parties can enforce the execution of the whole process. Therefore, there is no guarantee that the process will conform to the behavior agreed by the parties.

However, being able to reliably and continuously monitor such kind of processes is not a trivial task. Firstly, most monitoring techniques rely on a centralized execution log that contains high-level events, which explicitly indicate when activities in the process started and completed their execution. When a process is not automated, having such events cannot be taken for granted. Typically, the operator responsible for executing an activity has to send a notification. Therefore, operators may forget to send such notifications, they may anticipate or postpone the sending, or they may maliciously send notifications related to activities they never executed. Secondly, most of the conformance checking techniques, which are used to determine discrepancies in the execution flow of a process model with respect to the actual execution, rely on a static execution log generated after the process completed its execution. Thus, they are unsuited to detect deviations immediately after they happen.

© The Author(s), under exclusive license to Springer Nature Switzerland AG 2024
J. De Smedt and P. Soffer (Eds.): ICPM 2023 Workshops, LNBIP 503, pp. 475–486, 2024.
https://doi.org/10.1007/978-3-031-56107-8_36

To overcome such limitations and to achieve reliable and autonomous process monitoring, artifact-driven process monitoring has been proposed [8]. This technique relies on the E-GSM declarative language to model the process to monitor. In E-GSM, it is possible to specify rules to infer from the state of the artifacts (e.g., a freight container, an invoice, etc.) taking part in a process execution when each activity or process portion should start and terminate its execution. Therefore, as long as the conditions of the artifacts are made available to the monitoring platform (e.g., by using IoT smart devices), no user interaction is required. In addition, E-GSM allows to model execution flow dependencies that are descriptive rather than prescriptive. In this way, deviations can be identified without blocking the process or requiring the process to complete its execution.

One of the main challenges in adopting artifact-driven process monitoring is the complexity of i) modeling processes with E-GSM and ii) interpreting monitoring results. To address i), approaches to generate E-GSM models of the processes to monitor from imperative process models, such as BPMN, have been proposed [8]. In this way, the person in charge of configuring an artifact-driven monitoring platform does not need to know E-GSM. However, the person who needs to interpret the monitoring results still needs to know E-GSM. This paper aims at addressing ii) by proposing a method to map monitoring results back to the original BPMN process model. In this way, anyone who is familiar with BPMN will be able to interpret monitoring results.

This paper is structured as follows. Section 2 introduces an real-world process that will be used throughout the paper. Section 3 provides background information on E-GSM and a method to generate E-GSM models from BPMN diagrams. Section 4 presents our method to map monitoring results back to BPMN diagrams. Section 5 explains how the effectiveness of the approach has been evaluated. Section 6 surveys the state of the art for related work. Finally, Sect. 7 concludes this paper outlining future work.

2   Running Example

To better understand the challenges that non-automated processes pose, we focus on a real scenario taken from the logistics domain, which will be used throughout this paper. A manufacturer has to deliver several goods to one of its customers. To this aim, it resorts to a carrier. The shipment process is expected to start when the manufacturer receives the list of goods to be shipped from the customer. Then, the manufacturer has to fill in a shipping container with the goods. At the same time, the manufacturer has to wait for the carrier to inform him about when he will come to pick the container up. After that, the carrier has to pick the container up and start driving to the customer. Finally, the carrier has to inspect the goods, and then notify the manufacturer that the shipment is complete. Figure 1 shows the aforementioned process modeled with BPMN. Note that all the activities are manually executed by an operator, and require some interaction with the container, changing its conditions.

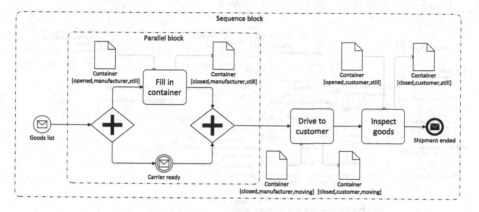

Fig. 1. Example delivery process modeled in BPMN.

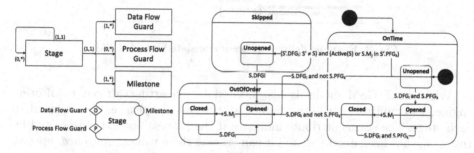

Fig. 2. Metamodel (top left), notation (bottom left) and lifecycle (right) of E-GSM.

3   E-GSM

E-GSM is an extension of the Guard-Stage-Milestone artifact-centric language [4] specifically designed for process monitoring. Its graphical representation and metamodel are represented in the left portion of Fig. 2[1]

E-GSM represents the elements of a process with **stages**, which can be either atomic, or they can nest other stages. To indicate under which condition a process element is executed, the corresponding stage is decorated with **data flow guards**. Similarly, to indicate under which condition the process element completes its execution, the stage is decorated with **milestones**. To specify the execution flow dependencies that a process model should fulfill, the corresponding stage is decorated with a **process flow guard**. Process flow guards, data flow guards and milestones are expressions that predicate on external events (e.g., a message indicating that the carrier is ready), on the elements in the model (e.g., on the milestone of another stage), or on the conditions of one or more artifacts (e.g., the container being open and standing still at the manufacturer's premises).

---

[1] Elements of E-GSM not relevant for this paper (e.g., fault loggers) are omitted.

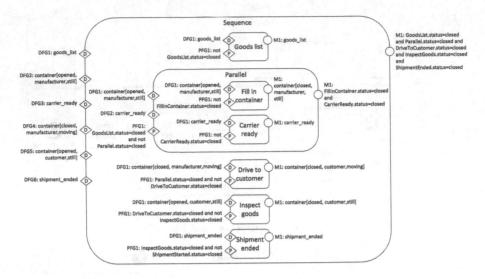

Fig. 3. Example delivery process translated into E-GSM.

When an E-GSM model is instantiated by an artifact-driven monitoring engine, two runtime attributes, named **status** and **compliance**, are assigned to each stage. The status attribute indicates if the process portion represented by that stage has been executed, and it can assume three values: *unopened*, *opened*, and *closed*. The compliance attribute indicates if the process portion represented by that stage conforms to the execution flow dependencies specified in the model, and it can assume three values: *onTime*, *skipped*, or *outOfOrder*. The right portion of Fig. 2 shows the lifecycle of these attributes.

Initially, all stages have *unopened* status and *onTime* compliance, indicating that they were never executed and they conform with the execution flow. When a data flow guard holds and the associated stage has *unopened* or *closed* status, its status becomes *opened*. When a milestone holds and the associated stage has *opened* status, its status becomes *closed*. Also, if that stage has any child stages with *opened* status, their status becomes *closed* too. When one of the data flow guards of a stage holds, its process flow guard does not, and the associated stage has *unopened* or *closed* status and *onTime* compliance, its compliance becomes *outOfOrder*, indicating that it violated the execution flow. In addition, if the process flow guard predicated on another stage having *opened* or *closed* status, and that stage has *unopened* status, then the compliance of that stage becomes *skipped*, indicating that it should have been executed before the current stage. When one of the data flow guards of a stage holds, and the associated stage has *unopened* status and *skipped* compliance, its compliance becomes *outOfOrder*.

3.1   From BPMN to E-GSM

One of the main issues of E-GSM - and, more in general, of declarative process modeling languages - is the higher cognitive load it requires. Compared to imperative languages, such as BPMN, modeling and understanding an E-GSM model can be much more difficult [6]. To address this issue, a method to automatically transform BPMN process models into E-GSM models has been defined in [8]. This method, which requires the BPMN process model to be block structured [11], decomposes the process into a set of nested blocks. Then, a set of transformation rules is applied to generate the E-GSM model. Figure 3 shows the E-GSM model obtained by applying this method to the BPMN process model shown in Fig. 1. To make this paper self-contained, a simplified version of the transformation rules is provided below:

- **R1:** Events and Activities are translated into atomic stages. For example, activity Fill in container is translated into an atomic stage Fill in container. Event Carrier ready is translated into an atomic stage Carrier ready.
- **R2:** Each process block is translated into a parent stage, which contains the stages derived from the inner process blocks. For example, the parallel block containing the activity Fill in container and the event Carrier ready is translated into a parent stage Parallel, which contains the atomic stages Fill in container and Carrier ready.
- **R3:** For each stage, with the exception of stages with no parent stage, a process flow guard is produced and attached to that stage. Its expression depends on the type of process block translated into the parent stage that contains the stage. For example, the parent stage of Fill in container is Parallel, which is translated from a parallel block. Therefore, the process flow guard of Fill in container requires Fill in container to be executed only once (i.e., its status not to be closed). Conversely, the parent stage of Inspect goods is Sequence, which is translated from a sequence block. Therefore, the process flow guard of Inspect goods requires its predecessor, i.e., Drive to customer, to complete its execution (i.e., its status to be closed).
- **R4:** For each stage, a set of data flow guards is produced and attached to that stage.
  For an activity stage, the set contains a data flow guard requiring the artifacts represented by the input data objects of the corresponding activity to be in the specified data state. For example, stage Fill in container has a data flow guard requiring the container to be at the manufacturer closed and standing still.
  For an event stage, the set contains data flow guard requiring the event to happen. For example, stage Carrier ready has a data flow guard requiring the *carrier ready* message to be sent.
  For a parent stage, the set contains the union of the data flow guards of its child stages. For example, stage Parallel has two data flow guards identical to ones of Fill in container and Carrier ready.
- **R5:** For each stage, a milestone is produced and attached to that stage.
  For an activity stage, that milestone requires the artifacts represented by the output data objects of the corresponding activity to be in the specified data state. For example, stage Fill in container has a data flow guard requiring the container to be at the manufacturer closed and standing still.

Table 1. Values of the status and compliance attributes reported by an artifact-driven monitoring platform during an execution of the delivery process.

Stage	Status	Compliance
Goods list	closed	onTime
Fill in container	closed	outOfOrder
Carrier ready	unopened	onTime
Drive to customer	closed	outOfOrder
Inspect goods	unopened	skipped
Shipment ended	closed	outOfOrder
Parallel	opened	onTime
Sequence	opened	onTime

For an event stage, that milestone requires the event to happen. For example, stage Carrier ready has a data flow guard requiring the *carrier ready* message to be sent.

For a parent stage, its expression depends on the type of process block translated into that stage. For example, the milestone of Parallel requires the status of Fill in container and Carrier ready to be closed.

This method is effective for generating an E-GSM model suitable for configuring an artifact-driven monitoring platform. However, it does not simplify the interpretation of the monitoring results. Indeed, when the generated E-GSM model is used by an artifact-driven monitoring platform, the platform will determine the status and compliance attributes of each stage based on how the process was executed. To understand the meaning of these attribute values (e.g., that one activity was executed before its predecessor), the person in charge of interpreting these results still needs to understand E-GSM.

To better understand this issue, consider the following execution of the previously introduced logistics process. After the process starts, the manufacturer fills the container in. However, after closing the container, he realizes that part of the goods is missing. Therefore, the manufacturer opens the container again, puts the missing goods, and closes it. Instead of notifying the manufacturer that he is ready to pick the container up, the carrier picks the container up and delivers it to the customer. Also, when he reaches the customer, he notifies that the shipment is complete, without inspecting the goods first. If the E-GSM model in Fig. 3 is used, an artifact-driven monitoring platform would produce the output shown in Table 1. Therefore, to understand what happened, one should understand the E-GSM model, and in particular the process flow guards, and the implications of the status and compliance attributes of each stage.

4   Approach

To address the issues discussed in Sect. 3.1, we define a method to map monitoring results obtained with an E-GSM model generated from a BPMN process

---

Algorithm 1: getIncompleteBlock

---

input : Stage S_current: current stage, Model model: E-GSM model

output: Stage S_incomplete: stage representing an incomplete block

S_pred = getPredecessor(model,S_current);

if *S_pred == null **or** (S_pred.status == opened **and** S_pred.compliance == onTime)* **then**

  | **return** *S_pred*;

else if *S_pred.status == closed* **then**

  | **return** *null*;

else

  | **return** *getIncompleteBlock(S_pred,model)*;

---

model back to the original BPMN model. To this aim, for each element in the BPMN model, we identify a set of deviations based on the status and compliance attributes of the stage translated from this element, as well as its child stages (if any). For each deviation, we then define rules to determine the BPMN process elements affected by that deviation. In particular, the rules take as input the original BPMN diagram, the E-GSM model derived from that diagram, and the information obtained from an artifact-driven monitoring platform using the E-GSM model. The result is a set of annotations indicating, for some elements in the BPMN diagram, if they were executed and what kind of deviation they caused, if any. Rules can be invoked whenever a change in the status or compliance attributes of a stage in the E-GSM model changes. In this way, real-time information on the execution of the process can be shown on the original BPMN diagram.

Activities. By looking at the status attribute of a stage translated from an activity, it is possible to know if the activity has not been executed (i.e., its status is *unopened*), it is being executed (i.e., its status is *opened*), or it has already been executed (i.e., its status is *closed*). Based on this information, the activity is annotated as *not executed*, *being executed*, or *completed*.

Events. By looking at the status attribute of a stage translated from an event, it is possible to know if the event happened (i.e., its status is *closed*) or not (i.e., its status is *unopened*). Based on this information, the event is annotated as *not happened* or being *happened*.

Sequence Blocks. By looking at the status and compliance attributes of a stage translated from a sequence block (i.e., a sequence stage) and its child stages, it is possible to identify the following classes of deviations:

– **Incomplete process blocks.** This deviation indicates that one or more of the process blocks translated into the child stages should have completed their execution, but they did not. This may happen in two cases: i) if the sequence

---

Algorithm 2: getSkippedBlocks

---

input : Stage S_current: current stage, Model model: E-GSM model
output: Set Skipped_set: set of stages representing skipped blocks
Skipped_set = {S_current};
S_pred = getPredecessor(model, S_current);
if *S_pred == null **or** S_pred.status != unopened* **then**
  ⌊ **return** *Skipped_set*;
else
  ⌊ **return** *Skipped_set.add(getSkippedBlocks(S_pred, model))*;

---

stage contains a child stage with *outOfOrder* compliance, or ii) if the process block translated into the sequence stage is incomplete.

To identify an incomplete process block when i) occurs, Algorithm 1 is invoked by passing the child stage with *outOfOrder* compliance and the E-GSM model, respectively, as input parameters *S_current* and *model*. The algorithm identifies from *model* the child stage *S_pred*, which is translated from the process block that is the predecessor of the block translated into *S_current*. If *S_pred* does not exist or its status is *closed*, no incomplete process block exists (hence *null* is returned). If the status of *S_pred* is *opened* and the compliance of *S_pred* is *onTime*, the process block translated into *S_pred* is incomplete (hence *S_pred* is returned). Otherwise, Algorithm 1 is recursively invoked by passing *S_pred* as input parameter.

To identify incomplete process blocks when ii) occurs, the status and compliance of all child stages of the sequence stage are inspected. If a child stage has *opened* status and *onTime* compliance, then the process block translated into that stage is incomplete.

- **Skipped process blocks.** This deviation indicates that one or more of the process blocks translated into the child stages were not executed, although they should have been. This may happen in two cases: i) if the sequence stage contains a child stage with *skipped* compliance, or ii) if the process block translated into the sequence stage is incomplete.

  To identify skipped process blocks when i) occurs, Algorithm 2 is invoked by passing the child stage with *skipped* compliance and the E-GSM model, respectively, as input parameters *S_current* and *model*. The algorithm creates the set *Skipped_set* containing *S_current*. The child stage *S_pred*, which is translated from the process block that is the predecessor of the block translated into *S_current*, is then identified from *model*. If *S_pred* does not exist, or its status is not *unopened*, *Skipped_set* is returned. Otherwise, Algorithm 2 is recursively invoked by passing *S_pred* as input parameter, its output set is added to *Skipped_set*, which is finally returned. By inspecting the contents of *Skipped_set*, it is then possible to determine which process blocks were skipped.

  To identify skipped process blocks when ii) occurs, the status of all child stages of the sequence stage is inspected. If a child stage has *unopened* status, then the process block translated into that stage was skipped.

- **Non-sequential process blocks.** This deviation indicates that one or more of the process blocks translated into the child stages did not respected the sequential ordering. This may happen because a process block was executed before their predecessor completed its execution, or because the process block was executed multiple times.

  To identify non-sequential process blocks, the compliance of all child stages of the sequence stage is inspected. If a child stage has *outOfOrder* compliance, then the process block translated into that stage is non-sequential.

Once a process block has been identified as *incomplete*, *skipped* or *non-sequential*, it will be annotated accordingly. In particular, for a block consisting in a single activity or an event, the annotation will be applied to this element. For a block consisting in a process portion, a BPMN group element containing the process portion will be created, and the annotation will be applied to this new element.

Exclusive, Inclusive, and Parallel Blocks. By looking at the status and compliance attributes of a stage translated from an exclusive, inclusive, or parallel block (i.e., an exclusive, inclusive, or parallel stage) and its child stages, it is possible to identify the following classes of deviations:

- **Incomplete branch.** This deviation indicates that the process block representing a branch should have completed its execution, but it did not. This may happen when the process block translated into the exclusive (or inclusive or parallel) stage is incomplete.

  To identify process blocks representing an incomplete branch, the status and compliance of all child stages of the exclusive (or inclusive or parallel) stage are inspected. If a child stage has *opened* status and *onTime* compliance, then the process block translated into that stage is incomplete.
- **Incorrect branch.** This deviation indicates that the process block representing a branch was or is being executed, although the branch condition did not hold, or that a branch was taken multiple times.

  To identify process blocks representing an incorrect branch, the compliance of all child stages of the exclusive (or inclusive or parallel) stage is inspected. If a child stage has *outOfOrder* compliance, then the process block translated into that stage represents an incorrect branch.
- **Skipped branch.** This deviation indicates that the process block representing a branch was not taken, although the branch condition did hold. This may happen when the process block translated into the exclusive (or inclusive or parallel) stage is incomplete.

  To identify a process block representing a skipped branch, the status of all child stages of the exclusive (or inclusive or parallel) stage are inspected, as well as the condition of the corresponding branch. If a child stage has *unopened* status and the branch condition holds, then the process block translated into that stage was skipped.

Once a process block has been identified as *incomplete*, *incorrect* or *skipped*, the corresponding branch will be annotated accordingly.   □

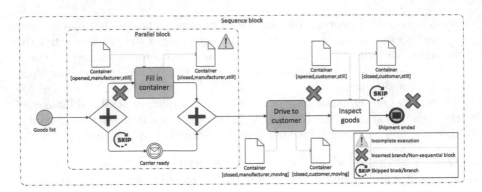

Fig. 4. Monitoring results mapped back to the BPMN process model.

Figure 4 shows the results of applying the method to the running example presented in Sect. 2. In particular, rules take as input the BPMN diagram shown in Fig. 1, the E-GSM model shown in Fig. 3, and the monitoring information related to the incorrect execution described at the end of Sect. 3.1 (shown in Table 1).

To show which portions of the process were executed, the method annotates activities Fill in container and Drive to customer as *completed*, since they were executed, and Inspect goods as *not executed*. The method also annotates event Goods list and Shipment ended as *happened*, since these events took place, and Carrier ready as *not happened*.

To show which portions of the process did not conform to the execution flow, the method annotates the branch in the parallel block containing the activity Fill in container as *incorrect*, since the manufacturer has executed that activity twice, implicitly violating the branch condition. The method also annotates the branch in the parallel block containing the event Carrier ready as *skipped*, the parallel block as *incomplete* and the activity Drive to customer as *non-sequential*. Indeed, the carrier started driving without notifying that he was ready first. Thus, he violated the execution flow constraint for Drive to customer by skipping the branch containing Carrier ready and, consequently, not waiting for the two parallel branches to converge. In addition, the method annotates the activity Inspect goods as *skipped* and the event Shipment ended as *non-sequential*. Indeed, the carrier notified the manufacturer that the shipment was complete without inspecting the container first. Thus, he violated the execution flow constraint for Shipment ended by skipping Inspect goods.

5   Evaluation

To evaluate the effectiveness of our approach, we extended the SMARTifact artifact-driven monitoring platform [1] by i) storing the original BPMN process model, along with the E-GSM model translated from that model and, for each element in the BPMN model, the type of deviation affecting that element (if any) in a database, ii) implementing the rules discussed in Sect. 4, iii) implementing a front-end module to display the monitoring results on the BPMN process model. To get up-to-date monitoring results, the module implementing ii) is called every time the status and compliance attributes of one of the stages in the E-GSM model change, and updates the database with information on the deviations and the affected elements. To visualize the monitoring results, iii) pulls the elements affected by a deviation from the database, and makes use of the BPMN.js library[2] to overlay an icon on the corresponding element in the BPMN model. Source code of the extended version of SMARTifact is available at https://github.com/eGSM-platform.

We then tested the extended platform with the process models and traces of the LHR-AMS process, which was originally used in [8] to validate the artifact-driven monitoring approach. When the execution conformed to the process model, no deviation was shown in the BPMN model. Conversely, when a deviation occurred, only the elements in the BPMN model that were affected by that deviation were marked as such.

6   Related Work

To achieve runtime process monitoring, [3] derives from an imperative process model a set of rules which are fed into a Complex Event Processor. In this way, one can infer if a process execution deviates from the modeled behavior. [9,12] and [10] rely on prefix alignment techniques identify deviations as soon as new events are received. All these approaches require the process to monitor to be modeled as a Petri Net, which is typically more complex for end users to interpret than BPMN. Additionally, they do not show how to map the effects of a deviation in the process model. Finally, they rely on high-level events explicitly indicating when activities are executed, which must be sent by human operators in case of manual activities.

To autonomously monitor processes involving manual activities, [7] and [2] rely on IoT data to determine when activities are run. They also use BPMN process diagrams to represent the process to monitor. However, these approaches require the process to conform with the model. Thus, they cannot be used for runtime conformance checking.

7   Conclusion

In this paper, we presented a method to map the results obtained from an artifact-driven monitoring platform back to the original BPMN process diagram. In this way, users are not required to understand E-GSM models and to interpret artifact-driven monitoring results. Although the results look promising, this method still suffers from several limitations. Firstly, it can be used only if the E-GSM model has been derived from a BPMN process diagram. Therefore, it is not applicable when the E-GSM model is designed from scratch or derived from

---

[2] See https://bpmn.io/toolkit/bpmn-js/.

other process models. Secondly, it considers only the current values assumed by the status and compliance attributes of each stage. Finally, this approach considers only one process execution at a time. Showing aggregate results (e.g., the most frequent deviations) is therefore not possible at the moment.

We plan to tackle these limitations in the future by investigating how to map monitoring results back to other modeling languages (e.g., Petri Nets or Direct-Follow-Graphs). We also plan to consider the history of the status and compliance attributes, which would make possible to identify more classes of deviations (e.g., to determine if a non-sequential process block is caused by an overlapping execution or a permutation).

References

1. Baresi, L., Di Ciccio, C., Mendling, J., Meroni, G., Plebani, P.: mArtifact: an artifact-driven process monitoring platform. In: BPM Demo Track 2017, vol. 1920. CEUR-WS.org (2017)
2. Beyer, J., Kuhn, P., Hewelt, M., Mandal, S., Weske, M.: Unicorn meets chimera: integrating external events into case management. In: BPM Demo Track 2016, pp. 67–72 (2016)
3. Burattin, A., van Zelst, S.J., Armas-Cervantes, A., van Dongen, B.F., Carmona, J.: Online conformance checking using behavioural patterns. In: Weske, M., Montali, M., Weber, I., vom Brocke, J. (eds.) BPM 2018. LNCS, vol. 11080, pp. 250–267. Springer, Cham (2018). https://doi.org/10.1007/978-3-319-98648-7_15
4. Damaggio, E., Hull, R., Vaculín, R.: On the equivalence of incremental and fixpoint semantics for business artifacts with guard-stage-milestone lifecycles. Inf. Syst. **38**(4), 561–584 (2013)
5. Dumas, M., La Rosa, M., Mendling, J., Reijers, H.A.: Fundamentals of Business Process Management. Springer, Heidelberg (2013). https://doi.org/10.1007/978-3-662-56509-4
6. Fahland, D., et al.: Declarative versus imperative process modeling languages: the issue of understandability. In: Halpin, T., et al. (eds.) BPMDS/EMMSAD -2009. LNBIP, vol. 29, pp. 353–366. Springer, Heidelberg (2009). https://doi.org/10.1007/978-3-642-01862-6_29
7. Gallik, F., Kirikkayis, Y., Reichert, M.: Modeling, executing and monitoring IoT-aware processes with BPM technology. In: ICSS 2022, pp. 96 103. IEEE (2022)
8. Meroni, G.: Artifact-Driven Business Process Monitoring - A Novel Approach to Transparently Monitor Business Processes, Supported by Methods, Tools, and Real-World Applications, vol. 368. Springer, Cham (2019). https://doi.org/10.1007/978-3-030-32412-4
9. Raun, K., Tommasini, R., Awad, A.: I will survive: An event-driven conformance checking approach over process streams. In: DEBS 2023. pp. 49–60 (2023)
10. Schuster, D., Kolhof, G.J.: Scalable online conformance checking using incremental prefix-alignment computation. In: Hacid, H., et al. (eds.) ICSOC 2020. LNCS, vol. 12632, pp. 379–394. Springer, Cham (2021). https://doi.org/10.1007/978-3-030-76352-7_36
11. Vanhatalo, J., Völzer, H., Koehler, J.: The refined process structure tree. Data Knowl. Eng. **68**(9), 793–818 (2009)
12. van Zelst, S.J., Bolt, A., Hassani, M., van Dongen, B.F., van der Aalst, W.M.P.: Online conformance checking: relating event streams to process models using prefix-alignments. Int. J. Data Sci. Anal. **8**(3), 269–284 (2019)

An Approach for Discovering Inter-organizational Collaborative Business Processes in BPMN 2.0

Leonel Peña, Daniela Andrade, Andrea Delgado(✉)[iD], and Daniel Calegari[iD]

Instituto de Computación, Facultad de Ingeniería, Universidad de la República, Montevideo, Uruguay
{lpena,dandrade,adelgado,dcalegar}@fing.edu.uy

Abstract. Inter-organizational collaborative business processes involve at least two participants from different organizations who interact with each other. Discovering and analyzing this kind of process adds several challenges to process mining initiatives, mainly due to traces spread across organizations with heterogeneous infrastructures, technologies, and data models. This paper presents a process mining approach for discovering inter-organizational collaborative business processes, which takes as input an extended XES event log with information on participants and messages exchanged to discover a BPMN 2.0 collaboration process model and corresponding choreography. We evaluated our approach using collaborative business process data from selected related work, discussing and comparing our results within different scenarios.

Keywords: Process mining · inter-organizational collaborative processes · process discovery · BPMN 2.0 collaboration and choreography

1 Introduction

Process Mining (PM) [1] is a powerful approach for organizations to be aware of the actual execution of their business processes (BPs) and discover improvement opportunities. However, it usually focuses on intra-organizational BPs, i.e., processes within a single participant (orchestration).

Inter-organizational collaborative BPs involve several organizations interacting to carry out a global process integrating single processes from each participant organization. These BPs present two complementary views in BPMN 2.0: the **collaboration**, which shows the participants, the orchestration of the activities of each participant, and the messages they exchange; and the **choreography**, which shows only the messages exchanged between participants. Collaborative processes present various challenges for their implementation, and the analysis of their execution, i.e., the execution traces of collaborative processes are spread in several organizations with heterogeneous data models and technologies, making the collection and preparation of process data complex.

J. De Smedt and P. Soffer (Eds.): ICPM 2023 Workshops, LNBIP 503, pp. 487–498, 2024.
https://doi.org/10.1007/978-3-031-56107-8_37

When discovering BPMN 2.0 collaborative BPs, the expected model should include participants from different organizations, their activities, and events in separate pools, also making explicit the messages they exchange. This collaborative view is of utmost importance for business people to provide a direct view of the participants and roles involved in performing the activities within the control flow of the BP model and the messages between participants, not only to analyze the collaborative process as a whole but also be able to analyze each organization separately. Also, the choreography analysis could be critical in some domains, e.g., e-Government, for compliance evaluation [8] of normative and regulations that apply to participant interactions.

Most existing discovery approaches do not include participants or interactions between them (e.g., Petri Nets and Disco process maps) or provide a basic view of them (e.g., BPMNminer [3]), which limits the comprehension and utility of the discovered models for business people to understand and further analyze. Recently, a few proposals appeared [6,9,11] about discovering collaborative BPs. Different levels of requirements for collaborative event logs are imposed within each proposal, apart from knowing the participant executing each event and the messages sent/received by each participant. This includes having an identifier for the messages exchanged, which is not always the case, or knowing the type of message exchange (set of messages allowed).

This work presents an alternative approach for PM discovery of inter-organizational collaborative BPs in BPMN 2.0, based on existing orchestration discovery algorithms and with fewer requirements than related approaches. We provide both BPMN 2.0 collaboration and choreography views. As with most PM approaches, we use as input event logs in the eXtensible Event Stream (XES) [10] format. This format was extended in previous work [8] for expressing collaborative information, including participants and the messages they exchanged. We provide supporting tools [2,12] as ProM plug-ins to show the proposal's feasibility. We evaluated our approach using collaborative BP data from selected related work and discussing and comparing our results within different scenarios.

The rest of the paper is structured as follows. In Sect. 2, we discuss related work. In Sect. 3, we present the approach for discovering inter-organizational collaborative BPs in BPMN 2.0. Then, in Sect. 4, we present an assessment of our approach, comparing our results with selected related work. Finally, in Sect. 5, we provide conclusions and an outline of future work.

2   Related Work

Recent proposals focus on inter-organizational collaborative PM. Each approach profits from different information levels, so using one or the other could depend on the information context.

In [11], an extension of Petri nets is presented that, similarly to ours, also includes elements for messages exchanged and organizations of the collaborative process. Each participant's BP is discovered using an extension of the Inductive Miner. A set of collaboration patterns is defined and used along with each participant's process to build the collaborative model as an extended Petri net. This pattern discovery complements ours but requires knowing a unique message name for correlating message activities from different participants.

In [9], BPMN 2.0 is used. The approach is based on identifying the correlation between events at the case and activity levels. The discovery of each participant's process model is then carried out using the Split Miner algorithm. A set of rules is defined to identify and mark messages within the discovered models, and message flows are added. Unlike this approach, we are not limited to collaborations involving only two participants. Moreover, in [9], message types (sending, receiving) are discovered based on the activities' names, which is not required in our case. As with the first proposals, the approach's implementation is neither accessible nor integrated into the ProM tool.

In [6], BPMN 2.0 is also used, including participants and messages sent/received within each other and an identifier of each message. The discovery approach is carried out for each participant and a messages analyzer uses the identifier of messages to pair the sent/received messages between them. Also, a correction step is provided to deal with problems in the output collaborative process model. The authors provides a PM4Py-based tool. Although it does not rely on a collaborative case identifier, it requires a unique message ID to connect the sent/received messages between participants with the corresponding message flow. Differently, we do not depend on a unique ID or rely on message names but send/receive messages and identifiable collaborative process cases. Our log format and the one in [6] can be transformed from one to another.

Some proposals for inter-organizational processes focus on constructing an event log containing cases merged from the collaborative process within different organizations, e.g., [5,7]. In these cases, the integrated event log represents the choreography of the collaborative process, not the collaboration, seen as the orchestration of events exchanged between participants. We also discover the choreography model in BPMN 2.0 for the messages exchanged, including the participants, and sent/received information as an orchestration. To the best of our knowledge, no proposals provide the messages interaction model as a BPMN 2.0 choreography using the constructs of the language, as we do.

3   Discovery Approach

We have defined a discovery approach for inter-organizational collaborative BPs in BPMN 2.0, as shown in Fig. 1. The input in each case is an extended event log, which includes information regarding the participants involved in the collaborative BP and the messages they exchange. The output is the corresponding BPMN 2.0 collaboration or choreography diagram, showing the participants and the message interactions or message flow interactions, respectively.

Traditional event logs only sometimes register data regarding which participant enacts the activity of the corresponding role/person. It does not represent a problem for intra-organizational process discovery but adds several challenges for inter-organizational collaborative process discovery. To cope with this limitation, we have defined an extension [8] of the XES format for collaborative

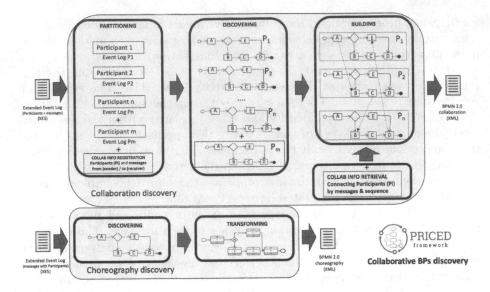

Fig. 1. General approach for BPMN 2.0 collaborative BPs discovery

BPs to include new specific attributes regarding participants involved and the messages exchanged. Although there is a single extension, the two scenarios, i.e., collaboration and choreography, have different information requirements, e.g., a choreography does not require knowing the events of each participant but only the message interactions between them. In this context, it is possible to define the mandatory content of each kind of event log.

A **collaboration event log** (CL) comprises collaborative cases involving several participants whose events come from different participants and include mandatory attributes: `participant` to identify the participant that enacts the event, `elemType` with the type of the event (user, message), and if the event is of type `message`, from which participant it is being received (`fromParticipant`) or to which participant it is being sent (`toParticipant`).

A **choreography event log** (ChL) comprises events that correspond only to the messages exchanged between participants in collaborative cases and includes mandatory attributes: `elemType` with the type of event `message`, which participant sends the message (`fromParticipant`), and which participant receives the message (`toParticipant`).

A collaboration event log can be built from the participants' logs by merging them, which could be performed as a first step of the discovery approach. A choreography event log can be generated from a collaboration event log by only extracting the message interactions as events and registering both the sender and receiver of such messages. The other way around is only sometimes possible since a choreography scenario could have less information, as mentioned before.

In Fig. 2, a simple collaborative BP from [13] is presented (2a) to show the concepts and extensions we propose, with example event logs (2b) for each par-

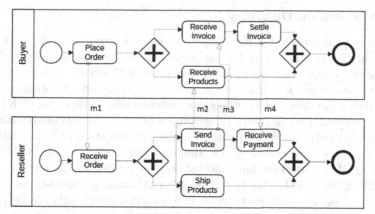

(a) Example collaborative BP with messages from [13]

Buyer event Log	
Event = Place Order	
* timestamp = 01/04/23 10-07-22	
Receive Invoice	
* timestamp = 01/04/23 12-21-05	
Receive Products	
* timestamp = 05/04/23 18-11-02	
Settle Invoice	
* timestamp = 06/04/23 09-10-01	

Reseller event Log	
Receive Order	
* timestamp = 01/04/23 10-10-09	
Send Invoice	
* timestamp = 01/04/23 12-11-06	
Ship Products	
* timestamp = 05/04/23 16-12-03	
Receive Payment	
* timestamp = 07/04/23 13-08-03	

(1)

Collaboration event Log
Event = Place Order
* Participant = Buyer
* toParticipant = Reseller
* timestamp = 01/04/23 10-07-22
Event = Receive Order
* Participant = Reseller
* fromParticipant = Buyer
* timestamp = 01/04/23 10-10-09
Event = Send Invoice
* Participant = Reseller
* toParticipant = Buyer
* timestamp = 01/04/23 12-11-06
Event = Receive Invoice
* Participant = Buyer
* fromParticipant = Reseller
* timestamp = 01/04/23 12-21-05
...

(2)

Choreography event Log
Event = Place Order (m1)
* fromParticipant = Buyer
* toParticipant = Reseller
* timestamp = 01/04/23 10-07-22
Event = Send Invoice (m2)
* fromParticipant = Reseller
* toParticipant = Buyer
* timestamp = 01/04/23 12-11-06
Event = Ship Products (m3)
* fromParticipant = Reseller
* toParticipant = Buyer
* timestamp = 05/04/23 16-12-03
Event = Settle Invoice (m4)
* fromParticipant = Buyer
* toParticipant = Reseller
* timestamp = 06/04/23 09-10-01

(3)

(b) Example of (1) reduced event log for each Participant (orchestration), and extended event logs for (2) collaboration and (3) choreography

Fig. 2. Example collaborative BP and associated event logs

ticipant and extended event logs for collaboration and choreography. It can be seen that the collaboration event log merges each participant's event log, considering the timestamp to maintain the order of execution in the general view of the collaborative case. For the choreography, each event corresponds with a message interaction; we take the name of the send message task as the event name. Defining a formal XES extension for including these mandatory attributes, instead of using a generic attribute, provides the conceptual elements to manage collaborative BPs and corresponding collaborative event logs. A complete example of the extended event logs and their use in BP compliance is in [8].

3.1   Collaboration Discovery

The discovery approach for the collaboration view comprises three steps, as depicted in Fig. 1. The input for the approach is the extended event log for collaboration, where cases are collaborative cases with events from every participant in the collaboration. Each event adds the participant's information about the activity's execution and identifies their interactions as messages with the role sender or receiver. The output of the approach is a BPMN 2.0 collaboration diagram, showing participants as pools with the orchestration of each participant and the messages they exchange. The diagram can be exported in XML format for input in BPMS tools for implementation as a process-aware system.

As shown in Fig. 1, the first step (`Partitioning`) consists of extracting an event log for each participant P_i (namely $Participant_1$, $Participant_2$, .. $Participant_n$), where each case consists of only those events corresponding to that participant, as were originally. A key extra participant is also extracted consisting only of events with the extension attribute *elemType* equal to the message, along with information regarding the Participant that sends/receives each message. All information regarding the Participants, their events, and their exchange messages are registered. The extra event log of messages will be used to discover the process model representing the messages flow between participants, which is then taken as input to add the messages interaction between participants when building the collaboration BP (see step `Building`).

In the second step (`Discovering`), each participant log P_i is used as input to discover the process model for each participant orchestration, and also the one corresponding to messages in P_m. Since our goal is to provide a BPMN 2.0 model, we selected the BPMN Miner [3] as a wrapper for the Inductive Miner algorithm that already transforms its output process tree into a structured BPMN 2.0 model. Although the BPMN Miner provides other algorithms, an existent benchmark [4] shows that the Inductive Miner is the one that offers better results. The discovered process model participant P_m contains the control flow between messages exchanged by participants, i.e., the paths representing the order and occurrence of messages within the collaboration, only for events of type message. An simple example is shown in Fig. 3. The collaborative process (a) (yet to be discovered) has four messages occurrences within the collaborative event log (b): message m1 composed of send task m1.1 in participant P1 and receive task m1.2 in participant P2, then either message m2 or message m3 occurs, with an XOR in participant P2 for sending tasks m2.1 and m3.1, and receive tasks m2.2 in participant P3 and m3.2 in participant P1. Finally, participant P3 sends the message m4 with sending task m4.1 and receiving task m4.2 in participant P1. The discovered model of messages Pm shows only the messages within the collaborative BP, i.e., associated tasks for m1, m2, m3, and m4.

Finally, in the third step (`Building`), we build the collaboration BP in BPMN 2.0. We use the discovered process models for each participant and the process model of the exchanged messages. We generate a pool for each participant and place each BPMN element in its corresponding pool and lane of the final BPMN diagram. After traveling the discovered process model for the messages partici-

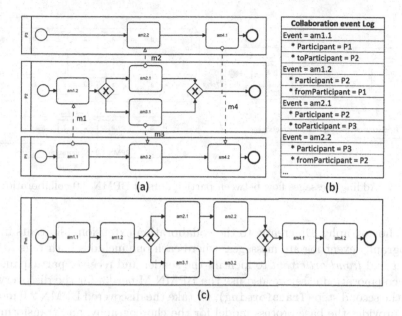

Fig. 3. Example discovered process model for Participant messages P_m

pant (P_m), we obtain the information of the message flow between participants to link the corresponding pair of activities from different pools.

For every activity (a_m) in the discovered model for messages Pm we look for the **first following** activity (a_n) in the discovered model for messages Pm, such that $a_n \rightarrow$Participant equals $a_m \rightarrow toParticipant$ and $a_n \rightarrow fromParticipant$ equal $a_m \rightarrow$Participant. If we find a match, a message flow is added between activities a_m and a_n from each pool of each corresponding participant of the collaboration diagram we generated. We continue traversing the discovered process model for messages Pm with the following activity (a_{m+1}) until we have checked all the activities in the participant Pm. For completeness, all activities without a matching generate a message flow between the activity and the "from" or "to" participant. In Fig. 4, we show the example of the matching between activities from different participants and the corresponding message flow between them in the BPMN 2.0 collaboration.

3.2   Choreography Discovery

The discovery approach for the choreography view comprises two main steps, as depicted in Fig. 1. The input for the approach is the extended event log for choreography, where events correspond to the messages exchanged by the participants involved, with the send or receive Participant information for each one. Since the choreography of messages exchanged between participants in a collaborative BP can be viewed as an orchestration of those messages, in the first step (Discovering), we discover the process model corresponding to the messages

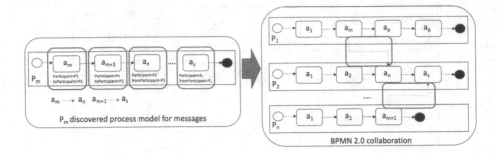

Fig. 4. Adding messages flow between participants in BPMN 2.0 collaboration

in the choreography. Differently to the collaboration extension, all events in the choreography event log are messages, where each one includes both tags *toParticipant* and *fromParticipant* to identify the sender and receiver participant. As in the collaboration case, we also use the BPMN Miner [3] for the discovery.

In the second step (`Transforming`), we take the discovered BPMN 2.0 model, which provides the base process model for the choreography, and transform the orchestration elements to the ones defined in the choreography language, leaving as is the common ones, e.g., gateways. That is, activities are changed to choreography activities type, adding the corresponding initiator and receiving participants, whilst sequence flows between them and gateways are left the same.

4   Evaluation

In what follows, we present a comparative evaluation of the collaborative discovery approach and an example of the choreography discovery approach. A comparison with related work in the second case is left for future work.

4.1   Practical Assessment (Collaboration Discovery)

The approaches in [6,11] are the most similar to ours. However, [11] has no available logs or tools. Thus, we conducted a comparative evaluation using the available event logs, both artificial and real, defined in [6], and the healthcare example.

The dataset consists of artificial and realistic collaboration models with the following characteristics: number of participants (2 to 4), size (16 to 42), and number of messages (2 to 8). Also, some models present undesirable characteristics, such as being unsound, unsafe, or unstructured; some models also have loops. In Table 1, we present the dataset for the evaluation and a summary of the discovery results comparison, which is discussed in the following.

Since we rely on the BPMN Miner's output for discovering each participant's BP, we can only retrieve the BPMN constructs it supports. For the collaboration view, we can only use AND, XOR gateways, and we set the type of activity for

Table 1. Dataset of process models for evaluation and discovery results

Model	#Parts	Size	#Msgs	Discovery results comparison
Artificial 1	2	16	2	Same as original
Artificial 2	2	31	3	Same as original but messages CC->F and EE->D changed to CC->D and EE->F
Artificial 3	3	39	5	Same as original but messages CC->F and EE->D changed to CC->D and EE->F
Artificial 4	2	16	2	Same as original but event based gateway changed to XOR
Artificial 5	4	42	6	Same as original but messages CC->F and EE->D changed to CC->D and EE->F
Real 1	2	11	2	Same as original for elements but no messages flow in original to compare
Real 2	2	18	5	Same as original for elements, differences with loops (missing XOR gateways)
Real 3	3	28	6	Same as original for elements, differences with loops (missing XOR or loop in tasks)
Real 4	3	29	4	Same as original for elements, differences in order and missing AND gateway join
Real 5	3	35	5	Same as original for elements, differences in order and XOR gateways for loops
Healthcare	4	34	8	Same as original

messages as send/receive. A general observation that deserves further work is that discovery algorithms mostly ignore other BPMN elements, such as events and task types. Execution logs do not usually store the data to discover such business information. Considering its role in synchronization in collaborative scenarios, the lack of an event-based gateway is a relevant limitation.

We mainly discover the same collaborative process models as [6] for the main elements: participants, tasks, gateways, and control flow for each orchestration (in the Inductive Miner case). Regarding messages, we found differences in the discovery of models Artificial 2, 3, and 5. Some receiving messages are not in the same sequence as the sending messages, for which, without adding some matching of names, IDs, or types of messages (domain), we discovered a different pair. We also found problems with loops, which are also challenging in the original discovery. Some process models of the original discovery also present issues (e.g., Real 1 has no message flows). For the real event logs Real 2, 3, 4, and 5, we have issues with missing XOR/AND gateways and swap in some tasks order.

As an example of our discovery approach for the BPMN 2.0 collaboration, we present in Fig. 5 the resulting process model for the Healthcare process introduced in [6], which is the same as ours. Event logs and models are in [12].

We decided not to change the message type activities for messages events (as done in [6]), but we could easily change it with post-processing. For the choreography, as mentioned, we transform the type of activities into choreography activities. Further post-processing could be done to improve the semantics of the discovered BPMN processes, which is left for future work. For example, it could be possible to identify when a process is triggered by an input message, e.g., Reseller in Fig. 2a, and P2/P3 in Fig. 3, and change the first receiving task by a message start event. Moreover, in some cases, it could be possible to identify potential event-based gateways when XOR gateways are followed by message tasks, e.g., in the Patient process of Fig. 5. However, this decision may not be entirely correct since data required to reconstruct the original semantics is usually absent in event logs, e.g., data-based decisions attached to gateways and other events that can be connected to gateways, such as time events.

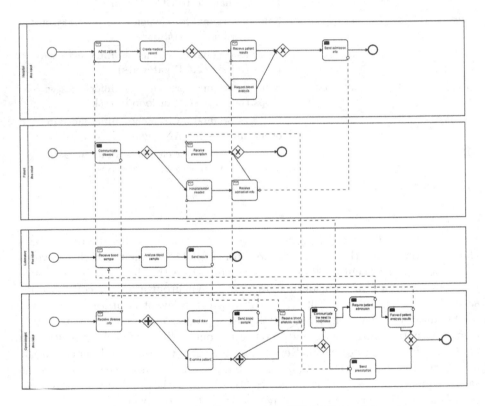

Fig. 5. Healthcare process discovered as BPMN 2.0 collaboration

4.2   Practical Assessment (Choreography Discovery)

In Fig. 6, we present the resulting process model for the BPMN 2.0 choreography corresponding to the Healthcare collaboration shown in Fig. 5 (event logs and models are in [2]). The messages involved have the initiator and receiver participants, as shown in the collaboration, and the control flow of the choreography corresponds to the paths that can be followed within the participant's message interactions in the collaboration. The discovery of choreography could be used to strengthen collaboration discovery since it can potentially discover complex behaviors, which requires further research. In particular, it could help address sequencing problems, e.g., those of the Artificial 2, 3, and 5 logs.

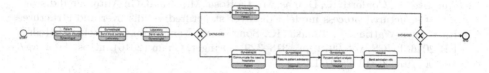

Fig. 6. Healthcare process discovered as BPMN 2.0 choreography

5 Conclusions

This work describes an approach for PM discovery of inter-organizational collaborative BPs in BPMN 2.0. It only requires information on the participants executing each event and the messages (send/receive) they exchange. As a result of the discovery approach, we generate a BPMN 2.0 collaboration diagram, showing participants as pools, the orchestration of each participant within each pool, and the messages they exchange. This diagram can be exported in XML format for input in BPMS tools for implementation as a process-aware system. Also, the collaboration event log can be transformed into a choreography event log from which a BPMN 2.0 choreography diagram is also discovered.

We have evaluated and compared our collaboration discovery approach to selected related work based on available collaborative event logs. We showed how it is possible to discover the collaboration and choreography diagrams for most processes, while some limitations appear when dealing with some exceptional scenarios, which we need to further analyze. Also, further improvements and a more rigorous experimental evaluation of the tool are necessary in terms of efficacy in discovery and execution performance.

We believe that a collaborative view based on BPMN 2.0 is of utmost importance for business people to analyze their processes with complete information. Nevertheless, performing a user validation that provides evidence about the proposal's benefits could be helpful. Also, using the process model discovered in other BPMN 2.0 compliant tools for further implementation or analysis, e.g., with BP simulation, will benefit the organization. Finally, we are analyzing the addition of organizational data to the extended event log as we already have in place for orchestrations (related to the OCED[1] standard initiative).

Acknowledgment. Supported by project "Minería de procesos y datos para la mejora de procesos colaborativos aplicada a e-Government" funded by Agencia Nacional de Investigación e Innovación (ANII), Fondo María Viñas (FMV) "Proyecto ANII N° FMV_1_2021_1_167483", Uruguay.

---

[1] https://www.tf-pm.org/resources/oced-standard.

References

1. van der Aalst, W.M.P.: Process Mining - Data Science in Action, 2nd edn. Springer, Heidelberg (2016). https://doi.org/10.1007/978-3-662-49851-4
2. Andrade, D., Delgado, A., Calegari, D.: BPMN 2.0 choreo.process discovery ProM plugin (2023). https://gitlab.fing.edu.uy/open-coal/bpmnchoreographypm
3. Augusto, A., Conforti, R., Dumas, M., La Rosa, M., Bruno, G.: Automated discovery of structured process models: discover structured vs. discover and structure. In: Comyn-Wattiau, I., Tanaka, K., Song, I.-Y., Yamamoto, S., Saeki, M. (eds.) ER 2016. LNCS, vol. 9974, pp. 313–329. Springer, Cham (2016). https://doi.org/10.1007/978-3-319-46397-1_25
4. Augusto, A., et al.: Automated discovery of process models from event logs: review and benchmark. IEEE Trans. Know. and Data Eng. **31**(4), 686–705 (2019)
5. Claes, J., Poels, G.: Merging event logs for process mining: a rule based merging method and rule suggestion algorithm. Expert Syst. Appl. **41**(16), 7291–7306 (2014)
6. Corradini, F., Re, B., Rossi, L., Tiezzi, F.: A technique for collaboration discovery. In: Augusto, A., Gill, A., Bork, D., Nurcan, S., Reinhartz-Berger, I., Schmidt, R. (eds.) BPMDS EMMSAD 2022. LNBIP, vol. 450, pp. 63–78. Springer, Cham (2022). https://doi.org/10.1007/978-3-031-07475-2_5
7. Engel, R., van der Aalst, W.M.P., Zapletal, M., Pichler, C., Werthner, H.: Mining inter-organizational business process models from EDI messages: a case study from the automotive sector. In: Ralyté, J., Franch, X., Brinkkemper, S., Wrycza, S. (eds.) CAiSE 2012. LNCS, vol. 7328, pp. 222–237. Springer, Heidelberg (2012). https://doi.org/10.1007/978-3-642-31095-9_15
8. González, L., Delgado, A.: Compliance requirements model for collaborative business process and evaluation with process mining. In: XLVII Latin American Computing Conference (CLEI). IEEE (2021)
9. Hernandez-Resendiz, J.D., Tello-Leal, E., Marin-Castro, H.M., Ramirez-Alcocer, U.M., Mata-Torres, J.A.: Merging event logs for inter-organizational process mining. In: Zapata-Cortes, J.A., Alor-Hernández, G., Sánchez-Ramírez, C., García-Alcaraz, J.L. (eds.) New Perspectives on Enterprise Decision-Making Applying Artificial Intelligence Techniques. SCI, vol. 966, pp. 3–26. Springer, Cham (2021). https://doi.org/10.1007/978-3-030-71115-3_1
10. IEEE: IEEE standard for extensible event stream (XES) for achieving interoperability in event logs and event streams. IEEE Std 1849-2016, pp. 1–50 (2016)
11. Liu, C., Li, H., Zeng, Q., Lu, T., Li, C.: Cross-organization emergency response process mining: an approach based on petri nets. Math. Probl. Eng. **2020**, 1–12 (2020). https://doi.org/10.1155/2020/8836007
12. Peña, L., Delgado, A., Calegari, D.: BPMN 2.0 collab. Process discovery ProM plugin (2022). https://gitlab.fing.edu.uy/open-coal/bpmncollaborativepm
13. Weske, M.: Business Process Management - Concepts, Languages, Architectures, 3rd edn. Springer, Heidelberg (2019). https://doi.org/10.1007/978-3-662-59432-2

Breaking Down Barriers with Knowledge Graphs: Data Integration for Cross-Organizational Process Mining

Julian Rott[1,2](✉) [ID], Rene Dorsch[3], Michael Freund[3], Markus Böhm[4] [ID], Andreas Harth[3] [ID], and Helmut Krcmar[2] [ID]

[1] Munich Airport, Munich, Germany
julian.rott@munich-airport.de
[2] Technical University of Munich, Garching, Germany
[3] Fraunhofer IIS, Nürnberg, Germany
[4] University of Applied Sciences Landshut, Landshut, Germany

Abstract. Cross-organizational process mining (coPM) with data from at least two organizations assists cooperating organizations in optimizing their operations by enabling an in-depth and continuous process analysis. As coPM faces unique challenges and is rarely applied, we followed a design science-based approach and developed a three-step extension to the PM project methodology to integrate data across organizational boundaries. Each organization first creates a local event data knowledge graph (KG). Second, a trusted third party integrates all local KGs into a global KG. Third, a federated event log and process knowledge are retrieved for coPM analysis. Overall, we present the first version of a methodology to support data integration for coPM, thereby assisting researchers and practitioners in unlocking value potentials from coPM analysis.

Keywords: Cross-organizational process mining · Data integration · Knowledge graphs · Methodology

1 Introduction

Process mining (PM) is increasingly implemented by organizations across different industries, such as Bayer, BMW, and Siemens to analyze and improve operations [1]. Many of these collaborate with other firms during the execution of their business (e.g., BMW purchases various parts from suppliers). However, the application of PM is mainly focused on use cases within one organization or is based on data from a single system [2]. As a result, significant value potential from cross-organizational PM (coPM) adoption – PM building upon data from at least two organizations – remains hidden [3]. Several reasons cause this situation. On the one hand, PM builds upon event-log data, which is retrieved from information systems [4]. To enable coPM, this data needs to be shared and integrated between multiple companies, leading to data privacy, information security, and data interoperability issues [5]. On the other hand, organizations may pursue different objectives, leading to conflicts of interest [6].

J. De Smedt and P. Soffer (Eds.): ICPM 2023 Workshops, LNBIP 503, pp. 499–512, 2024.
https://doi.org/10.1007/978-3-031-56107-8_38

Looking at the data integration literature, we find that knowledge graphs (KGs) are a promising solution to overcome some of the hurdles described above. They are already applied in various organizations, e.g., at Google and Microsoft, to increase the interoperability across multiple data sources and support with data provenance tracking [7]. In addition, KGs provide human and machine-readable descriptions of metadata [8], which can enhance PM analysis. The literature on applying KGs to support PM analysis, however, is scarce (see Sect. 2.2). Against this background, we aim to support the process of integrating data from multiple organizations for coPM by enriching the well-established PM^2 methodology with a KG-based data integration step [9]. Thus, we enable the integration of data across organizational boundaries for coPM as the basis for unlocking currently hidden value potentials of cross-organizational business process analysis and improvement.

The rest of the article is structured as follows. Section 2 describes the theoretical background on PM^2, coPM, KGs, and the application of KGs for PM. Section 3 elaborates on our research approach, while the results are described in Sect. 4. Section 5 discusses the results. Finally, Sect. 6 concludes the article.

2 Theoretical Background

2.1 PM Project Methodology (PM^2) and coPM

PM was developed with the aim of harnessing the potential of event-log data stored in information systems. According to the PM^2 methodology [9], a PM project typically consists of six phases. First, the project is planned, which includes defining the process to analyze, the hypothesis to investigate, the questions to answer, the information systems storing the required data, and assembling the project team. Second, event data is extracted from the source systems considering the required scope (e.g., data granularity, time periods, and attributes), while knowledge is transferred between the business experts and the process analysts to enable effective analysis. Third, the data is processed to produce event log data for the subsequent phases. Fourth, the process is mined and analyzed by discovering an actual process model, checking behavioral conformance, enriching a process model with additional information (e.g., performance), or applying generic data analytics techniques (e.g., visual analytics). Fifth, the results are evaluated by diagnosing, verifying, and validating the hypotheses and questions to determine process improvement actions. Finally, the process is improved, and its execution is continuously supported with live analysis. As the projects' objectives evolve, it may be necessary to iterate between phases multiple times to realize the desired outcome.

CoPM arises when data from at least two organizations are gathered and analyzed, offering two distinct scenarios: collaboration on business process execution (e.g., within supply chains or at airports), and exploiting commonalities in the execution of similar business processes across different organizations (e.g., comparing patient handling between two hospitals) [10]. In this context, unique challenges arise, such as integrating data from different sources [11], aligning event data from different levels of granularity with different identifiers for cases and process objects [5, 12–14], preserving privacy and confidentiality [5], and ensuring semantic interoperability [12]. Furthermore, convergence (one event relates to multiple cases and is therefore duplicated when a flattened, non-object-centric event log is created) and divergence (events are erroneously interpreted as causally related) issues need to be handled when analyzing an inter-organizational process [5]. Looking at current coPM literature, some of these challenges are addressed as [14] presented a solution to transform event logs into Petri-Nets to address privacy and confidentiality concerns, while [15] developed a toolset to enable PM on electronic data interchange (EDI) messages exchanged between organizations. In addition, [5] developed a formal framework for creating a federated event log (an event log based on merging multiple event logs from different organizations), while [16] presented a procedure for defining and comparing metrics usable in coPM analysis.

2.2 Knowledge Graphs for PM

KGs employ a directed, edge-labeled graph structure composed of nodes and edges to form statements that capture knowledge [17]. Nodes in the graph represent abstract concepts (e.g., *:MetalSheetCuttingEvent*, see Fig. 1) or specific entities (e.g., *:event#1*), while the edges establish relationships between these nodes (e.g., *:hasTimestamp*). To express connections between nodes, KGs use a triple structure, where one node is linked to another via an edge (see Fig. 1(1)).

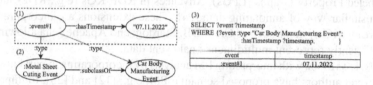

Fig. 1. RDF graph structure (1), ontology (2), and SPARQL query (3)

KGs use terms, such as *:type* and *:hasTimestamp*, to represent the meanings and logical constraints of concepts that are defined in an ontology. An ontology creates a shared understanding of the represented entities and relationships understandable for humans and software agents. Thus, enhancing the reusability of integrated data and promoting interoperability between KGs [18]. Figure 1(1–2) illustrates an ontology. Information about *:event#1*, such as the concrete event type, can be added to the graph with the statement *:event#1 :type :MetalSheetCuttingEvent*, where the class *:MetalSheetCuttingEvent* is defined in an ontology as a subclass of *:CarBodyManufacturingEvent*. KGs often leverage Semantic Web technologies, such as Uniform Resource Identifiers (URIs) for global identification of entities and relationships[1], the Resource Description Framework (RDF) and RDF Schema[2] for data representation and ontology definition[3]. RDF KGs can be created from existing datasets by directly converting the data to RDF format or by creating a virtual KG [19]. A virtual KG provides an additional graph-based abstraction layer for legacy databases (e.g., relational databases). To validate RDF data

---

[1] https://www.ietf.org/rfc/rfc2396.txt.

[2] https://www.w3.org/TR/2014/REC-rdf11-concepts-20140225/.

[3] https://www.w3.org/TR/2012/REC-owl2-overview-20121211/.

against syntactic, structural, and semantic rules, the technology SHACL[4] can be used, while data access and modification in RDF-based KGs is performed using SPARQL[5].

To support coPM, data from multiple organizations need to be integrated with the goal of achieving interoperability between all sources [20]. However, challenges related to the structure (e.g., attributes in different databases may have different structures), content (e.g., the same type of data may be stored in different forms), syntax (e.g., different attribute names may be used to identify the same values), and semantics of the data (e.g., there may be no common definition of terms used) need to be addressed [20]. RDF KGs and their underlying technologies assist with addressing these challenges by unifying the structure, content, and syntax of the data with RDF and enabling semantic interoperability through ontologies [20, 21]. Hence, the onprom system was developed, transforming event data from legacy systems into virtual KGs. Also, it maps data from relational databases and matches it to a business process ontology to generate a KG that can be queried to extract event data in XES or OCEL format [21].

Furthermore, graph-based data models assist coPM with representing multi-dimensional event data (event data with process events involving various entities sharing one or more case identifiers) [22]. Thereby, convergence and divergence can be prevented by annotating event data with directly follows relationships between pairs of events that are related to specific entities [23]. An approach which is demonstrated by [22] and [23] using Labeled Property Graphs (LPGs). Advances in RDF KGs (e.g., RDF-Star) have enabled a similar way of annotating data [24]. These extensions are incorporated into industry-ready KG systems such as GraphDB, Stardog, and Apache Jena allowing RDF KGs to efficiently represent multidimensional event data.

Finally, KGs assist with interpreting PM analysis by incorporating expert knowledge. Hence, several authors have proposed semantic PM, e.g., [12] and [25], to improve the interoperability and analytical capabilities of PM methods. In semantic PM, event logs are transformed from a string-based format to an entity-based format (e.g., RDF). These entities (e.g., events or activities) are mapped to concepts in an ontology to model different levels of abstraction of the event logs, allowing different views of the event data and complementing event data with process knowledge [25].

In summary, RDF KGs are suitable for coPM data integration and analysis interpretation. They can represent multidimensional event datasets and allow for a flexible extension of data schemas over the course of a coPM project. In addition, RDF KGs can handle data from multiple sources by using existing Web standards and enrich existing data with additional metadata to create different levels of abstraction for coPM.

3   Research Approach

As design science research "creates and evaluates [...] artifacts intended to solve identified organizational problems." [26], we followed this approach to develop a methodology (our artifact) assisting practitioners and researchers with data integration for coPM (our problem). We started with analyzing the literature on cross-organizational and semantic

---

[4] https://www.w3.org/TR/shacl/.

[5] https://www.w3.org/TR/2008/REC-rdf-sparql-query-20080115/.

PM (see Fig. 2), which revealed various requirements: Integrating data from different sources, representing event datasets with multiple entities, and supporting data interoperability (see Sect. 2.2). Subsequently, we identified different KG types (e.g., RDF and LPG), including advantages and disadvantages. Among them, we chose RDF due to its ability to include metadata (e.g., process knowledge), its flexibility, openness, standardized implementation, and its broad applicability for data integration use cases [27, 28]. During our first evaluation cycle, we applied this approach to a fictional dataset[6] for an assembly process in the automotive industry with three organizations (Org.), each with its own product identifiers: car frame (Org. 1), suspension (Org. 2), and chassis manufacturer (Org. 3). Also, we evaluated the approach partially (step 3.1 according to Fig. 3) – due to data availability – to a real dataset from the baggage handling process at Munich Airport involving airlines and ground handlers.

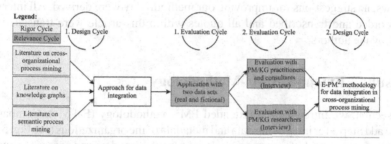

Fig. 2. Design science-based research approach

Table 1. Overview of Conducted Expert Interviews

ID	Job description	Role in E-PM^2 (see Fig. 3)	Experience (in years)			Date	Duration
			DA	PM	KG		
P1	PM Consultant	Process Analyst	5	3	<1	27/10/2022	41 min
P2	KG Consultant	KG Expert	2	<1	2	31/10/2022	46 min
P3	Team Lead Dataspaces	Business Expert	10	<1	<1	02/11/2022	28 min
R1	Research Associate	KG Expert	3.5	<1	2	02/11/2022	51 min
P4	Manager for Data, Processes, and Strategy	Business Expert	10	1	<1	04/11/2022	50 min
R2	Research Associate	Process Analyst	3.5	2.5	<1	07/11/2022	43 min
R3	Senior Researcher	Process Analyst	6	6	<1	08/11/2022	35 min
Legend:	P (Practitioner)	R (Researcher)	DA (Data Analytics)		PM (Process Mining)	KG (Knowledge Graph)	

To further evaluate our methodology and extend its generalizability, we conducted seven semi-structured expert interviews [29] with PM/KG researchers and practitioners

---

[6] The example is publicly available in a GitHub repository (https://anonymous.4open.science/r/e-pm2-data-5D3B).

(see Table 1). We included these experts in our evaluation, as it allowed us to incorporate different views on our approach and challenge, discuss and improve it based on different backgrounds. Following [30], we constructed the interview guide based on our research objective and the interviewees' experience. The applicability and comprehensiveness of our methodology were focused within the interviews with PM researchers and practitioners, while the thoroughness and correctness were primarily discussed with the KG experts. Further, we asked the interviewees about the challenges of coPM, and the advantages and challenges of our approach, which we discuss in Sect. 5. After each interview, the first three authors discussed the interview results to decide on improvements for the methodology, which were incorporated for the next interview. Following this procedure, role definitions for the tasks (Process analyst, Business expert, and KG expert), knowledge transfer relations between complementing steps, outcomes of each step, and a step for data quality assurance were added. During the sixth and seventh interviews, no suggestions for improving our methodology were derived. All interviews were recorded and transcribed and all quotes within this article were translated from German by the authors.

4   Results – Extended PM^2-Methodology

In this section, we introduce the Extended PM^2 methodology (E-PM^2). Compared to PM^2, we add Step 3 for integrating data and metadata of the organizations (see Fig. 3). The data integration primarily focuses on combining local event data and process knowledge from intra-organizational sub-processes to cross-organizational (global) data using RDF KGs. Therefore, we incorporate the new role of a KG expert, proficient in data and knowledge modeling and integration.

Step 3.1: Creation of local event data KGs: The successful execution of the Extraction step of the PM^2 methodology results in two retrieved data sources for each involved organization: (1) event data from relevant internal information systems and (2) process knowledge (e.g., semantic and descriptive metadata) about the sub-process performed in the organization (e.g., obtained through interviews) [9]. From both data sources, each organization builds its own local event data KG that links the process knowledge and event data. To create the local event data KG, the selected internal data sources and the acquired process knowledge must be transformed into RDF triples. This can either be done manually or be supported by applying tools like RMLMapper[7]. The data transformation is based on mapping rules that relate the available data and process knowledge to the structure provided by the ontology. An organization is free to choose the ontologies used for data integration, or to develop a new organization-specific ontology. In general, however, the reuse of existing ontologies is preferred to facilitate interoperability between the KGs of different organizations [18]. Selected existing ontologies to consider are, for example, the Semantic Utilised for Process Management within and between Enterprises (SUPER) ontology stack [31] and the SEM ontology [32]. Onprom [33] can be used to create RDF triples based on the created mapping rules or to align different ontologies. To enforce data quality policies across organizations, the generated RDF

---

[7] https://github.com/RMLio/rmlmapper-java.

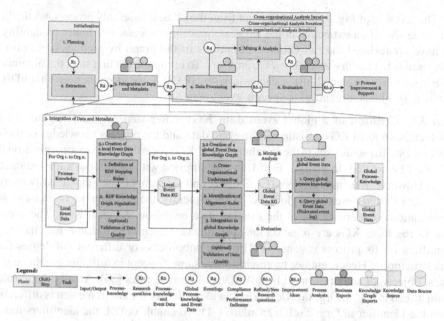

Fig. 3. Flowchart of the Extended-PM^2 (E-PM^2) methodology

data can optionally be validated using SHACL (see Sect. 2.2). In the examples shown in Fig. 4, we used the SEM ontology to structure the event data because of its simplicity. To model multidimensional event data (see Sect. 2.2) and include domain-specific knowledge, we extended the SEM ontology with additional terms, e.g., to provide a directly follows relation (*ex:directlyFollows*) [23]. In addition, we used the PROV ontology[8] and the SKOS ontology[9] to represent further metadata.

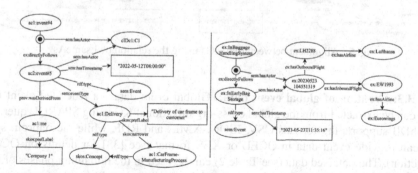

Fig. 4. Extract of the local event data KG for a chassis assembly process (left side) and a baggage handling process (right side)

[8] https://www.w3.org/TR/2013/REC-prov-O-20130430/.

[9] https://www.w3.org/TR/2008/WD-skos-reference-20080829/skos.html.

The left side of Fig. 4 shows an extract from the chassis assembly process, while the right side shows an extract from the baggage handling process. For better readability, we have abbreviated the full URIs of all entities in the graph by prefixes (e.g., prov: corresponds to https://www.w3.org/TR/prov-o/). To complete the first step, the obtained RDF data must be loaded into a database with SPARQL service, such as GraphDB, resulting in a local, organization-specific event data KG.

Step 3.2: Creation of a global event data KG: After step 3.1, each organization involved has a local KG consisting of the event data and the process knowledge of their sub-process. To use the data in the distributed local KGs for coPM, a cross-organizational KG must be created. In general, E-PM^2 can be applied with or without a trusted third party. However, four interviewees (P3, P4, R2, and R3) emphasized that a trustworthy third party should develop the global KG. Consequently, the first step is to gain a cross-organizational understanding of the existing data based on the local KGs. The event data in the local KGs are organization-specific, i.e., each organization uses its own identifiers for its process instances [34] of the subprocess or different ontologies for data structuring. Hence, entities representing the same concept in different graphs (e.g., cases, objects, or activities) must be linked via alignment rules [35]. An alignment rule is illustrated in Fig. 5: Org. 1 (cIDc1:1) has an identifier for the car frame that is different from the identifier of Org. 2 (cIDc2:OrderC1-1). To enable coPM, the identifiers must be marked as an entity with two different identifiers using the *owl:sameAs* property. SPARQL queries of type INSERT to each organization's local KGs can be used to retrieve local event data and process knowledge, and insert the results into the global KG. SHACL rules can be applied to validate the results from multiple KGs. The query results, alignment rules, and additional metadata are linked in a cross-organizational global KG, which needs to be stored in an RDF graph database and consists of global event data, process knowledge, and metadata.

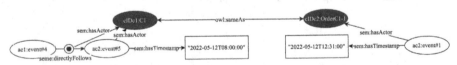

Fig. 5. Alignment between two KGs using the relation owl:sameAs

Step 3.3: Creation of global event data: Global event data – a federated event log [5] – can be extracted from the global cross-organizational KG using SPARQL queries. GraphDB supports the formats CSV, JSON, XML, and RDF, while the onprom system can provide event data in OCEL or XES format (see [33] for details on OCEL extraction). The obtained data (see Table 2) can be used in the remaining phases of the E-PM^2 methodology with available commercial or open-source PM tools, for example, to discover cross-organizational process models (see Fig. 6, generated with PM4py) or to pursue cross-organizational conformance checking, performance analysis, and process improvement. In addition, process knowledge and other metadata stored in the KG can be queried with SPARQL and assist in steps 5–7 of the E-PM^2 methodology with verifying and understanding the analysis results.

Table 2. Global event data and global process knowledge

Global Event Data			Global Process Knowledge			
Activity	Timestamp	Entities	Activity	Broader Activity	Description	Responsibility
ac1:HS	2022-05-11T 13:00:00	C1	ac1:HS	ac1:CarFrameManufacturingProcess	Heats a steelsheet to a temperature of 1000° Celsius	Organization 1
ac1:PS	2022-06-11T 08:00:00	C1	ac1:PS	ac1:CarFrameManufacturingProcess	Hot Forming of a frame	Organization 1
ac3:RO	2022-05-11T 11:33:00	C1	ac3:RO	ac3:ChassisAssembly-Process	Received the order of a supplier	Organization 3
ac3:MSonF	2022-05-13T 13:55:00	C1	ac3:MSonF	ac3:ChassisAssembly-Process	Mount suspension system to car chassis	Organization 3
ac3:CID	2022-05-13T 13:35:30	C1	ac3:CID	ac3:ChassisAssembly-Process	Create a unique identifier for the chassis	Organization 3

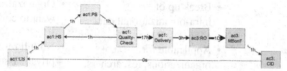

Fig. 6. Process Model for the Chassis Assembly Process with Org. 1 (yellow) and Org. 3 (blue) (Color figure online)

5 Discussion

We discussed the E-PM² methodology within our expert interviews and revealed challenges of coPM, and advantages and challenges of adopting E-PM² (see Table 3).

Without E-PM², organizations may suffer from a limited overview: "Depending on the information, I have a lot of black holes before or after my process. Then I don't care, and I don't try to make it better, because I don't know what happens afterward." (P4) Hence, we enable data integration from multiple organizations through KGs. We propose to use the RDF data model to represent data and metadata in a KG, allowing organizations to use different systems as "across organizations, it is difficult or impossible to define a single platform for data exchange". (P4) Compared to existing coPM techniques, e.g., PM based on EDI messages [15], our approach does not require organizations to exchange pre-defined messages with each other or to agree on storing data in a specific,

Table 3. Challenges of coPM, Advantages and Challenges of the E-PM2 Methodology

Challenges of cross-organizational PM	Advantages of E-PM^2	Challenges of E-PM^2
• Integration of dispersed expert knowledge (P1, P4) • Definition of a secure data exchange platform (P3, P4) • Lack of standards for data integration (P3, P4) • Data granularity of cases and activities (P4, R2, R3) • Lack of tool support for analyzing process networks (R3) • Rights and role concept (P1, R3) • Availability of business experts (P1, P4) • Organizational motivation to create data and analytical transparency (P3) • Fear of transparency (R2) • Data privacy (P1, P4, R3) • Legal aspects (R1)	• Analysis and display of cross-organizational business processes and process networks (P2, R1, P4, R3) • "Step-by-step" approach, including feedback loops (P1, P4) • Usage of metadata, assisting with data understanding and analysis (P1, P2, P3, R3) • Integration of data from multiple organizations (P1, R1, P4, R3) • Fine granular sharing of data (P3) • Definition of responsibilities for certain steps (P1) • Representation of internal knowledge in the data (P1, P2, P3) • Break up of intra-organizational data silos (P4, R3) • Applicable for organizations, researchers, and consultancies (P3, P4, R2) • Data sovereignty stays with the organization (P3) • Integration of external knowledge and data (P1, P4) • Assistance with data privacy and security aspects (P3, R3)	• Lack of standard tool support (R3) • Regular updating of data (P4) • KG is not the most efficient technology for storing large volumes of data (P2) • Risk of high complexity within the large global KG (R2) • Know-How regarding KGs required (P2, P3, R1, P4) • Need to determine responsibility for global KG (P4, R2) • Determination of rights and role concept (P4) • High effort for KG development • Slowdown of initial project speed (P2, P3, R1, R2) • Organizations still need to want to collaborate (P2, R3) • No full resolution of data privacy issues (P1, P2)

unified format. In contrast, E-PM^2 enables organizations to integrate their existing data sources by building KGs that are linked through alignment rules. Hence, legacy systems and databases don't need to be modified. Compared to relational databases, it is further not necessary to join numerous tables with each other during data-preprocessing [22] as the data is linked in a global KG, which allows for multiple views on the process. Hence, different parts can be extracted based on questions to be answered or confidentiality and privacy requirements. Further, convergence and divergence issues (see Sect. 2.1) can be handled if the data is not "flattened" during export in step 3.3 but exported in OCEL format. In addition, E-PM^2 allows for connecting the same entities from different organizations: "When some organizations share the same entity but call them differently. That's where I see a big advantage in the methodology" (R3). Further, our approach enables end-to-end transparency and an impact analysis for cross-organizational business processes: "Dependency analyses [...] are meanwhile really not so well possible, [...] are actually almost a bit of the holy grail [...] because it's really expensive if something fails somewhere, something goes wrong, and if I can then quickly show what the impact is, [...] then I think it's very helpful" (R3). In addition, we suggest incorporating metadata (e.g., process inefficiencies) within the KG, which can be leveraged during the analysis iterations, e.g., for interpreting deviations in conformance checking, or deriving process improvement recommendations: "I think it's really helpful to have not only the data but also additional process models where you've already incorporated expert knowledge; especially for the familiarization" (P1). Hence, we also support the challenge of semantic interoperability in coPM (see Sect. 2.1).

Limitations. E-PM^2 builds upon event data (including cases or objects) provided by the organizations. Thus, issues of case correlation are so far not considered. Also, building the KGs requires a high initial effort and, to some extent, organizations willing to collaborate and increase each other's transparency: "It must be clear that it is a lot of work [...] manual work. You have to make these mapping rules, and then you have to somehow agree on how the data from the different companies go together." (R1). In addition, specific questions need to be clarified between the organizations during the application, e.g., "Who develops and manages a rights and role concepts?", "Which software tools are used within each step of the E-PM^2 methodology?", and – if necessary – "How can a trusted third party be formed or identified?".

Future Research. Supporting and detailing these questions is a matter of future research, which also requires to improve E-PM^2 through additional evaluation with complex, real-world cross-organizational datasets and real-time data. As we focused on creating a general, non-tool-specific approach, we performed steps 3.1–3.3 of E-PM^2 manually within our evaluations, suggested various tools to apply but did not systematically compare all existing tools. Hence, future research can improve tool support, develop standard ontologies for a more automatized and guided implementation of E-PM^2, and work on ways to overcome the need for a trusted third party.

6 Conclusion

Our article provides the first step towards a coPM project methodology by presenting the E-PM^2 methodology including instructions, tools and ontologies for cross-organizational data integration: First, each organization creates a local event data KG. Second, a trusted third party integrates all local KGs into a global event data KG. Third, a federated event log and process knowledge are retrieved for coPM analysis. Thereby, E-PM^2 enables integrating data from multiple sources across organizations and representing event datasets with multiple entities. In addition, E-PM^2 enables the storage and retrieval of metadata (e.g., process knowledge), which supports and enhances coPM analysis. Thereby, we also contribute to solving one of the most important BPM problems: "Augmenting process mining with common sense and domain knowledge" [36].

Acknowledgments. This work was supported by the Bayerisches Verbundforschungsprogramm (BayVFP) through the KIWI project (grant no. DIK0318/03).

References

1. Reinkemeyer, L.: Process Mining in Action - Principles, Use Cases and Outlook. Springer, Cham (2020)
2. Thiede, M., Fuerstenau, D., Bezerra Barquet Ana, P.: How is process mining technology used by organizations? A systematic literature review of empirical studies. Bus. Process Manag. J. **24**(4), 900–922 (2018)
3. Rott, J., Böhm, M.: Value distribution in cross-organizational process mining: insights from related literature. In: Pacific Asia Conference for Information Systems (PACIS), pp. 1–17. Virtual Conference (2022)
4. Van Der Aalst, W.: Process Mining - Data Science in Action. Springer, Heidelberg (2016)
5. Van Der Aalst, W.: Federated process mining: exploiting event data across organizational boundaries. In: 2021 IEEE International Conference on Smart Data Services (SMDS), pp. 1–7. Virtual Conference (2021)
6. Buijs, J.C.A.M., Reijers, H.A.: Comparing business process variants using models and event logs. In: Bider, I., et al. (eds.) BPMDS/EMMSAD -2014. LNBIP, vol. 175, pp. 154–168. Springer, Heidelberg (2014). https://doi.org/10.1007/978-3-662-43745-2_11
7. Noy, N., Gao, Y., Jain, A., Narayanan, A., Patterson, A., Taylor, J.: Industry-scale knowledge graphs: lessons and challenges. Commun. ACM **62**(8), 36–43 (2019)
8. Jeffery, K.: Metadata: an overview and some issues. Ercim News **35**, 1–6 (1998)
9. Van Eck, M.L., Lu, X., Leemans, S.J.J., van der Aalst, W.M.P.: PM^2: a process mining project methodology. In: Zdravkovic, J., Kirikova, M., Johannesson, P. (eds.) CAiSE 2015. LNCS, vol. 9097, pp. 297–313. Springer, Cham (2015). https://doi.org/10.1007/978-3-319-19069-3_19
10. Van der Aalst, W.: Intra- and inter-organizational process mining: discovering processes within and between organizations. In: Johannesson, P., Krogstie, J., Opdahl, A.L. (eds.) PoEM 2011. LNBIP, vol. 92, pp. 1–11. Springer, Heidelberg (2011). https://doi.org/10.1007/978-3-642-24849-8_1
11. Golshan, B., Halevy, A., Mihaila, G., Tan, W.-C.: Data integration: after the teenage years. In: Proceedings of the 36th ACM SIGMOD-SIGACT-SIGAI Symposium on Principles of Database Systems, pp. 101–106 (2017)
12. Pereira Detro, S., Morozov, D., Lezoche, M., Panetto, H., Portela Santos, E., Zdravkovic, M.: Enhancing semantic interoperability in healthcare using semantic process mining. In: 6th International Conference on Information Society and Technology, ICIST 2016, pp. 80–85 (2016)
13. Suriadi, S., Mans, R.S., Wynn, M.T., Partington, A., Karnon, J.: Measuring patient flow variations: a cross-organisational process mining approach. In: Ouyang, C., Jung, J.-Y. (eds.) AP-BPM 2014. LNBIP, vol. 181, pp. 43–58. Springer, Cham (2014). https://doi.org/10.1007/978-3-319-08222-6_4

14. Zeng, Q., Sun, S.X., Duan, H., Liu, C., Wang, H.: Cross-organizational collaborative workflow mining from a multi-source log. Decis. Support. Syst. **54**(3), 1280–1301 (2013)
15. Engel, R., et al.: Analyzing inter-organizational business processes. IseB **14**(3), 577–612 (2016)
16. Aksu, Ü., Schunselaar, D.M.M., Reijers, H.A.: A cross-organizational process mining framework for obtaining insights from software products: accurate comparison challenges. In: 2016 IEEE 18th Conference on Business Informatics (CBI), Paris, France, pp. 153–162 (2016)
17. Yan, J., Wang, C., Cheng, W., Gao, M., Zhou, A.: A retrospective of knowledge graphs. Front. Comput. Sci. **12**(1), 55–74 (2018)
18. Noy, N.F., Mcguinness, D.L.: Ontology Development 101: A Guide to Creating Your First Ontology. https://corais.org/sites/default/files/ontology_development_101_aguide_to_creating_your_first_ontology.pdf. Accessed 25 Aug 2023
19. Xiao, G., Ding, L., Cogrel, B., Calvanese, D.: Virtual knowledge graphs: an overview of systems and use cases. Data Intell. **1**(3), 201–223 (2019)
20. Asgari, R., Moghadam, M.G., Mahdavi, M., Erfanian, A.: An ontology-based approach for integrating heterogeneous databases. Open Comput. Sci. **5**(1), 41–50 (2015)
21. Calvanese, D., Kalayci, T.E., Montali, M., Tinella, S.: Ontology-based data access for extracting event logs from legacy data: the onprom tool and methodology. In: Abramowicz, W. (ed.) BIS 2017. LNBIP, vol. 288, pp. 220–236. Springer, Cham (2017). https://doi.org/10.1007/978-3-319-59336-4_16
22. Esser, S., Fahland, D.: Multi-dimensional event data in graph databases. J. Data Semant. **10**(1), 109–141 (2021)
23. Fahland, D.: Process mining over multiple behavioral dimensions with event knowledge graphs. In: van der Aalst, W., Carmona, J. (eds.) Process Mining Handbook, pp. 274–319. Springer, Cham (2022). https://doi.org/10.1007/978-3-031-08848-3_9
24. Hartig, O.: RDF* and SPARQL*: an alternative approach to annotate statements in RDF. In: International Semantic Web Conference 2017, Vienna, Austria, pp. 1–4 (2017)
25. Ingvaldsen, J.E., Gulla, J.A.: Industrial application of semantic process mining. Enterp. Inf. Syst. **6**(2), 139–163 (2012)
26. Hevner, A.R., March, S.T., Park, J., Ram, S.: Design science in information systems research. MIS Q. **28**(1), 75–105 (2004)
27. Angles, R., Thakkar, H., Tomaszuk, D.: Mapping RDF databases to property graph databases. IEEE Access **8**, 86091–86110 (2020)
28. Spanos, D.-E., Stavrou, P., Mitrou, N.: Bringing relational databases into the semantic web: a survey. Semant. Web **3**(2), 169–209 (2012)
29. Österle, H., et al.: Memorandum on design-oriented information systems research. Eur. J. Inf. Syst. **20**(1), 7–10 (2011)
30. Gläser, J., Laudel, G.: Experteninterviews und qualitative Inhaltsanalyse. VS Verlag für Sozialwissenschaften Wiesbaden (Germany) (2010)
31. Pedrinaci, C., Domingue, J.: Towards an ontology for process monitoring and mining. In: CEUR Workshop Proceedings, Innsbruck, Austria, pp. 76–87 (2007)
32. Van Hage, W.R., Ceolin, D.: The simple event model. In: van de Laar, P., Tretmans, J., Borth, M. (eds.) Situation Awareness with Systems of Systems, pp. 149–169. Springer, New York (2013). https://doi.org/10.1007/978-1-4614-6230-9_10
33. Xiong, J., Xiao, G., Kalayci, T.E., Montali, M., Gu, Z., Calvanese, D.: A virtual knowledge graph based approach for object-centric event logs extraction. In: Montali, M., Senderovich, A., Weidlich, M. (eds.) ICPM 2022. LNBP, vol. 468, pp. 466–478. Springer, Cham (2023). https://doi.org/10.1007/978-3-031-27815-0_34
34. Van der Aalst, W.: Decomposing process mining problems using passages. In: Haddad, S., Pomello, L. (eds.) PETRI NETS 2012. LNCS, vol. 7347, pp. 72–91. Springer, Heidelberg (2012). https://doi.org/10.1007/978-3-642-31131-4_5

35. Zhu, L., Ghasemi-Gol, M., Szekely, P., Galstyan, A., Knoblock, C.A.: Unsupervised entity resolution on multi-type graphs. In: Groth, P., et al. (eds.) ISWC 2016. LNCS, vol. 9981, pp. 649–667. Springer, Cham (2016). https://doi.org/10.1007/978-3-319-46523-4_39
36. Beerepoot, I., et al.: The biggest business process management problems to solve before we die. Comput. Ind. **146**(103837) (2023)

Author Index

J. De Smedt and P. Soffer (Eds.): ICPM 2023 Workshops, LNBIP 503, pp. 513–514, 2024.
https://doi.org/10.1007/978-3-031-56107-8

Printed in the United States
by Baker & Taylor Publisher Services

Printed in the United States
by Baker & Taylor Publisher Services